Hemolytic Uremic Syndrome and Thrombotic Thrombocytopenic Purpura

KIDNEY DISEASE

Editors

J. Stewart Cameron
Professor in Renal Medicine
Clinical Science Laboratories, Guy's Hospital
London, England

Richard J. Glassock
Professor and Chairman, Department of Medicine
University of Kentucky College of Medicine
Lexington, Kentucky

Andrew Whelton
Associate Professor of Medicine
The Johns Hopkins University School of Medicine
Baltimore, Maryland

1. Proteinuria: An Integrated Review, *Amadeo J. Pesce and Martin Roy First*
2. The Aminoglycosides: Microbiology, Clinical Use, and Toxicology, *edited by Andrew Whelton and Harold C. Neu*
3. Hepatorenal Disorders, *S. P. Wilkinson*
4. Acute Renal Failure: Correlations Between Morphology and Function, *edited by Kim Solez and Andrew Whelton*
5. Renal Tubular Disorders: Pathophysiology, Diagnosis, and Management, *edited by Harvey C. Gonick and Vardaman M. Buckalew, Jr.*
6. Potassium in Cardiovascular and Renal Medicine: Arrhythmias, Myocardial Infarction, and Hypertension, *edited by Paul K. Whelton, Andrew Whelton, and W. Gordon Walker*
7. Kidney Transplant Rejection: Diagnosis and Treatment, *edited by G. Melville Williams, James F. Burdick, and Kim Solez*
8. The Nephrotic Syndrome, *edited by J. Stewart Cameron and Richard J. Glassock*
9. Kidney Transplant Rejection: Diagnosis and Treatment, Second Edition, *edited by James F. Burdick, Lorraine C. Racusen, Kim Solez, and G. Melville Williams*
10. Hemolytic Uremic Syndrome and Thrombotic Thrombocytopenic Purpura, *edited by Bernard S. Kaplan, Richard S. Trompeter, and Joel L. Moake*

ADDITIONAL VOLUMES IN PREPARATION

Hemolytic Uremic Syndrome and Thrombotic Thrombocytopenic Purpura

edited by

Bernard S. Kaplan

Children's Hospital of Philadelphia and
The University of Pennsylvania
Philadelphia, Pennsylvania

Richard S. Trompeter

Hospitals for Sick Children
London, England

Joel L. Moake

Baylor College of Medicine and
Rice University
Houston, Texas

Marcel Dekker, Inc. New York • Basel • Hong Kong

Library of Congress Cataloging-in-Publication Data

Hemolytic uremic syndrome and thrombotic thrombocytopenic purpura /
edited by Bernard S. Kaplan, Richard S. Trompeter, Joel L. Moake.
p. cm. -- (Kidney disease ; v.10)
1. Hemolytic-uremic syndrome. 2. Thrombotic thrombocytopenic
purpura. I. Kaplan, Bernard S. II. Trompeter, Richard S. III.
Moake, Joel L. IV. Series.
[DNLM: 1. Hemolytic-Uremic Syndrome--in infancy & childhood.
2. Purpura, Thrombotic Thrombocytopenic--in infancy & childhood.
W1 KI586R v. 10 / WJ 348 H489]
RC647.H44H46 1992
616.6'1--dc20
DNLM/DLC
for Library of Congress 92-18548
CIP

This book is printed on acid-free paper.

MARCEL DEKKER, INC.
270 Madison Avenue, New York, New York 10016

Current printing (last digit):
10 9 8 7 6 5 4 3 2 1

PRINTED IN THE UNITED STATES OF AMERICA

About the Series

This book is the tenth in a series of texts on nephrology intended to cover all aspects of that discipline. Nephrology has grown at a great rate over the past decade, and the available knowledge has outstripped the texts available. The discipline has, however, attained such maturity that a description of any one of its parts becomes more than ephermeral—or worse, outdated before it even appears. We aim to fill some of the many gaps that exist, not only for the specialist in nephrology, but also for the general physician interested in nephrology. In this description, we include the study and management of hypertension, since these two are interwoven at so many points. We welcome comments on the series as it evolves, or suggestions for topics that might be considered for future volumes.

J. Stewart Cameron
London, England
Richard J. Glassock
Lexington, Kentucky
Andrew Whelton
Baltimore, Maryland

Preface

Hemolytic uremic syndrome (HUS) occurs all over the world and has become the most important cause of acute renal failure in children. HUS and the related disorder thrombotic thrombocytopenic purpura (TTP) have been the subject of much interest and research, individual reports and epidemiological studies contributing more than 2000 case histories to the literature since the disorder was characterized more than a quarter of a century ago. The triad of microangiopathic hemolytic anemia, thrombocytopenia, and renal failure by which HUS is defined and its extension to include neurological involvement and fever, the pentad of TTP, are clinical end points that may be reached by numerous pathways. The etiology of HUS is unknown. Some patients may have a genetic predisposition to develop the disorder; in others, an initiating agent such as a virus or bacteria has been identified. The primary site of injury may be the erythrocyte, platelet, endothelium, or coagulation system, yet the end result is a similar clinical presentation.

HUS is predominantly a disease of infants and young children. Epidemic foci are endemic to parts of South America, the low countries of Europe, and the western United States. Elsewhere the disease occurs in mini-epidemics. HUS in adults is usually associated with an underlying systemic disorder such as pregnancy or a collagen vascular disease; in children, however, this type of association is extremely rare. The evidence for such heterogeneity is to be found in the epidemiological, histopathological, and pathophysiological studies that have provided a basis for a tentative classification of the disorder.

With justification we have avoided the need to include a section covering the management of the patient with HUS. Dialysis, after all, is the standard treatment for acute renal failure, and complications of the syndrome have been individually addressed. We hope this book will, for the first time, gather together the wide and varied clinical and experimental experience of the many doctors who have made valuable contributions to the understanding and treatment of HUS, and provide a useful source of reference for pediatricians, internists, nephrologists, and pathologists.

Bernard S. Kaplan
Richard S. Trompeter
Joel L. Moake

Contents

PART VII TREATMENT

PART VIII THROMBOTIC THROMBOCYTOPENIC PURPURA

Contributors

Sharon Phillips Andreoli, M.D. Associate Professor, Department of Pediatric Nephrology, Indiana University Medical Center, Indianapolis, Indiana

Yujiro Asada, M.D. First Department of Pathology, Miyazaki Medical College, Miyazaki, Japan

T. Martin Barratt, FRCP Professor, Department of Pediatric Nephrology, Institute of Child Health, London, England

Jerry Michael Bergstein, M.D. Professor and Head, Section of Nephrology, Department of Pediatrics, Indiana University School of Medicine, Indianapolis, Indiana

Jeffrey S. Berns, M.D. Clinical Assistant Professor of Medicine, Division of Nephrology and Hypertension, University of Pennsylvania School of Medicine, and The Graduate Hospital, Philadelphia, Pennsylvania

Kenneth M. Brinkhous, M.D. Alumni Distinguished Professor Emeritus, Department of Pathology, University of North Carolina, Chapel Hill, North Carolina

S.-H. Chen, M.D. Fellow, Department of Medicine, Veterans Administration Medical Center, and University of Miami School of Medicine, Miami, Florida

Russell W. Chesney, M.D. Le Bonheur Professor and Chairman, Department of Pediatrics, The University of Tennessee, and Vice President for Academic Affairs, Le Bonheur Children's Medical Center, Memphis, Tennessee

Thomas G. Cleary M.D. Professor, Department of Pediatrics, University of Texas Medical School, Houston, Texas

Jean-Michel Descamps, M.D. Centre Hospitalier Georges Renon, Niort, France

Michael J. Dillon Department of Nephrology, Institute of Child Health, London, England

Josée Doyon, M.D. Resident, Department of Pathology, Université de Montréal, Montreal, Quebec, Canada

Roger Eeckels, M.D., D.T.M.&H. Professor, Department of Pediatrics, Leuven University Hospital, Leuven, Belgium

L.-M. Feng, M.D. Fellow, Department of Medicine, Veterans Administration Medical Center and University of Miami School of Medicine, Miami, Florida

Margaret M. Fitzpatrick, B.Sc., MRCP Lecturer in Pediatric Nephrology, Department of Nephrology, Institute of Child Health, London, England

Yaacov Frishberg, M.D. Fellow, Pediatric Nephrology, Children's Hospital of Philadelphia, and University of Pennsylvania, Philadelphia, Pennsylvania

E. Gautier, M.D. Professor Emeritus, Department of Pediatrics, Centre Hospitalier Universitaire Vaudois, Lausanne, Switzerland

Carlos A. Gianantonio, M.D. Chairman and Honorary Professor of Pediatrics, Department of Pediatrics, Hospital Italiano, Buenos Aires, Argentina

Jean-Pierre Grünfeld, M.D. Professor, Department of Nephrology, Hôpital Necker, Paris, France

Lorence A. Gutterman, M.D. Department of Hematology/Oncology, Riverside Methodist Hospital, Columbus, Ohio

Renée Habib, M.D. Director of Research, Research Unit of Pediatric Nephrology, INSERM U192, Hôpital Necker-Enfants Malades, Paris, France

Diane Hébert, M.D., FRCP(C). Assistant Professor, Department of Pediatrics, The Hospital for Sick Children, University of Toronto, Toronto, Ontario, Canada

Michel Hecht, M.D. Centre Hospitalier Henri Duffaut, Avignon, France

Bernard S. Kaplan, M.B., B.Ch., F.C.P.(SA) Director of Nephrology and Professor of Pediatrics and Medicine, Department of Pediatrics, Children's Hospital of Philadelphia, and University of Pennsylvania, Philadelphia, Pennsylvania

Paige Kaplan, M.B.B.Ch., FRCP(C) Associate Professor, Department of Pediatrics, Division of Metabolism and Genetics, Children's Hospital of Philadelphia, and University of Pennsylvania, Philadelphia, Pennsylvania

Mohamed A. Karmali, M.B.Ch.B., FRCP. Microbiologist-in-Chief and Professor of Microbiology, Department of Microbiology, The Hospital for Sick Children, The University of Toronto, Toronto, Ontario, Canada

Christophe Legendre, M.D. Professor, Department of Nephrology, Hôpital Necker, Paris, France

J.-Z. Li, M.D. Professor, Institute of Hematology, Chinese Academy of Medical Sciences, Tianjing, China

Eric C.-Y. Lian, M.D. Professor, Department of Medicine, Veterans Administration Medical Center and University of Miami School of Medicine, Miami, Florida

Chantal Loirat, M.D. Professor, Department of Pediatric Nephrology, Hôpital Robert Debré, Paris, France

Eduardo L. Lopez, M.D. Chief of Infectious Diseases, Department of Pediatrics, Hospital de Niños "Ricardo Gutierrez," Buenos Aires, Argentina

Aaron J. Marcus, M.D. Professor of Medicine in Pathology, Departments of Medicine and Pathology, Cornell University Medical College; Chief, Division of Hematology-Oncology, and Attending Physician, Department of Veterans Affairs Medical Center; Attending Physician, New York Hospital, New York, New York

S. Michael Mauer, M.D. Professor, Department of Pediatrics, University of Minnesota, Minneapolis, Minnesota

Peter N. McLaine, M.D., FRCP(C) Associate Professor, Department of Pediatrics, University of Ottawa, and the Children's Hospital of Eastern Ontario, Ottawa, Ontario, Canada

David Milford, B.M., MRCP Senior Registrar, Department of Nephrology, The Children's Hospital, Birmingham, England

Joel L. Moake, M.D. Professor of Medicine and Director, Hematology Section, Baylor College of Medicine, and Associate Director, Biomedical Engineering Laboratory, Rice University, Houston, Texas

Anthony J. Murgo, M.D. Medical Officer, Division of Oncology Drug Products, Center for Drug Evaluation and Research, Food and Drug Administration, Rockville, Maryland

Tom G. Obrig, Ph.D. Senior Scientist, Department of Microbiology and Immunology, University of Rochester Medical Center, Rochester, New York

Hélène Ogier, Ph.D. Praheun Hospitalier, Service d'endocrinologie, diabétologie et métabolisme, Hôpital Robert Debre, Paris, France

Elaine Orrbine Research Coordinator, Canadian Pediatric Kidney Disease Reference Centre, Department of Pediatrics, Children's Hospital of Eastern Ontario, University of Ottawa, Ottawa, Ontario, Canada

Martin D. Phillips, M.D. Assistant Professor, Section of Hematology, Department of Medicine, Baylor College of Medicine, and Adjunct Assistant Professor, Biomedical Engineering Laboratory, Rice University, Houston, Texas

H. R. Powell, FRACP Director of Renal Unit, The Royal Children's Hospital, Melbourne, Australia

Willem Proesmans, M.D. Professor, Renal Unit, Department of Pediatrics, Leuven University Hospital, Leuven, Belgium

Marjorie S. Read, Ph.D. Research Assistant Professor, Department of Pathology, University of North Carolina, Chapel Hill, North Carolina

Giuseppe Remuzzi, M.D. Head, Laboratory of Kidney Diseases, and Director, Negri Bergamo Laboratories, Mario Negri Institute for Pharmacological Research, Bergamo, Italy

Horacio A. Repetto, M.D. Professor, Department of Pediatrics, University of Buenos Aires, and Head, Pediatric Service, Hospital Nacional A. Posadas, Buenos Aires, Argentina

Peter C. Rowe, M.D. Assistant Professor, Department of Pediatrics, The Johns Hopkins Hospital, Baltimore, Maryland

Pierre A. Russo, M.D. Assistant Clinical Professor of Pathology, Department of Pathology, Hôpital Ste-Justine, Université de Montréal, Montreal, Quebec, Canada

Claudine Saltiel, M.D. Department of Nephrology, Hôpital Necker, Paris, France

William E. Sanders, M.D. Cardiology Fellow, Division of Cardiology, Department of Medicine, Duke University, Durham, North Carolina

Jean-Marie Saudubray, M.D. Professeur agrégé, Chef de service de génétique médicale, Hôpital Necker-Enfants Malades, Paris, France

Farooq A. Siddiqui, Ph.D. Assistant Professor, Department of Medicine, University of Miami School of Medicine, and Veterans Administration Medical Center, Miami, Florida

R. E. Siebenmann, M.D. Professor Emeritus, Zurich, Switzerland

Richard L. Siegler, M.D. Professor and Division Chief, Division of Nephrology and Hypertension, Department of Pediatrics, University of Utah School of Medicine, Salt Lake City, Utah

Elise Sonsino, M.D. Laboratoire d'Anatomie Pathologique, Hôpital Robert Debre, Paris, France

Rajendra N. Srivastava, FRCP Professor, Department of Pediatrics, All India Institute of Medical Sciences, New Delhi, India

Akinobu Sumiyoshi, M.D. First Department of Pathology, Miyazaki Medical College, Miyazaki, Japan

C. M. Taylor, FRCP, DCH. Consultant Pediatric Nephrologist, Department of Nephrology, The Children's Hospital, Birmingham, England

Peter D. Thomson, M.B., B.Ch., F.C.P.(SA) Associate Professor and Head of the Division of Pediatric Nephrology, University of the Witwatersrand, and Johannesburg Hospital, Johannesburg, South Africa

John E. Tomaszewski, M.D. Associate Professor, Department of Pathology and Laboratory Medicine, University of Pennsylvania Medical Center, Philadelphia, Pennsylvania

Richard S. Trompeter, M.B., FRCP Consultant Pediatric Nephrologist, Renal Unit, Hospitals for Sick Children, London, England

Peter F. Whitington, M.D. Associate Professor of Pediatrics and Medicine, Section of Gastroenterology, Hepatology and Nutrition, Department of Pediatrics, The University of Chicago, Chicago, Illinois

Kenneth K. Wu, M.D. Professor of Medicine and Pathology and Director, Division of Hematology/Oncology and Vascular Biology Research Center, Department of Internal Medicine, University of Texas Medical School, Houston, Texas

Carla Zoja, Biol. Sci.D. Head, Unit of Experimental Modeling for Human Renal Diseases, Mario Negri Institute for Pharmacological Research, Bergamo, Italy

Introduction

Bernard S. Kaplan *Children's Hospital of Philadelphia and University of Pennsylvania, Philadelphia, Pennsylvania* **Richard S. Trompeter** *Hospitals for Sick Children, London, England* **Joel L. Moake** *Baylor College of Medicine and Rice University, Houston, Texas*

This introduction is divided into two main sections. Although thrombotic thrombocytopenic purpura (TTP) was first described many years before hemolytic uremic syndrome (HUS), we have chosen to present reviews on HUS before TTP, because the former is so much more common.

In 1965, Dr. Maurice Kibel from Bulawayo offered a commentary (1) on a report of an outbreak of hemolytic uremic syndrome in North Wales (2):

> There are still a few skeptics who would doubt the existence of a malady of undetermined but uniform pathogenesis, occurring in outbreaks, affecting young children and characterized by hemolytic anemia and nephropathy of varying degrees.
>
> The occurrence of bilateral cortical necrosis . . . in infants dying from gastroenteritis due to *E. coli* type 0-111 [*Lancet* 2: 1199 (1954). (Fig 1)] suggests that the causation of the hemolytic-uremic syndrome may be on a similar basis. Perhaps the priming mechanism is a virus and the trigger the *E. coli*. There is no doubt that this fascinating syndrome has not engendered the interest it deserves, presumably because the Great Seats of Learning, other than Johannesburg and Buenos Aires, have not experienced outbreaks. So, put an end to this torpor, Mr. Editor, Sir. Step out . . . and proclaim an International conference on Gasser's Syndrome! . . .

The editor's comment: "That Kibel is a gasser."

Kibel displayed remarkable foresight. Only 10 years previously Conrad von Gasser and his co-workers Gautier, Steck, Siebenman, and Oeschlin, had delineated the features of what they initially called the hemolytic uremic syndromes (*Hamolytiche uramiche syndrome*) (3). Gasser (Fig. 2) was a Swiss hematologist who, while he was examining numerous peripheral blood films as part of a thesis on the hemolytic

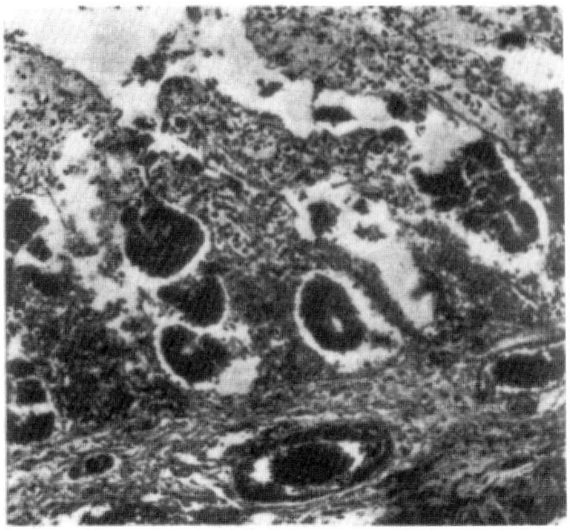

Figure 1 McKay et al., *Lancet* 2: 1199 (1954).

anemias, noted that some contained bizarre-shaped erythrocytes. Five cases were selected who, in addition to evidence of hemolysis, were severely ill with thrombocytopenia, acute renal failure, and cerebral symptoms. The features of these cases were published under the heading of the hemolytic uremic syndromes (Fig. 3). The series of events that led him and his co-workers to define the syndrome that initially bore his name is described by his close collaborators and coauthors in Chapter 1. It was their opinion that the essential features distinguishing hemolytic uremic syndromes from thrombotic thrombocytopenic purpura were the severe renal involvement in the former and the multiorgan involvement in the latter. He meticulously detailed the points of difference in subsequent papers (4,5). He continued to follow the literature on his syndrome until his death in 1982. Kaplan met him when he visited

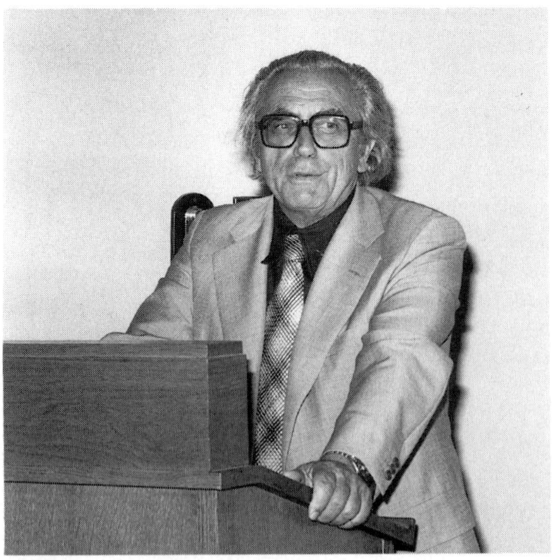

Figure 2 Conrad von Gasser giving Grand Rounds in The Montreal Children's Hospital, 1980.

Hämolytisch-urämische Syndrome:
Bilaterale Nierenrindennekrosen bei akuten erworbener hämolytischen Anämien

Von C. Gasser, E. Gautier und Annemarie Steck (klinischer Teil) und R. E. Siebenmann und R. Oechslin (pathologisch-anatomischer Teil)

Hiezu 4 Abbildungen Seite 929

Aus einer Gruppe von 10 letal verlaufenen Krankheitsbildern, die mit Urämie und hämolytischer Anämie einhergingen, werden 5 akute Fälle beschrieben, die charakterisiert sind durch eine aus unbekannter Ursache plötzlich einsetzende akute intravasale Hämo-

Figure 3 Gasser, C., Gautier, C., Steck, A., Siebenmann, R. E., and Oechslin, R., Hamolytisch-uramische syndrome: Bilaterale nierenindennekrosen bei akuten erworbenen hamolytischen anamien. *Schweiz. Med. Woschenschr.*, 85:905–909 (1955).

Montreal in 1980. He was full of vitality and delivered a memorable Grand Rounds on Hemolytic Uremic Syndrome. He was au fait with the most recent developments on the subject and had an acute awareness of what were and what were not worthwhile contributions. He presented Kaplan with a Swiss cow bell and asked him to ring it at an International Symposium on Gasser's syndrome. Despite Kibel's exhortation, the first symposium on hemolytic uremic syndrome at an international meeting did not take place until 1982 in Hanover, West Germany at the sixth *International Congress of Pediatric Nephrology*. As chairman of that symposium, Kaplan complied with Conrad von Gasser's wishes and rang the bell in his memory.

Between 1957 and 1960, Rénee Habib and her colleagues wrote five papers on HUS (6–10). Their first case was presented to la Société de Pediatrie in May 1957 and was subsequently reported in *la Presse Medicale* (Fig. 4) (6). The name *purpura thrombotique thrombocytopenique* was given to this condition by her hematologist colleague, in spite of the fact that [she] told him that the arteriolar and glomerular

2144 LA PRESSE MEDICALE, N° 94.

Purpura thrombotique thrombocytopénique
(MALADIE DE MOSCHCOVITZ)
chez une enfant de dix mois

Par MM.

Robert CLEMENT, Jean BERNARD, A. PAPAIOANNOU, G. MATHÉ, R. HABIB et M. DESIGNOLLE (Paris)

L'ANÉMIE hémolytique aiguë fébrile décrite sous le nom de « maladie de Moschcovitz » ou de « purpura thrombotique thrombo-cytopénique », mérite une place à part en nosologie en raison de la gravité de son pronostic, des nombreuses thromboses artériolaires et capillaires par nécrose fibrinoïde des parois vasculaires qui, suivant le siège, entraînent des signes cliniques rénaux ou nerveux, alors que les manifestations purpuriques sont relativement discrètes.

L'étiologie de cette affection est encore imprécise. Elle a été jusqu'à présent observée chez l'adulte ; il n'existe à notre connaissance que deux observations concernant des enfants âgés respectivement de 7 et 10 mois (C. Gasser et coll., S. A. Wile et Ph. Sturgeon).

Figure 4 Clement, R., Bernard, J., Papainnou, A., Mathe, G., Habib, R., and Designolle, M., Purpura thrombotique thrombocytopenique (maladie de Moschcovitz) chez un enfant de dix mois. *Press. Med.*, 65: 2144–2146 (1957).

lesions were extremely special and probably similar to what Moschcowitz had described (which in fact was a case of HUS), but totally different from what Gasser had described (cortical necrosis) (R. Habib, personal communication, 1990). While working in the pathology laboratory of Professor Debre, Habib undertook a retrospective survey of his records of 60 infants who had died with acute renal failure. Six of these had the same pathological features that she had observed in her first case. These findings were published under the title *Maladie Thrombotique Arteriolocapillaire du Rein* (Fig. 5) (7). In 1959 Mme. Habib first used the term *microangiopathie thrombotique du rein* (9). Habib continued to define and redefine our understanding of the pathology of HUS for more than 30 years (11, 12). One of her most important contributions was the recognition that the severity of the renal clinical findings could be correlated with the predominant histopathological lesion. She and her co-workers described three main groups of renal injury: cortical necrosis, predominance of glomerular injury, and predominance of arteriolar injury. A mixture of glomerular and arteriolar lesions also occur. They also demonstrated that the severity of the clinical disease and its prognosis correlated with this classification (12).

Was HUS a "new" syndrome or had unrecognized cases either been seen or published before 1954? Fluge and Moe (13) attempted to answer this question by reviewing the records of infants with acute gastroenteritis who had presented during the years 1950–1955, and they were able to retrospectively diagnose 2 out of 104 as having had HUS. It is of interest that urine culture grew *Escherichia coli* in one of these patients (13). Joan Wagner may have reported a case of HUS under the heading of *Acute Tubular Necrosis with Anaemia* from The Hospitals for Sick Children, Great Ormond Street, in 1954 (Fig. 6) (14). Although the patient had hemolytic anemia, thrombocytopenia, acute renal failure, and seizures, a definitive diagnosis of HUS is difficult to make because, unfortunately, there is no mention of the presence or absence of fragmented erythrocytes. Familial, probably autosomal recessive, hemolytic uremic syndrome was first reported by Fison in 1956 as *Acute Glomerulonephritis in Infancy* (15). Also in 1954, there appeared, what seems to be in

MALADIE THROMBOTIQUE ARTÉRIOLOCAPILLAIRE DU REIN CHEZ L'ENFANT

par R. HABIB, H. MATHIEU et P. ROYER *

(Centre d'étude des maladies du métabolisme chez l'enfant, Directeur : P. Royer, Hôpital des Enfants-Malades, Paris.)

Le problème de la classification nosologique des néphropathies aiguës graves du jeune enfant n'est pas encore résolu. Ce travail a été entrepris en fonction de ce fait, et il nous a conduit à l'isolement d'une variété particulière de néphropathie aiguë dont les liens avec le syndrome de Gasser et avec la maladie de Moschowitz restent à préciser.

* Travail effectué avec l'aide de l'Institut National d'Hygiène.

MÉTHODE

Nous avons repris l'étude anatomique de 60 cas de néphropathies infantiles décédées en 16 ans à l'Hôpital des Enfants-Malades. Dans 6 cas, nous avons pu mettre en évidence une lésion rénale très particulière survenue chez des enfants dont l'âge s'échelonnait entre 9 mois et 11 ans.

L'étude à posteriori des observations cliniques nous

REV. FRANÇ. ÉTUDES CLIN. ET BIOL. 1958, III, 891-894.

Figure 5 Habib, R., Mathieu, H., and Royer, P., Maladie thrombotique arteriocapillaire du rein chez l'enfant. *Rev. Fr. Etud. Clin. Biol.*, 8: 891–894 (1958).

ACUTE TUBULAR NECROSIS WITH ANÆMIA

BY

JOAN WAGNER, M.B., M.R.C.P.

Introduction

This case is presented as a problem of diagnosis and an example of the changes that may occur in the various stages of acute tubular necrosis with ultimate recovery. The relationship of anæmia to the kidney lesion and the possible cause of anæmia will be discussed.

Figure 6 Wagner, J., Acute tubular necrosis with anaemia. *Great Ormond Street J.*, 7: 66–72 (1954).

retrospect, a remarkable report by McKay and Wahle from Virginia, in *The Lancet* (16). These pathologists described an epidemic of severe gastroenteritis in neonatal infants (no ages were given) caused by *E. coli* 0–111, B4. Thrombi were noted in many organs, and "The amount of thrombosis varied from case to case, but in the more severely affected kidneys every glomerular tuft was completely occluded by a fibrin thrombus." There is insufficient evidence to characterize these patients as having had HUS, but the report is of historical interest.

No one in the world has seen and treated more cases of HUS than Carlos Gianantonio from Buenos Aires, Argentina (Fig. 7). His contributions are all the more noteworthy when one takes into consideration the difficult circumstances under which he has worked and studied. Everything was in short supply—facilities, money, contact with the outside world. Indeed, for a time, he was unable to have access to current medical journals. His significant contributions (17–22), which now span nearly 30 years, were made despite a very heavy working load as a pediatrician. Among Gianantonio's important contributions is the recognition that some patients with HUS who recover from the acute episode may go on to develop end-stage renal failure many years later (19). In 1973, Gianantonio et al. described the clinical and pathological characteristics of the acute stage of HUS, drawn from a series of 678 patients (20).

The first report of a small epidemic of HUS was published in 1966. McClean et al. presented ten histories of patients whose illness all occurred within a 6-month period in North Wales (2). The first major epidemiological studies on HUS were reported from southern Africa by Kibel and Barnard (23, 24). These workers were the first to note that HUS was (and remains) an uncommon occurrence in blacks.

Hemolytic uremic syndrome seemed initially to be largely confined to infants and children, and it was not until 1966, that the syndrome was first described in adults as HUS (25), rather than as TTP (26). There has been much discussion and a great deal of confusion and disagreement concerning the relation between HUS and TTP. Several different points of view have been expressed in this volume, and the subject has been reviewed in Chapter 3. Kaplan et al. (27) recognized, in 1975, that there were two patterns of familial involvement of HUS, in that some sibs seemed to have developed HUS as a result of exogenous exposure to an infective agent, and a second group of sibs seemed to have had a genetic predisposition to develop HUS. This speculation was followed by the observation of Trompeter et al. that most cases

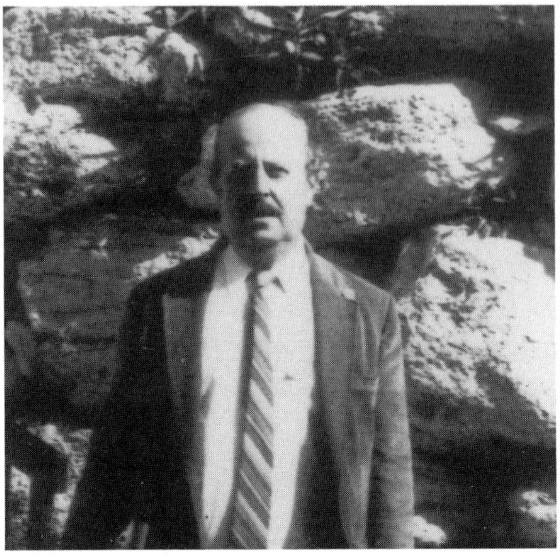

Figure 7 Carlos Gianantonio in Bal Harbour, Florida, 1983. Jose Strauss had invited Kaplan, Gianantonio, Alan Gruskin, and J. J. Byrnes to participate in a seminar on HUS at his 10th Pediatric Nephrology course.

of HUS can be divided into two groups on the basis of whether a diarrheal prodrome was present (D+) or not (D–) (28). The D– patients tend to have a poorer outcome, as described in Chapter 14.

Karmali's recognition that a majority of patients with HUS have evidence of exposure to verotoxin (Shiga toxin)-producing *E. coli* has been the most important contribution to understanding the etiology, pathogenesis, and epidemiology of typical HUS (28–31). During the fall of 1980, an infant died suddenly at home in Toronto after a bloody diarrheal illness. A diagnosis of HUS was made by Dr. L. Becker, who did a coroner's autopsy at The Hospital for Sick Children. Karmali cultured an *E. coli* from this patient's stool that produced verotoxin, a toxin about which little was known. Many microbiologists had never heard of it. Disappointingly, the organism could not be isolated from any of the next five patients with HUS whom they investigated. In the sixth case they not only isolated the *E. coli,* but also found large quantities of the verotoxin in the feces. When they retested the other five cases, they were able to demonstrate verotoxin in the stools of two (Fig. 8). The work and observations of Karmali's team culminated in an international symposium, which was held in Toronto in 1987 (Fig. 9). It is now becoming increasingly evident that patients with Shigatoxin-associated HUS correspond to the first group of sibs with environmentally induced HUS, as described by Kaplan et al. (27), and to most of the patients with D+ HUS, as reported by Barratt et al. (32). It is also becoming apparent that patients with Shiga toxin-associated HUS have a **disease** called *Shiga toxin-associated hemolytic uremic syndrome*, whether they are children or adults, and whether they are labeled as HUS or TTP.

Some landmarks of interest and important contributions to our understanding of HUS are presented in chronologic order:

Preliminary Communication

SPORADIC CASES OF HAEMOLYTIC-URAEMIC SYNDROME ASSOCIATED WITH FAECAL CYTOTOXIN AND CYTOTOXIN-PRODUCING ESCHERICHIA COLI IN STOOLS

MOHAMED A. KARMALI BRIAN T. STEELE*
MARTIN PETRIC CORAZON LIM

Departments of Bacteriology and Virology; Research Institute; and Division of Nephrology, Department of Pediatrics, Hospital for Sick Children, Toronto, Ontario, Canada M5G 1X8 and Department of Microbiology, University of Toronto

Summary A cytotoxin active on Vero cells, less active on hela cells, and inactive on WI38 cells (Vero toxin [VT]) was detected in stool isolates of *Escherichia*

Figure 8 Arguably the most important paper ever published on HUS. Karmali, M. A., Steele, B. T., Petric, M., and Lim, C., Sporadic cases of haemolytic-uraemic syndrome associated with faecal cytotoxin and cytotoxin-producing *E. coli* in stools. *Lancet, 1*: 619–620 (1983).

Description of *the syndrome*, by Gasser et al. in 1955 (3).
Recognition of the unique nature of *the renal histopathological features*, by Habib et al. in 1958 (7–11).
Definition of the concept of *microangiopathic hemolytic anemia*, by Brain et al. in 1962 (Fig. 10) (33).
Demonstration of improved survival by using *early peritoneal dialysis*, by Gianantonio et al. in 1964 (18).
The suggestion by Barnard and Kibel, in 1965, that *enteropathogenic E. coli* may be the causative agent of HUS (24).
The first report of an *epidemic of HUS* in 1966, by McLean et al. (2).
The first authoritative and *comprehensive review* of HUS, by Brain in 1969 (34).
The recognition of a subset of HUS with *autosomal recessive inheritance*, by Kaplan et al., in 1975 (27).
The recognition of a subset with *autosomal dominant inheritance*, by Farr et al., in 1975 (35).
Recognition of the importance of *recurrent HUS*, by Kaplan, in 1977 (36).
Demonstration of a role for *S. pneumoniae* in the pathogenesis of a small subset of HUS, by Klein et al., in 1977 (37).
Recognition of a role for *prostanoids* in the pathogenesis of HUS, by Remuzzi et al., in 1978 (38).
Demonstration of a role for *verotoxin (Shiga-like toxin)*, by Karmali et al., in 1983 (28).
Delineation of *D+ and D– forms* of HUS, by Barratt et al., in 1987 (29).

Thrombotic thrombocytopenic purpura, which was first described by Moschcowitz in 1924 (39), has fascinated physicians with its dramatic clinical presentations, high mortality rate and, during the last 10–15 years, increasingly effective empirical

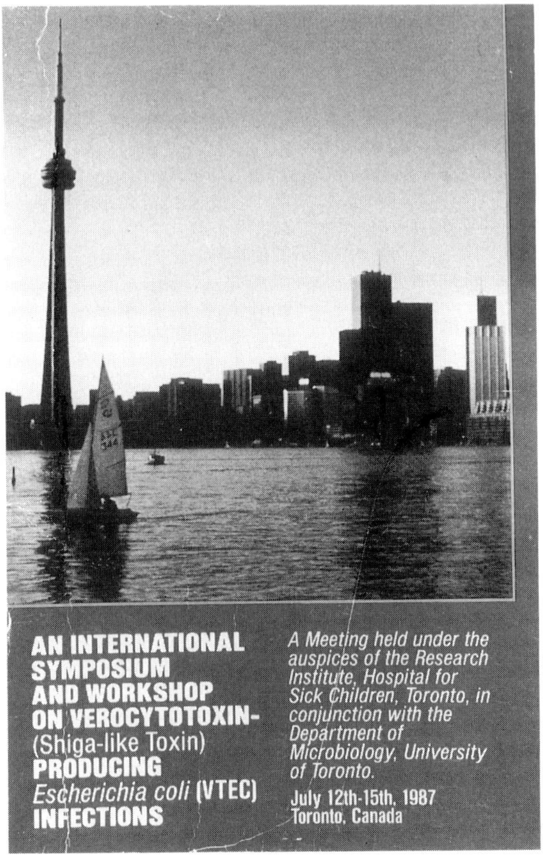

Figure 9 The view of Toronto from Lake Ontario.

treatment (40). The platelet aggregates in TTP produce fluctuating ischemia or infarction in various organs, including the brain in 50–71% of episodes (41, 42). In the closely related disorder, the hemolytic uremic syndrome, the ischemia primarily occurs in the kidneys (40). The most important advance, since the initial description of TTP, has been the discovery by Byrnes (43), Bukowski (44), and their colleagues, that plasma infusion or exchange allows most patients to survive an episode of TTP. This has recently been confirmed in studies of more than 200 patients (41, 42). In most of these patients, the disorder neither recurs nor produces persistent organ damage (42).

Truly recurrent TTP [as opposed to a protracted single episode with periods of incomplete remission (42)] occurs in about 11–28% of TTP patients (41, 42). Thrombotic thrombocytopenic purpura is possibly the result of the intrusion of platelet-aggregating agents into the systemic circulation. This probably accounts for observations that TTP can often be aggravated by platelet transfusions (40, 42). The putative platelet-aggregating substance has variously been reported to be one of several small proteins (45), a calcium-activated cysteine protease capable of cleaving von Willebrand factor (vWF) multimers into more active aggregating forms (46), or "unusually large" vWF multimers (57, 48).

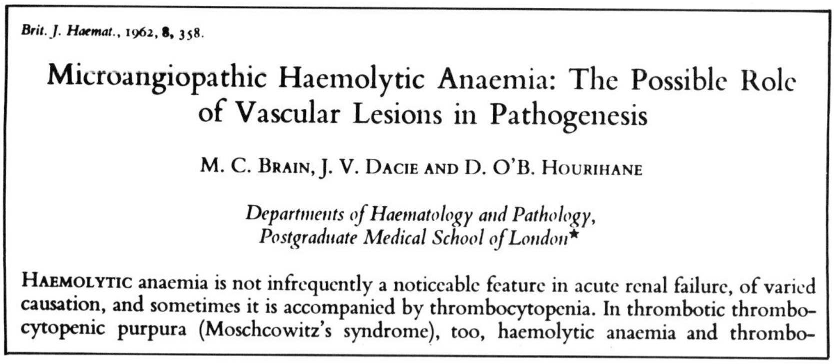
Brit. J. Haemat., 1962, 8, 358.

Microangiopathic Haemolytic Anaemia: The Possible Role of Vascular Lesions in Pathogenesis

M. C. BRAIN, J. V. DACIE AND D. O'B. HOURIHANE

*Departments of Haematology and Pathology, Postgraduate Medical School of London**

HAEMOLYTIC anaemia is not infrequently a noticeable feature in acute renal failure, of varied causation, and sometimes it is accompanied by thrombocytopenia. In thrombotic thrombocytopenic purpura (Moschcowitz's syndrome), too, haemolytic anaemia and thrombo-

Figure 10 Brain et al. introduced the concept of microangiopathic hemolytic anemia.

Some landmarks of interest and important contributions to our understanding of TTP are presented in chronologic order:

Description of *the syndrome*, by Eli Moschcowitz, in 1924 (39).
Definition of the typical, *fully developed case* of TTP, in 1952 (49).
Effective *treatment with fresh plasma*, by Byrnes et al., 1977 (43).
Detection of *abnormal vWF multimers* in relapsing TTP, by Moake et al., in 1982 (50).

Detailed discussions of the history, pathology, possible pathohysiology, and approaches to treatment of HUS and TTP are presented in this monograph. Because these subjects are still in a state of great flux, no attempt has been made to impose the editors' views on areas of disagreement. Therefore, a number of conflicting points of view will be apparent.

References

1. Kibel, M. A., Commentary. In: *The Year Book of Pediatrics* (S. S. Gellis, ed.), Year Book Medical Publishers, Chicago, pp. 301–302 (1967).
2. McLean, M. M., Jones, C. H., and Sutherland, D. A. Haemolytic-uraemic syndrome. A report of an outbreak. *Arch. Dis. Child.*, *41*: 76–81 (1966).
3. Gasser, C., Gautier, C., Steck, A., Siebenmann, R. E., and Oechslin, R., Hamolytisch-uramische syndrome. Bilaterale nierenindennekrosen bei akuten erworbenen hamolytischen anamien. *Schweiz. Med. Woschenschr.*, *85*: 905–909 (1955).
4. Gasser, C., Hamolyticsh-Uramisches Syndrom. In *Handbuch Der Kinderheilkunde* (H. Opitz and F. S. Schmid, eds.), Springer-Verlag, Berlin, pp. 951–963 (1967).
5. Gasser, C., Hamolytisch-uramisches syndrom (HUS) (Gasser) und thrombotish-thrombozytopenische purpura (TTP) (Moschcowitz). In *Niere Blutgerinnung und Hamoatse* (R. Marx and H. A. Thies, eds.), F. K. Schattauer Verlag, Stuttgart, pp. 161–178 (1978).
6. Clement, R., Bernard, J., Papainnou, A., Mathe, G., Habib, R., and Designolle, M., Purpura thrombotique thrombocytopenique (maladie de Moschcovitz) chez un enfant de dix mois. *Press. Med.*, *65*: 2144–2146 (1957).
7. Habib, R., Mathieu, H., and Royer, P., Maladie thrombotique arteriocapillaire du rein chez l'enfant. *Rev. Fr. Etud. Clin. Biol.* *8*: 891–894 (1958).

8. Debre, R., Mozziconacci, P., Brissaud, H.–E., Lagrue, G., and Habib, R., Purpura thrombopenique et nephropathies. *Arch. Fr. Pediatr.* *15*: 289–301 (1958).
9. Royer, P., Habib, R., and Mathieu, H., La microangiopathie thrombotique du rein chez l'enfant. *J. Urol.*, *65*: 169–177 (1959).
10. Royer, P., Habib, R., and Mathieu, H., La microangiopathie thrombotique du rein chez l'enfant. *Ann. Pediatr.*, *36*: 1–16 (1960).
11. Habib, R., Mathieu, H., Royer, P., Le syndrome hemolytique et uremique de l'enfant. Aspects cliniques et anatomiques dans 27 observations. *Nephron*, *4*: 139–172 (1967).
12. Habib, R., Levy, M., Gagnadoux, M. F., and Broyer, M., Prognosis of the hemolytic uremic syndrome in children. *Adv. Nephrol.*, *11*: 109–128 (1982).
13. Fluge, G., and Moe, P. J., Hemolytic-uremic (nephropathic) syndrome. A clinical picture unrecognized in the past? *Acta Pediatr. Scand.*, *56*: 665–670 (1967).
14. Wagner, J., Acute tubular necrosis with anaemia. *Great Ormond Street J.*, *7*: 66–72 (1954).
15. Fison, T. N., Acute glomerulonephritis in infancy. *Arch. Dis. Child.*, *3*: 101–109 (1956).
16. McKay, D. G., and Wahle, G. H., Shwartzman phenomenon in fatal infantile diarrhoea due to *Escherichia coli* 0-111,B4. *Lancet*, *2*: 1199–1200 (1954).
17. Gianantonio, C. A., Vitacco, M., Mendilaharzu, J., Mendilaharzu, F., and Rutty, A., Acute renal failure in infancy and childhood. Clinical course and treatment of forty-one patients. *J. Pediatr.*, *61*: 660–678 (1962).
18. Gianantonio, C., Vitacco, M., Mendilaharzu F., and Rutty, A., The hemolytic-uremic syndrome. *J. Pediatr.*, *64*: 478–490 (1964).
19. Gianantonio, C., Vitacco, M., Mendilaharzu, F., and Gallo, G., The hemolytic-uremic syndrome. *J. Pediatr.*, *72*: 757–765 (1968).
20. Gianantonio, C., Vitacco, M., Mendilaharzu, F., Gallo, G., and Sojo, E. T. The hemolytic-uremic syndrome. *Nephron*, *11*: 174–192 (1973).
21. Avalos, J. S., Vitacco, M., Molinas, F., Penalver, J., and Gianantonio, C., Coagulation findings in the hemolytic-uremic syndrome. *J. Pediatr.*, *76*: 538–548 (1970).
22. Grunfeld, B., Gimenez, S., Liapchuc, S., Mendilaharzu, J., and Gianantonio, C., Systemic hypertension and plasma renin activity in children with the hemolytic-uremic syndrome. *Int. J. Pediatr. Nephrol.*, *3*: 211–214 (1982).
23. Barnard, P. J., and Kibel, M., The haemolytic-uraemic syndrome of infancy and childhood. A report of eleven cases. *Cent. Afr. J. Med.*, *11*: 4–11; 31–34, (1965).
24. Kibel, M., and Barnard, P. J., The haemolytic-uraemic syndrome: A survey in southern Africa. *S. Afr. Med. J.*, *42*: 692–698 (1965).
25. Waddell, A. J. H., and Matz, L. R., Haemolytic-uremic syndrome: A report of two cases in adults. *Med. J. Aust.*, *2*: 893–897 (1966).
26. Dunea, G., Muehrcke, R. C., Nakamoto, S., et al., Thrombotic thrombocytopenic purpura with acute renal failure. *Am. J. Med.*, *41*: 1000–1006 (1966).
27. Kaplan, B. S., Chesney, R. W., and Drummond, K. N., Hemolytic uremic syndrome in families. *N. Engl. J. Med.*, *292*: 1090–1093 (1975).
28. Karmali, M. A., Steele, B. T., Petric, M., and Lim, C. Sporadic cases of haemolytic-uraemic syndrome associated with faecal cytotoxin and cytotoxin-producing *E. coli* in stools. *Lancet*, *1*: 619–620 (1983).
29. Lingwood, C. A., Law, H., Richardson, S., Petric, M., Brunton, L., Degrandis, S., and Karmali, M., Glycolipid binding of purified and recombinant *E. coli* produced verotoxin in vitro. *J. Biol. Chem.*, *262*: 8834–8839 (1987).
30. Head, S. C., Karmali, M. A., Roscoe, M. E., Petric, M., Strockbine, N. A., and Wachsmuth, I. K., Serologic differences between verocytotoxin 2 and Shiga-like toxin II. *Lancet*, *2*: 751 (1988).
31. Richardson, S. E., Karmali, M. A., Becker, L. E., and Smith, C. R., The histopathology of the hemolytic uremic syndrome associated with verocytotoxin-producing *E. coli*. *Hum. Pathol.*, *19*: 1102–1108 (1988).

32. Barratt, T. M., Dillon, M. G., Hardisty, R. M., Levin, M., Nokes, T. J. C., Stroobant, P., and Walters, M. D. S., The role of platelets and platelet-derived growth factors in the pathogenesis of haemolytic-uraemic syndrome. In *Recent Advances in Pediatric Nephrology*, (K. Murakami, T. Kitagawa, K. Yabuta, et al., eds.), Excerpta Medica, Amsterdam, pp. 577–580 (1987).
33. Brain, M. C., Dacie, J. V., and Hourihane, D. O., Microangiopathic haemolytic anaemia: Possible role of vascular lesions in pathogenesis. *Br. J. Haematol.*, *8*: 358–374 (1962).
34. Brain, M., The haemolytic-uraemic syndrome. *Semin. Hematol.*, *6*: 162–180 (1969).
35. Farr, M. J., Roberts, S., Morley, A. R., Dewar, P. J., Roberts, D. F., and Uldall, P. R., The haemolytic-uraemic syndrome—a family study. *Q. J. Med.*, *44*: 161–188 (1975).
36. Kaplan, B. S., Hemolytic uremic syndrome with recurrent episodes: An important subset. *Clin. Nephrol.*, *8*: 495–498 (1977).
37. Klein, P. J., Bulla, M., Newman, R. A., Muller, P., Uhlenbruck, G., Schaefer, H. E., Kruger, G., and Fisher, R., Thomsen–Friedenreich antigen in haemolytic uraemic syndrome. *Lancet*, *2*: 1024–1025 (1977).
38. Remuzzi, G., Misiani, R., Marchesi, D., Livio, M., and de Gaetano, G., Haemolytic-uraemic syndrome: Deficiency of plasma factor(s) regulating prostacyclin activity? *Lancet*, *2*: 871–872 (1978).
39. Moschcowitz, E., Hyaline thrombosis in the terminal arterioles and capillaries: A hitherto undescribed disease. *Proc. N. Y. Pathol. Soc.*, *24*: 21–24 (1924).
40. Moake, J. L., Thrombotic thrombocytopenic purpura and the hemolytic-uremic syndrome. In *Hematology: Basic Principles and Practice*, (R. Hoffman, E. Benz, S. Shattil, B. Furie, and H. Cohen, eds.), Churchill-Livingstone, New York, pp. 1495–1501 (1991).
41. Rock, G. A., Shumak, K. H., Buskard, N. A., et al., Comparison of plasma exchange with plasma infusion in the treatment of thrombotic thrombocytopenic purpura. *N. Engl. J. Med.*, *325*: 393–397 (1991).
42. Bell, W. R., Braine, H. G., Ness, P. M., and Kickler, T. S., Improved survival in thrombotic thrombocytopenic purpura-hemolytic uremic syndrome—clinical experience in 108 patients. *N. Engl. J. Med.*, *325*: 398–402 (1991).
43. Byrnes, J. J., and Khurana, M., Treatment of thrombotic thrombocytopenic purpura with plasma. *N. Engl. J. Med. 297*: 1386–1389 (1977).
44. Bukowski, R. M., Hewlett, J. S., Reimer, R. R., et al., Therapy of thrombotic thrombocytopenic purpura: An overview. *Semin. Thromb. Hemost.*, *7*: 1–8 (1981).
45. Lian, E. C., Thrombotic thrombocytopenic purpura. *Annu. Rev. Med.*, *39*: 203–212 (1988).
46. Moore, J. C., Murphy, W. G., and Kelton, J. G., Calpain proteolysis of von Willebrand factor enhances its binding to platelet membrane glycoprotein IIb/IIIa: An explanation for platelet aggregation in thrombotic thrombocytopenic purpura. *Br. J. Haematol.*, *74*: 457–464 (1990).
47. Moake, J. L. and McPherson, P. D., Abnormalities of von Willebrand factor multimers in thrombotic thrombocytopenic purpura and the hemolytic-uremic syndrome. *Am. J. Hematol.*, *74*: 457–464 (1990).
48. Moake, J. L., Turner, N. A., Stathopoulos, N. A., Nolasco, L., and Hellums, J. D., Shear-induced platelet aggregation can be mediated by vWF released from platelets, as well as by exogenous large or unusually large vWF multimers, requires adenosine diphosphate, and is resistant to aspirin. *Blood*, *71*: 1366–1374 (1988).
49. Symmers, W. S. C., Thrombotic microangiopathic haemolytic anaemia (thrombotic microangiopathy). *Br. Med. J.*, *2*: 897–903. (1952).
50. Moake J. L., Rudy, C. K., Troll, L. H., Weinstein, M. J., Colaninno, N. M., Azacar, J., Seder, R. H., Hong, S. L., and Deykin, D., Unusually large plasma factor VIII:von Willebrand factor multimers in chronic relapsing thrombotic thrombocytopenic purpura. *N. Engl. J. Med.*, *307*: 1432–1435 (1982).

I
Historical Review

1
The Birth of the Hemolytic Uremic Syndrome

E. Gautier *Centre Hospitalier Universitaire Vaudois, Lausanne, Switzerland*
R. E. Siebenmann *Zurich, Switzerland*

CLINICAL ASPECTS

Conrad Gasser (Fig. 1) obtained his M.D. degree in 1937 and then trained in microbiology, morbid anatomy, and internal medicine. In 1941 he became a resident at the Zurich Kinderspital under the prestigious leadership of Guido Fanconi. From 1945–1956, Gasser was Oberarzt (chief resident). Besides a heavy load of clinical responsibilities and teaching, he pursued intensive research activities in hematology. Gasser described a form of anemia in premature babies with spontaneous formation of Heinz bodies (1948) and acute erythroblastopenia (1949). His monograph *Die Hämolytischen Syndrome des Kindesalters* was published in 1951. It contained a wealth of carefully documented observations which earned him his venia legendi and established his international reputation. As Oberarzt, Conrad Gasser was the tutor of the incoming residents who worked initially in a large ward called Saal 4. He was an astute, original clinician with vast experience. He guided residents through their clinical apprenticeship and in the absorbing and fascinating field of hematology wherein they did all the blood counts and examined blood smears and bone marrow aspirates.

Emile Gautier entered the Kinderspital of Zurich in the fall of 1952, after 2 years in physiology in Bern with Alexandre von Muralt, 2 years as research fellow with Alan Butler of the Massachusetts General Hospital, and one year of internal medicine in Geneva. While in Boston, he had been exposed to John Merrill's work on acute renal insufficiency.

The first patient described in the original paper of 1955 was seen in May 1953. Cases 4, 2, and 3 were admitted in January, February, and July 1954. A retrospective search identified case 5, who was seen in 1952. All patients died. Gautier remembers admitting cases 1 and 2. The medical records of four of those five patients were retrieved from the files of the Kinderspital in 1989. Figure 2 shows the upper part of

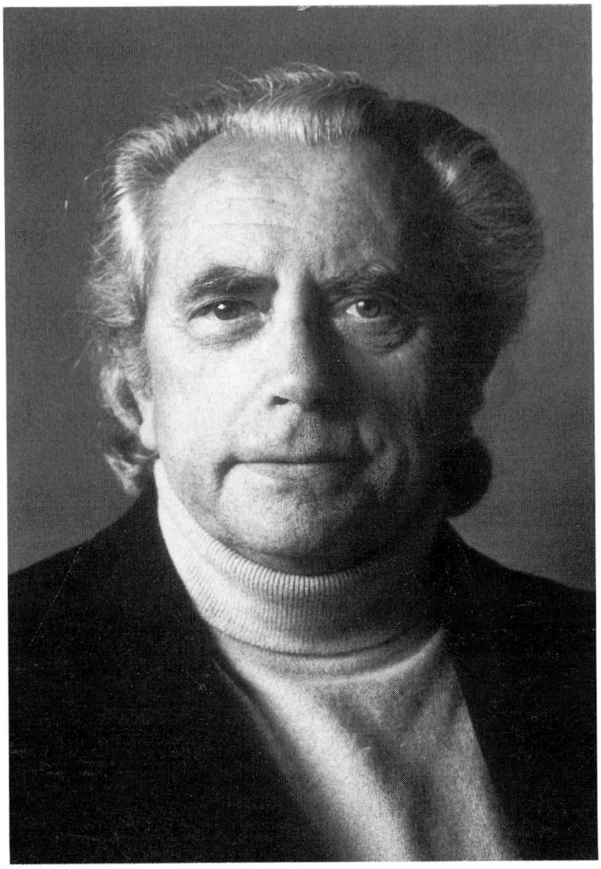

Figure 1 Professor Conrad Gasser, 1912–1982.

the front page of these records. The diagnoses are descriptive, and the numerous question marks attest to the perplexity of the house staff. The handwritten annotations were added by Conrad Gasser as the results of the postmortem examination became available. The diagnosis "hemolytic uremic syndrome" was made on clinical grounds in patient 3.

Figure 3 shows the transcription, carried out by Gasser, of the emergency status of case 2; Figures 4 and 5 show the evaluation of her blood and bone marrow aspirate on admission. It was also possible to look back to the slides of the peripheral blood and bone marrow aspirates of all patients. Mrs. S. Adank-Stahel, laboratory technician at the Kinderspital at the time the patients were observed, kindly reviewed each slide this year. She confirmed that megacaryocytes are present in the bone marrow, sometimes in increased and sometimes in decreased numbers. Platelet-forming megacaryocytes are either decreased or absent. Figure 6 shows the bone marrow smear of patient 1. She saw schizocytes in every blood smear, although this finding was not mentioned in the original paper in regard to patient 1.

The Pathology Institute is situated in the Kantonsspital area at a distance from the Kinderspital. Every week Guido Fanconi and his Oberärzte and residents paced rapidly along the Freiestrasse to attend the clinicopathological confrontations. Cases

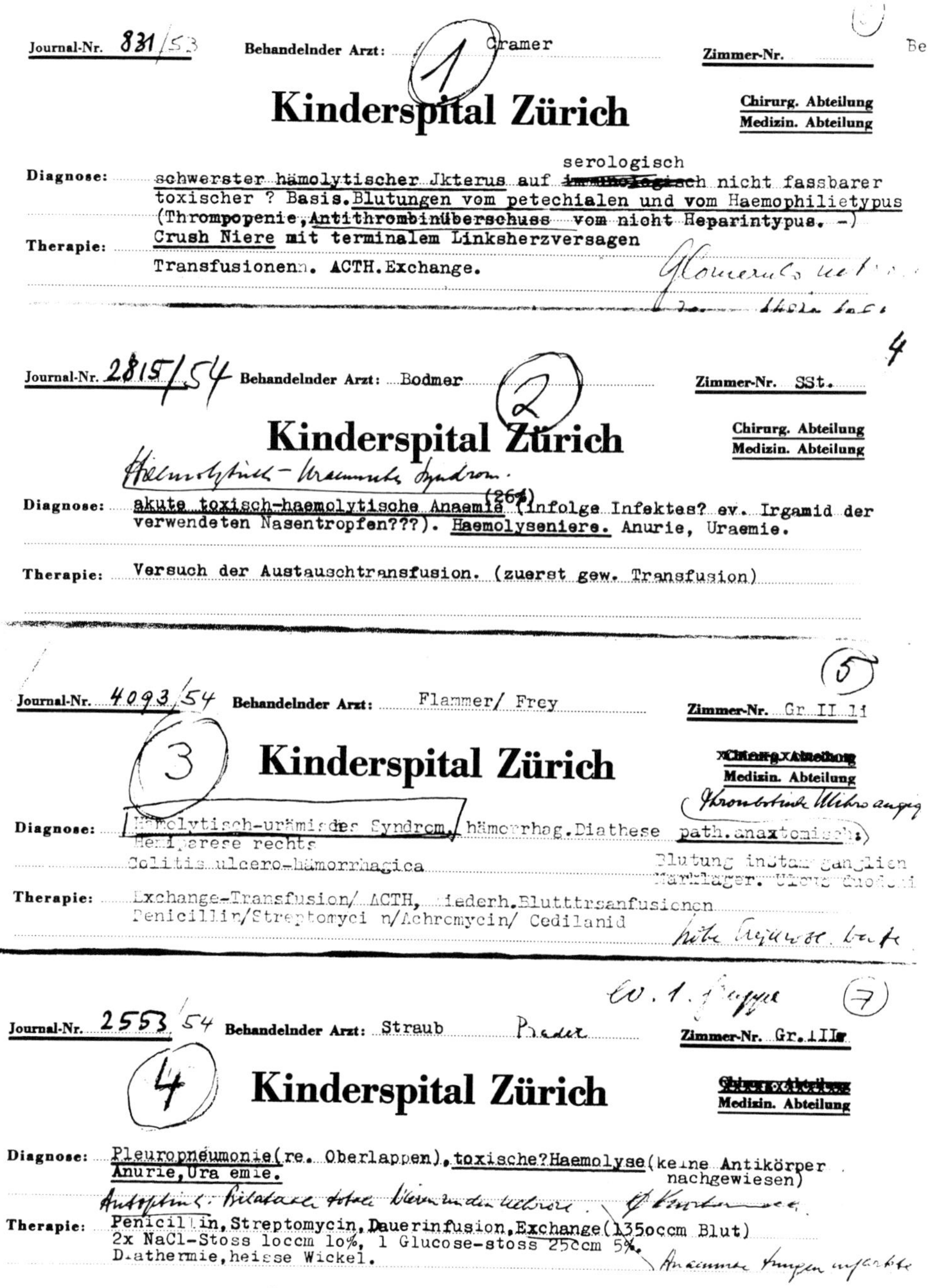

Journal-Nr. 831/53 Behandelnder Arzt: Cramer Zimmer-Nr. Be

Kinderspital Zürich

Chirurg. Abteilung
Medizin. Abteilung

Diagnose: schwerster hämolytischer Jkterus auf serologisch nicht fassbarer toxischer ? Basis. Blutungen vom petechialen und vom Haemophilietypus (Thrompopenie, Antithrombinüberschuss vom nicht Heparintypus. –) Crush Niere mit terminalem Linksherzversagen

Therapie: Transfusionen. ACTH. Exchange.

Journal-Nr. 2815/54 Behandelnder Arzt: Bodmer Zimmer-Nr. SSt.

Kinderspital Zürich

Chirurg. Abteilung
Medizin. Abteilung

Diagnose: akute toxisch-haemolytische Anaemia (infolge Infektes? ev. Irgamid der verwendeten Nasentropfen???). Haemolyseniere. Anurie, Uraemie.

Therapie: Versuch der Austauschtransfusion. (zuerst gew. Transfusion)

Journal-Nr. 4093/54 Behandelnder Arzt: Flammer/ Frey Zimmer-Nr. Gr. II 11

Kinderspital Zürich

Medizin. Abteilung

Diagnose: Hämolytisch-urämisches Syndrom, hämorrhag. Diathese path. anatomisch: Hemiparese rechts Blutung in Stammganglien Colitis ulcero-hämorrhagica Marklager. Ulcus duodeni

Therapie: Exchange-Transfusion/ ACTH, wiederh. Bluttransfusionen Penicillin/Streptomycin/Achromycin/ Cedilanid

Journal-Nr. 2553/54 Behandelnder Arzt: Straub Zimmer-Nr. Gr. III

Kinderspital Zürich

Medizin. Abteilung

Diagnose: Pleuropneumonie (re. Oberlappen), toxische? Haemolyse (keine Antikörper nachgewiesen) Anurie, Uraemie.

Therapie: Penicillin, Streptomycin, Dauerinfusion, Exchange (1350ccm Blut) 2x NaCl-Stoss 10ccm 10%, 1 Glucose-stoss 250ccm 5%. Diathermie, heisse Wickel.

Figure 2 Front pages of the medical records of four patients admitted to the Kinderspital of Zurich.

Name: Einlagebogen Nr.

Datum

2.2.54 Notfall Status (Dr Gasser)

Kind ist sehr blass, mit einem grünen Kolorit der Skleren. Kein Ikterus.
Schreit noch lebhaft, schaut herum , scheint nicht benommen zu sein. Ist durstig und trinkt gut. bricht nicht. gähnt.
Turgor nicht schlecht. Mundschleimhaut noch feucht.
Am Gesäss einige erodierte Hautstellen infolge des Durchfalles.
keine Drüsenschwellung.
Abdomen, weich, Milzkuppe kaum unter dem RB, dagegen Leber vergrössert, 1 1/2 QF unter dem RB.

Lungen Herz oB. (Durchleuchtung in dr P Schule: normaler Befund, aber Herz kelin)
Fontanelle nicht gespannt, nicht eingesunken.

Coombs Test neg. warscheinl ch handelt sich mit der Anamnese und dem neg. Coombstest um eine toxische hemolytische Anaemie.

(Das Fehlen der Splenomegalie spricht auch gegen Antigen Antikörper Prozess.

Urin: makroskopisch braunlich, gegen eine Lichtquelle gesehen, zeigt eine rötliche Komponente.
Überschicht nach Zentrifugation ungefähr gleich gefärbt.
Benz +++
Sediment: massenhaft Rote, viele Leuko, und Erythrocaten Zylinder, Benz +++
E ++
Ubg -
Cl vermindert.

.. Das Rest des Urins wurde zur Spektrometrie behalten.

Blutbild
Hb um 22U 38% Rek 84 ‰.
Rote 2,2, Index 0,86
Leuko leider verunglückt.
Diff: 1,5 halbreife Myelocyten
0,5 reife Myelocyten
1 Metamyelocyten
21 Stab
12,5 Seg,
1,5 Eos
9,5 Mono
52 Lympho
0,5 plasmatelle

Zeichen einer starken Regeneration, keine Innenkörper
enorme Anisocytose, mit Fragmentocyten und winzigen Mikrocyten

Dr Gasser: bis Morgen für die Transfusion warten.

3.2.54. Kind sieht heute morgen sehr blass aus:
Hgb. 26%.

XXXXXXXXXXXXXXXXXXXXXXXXXXXXXX Heute fällt auf, dass das Kind am ganzen Körper eigenartig steif ist: Arme gebeugt, Beine gant gestreckt, auch beim Schreien. PSR +++/+++, mit nach oben und unten stark erweiterter reflexogener Zone.

Ist wohl hinter dem Ganzen noch eine cerebrale Störung? Oder ist diese nur die Folge der schweren Anaemie? Babinski bds. kaum angedeutet.

244 ✉ X. 52. 3000

Figure 3 Emergency physical examination of case 2 by Dr. Gasser.

were reviewed and the pertinent slides were available for microscopic examination. At one of those confrontations, they learned that case 1 did not present with a shock-kidney but a glomerulonephritis necroticans acuta, which could be viewed as a minimal form of cortical necrosis. Case 2 was discussed with the pathologist in May

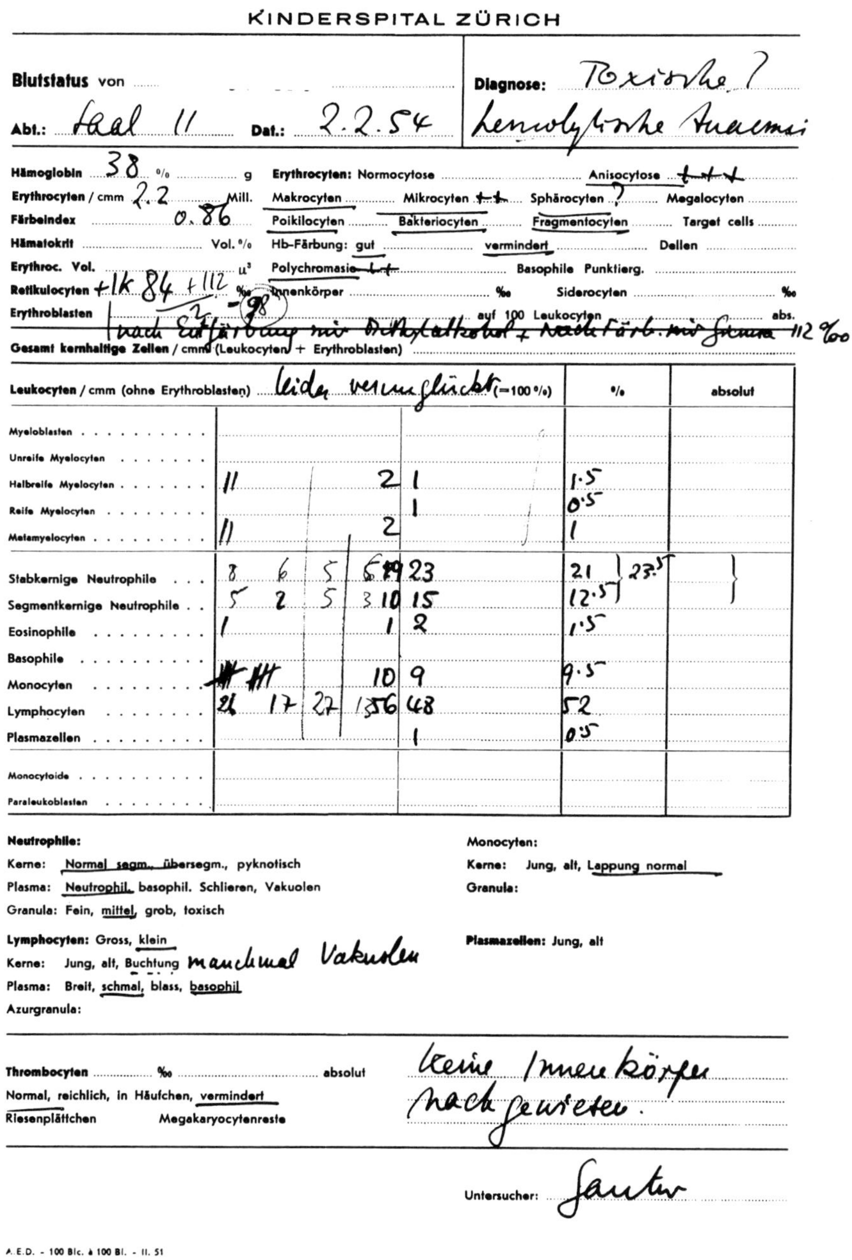
KINDERSPITAL ZÜRICH

Blutstatus von ..... Diagnose: Toxicose ?
Abt.: Saal 11 Dat.: 2.2.54 hemolytische Anaemie

Hämoglobin 38 % g Erythrocyten: Normocytose Anisocytose +++
Erythrocyten / cmm 2.2 Mill. Makrocyten Mikrocyten ++ Sphärocyten ? Megalocyten
Färbeindex 0.86 Poikilocyten Bakteriocyten Fragmentocyten Target cells
Hämatokrit Vol. % Hb-Färbung: gut vermindert Dellen
Erythroc. Vol. u³ Polychromasie ++ Basophile Punktierg.
Retikulocyten +1k 84 +112 ‰ Innenkörper ‰ Siderocyten ‰
Erythroblasten auf 100 Leukocyten abs.
Gesamt kernhaltige Zellen / cmm (Leukocyten + Erythroblasten) 112 ‰

Leukocyten / cmm (ohne Erythroblasten) leider verunglückt (=100 %) % absolut

			%	absolut
Myeloblasten				
Unreife Myelocyten				
Halbreife Myelocyten	11	2 1	1.5	
Reife Myelocyten		1	0.5	
Metamyelocyten	11	2	1	
Stabkernige Neutrophile	8 6 5	6 19 23	21	23.5
Segmentkernige Neutrophile	5 2 5	3 10 15	12.5	
Eosinophile	1	1 2	1.5	
Basophile				
Monocyten	### ###	10 9	9.5	
Lymphocyten	26 17 27	56 48	52	
Plasmazellen		1	0.5	
Monocytoide				
Paraleukoblasten				

Neutrophile:
Kerne: Normal segm., übersegm., pyknotisch
Plasma: Neutrophil, basophil. Schlieren, Vakuolen
Granula: Fein, mittel, grob, toxisch

Monocyten:
Kerne: Jung, alt, Lappung normal
Granula:

Lymphocyten: Gross, klein
Kerne: Jung, alt, Buchtung manchmal Vakuolen
Plasma: Breit, schmal, blass, basophil
Azurgranula:

Plasmazellen: Jung, alt

Thrombocyten ‰ absolut keine Innenkörper
Normal, reichlich, in Häufchen, vermindert nachgewiesen.
Riesenplättchen Megakaryocytenreste

Untersucher: Sauter

A.E.D. - 100 Blc. à 100 Bl. - II. 51

Figure 4 Peripheral blood examination of case 2 on admission.

54, case 4 in June 54. The medical record of case 5 could not be retrieved, but his hemolytic anemia and anuria had occurred in the presence of a pneumonitis with pleural empyema. The Coombs' test was positive and, during the cross-matching, a polyagglutination had been noted.

By early May 1955, graphs were drawn in the typical style of Fanconi's Kinder-

KINDERSPITAL ZÜRICH

Name: 7 Wo. Abt.: S.St.

Präp. Nr. 4590

Klinische Diagnose: Haemolyt. Anaemie

Myelogramm ~~Sternum~~ Tibia ~~Becken~~ Dat.: 3. II. 54.

Reticuloendothel				Normal-Werte
Reticulumzellen:				
Makrophagen				—0,4
plasmazelluläre	0,3			—1,0
lymphoide				
Endothelzellen:				
Fettzellen:				

Plasmazell. Mitosen Besonderheiten:

Erythropoëse			Normal-Werte
Proerythroblasten	9,0	103,3	—1
Makroblasten	1,3		—1
Normoblast basophil	54,3		—5
polychrom	35,0		—15
orthochrom	3,7		—5 (10—20)

Erythrobl. Mitosen 3/310 Besonderheiten: Karyorrhexis 19/310

Retikulocyten

Leuko- und Lymphopoëse				Normal-Werte
Myeloblasten		0,3	auf 100 =	—4
unreife Myelocyten	6,0			-6
halbreife Myelocyten	14,3	21,0		-12 (-25)
reife Myelocyten	0,7			-12
Metamyelocyten	7,7			-15
Neutrophile stabk.	13,7	23,1		-40 (-60)
segmentk.	1,7			-10
Eosinophile I / II	3,0 / 2,0	5,0		—3 / —3 (—5)
Basophile		—		—1
Monocyten		8,0		—5
Lymphoide Zellen		42,6		8—20

Mitosen — Besonderheiten: Riesenneutrophile — Toxisch: — —

Unklare Zellen 88/610

Thrombopoëse					
Megakaryocyten: (Zahl)	vermindert		unreif (+)	Thrombocyten	spärlich vorhanden
	normal	++	halbreif +		
	vermehrt		reif	Riesenplättchen	

Zellgehalt: Zellreiche Präp. mit sehr viel zerstörten Zellen

Beurteilung:

Erythroblasten sehr stark vermehrt, einige in Karyorrhexis

Reifere Neutro in mässiger Zahl

Monozyten vermehrt

Lymphoide Zellen vermehrt

Megakaryozyten z.T. stark segmentiert

Figure 5 Bone marrow examination of case 2.

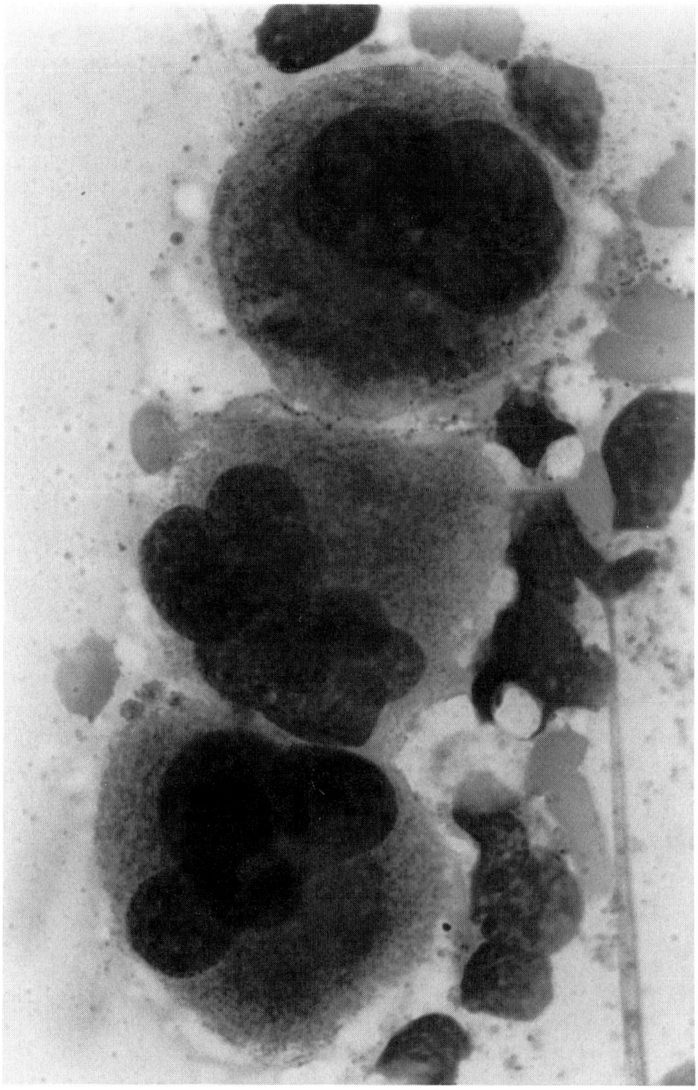

Figure 6 Three megacaryocytes in a bone marrow smear of case 1.

spital. These depicted the evolution of the different parameters for each patient. (Figures 7 and 8 concern patients 1 and 3.)

At the 10th annual meeting of the Swiss Society of Haematology in May 1955, Gasser and Siebenmann gave a paper entitled "Hämolytisch-urämische Syndrome, bilaterale Nierenrindennekrose bei akuten erworbenen hämolytischen Anämien."

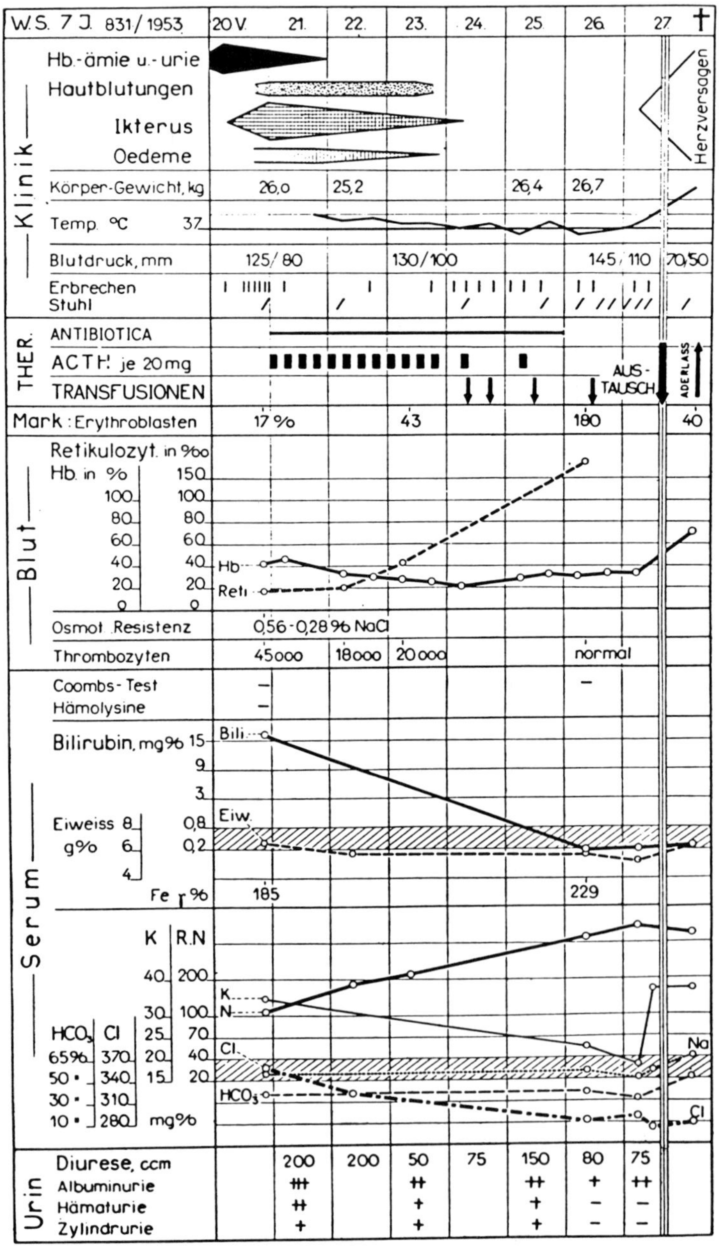

Abb. 1. Verlaufskurve zu Fall 1.

Figure 7 Graph of the evolution of case 1.

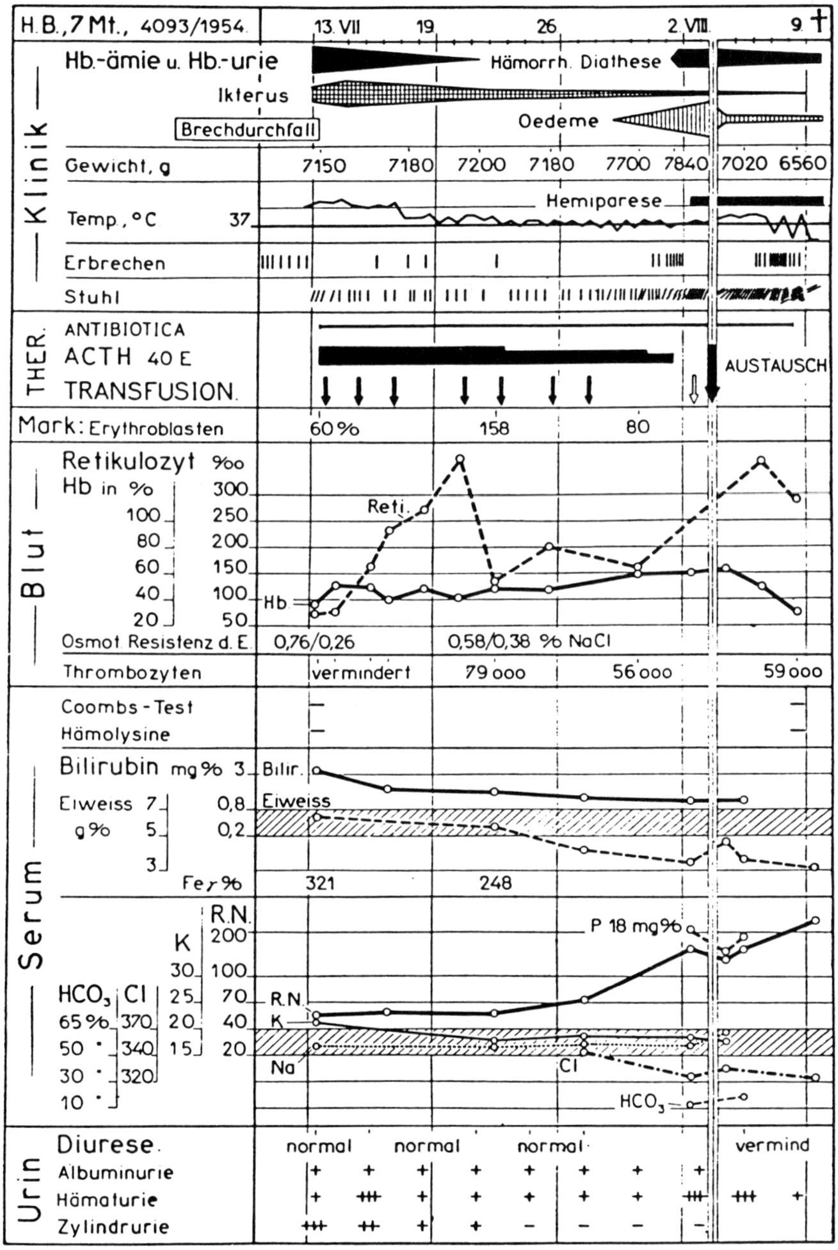

Abb. 4. Verlaufskurve zu Fall 3.

Figure 8 Graph of the evolution of case 3.

The striking appellation has become a classic. Gasser was extremely cautious. Not only did he use the term syndrome but applied the plural syndromes. Clearly certain characteristics were common to the five patients: the acquired hemolytic anemia, the renal failure (the cause of which was cortical necrosis), and the thrombocytopenia. On the other hand, the patients differed in age, course, involvement of other organs, and pathogenesis. Case 5 had a positive Coombs' test and is similar to those described by Klein et al. in 1977.

The text of the Geneva conference was published in the *Schweizerische Medizinische Wochenschrift* in 1955 (1) (Fig. 9). Without a doubt, the highlights of the publication are the graphs depicting the clinical evolution in two patients and the photographs of the renal histology and blood smears. It is of interest, in retrospect, that certain elements available to the authors were not taken into consideration. For example, no explanation was given for the thrombocytopenia. Bone marrow aspirates that had been evaluated showed the presence of megacaryocytes; this could have suggested increased peripheral destruction of platelets. The striking shape of erythrocytes with many egg shells is described without comment. Therapeutic attempts lacked clear indications: All the patients received antibiotics, even though infection was evident only in cases 4 and 5; three patients were given ACTH despite the fact that only one of them had evidence of immunopathology. Exchange transfusions were done late in the course of all patients, with little effect. Repeated transfusions were given, with prompt recurrence of anemia. Water balance was not maintained adequately.

Soon after the publication, other authors confirmed and extended the characteristics of the hemolytic-uremic syndrome. Gasser was fascinated. In 1959, at a symposium in Freiburg on hemolytic diseases, he broadened his approach and dealt with "Erworbene hämolytische Erkrankungen bei renaler Insuffizienz". Gasser reported four new cases; each recovered. Gasser suspected a constitutional predisposition in one of the patients who had a second episode 4 years later (2).

Until his death in 1982, Gasser followed with great interest the development of knowledge in this field to which his critical and original mind had made such a great contribution.

Sonderabdruck aus der Schweizerischen Medizinischen Wochenschrift
85. Jahrgang 1955, Nr. 38/39, Seite 905

Aus der Universitätskinderklinik (Direktor: Prof. G. Fanconi) und dem pathologisch-anatomischen Institut (Direktor: Prof. E. Uehlinger) Zürich

Hämolytisch-urämische Syndrome: Bilaterale Nierenrindennekrosen bei akuten erworbenen hämolytischen Anämien*

Von C. Gasser, E. Gautier und Annemarie Steck (klinischer Teil) und R. E. Siebenmann und R. Oechslin (pathologisch-anatomischer Teil)

Figure 9 Title of the original paper on the hemolytic-uremic syndrome.

PATHOLOGICAL ASPECTS

Rudolf E. Siebenmann was employed as Professor E. Uehlinger's second associate pathologist in January 1954. Uehlinger, chairman of the University Institute of Pathology in Zurich, asked Siebenmann to be responsible for the autopsy service for the University Children's Hospital of Zurich. This was directed by Professor Guido Fanconi, whose associates were C. Gasser, E. Rossi, and A. Prader. Siebenmann performed or supervised most of the autopsies for several years and found the task gratifying because the pediatricians were so interested in the findings. The clinical and laboratory aspects had been studied carefully and were frequently discussed at clinicopathological conferences.

In January 1954, Siebenmann performed the autopsy on Th. Ruth, age 13 months, who had simultaneously developed acute hemolytic anemia and anuria and died 12 days later. The clinical diagnosis was "bronchopneumonia, acute toxic hemolytic anemia and acute hemorrhagic nephritis." Massive *bilateral renal cortical necrosis* was found (Fig. 10). There were also unusual ischemic infarcts in a bronchopneumonic area of the right upper lobe (Figs. 11, 12). Widespread hyaline thrombi were revealed with special stains in the glomeruli and afferent arterioles of the necrotic cortex. The thrombosis extended into the arteries up to the margin of the necrosis. Only a few viable glomeruli remained; some were normal, others had hyalin thrombi. Thrombi were seen only in the necrotic arteries and veins within the infarcted bronchopneumonic areas of the lung. There were no other extrarenal thrombi or vascular lesions. This patient became case 4.

A second case was seen in August 1954. A girl aged 7 months presented with hemolysis, followed by uremia and hemiparesis. She died 30 days after the onset of illness and the clinical diagnosis was "hemiplegia and *hemolytic uremic syndrome*." The term was coined for the first time by Gasser in connection with this fatal case. In contrast to the first case, hyaline and granular thrombi were found in many organs in capillaries and arterioles. Some were occlusive, some bulged into the lumen and were covered by endothelium, and others seemed to be localized in the subintimal space. The changes were those of *thrombotic microangiopathy* described by Symmers in 1952 (3) as typical for *thrombotic thrombocytopenic purpura (TTP)* described by Moschcowitz (4). The cause of the uremia, however, was *bilateral renal cortical necrosis*. This was unusual in TTP; only one other instance had been reported in the literature up to that time. There were also myocardial and cerebral infarcts and multiple hemorrhages (Fig. 13). This was case 3. Because this autopsy had been performed by a skilled resident, Dr. R. Oechslin, he was included as an author of the publication and later became a practicing internist.

Toward the end of 1954, Gasser approached Siebenmann with a request to review the pathology of these two patients and that of *six other infants* who had died with what he considered to be the same clinical entity of a "hemolytic uremic syndrome". In three of these six cases, the histopathological diagnosis had been "glomerular necrosis," "glomerular thrombosis with necrosis," and necrotizing acute glomerulonephritis." Glomerulonephritis was excluded in three cases because of bilateral cortical necrosis. The thrombosis of capillaries, arterioles, and some arteries was restricted to the kidneys. In one case, however, Siebenmann found the same peculiar anemic pulmonary infarcts in a preexisting bronchopneumonia as in the first case mentioned. These three patients had the full-blown clinical syndrome. In the

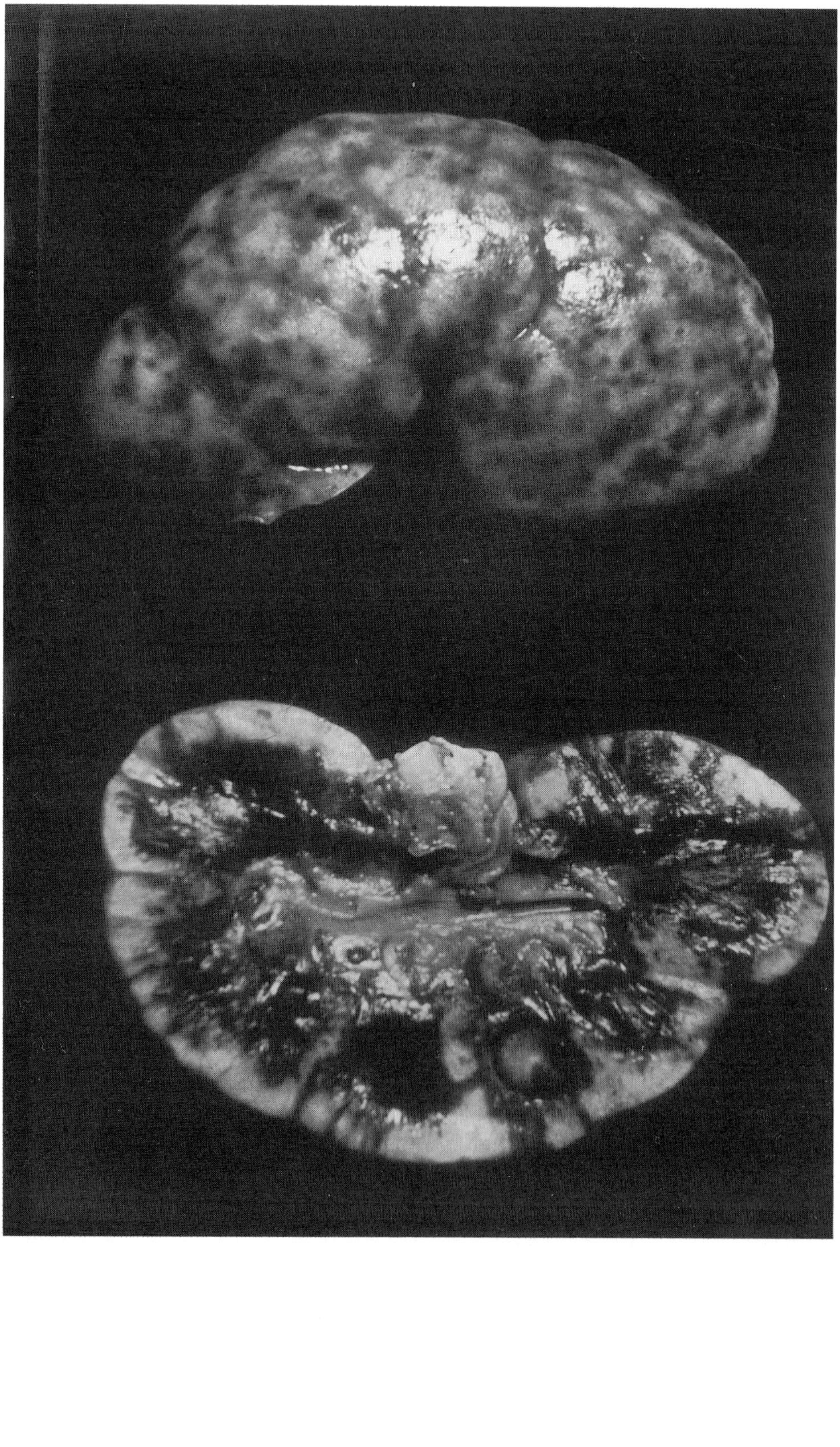

Figure 10 Massive bilateral cortical necrosis in case 4.

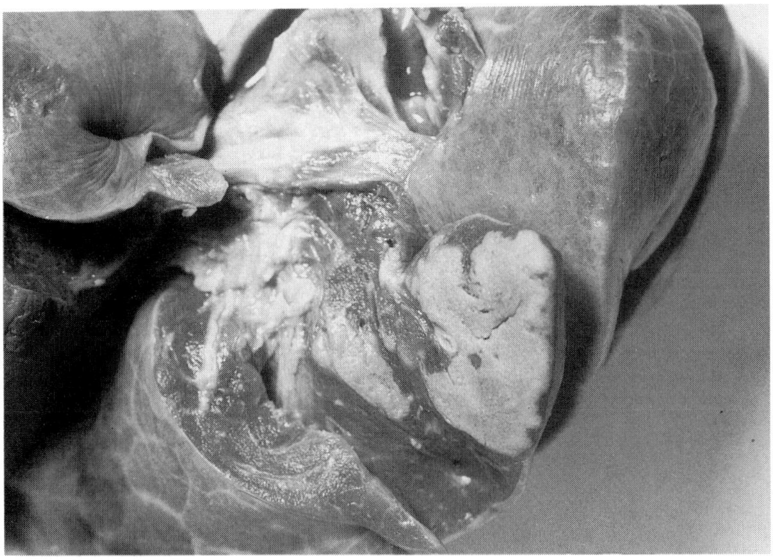

Figure 11 Ischemic infarcts in the lung of case 4.

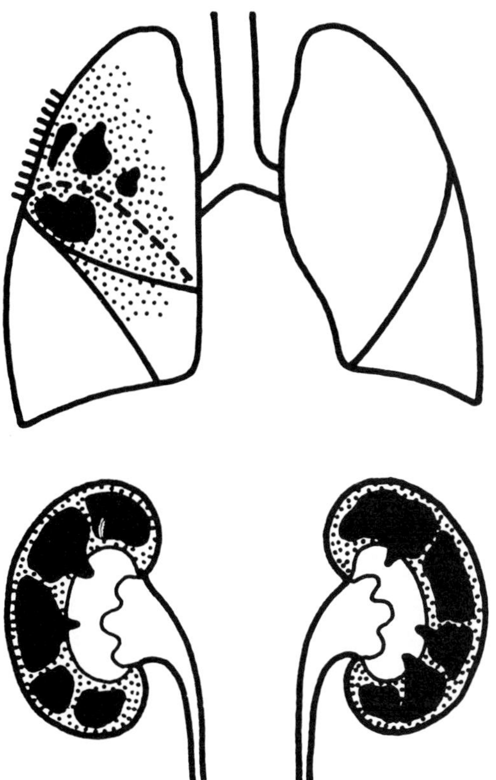

Figure 12 Drawing of the organs affected by infarcts in case 4.

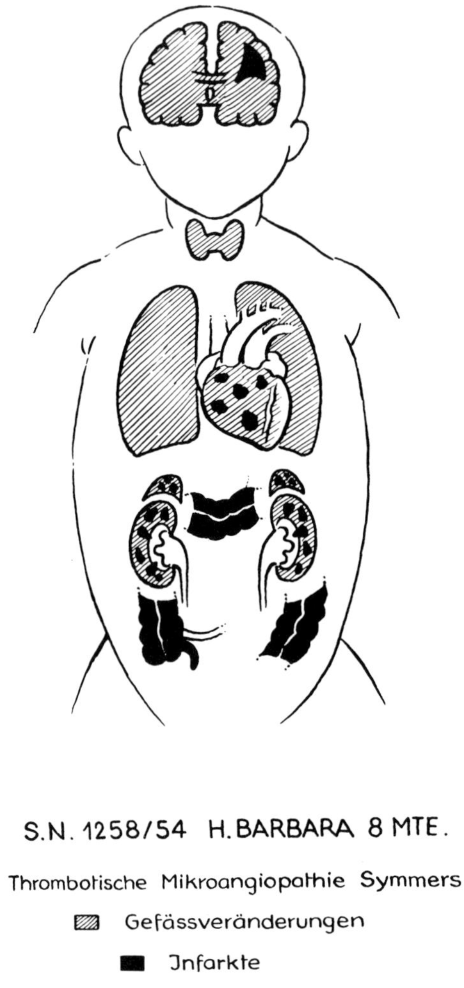

Figure 13 Drawing of the multiple lesions in case 3.

remaining three cases, however, the diagnosis of glomerulonephritis was confirmed and was not included in the original description of the syndrome. The five index cases all had variable *bilateral renal cortical necrosis* with glomerular necrosis, patchy necrosis, and massive confluent necrosis, as described by Sheehan and Moore in 1952 (5).

Siebenmann remembers one winter evening when he and Oechslin went to Gasser's office in the Children's Hospital to explain to him, Gautier, and Steck the pathology of renal cortical necrosis. They decided to prepare a paper based on these five selected cases.

Gasser and Siebenmann presented a joint paper at the 10th Annual Meeting of the Swiss Society of Haematology, in Geneva, in May 1955. Gasser described and discussed the clinical picture, and Siebenmann the pathological findings. As was traditional, the presentation was published, in abbreviated form with some of the illustrations, in the *Schweizerische Medizinische Wochenschrift* (1). They illustrated the findings, which ranged from glomerular necrosis in one case to more extensive patchy necrosis in two cases and to massive confluent necrosis in two others. The thrombosis of capillary loops, of afferent arterioles, of radiate arteries in cases with more extensive necrosis, is always found in cortical necrosis and is an element of the diagnosis. This was not mentioned in the text of the publication but is illustrated in it, and Siebenmann still has the text of their Geneva paper in which he described the occurrence of thrombi with microscopic slides.

With the exception of the one patient (of Moschcowitz) who had TTP, no generalized intravascular thrombosis was found. Therefore, of the five patients with the hemolytic uremic syndrome, two only had renal cortical necrosis, two also had peculiar pulmonary infarcts in preexisting bronchopneumonia, and one had renal cortical necrosis and generalized thrombotic microangiopathy.

Although the cause of uremia was easily explained by the morphologic findings, Siebenmann was unable to determine a basis for the acute hemolysis. He could see only minor consequences of the hemolytic process with pigmented tubule casts and hemosiderosis in spleen and bone marrow. They excluded hemolysis-induced renal damage, as seen in the crush-kidney. Siebenmann accepted the views of Sheehan and Moore on the pathogenesis of the cortical necrosis; these authors considered spasm as the cause of the thrombi in the small vessels. He had no explanation for the pulmonary infarcts except for an arteritis occurring in association with bronchopneumonia. He excluded an embolic process. The question of shock induced by hemolysis was raised at the Geneva meeting, and they agreed that the renal cortical necrosis could well have been the result of severe shock.

RE-EVALUATION

How does the body of knowledge we had assembled in 1955 look in retrospect, in light of subsequent findings by ourselves and others?

The first subsequent important finding was by Habib et al. in 1958 (6). They noted that the syndrome could be observed in infants who did not have cortical necrosis but had a thrombotic microangiopathy or arteriolocapillary thrombosis that was localized to the kidney. These authors later suggested, on the basis of electron microscopic studies of kidney specimens obtained by renal biopsy, that the vascular disease was the primary event and the thrombosis was a subsequent secondary phenomenon. Six of their 27 patients reviewed in 1967 survived (7).

Our first observations were therefore expanded and corrected:

1. The syndrome was not invariably fatal.
2. Renal cortical necrosis was not an invariable finding. On the contrary, localized renal thrombotic microangiopathy was more frequent, even in fatal cases.
3. The occurrence of cortical necrosis in the context of TTP (Moschcowitz), as in one of our cases, proved to be unusual.

A second important observation was the recognition of disseminated intravascular coagulation as an important pathogenetic mechanism (8, 9). It now seems that small-vessel thrombosis is not the consequence, but the cause of the renal cortical necrosis. McKay (8), however, still thought that spasm of the renal arteries was a local factor during the process of intravascular coagulation.

It was also claimed that the thrombotic microangiopathy might be the manifestation of a primary coagulation process with secondary changes in vessel walls. This theory is supported by the observation that paraneoplastic microthrombosis, which is not a primary vascular disease, leads to the same pathologic changes in vessels as idiopathic thrombotic microangiopathy (10). We still think that the concept that the deciding event is a primary intravascular coagulation has not been excluded (9). Fibrinolysis, which occurs very quickly in vessels and tissues, even postmortem, may lyse many thrombi and thereby render their detection impossible.

A third important finding was that acute hemolysis was the result of mechanical fragmentation of the erythrocytes (11). These workers showed that the typical changes of red blood cells observed by Gasser could be produced by fibrin strands or endothelial lesions. The erythrocyte fragmentation has been observed in other instances of renal cortical necrosis and shock and other causes of intravascular coagulation. Confirmation of this pathogenetic mechanism was not possible in our histological studies and has never been observed in tissue sections from cases of HUS. Interestingly, the fragmentation of erythrocytes was described by Rindfleisch, a professor of pathology in Zurich, in 1891. He thought it was due to mechanical impacts. Ehrlich (12), who mentions this in 1891, considered that it was caused by a chemical process.

CONCLUSION

In conclusion, it is not unusual that the detection and first description of a new syndrome is based on the observation of the most severe form of the disease, so that the less severe nonfatal forms, which fortunately occur more frequently, are noted only later. The observation of this unique clinical syndrome by Gasser triggered many important clinical, pathological, and experimental studies which were of a great importance in general pathology. Siebenmann is pleased that a pathologist contributed to the characterization and delimitation of the syndrome and has always thought that this work was a good example of fruitful clinicopathological cooperation.

REFERENCES

1. Gasser, C., Gautier, E., Steck, A., Siebenmann, R. E., and Oechslin, R. Hämolytisch-urämische Syndrome: Bilaterale Nierenrindennekrosen bei akuten erworbenen hämolytischen Anämien. *Schweiz. Med. Wochenschr*, *85*: 905 (1955).
2. Gasser, C. Erworbene hämolytische Erkrankungen bei renaler Insuffizienz. In: *Siebentes Freiburger Symposion über Hämolyse und hämolytische Erkrankungen*, Springer-Verlag, Berlin, Göttingen, Heidelberg, p. 259 (1961).
3. Symmers, W. St. C. Thrombotic microangiopathic haemolytic anaemia (Thrombotic microangiopathy). *Br. Med. J.*, *2*: 897 (1952).
4. Moschcowitz, E. An acute febrile pleiochromic anemia with hyaline thrombosis of the terminal arterioles and capillaries: An undescribed disease. *Arch. Intern. Med.*, *36*: 89 (1925).
5. Sheehan, H. L., Moore, H. C. *Renal Cortical Necrosis of the Kidney and Concealed Accidental Hemorrhage*, C. C. Thomas, Springfield, Ill. (1952).
6. Habib, R., Mathieu, H., Royer, P. Maladie thrombotique artériolocapillaire du rein chez l'enfant. *Rev. Fr. Etudes Clin. Biol.*, *3*: 891 (1958).
7. Habib, R., Mathieu, H., Royer, P. Le syndrome hémolytique et urémique de l'enfant. *Nephron*, *4*: 139 (1967).

8. McKay, D. G. *Disseminated Intravascular Coagulation. An Intermediary Mechanism of Disease.* Hoeber Medical Division, Harper & Row, New York, Evanston, London. (1965).
9. Hardaway, R. M. *Syndromes of Disseminated Intravascular Coagulation*, C. C. Thomas, Springfield, Ill. (1966).
10. Brain, M. C. Microangiopathic hemolytic anemia. *N. Engl. J. Med.*, *281*: 833 (1969).
11. Brain, M. C., Dacie, J. V., Hourihane, D. O. B. Microangiopathic haemolytic anaemia: the possible role of vascular lesions in pathogenesis. *Br. J. Haematol.*, *8*: 358 (1962).
12. Ehrlich, P. Beobachtungen am anaemischen Blut. Vortrag in der Gesellschaft der Charité-Aerzte in Berlin. *Berliner Klin. Wochenschr.*, *18*: 43 (1891).

2
Dr. Eli Moschcowitz

Aaron J. Marcus *Department of Veterans Affairs Medical Center, Cornell University Medical College, and New York Hospital, New York, New York*

The May–June 1945 volume of the *Journal of the Mount Sinai Hospital* (New York) was dedicated to Dr. Eli Moschcowitz upon the occasion of his 65th birthday (1). The list of friends, associates, and pupils who contributed to the assembly of the volume comprises individuals who had distinguished themselves in a broad range of worldly pursuits.

In the Foreword to this document, Dr. George Baehr, a distinguished physician and a founder of the Hospital Insurance Plan of N.Y. (HIP), stated: "This volume is dedicated to Dr. Eli Moschcowitz, physician, scientist, scholar, traveler, epicure, bibliophile, magician, and lover of music and the arts." Dr. Baehr said that "no member of the staff of The Mount Sinai Hospital in this generation has commanded the respect and devotion of his associates in quite the same degree." Continuing: "To many, his capacity for friendship and his worldly philosophy seem outstanding. To others, the freshness of his outlook upon life and his enjoyment of music and of books are most attractive. Undoubtedly, the combination of these qualities is responsible for the fact that the fertility of his mind and the youthfulness of his spirit continue undiminished, and give increasing promise for the future" (1).

In 1964, the obituary for Dr. Moschcowitz was published in the *Journal of the Mount Sinai Hospital*. It read: "On the morning of February 23, 1964, with the strains of his favorite music echoing softly in his room, the life of a beloved friend and colleague quietly slipped away. For over 60 years Eli Moschcowitz was intimately identified with The Mount Sinai Hospital and the loss of one who labored so diligently in its behalf, and who did so much to enhance its reputation, will be irreplaceable" (2).

Dr. Eli Moschcowitz was born in Giralt, Hungary, in 1879. His family emigrated to the United Stated when Eli was 2 years of age. His older brother, Alexis (1865–1933), later became a noted surgeon with a particular interest in abdominal surgery (3). The "Moschcowitz operation" for femoral hernia repair via an inguinal approach was named for him. Alexis inspired Eli to pursue a medical career.

Dr. Eli Moschcowitz received his M.D. degree from the College of Physicians and Surgeons of Columbia University in 1900. This was followed by 3 years of surgical internship at Mount Sinai Hospital. He then took postgraduate training in Berlin with Dr. Ludwig Pick, a leading figure in pathology and laboratory medicine. Dr. Pick was studying what is now known as Niemann-Pick's disease (a systemic accumulation of sphingomyelin in the reticuloendothelial system, characterized histologically by phospholipid-laden histiocytes). The training qualified him for the appointment of Pathologist to Beth Israel Hospital in New York City. He maintained this position for 20 years and at the same time developed a medical practice. He was also appointed to the Visiting Staff of Mount Sinai and was given the title of Consulting Pathologist to Beth Israel. Dr. Moschcowitz' written and personal contributions to the science and art of medicine began as early as 1906. The breadth and magnitude of the disciplines in which he developed expertise could hardly be equaled in this day and age.

THROMBOTIC THROMBOCYTOPENIC PURPURA

It was during his tenure at Beth Israel Hospital, when Dr. Moschcowitz was maintaining his home and office at 25 West 68th Street, that he admitted patient "K. Z." to Beth Israel Hospital (September 15, 1923). K. Z. was a 16-year-old female afflicted with what Dr. Moschcowitz termed "an acute febrile pleiochromic anemia with hyaline thrombosis of the terminal arterioles and capillaries (an undescribed disease)" (4). K. Z. had been clerically employed after attending business school. "There were no home difficulties, and poverty was not extreme." She had spent what was probably the Labor Day weekend at the seashore in Rockaway Beach. In those days, the Marine Park Bridge, which connects Brooklyn with Rockaway, was not present. The trip to Rockaway was more of a trek on the old "Sunrise Highway." On September 6, she noted weakness in the upper extremities with pain on mobility of the wrists and elbows. Marked pallor and constipation were also present. There was a progressive increase in these and other symptoms which mandated admission to Beth Israel Hospital on September 15. During the preceding days, her temperature ranged between 101° and 102° F. Dr. Moschcowitz described K. Z. as being pale, with a "café au lait" tinge. Petechiae were noted on the left arm, but the heart, lungs, spleen and liver were unremarkable upon physical examination.

The erythrocyte count was 1,330,000, hemoglobin 40%, leukocyte count 12,600 with 65% polymorphonuclear cells. Erythrocytes on smear demonstrated a central pallor and nucleated forms were not observed. Platelets were not enumerated or described. Blood culture revealed no growth. There was trace albuminuria with hyaline and granular casts. Blood chemistries were as follows: urea 21.2 mg/100 mL, creatinine 1.1 mg/100 mL. Tests for occult blood in gastric contents and feces were strongly positive. The chest radiograph was normal and the electrocardiogram demonstrated T wave inversion in Lead III. Blood pressure was 130/60.

Four days after admission, there was partial paralysis of the left arm and leg, and a slight facial paralysis. That evening, K. Z. developed pulmonary edema which responded to treatment, but was followed by coma, irregular respirations and demise (September 20). Dr. Emanuel Libman of Mount Sinai Hospital had been called to see the patient in consultation and commented that the condition appeared to be a new disease.

At autopsy, the body was described as "pale and poorly nourished." This deterioration took place between September 6 and 20; she had been in perfect health prior to that time. Otherwise, there were no specific or pathognomonic signs on gross inspection.

Upon microscopic examination of the tissues, almost every low-power field contained from 1–12 lesions which were thrombotic in nature. They were located in terminal arterioles or capillaries. On closer inspection, the lesions were in various stages of progression from an inflammatory response to that of organization. Early thrombi seemed to be plugging the vessel as a "hyaline mass" which partially or completely occluded the lumen. If the plugs were not in close proximity to the vessel wall, they were surrounded by "a layer of flat cells of the fibroblastic type." The latter were classifiable as endothelial intima. In plugs which appeared to be chronologically more advanced, fibroblasts penetrated the hyaline mass in quantities which paralleled the age of the lesion. This fibroblastic infiltration took place at the expense of the hyaline material. Dr. Moschcowitz considered the end-stage of these lesions to be a "small fibroblastic tubercle-like structure." These fibroblasts appeared to originate from the vessel endothelium. There was also a concentric fibroblastic proliferation around the outer wall of the vessel. In areas where hyaline masses did not completely fill the lumen, the spaces were occupied by erythrocytes.

Importantly, Dr. Moschcowitz observed that only the terminal arterioles and capillaries were involved. Vessels large enough to have a well-defined muscular coat were completely intact. All vascular sections examined from heart muscle were involved, and there was also moderate edema of cardiac parenchyma. The liver demonstrated moderate fatty infiltration with only a few hyaline thrombi. The spleen was enormously congested and, again, hyaline thrombi were not prominent. In the kidney, arterioles and capillaries of the middle zone, and the region of the vasa recta showed the same hyaline thrombi as observed in the heart. No bacteria or spirochetes were seen in any tissues.

Although not stressed in the original report, another important feature was the absence of perivascular inflammation around involved arterioles and capillaries. This subsequently has been considered to be an important histologic feature of the syndrome (5). The presence of microaneurysms has also been demonstrated in these lesions (5).

It should be mentioned that only a partial necropsy was carried out on K. Z. Later, detailed studies in other patients revealed the presence of hyaline microthrombi in the brain, pancreas, spleen, and adrenal glands, as well as the heart and kidney.

The above details of what is now known as thrombotic thrombocytopenic purpura (TTP) or Moschcowitz' disease have become what is probaby the most frequently presented Clinical Pathological Conference for medical students, academicians, and physicians in practice. This is because of the uniqueness of the disorder and the extensive systemic complications which accompany it. TTP (also referred to as thrombotic microangiopathy) can be regarded as the original occlusive vascular disease, and definitely has its own intellectual attraction.

It has been said that there are almost as many "experts" on this disease as there are patients. Articles or conferences on any aspect of TTP frequently give rise to a barrage of Letters to the Editor consisting of protests about not being quoted, anecdotal cases in almost everyone's practice, and, of course, new therapies. There may also be complaints that the respondent had originated the proposed therapeutic approach 10 years previously (6, 7).

Whenever new biologic substances are characterized (such as the eicosanoid prostacyclin), patients with thrombotic thrombocytopenic purpura are soon reported to have too little of the substance if it is beneficial or produce too much if it is harmful. This is not unusual in diseases wherein the precise etiology remains elusive (8). All "new explanations" for TTP should be taken seriously. As can be gleaned from this volume, thrombotic thrombocytopenic purpura is becoming more and more treatable and our concepts of its etiology are more scientific. In the years before 1960, less than 3% of patients with Moschcowitz' disease survived. Now, with plasma exchange and related modalities, survival rates are in the vicinity of 82% (9). Nevertheless, despite these highly significant advances in therapy, the disorder still has an overall fatality rate which is not acceptable—about 18% (9).

In the discussion section of the original report (4), Dr. Moschcowitz surveyed the literature on hyaline thrombi, since they were so widespread in patient K. Z. They were observed previously by investigators such as Klebs in burn cases and Kaufman in mercury poisoning. Schmorl noted them in stomach and liver as a toxic effect of abrin (a phytotoxin from the seed of *Abrus precatorius*, a medication used in eye disorders). Flexner reported hyaline lesions near typhoid ulcers in the ileum and lung. They have also been seen in the liver in eclampsia and the stomach after carbolic acid poisoning. Moschcowitz mentioned that Loeb and colleagues reported "red cell thrombi" in the lungs of animals who had received injections of "foreign serum." After injecting ricin into rabbits, Flexner concluded that the hyaline thrombi he observed originated from agglutinated erythrocytes.

From this literature survey (4), Dr. Moschcowitz concluded that the cause of death in K. Z. was "some powerful poison which had both agglutinative and hemolytic properties."

Of particular pertinence in the original article (4) was a personal communication which Dr. Moschcowitz rendered from Dr. Max Lederer, Pathologist-in-Chief at the Jewish Hospital of Brooklyn. Dr. Lederer informed Dr. Moschcowitz that he had seen four cases which were clinically identical to K. Z. Dr. Lederer did not know the cause of the disorder, but all four patients promptly recovered after administration of a single blood transfusion! Was this a harbinger of things to come (10)? This observation should be classified as more than hearsay, because Dr. Lederer was an experienced hematologist. In fact, "Lederer's anemia" was considered as an acute state of hemolysis of short duration and unknown etiology—possibly autoimmune. When originally described, it was one of the first clinical situations which led to the concept of acquired hemolytic anemia as contrasted to the congenital type. This is not to suggest that Lederer's anemia was TTP. Parenthetically, the erythrocyte osmotic fragility test in K. Z. was markedly abnormal. In any case, despite all of our recent advances, TTP still presents important clinical and therapeutic dilemmas—especially the chronic variants (11).

DR. ELI MOSCHCOWITZ AS A SCHOLAR

As already mentioned, Dr. Moschcowitz' contributions to the "science and art of medicine and related topics" began in 1906. Some of these represented observations made on patients and in the pathology laboratory. Others represented scholarly treatises on a variety of disease entities and their pathogenesis. In addition, Dr. Moschcowitz published a series of articles in the *Journal of the Mount Sinai Hospital* entitled "Essays on the Biology of Disease." I had the opportunity to read 12 essays in the series. The purpose of these articles was to interpret certain forms of chronic disease from the biologic viewpoint. This was theoretically in contrast to the trend of that time toward rigid classifications which implied concepts of disease as "a more or less static phenomenon." Typical titles were "The Biology of Graves' Disease," "Recent Advances in Psychosomatic Medicine," and "Arteriosclerosis." The latter included Dr. Moschcowitz' definition of this disorder: "Arteriosclerosis is a progressive and irreversible affection in which hyperplasia of one or more coats is a primary reaction, with deposition of collagenous, lipoid, hyaline and calcium as a secondary reaction, the totality of both components resulting in thickening, dilatation, deformity and loss of elasticity of the walls." There was also a scholarly tome on periarteritis nodosa.

Specific contributions to medical knowledge by Dr. Moschcowitz can be summarized from a bibliography which appeared in the volume of the *Journal of the Mount Sinai Hospital* which was dedicated to him (1):

Dr. Moschcowitz was the first observer to demonstrate that anaphylactic disorders in humans were accompanied by the appearance of eosinophils in blood (*N.Y. Med. J.*, January, 1911). He wrote an early article on the presence of thrombosis in the aorta and both iliac arteries following streptococcal sepsis (*Proc. N.Y. Pathol. Soc.*, vol. 14, January, 1914). He described vegetative endocarditis of the pulmonary valve in that same journal and volume. Invasion of nervous tissue by carcinomatous cells was described in 1914 (*Virchows Arch. f. Pathol. Anat.* 118:351). An article on William Withering appeared in 1915 (*Med. Pickwick.* 1:72).

In the *Annals of Surgery* (page 697, June, 1916), Dr. Moschcowitz published a paper on the pathological diagnosis of diseases of the appendix based on a study of 1,500 specimens. An article on ectopic and latent chorionepithelioma appeared in the *Proceedings of the New York Pathology Society* in 1917 (17:164). A critique of Banti's disease appeared in the *Journal of the American Medical Association* in 1917 (69:1045). In the *Johns Hopkins Medical Bulletin* in June, 1918, an article appeared entitled "John Hall: Shakespeare's Son-in-Law."

Another article was entitled "Hypertension: Its Significance, Relation to Arteriosclerosis and Nephritis and Etiology" (*Am. J. Med. Sci.* 158:668, 1919). In the *JAMA*, there appeared an article on "The Pathology of Hypertension" (vol. 79, 1922). A possible forerunner of future diseases was described in "Non-specific Granulomata of the Intestine" (*Am. J. Med. Sci.* 166:148, 1923). In 1927, Dr. Moschcowitz published the first description of the clinical syndrome of hypertension in the pulmonary circulation (*Am. J. Med. Sci.* 174).

Dr. Moschcowitz is considered to be the first investigator to link tobacco with heart disease in an article entitled "Tobacco Angina Pectoris" (*JAMA* 90:733, 1928). Apparently, he was also the first physician to note that the pathogenesis of brown induration of the lung was due to pulmonary hypertension with consequent pulmonary capillary sclerosis (*Am. Heart J.* 6:171, 1930).

Of interest to hematologists is Dr. Moschcowitz' article entitled "The Relation of Achlorhydria to Pernicious Anemia" (*Arch. Intern. Med.* 48:171, 1931). Dr. Moschcowitz demonstrated that achlorhydria was a constant symptom in pernicious anemia and preceded the development of this disorder by many years.

Other titles which should be cited are as follows: "A Biologic Concept of Disease" (*JAMA* 99:714, 1932); "A New Sign of Pericardial Effusion" (*JAMA* 100:1663, 1933); and "Hypoproteinemia" (*JAMA* 100:1086, 1933).

Two articles representing Dr. Moschcowitz' interest in psychosomatic medicine appeared in the *New England Journal of Medicine* in 1935 (212:603, and 213:617). These were entitled "Psychogenic Origin of Organic Disease" and "Allergy to Life: An Interpretation of the Neurotic Constitution."

Other titles included: "Superior Sulcus Tumor" (*J. Mt. Sinai Hosp.* 3:198, 1937); "The Simultaneous Association of Hiatus Hernia and Coronary Artery Disease" (*J. Mt. Sinai Hosp.* 4:272, 1937); "Causes of Painless Gastro-Duodenal Hemorrhage" (*Am. J. Med. Sci.* 202:52, 1941); and, later in that same journal, "The Hyperkinetic Diseases" (206:576, 1943).

THE 65TH BIRTHDAY VOLUME OF THE *JOURNAL OF THE MOUNT SINAI HOSPITAL*

This issue contained a listing of Dr. Eli Moschowitz' friends, associates, and pupils who had assembled the volume. In addition there were 75 research articles and reviews on major clinical and basic medical subjects. The authors, who were authorities on the subjects that appeared in the volume (1), included: Murray Bass, Director of Pediatrics at Mount Sinai Hospital, protegé of Bela Schick (of the Schick test), and father of the noted blood physiologist Marjorie B. Zucker; Lucrezia Bori, prima donna in the Metropolitan Opera; Samuel Chotzinoff, a pianist who accompanied Efrem Zimbalist and Jascha Heifetz and was later music critic for the *New York World* and *New York Post;* Burrill B. Crohn (Crohn's disease); Louis N. Katz, cardiologist; Emanuel Libman (Libman-Sacks Disease, or atypical verrucous endocarditis), who was also a consultant on the original case of TTP; Arthur M. Master, cardiologist and originator of the "2-step test;" Myron Prinzmetal, cardiologist (Prinzmetal's angina); Judge Proskauer; Nathan Rosenthal, the first practicing hematologist in New York City; Gregory Shwartzman (Shwartzman reaction); Isadore Snapper, renowned diagnostician and physician; Lawrence Valenstein, founding chairman (with Arthur C. Fatt) of the Grey Advertising Agency; and Paul Dudley White, eminent cardiologist. The years during which Dr. Eli Moschcowitz practiced medicine and carried out his clinical research represent an era in medicine that can never be paralleled or duplicated.

I am proud and privileged to belong to the same profession as Dr. Eli Moschcowitz.

TTP IN 1991: A DISORDER OF "THROMBOREGULATION"

The hallmark lesion of thrombotic thrombocytopenic purpura is small blood vessel occlusion by thrombi probably consisting mainly of platelets (5). This can be viewed as representing a breakdown of normal hemostatic and thrombotic control mechanisms (thromboregulation).

Experimental data from my laboratory as well as several others now indicate that there is an extensive and integrated group of intrinsic mechanisms that are capable of preventing and/or limiting the evolution of an occlusive platelet lesion. Two of these systems are fluid phase reactants [the eicosanoids (PGI_2 and PGD_2), and the endothelium-derived relaxing factor/nitric oxide (EDRF/NO)]. The third is a cell-associated ecto-ADPase system on the surface of vascular endothelium (12, 13). We have found that cultured human endothelial cells contain an ecto-ADPase activity that metabolizes ADP released from stimulated platelets in close proximity. This results in a loss of platelet reactivity in the fluid phase. It has not been sufficiently appreciated in the past that cells respond to perturbation or injury by releasing nucleotides, and these nucleotides serve to modulate many vascular phenomena (13, 14). We currently believe that this aspirin-insensitive, cell-associated nucleotidase system is a prime regulator of platelet reactivity. We suggest that a breakdown or destruction of the ADPase system in small blood vessels could be a major feature of the pathogenesis of TTP. Recent experimental evidence involving studies of ADPase in glomerular basement membrane of the rat kidney provide evidence in favor of this concept (15). It has been demonstrated that intravenous injection of doxorubicin or x-irradiation can result in reduction of glomerular ADPase activity. A consequence of this injury is intraglomerular platelet aggregation and immunologic evidence of platelet activation (increases in beta-thromboglobulin and platelet factor 4) following alternate perfusion with platelets and ADP. This did not occur in normal rat kidney controls perfused in the same manner in the absence of doxorubicin treatment. Thus, activity of ADPase in the glomeruli is involved in thromboregulation in the kidney (15).

The aforementioned phenomenon leads to another relatively recently recognized and completely inexplicable syndrome—the TTP that develops following chemotherapy for neoplastic disorders (16). Patients receiving chemotherapeutic agents that included cisplatin, bleomycin and a vinca alkaloid developed TTP at a time when they were either clinically free of tumor or found to have only a small quantity of necrotic tumor (16). I speculate that this chemotherapy-induced disorder (which can also be manifested as the hemolytic-uremic syndrome) is due to destruction or inactivation of ADPase activity in small blood vessels by the chemotherapeutic agent. This syndrome had been described earlier in relation to the use of mitomycin and doxorubicin. Renal complications were frequently superimposed upon a microangiopathic hemolytic anemia (16).

With regard to the chronic relapsing form of TTP, which is associated with large unprocessed von Willebrand factor (vWF) multimers (17), I speculate that these multimers interfere with the action of ecto-ADPases on small vessel endothelial cells. In addition, these large multimers agglutinate platelets, perhaps in association with some "in vivo form of ristocetin" (10) that might even be ADP (18).

CONCLUDING REMARKS

Dr. Moschcowitz said, "Death, in the case described, resulted from some powerful poison which had both agglutinative and hemolytic properties" (4). Based on recent experimental and clinical evidence cited above, I would add that the "powerful poison" transformed the syndrome from ordinary thrombocytopenia and hemolytic anemia into a total loss of thromboregulation, possibly by deletion of vascular ecto-ADPase activity. One reason why plasma administration has been so successful as a therapeutic modality in TTP may be that, in addition to other components, it contains ADPase activity to replenish that which has been lost during the development of TTP or during certain types of chemotherapy (19).

ACKNOWLEDGMENTS

I thank Ms. Lyn Kasner Morgan, Director of the library of the Mount Sinai Medical Center, and Ms. Barbara J. Niss, Archivist of the library, for the excellent biographical material concerning Dr. Moschcowitz. I also thank Ms. Lenore Safier for excellent discussions, and Ms. Evelyn M. Ludwig for preparation of the manuscript.

REFERENCES

1. *J. Mt. Sinai Hosp., 12*: 1–793 (1945).
2. Klingenstein, P. In Memoriam: Eli Moschcowitz. *J. Mt. Sinai Hosp., 31*(5): 366–369 (1964).
3. Moschowitz, A. V. The pathogenesis, anatomy, and cure of prolapse of the rectum. *Dis. Colon Rect., 26*(8): 553–565 (1983).
4. Moschcowitz, E. An acute febrile pleiochromic anemia with hyaline thrombosis of the terminal arterioles and capillaries. *Arch. Intern. Med., 36*(1): 89–93 (1925).
5. Orbison, J. L. Morphology of thrombotic thrombocytopenic purpura with demonstration of aneurysms. *Am. J. Pathol., 28*: 129–143 (1952).
6. Rosove, M. H., Ho, W. G., Goldfinger, D. Ineffectiveness of aspirin and dipyridamole in the treatment of thrombotic thrombocytopenic purpura. *Ann. Intern. Med., 96*(1): 27–33 (1982).
7. Zacharski, L. R., and others. Aspirin, dipyridamole, and thrombotic thrombocytopenic purpura. *Ann. Intern. Med., 96*(5): 679–681 (1982).
8. Schmidt, J. L. Thrombotic thrombocytopenic purpura: Successful treatment unlocks etiologic secrets. *Mayo Clin. Proc., 64*(8): 956–961 (1989).
9. Kwaan, H. C., Domer, P. H. Fatal thrombotic thrombocytopenic purpura despite plasmapheresis. *Haemostasis, 19*: 344–347 (1989).
10. Marcus, A. J. Moschcowitz revisited (editorial). *N. Engl. J. Med., 307*(23): 1447–1448 (1982).
11. Brain, M. C. An acute febrile pleichromic anemia with hyaline thrombosis of the terminal arterioles and capillaries (Moschcowitz 1925). *Thrombos. Haemostas., 40*: 9–10 (1978).
12. Marcus, A. J. New considerations in therapy for thrombotic diseases. In *Hematology: Basic Principles and Practice.* (E. J. Benz, H. J. Cohen, B. Furie, R. Hoffman, S. Shattil, eds.), Churchill Livingstone Ince., New York, pp. 1446–1464 (1990).
13. Coade, S. B., Pearson, J. D. Metabolism of adenine nucleotides in human blood. *Circ. Res., 65*: 531–537 (1989).
14. Marcus, A. J., Safier, L. B., Hajjar, K. A., Ullman, H. L., Islam, N., Broekman, M. J., and Eiroa, A. M. Inhibition of platelet function by an aspirin-insensitive endothelial cell ADPase. Thromboregulation by endothelial cells. *J. Clin. Invest., 88*: (November 1991), (in press).
15. Bakker, W. W., Willink, E. J., Donga, J., Hulstaert, C. E., and Hardonk, M. J. Antithrombotic activity of glomerular adenosine diphosphatase in the glomerular basement membrane of the rat kidney. *J. Lab. Clin. Med., 109*: 171–177 (1987).
16. Jackson, A. M., Rose, B. D., Graff, L. G., Jacobs, J. B., Schwartz, J. H., Strauss, G. M., Yang, J. P. S., Rudnick, M. R., Elfenbein, I. B., and Narins, R. G. Thrombotic microangiopathy and renal failure associated with antineoplastic chemotherapy. *Ann. Intern. Med., 101*: 41–44 (1984).
17. Moake, J. L., Turner, N. A., Stathopoulos, N. A., Nolasco, L. H., and Hellums, J. D. Involvement of large plasma von willebrand factor (vWF) multimers and unusually large vWF forms derived from endothelial cells in shear stress-induced platelet aggregation. *J. Clin. Invest., 78*: 1456–1461 (1986).

18. Moake, J. L., Turner, N. A., Stathopoulos, N. A., Nolasco, L., and Hellums, J. D. Shear-induced platelet aggregation can be mediated by vWF released from platelets, as well as by exogenous large and unusually large vWF multimers, requires adenosine diphosphate, and is resistant to aspirin. *Blood, 71*: 1366–1374 (1988).
19. Holmsen, H., Stormorken, H., and Goote, T. M. Kinetic studies on the breakdown of adenosine diphosphate in human plasma. *Scand. J. Clin. Lab. Invest., 17*: 138–150 (1965).

3
Commentary on the Relationships Between HUS and TTP

Bernard S. Kaplan *Children's Hospital of Philadelphia and University of Pennsylvania, Philadelphia, Pennsylvania*

INTRODUCTION

The difficulties encountered in differentiating the hemolytic uremic syndrome (HUS) from thrombotic thrombocytopenic purpura (TTP) have been discussed by Madame Renée Habib in Chapter 24. These attempts are constantly plagued by problems similar to those described in another context by Gould (1):

> [He] continually traps himself in borrowed conceptual schemes, escaping by good sense, but only with difficulty because language proves to be so restrictive. For example, the sequence . . . becomes a progressive continuum because tradition dictates this form of speech and iconography. Yet all [his] descriptions cry out for a completely different concept. . . . *We need a different iconography*. . . .

The notion that language can become very restrictive is embodied in the passage from Genesis (2) that "whatsoever Adam called every living creature, that *was* the name thereof" (Genesis 2:19).

That language can also become confusing is also well documented in the passage that says (2) "let us go down, and confound their language, that they may not understand one another's speech" (Genesis 11:7) (Table 1).

Once something has been given a name and the name gains widespread acceptance, the precise definitions are often forgotten. For example, HUS is usually characterized by a triad of features. Almost forgotten is the fact that the original definition contained four features (3). There is even a debate as to whether the original description of HUS was a description of what has now come to be accepted as HUS. Modifiers may be introduced, and these convey different messages and stir up

Table 1 A Babble of Names

TTP
Thrombocytic acrioangiothrombosis
Thrombocytopenic thrombocytic microangiothrombosis
Generalized blood platelet thrombosis
Platelet thrombosis syndrome
Moschcowitz' syndrome
Thrombotic thrombocytopenic purpura
Thrombotic microangiopathy
Thromobohemolytic thrombocytopenic purpura
HUS
Gasser's syndrome
Hemolytic-uremic syndrome
Hemolytic uremic syndrome
Hemolytic uremic syndromes
Classical HUS
Atypical HUS
Prototypic HUS
Endemic HUS
Epidemic HUS
D+ and D– HUS
Postenteropathic form of HUS
Sporadic HUS

new areas of controversy. Modifiers have included postdiarrheal (typical) HUS or HUS with recurrent episodes. Some prefer the designations D+ for diarrhea associated HUS and D– for nondiarrheal HUS (4,5). HUS is no longer merely HUS or even HUS's but has become combinations of classical, infantile, typical, prototypic, postdiarrheal, D+.

New discoveries are beginning to change the definition and designation of the syndrome(s). Verotoxin (or verocytotoxin)-associated HUS is, it would seem, as acceptable a designation as meningococcal meningitis. Unfortunately, verocytotoxin is giving way to Shiga-like toxin (SL-T)-associated HUS. The tradition established at the Tower of Babel lives on and reflects the dynamic nature of our languages as well as ongoing changes in our understanding of HUS.

It is also confusing when the definition of a new syndrome (HUS) is contained within that of the one from which it is being differentiated (TTP) (6). The use of abbreviations such as TTP and HUS may be followed by abbreviated thought and conceptual leaps, so that TTP and HUS beget HUS/TTP, which in their turn beget the idea that HUS = TTP (7). The problem becomes even more confusing when some authors accept both the idea that HUS and TTP are different entities *and* the apparently contradictory notion that HUS and TTP may be part of the spectrum of the same disease process (8). It's a little like thinking that lions and tigers are not only different kinds of animal, but also members of the cat family. Most people, however, know the difference between a lion and a tiger.

It is entirely possible (and the history of medicine is replete with numerous examples) that HUS and TTP can be defined as pure syndromes, that each has subsets, and that there are examples of patients with overlapping features. One only has to think of rickets and osteomalacia as an example. Rickets is osteomalacia in a child, and osteomalacia is rickets in an adult. Rickets itself has many subsets that include environmental and inherited causes. However, once a cause is known, the question of whether a patient has rickets or osteomalacia becomes of secondary importance—that is, X-linked hypophosphatemic rickets (XHPD) is XHPD whether it is occurring in an adult or a child. I am indebted to Charles Scriver for pointing out this concept so elegantly (9). If one extrapolates this idea to HUS and TTP, reports of verotoxin-associated HUS (10) and those of "TTP" in association with verotoxin (11) begin to confuse the subject more and more (11, 12).

A NEW ICONOGRAPHY

A new iconography, based on an etiologic classification, has been proposed for the hemolytic uremic syndromes (13, 14). This approach is gradually gaining acceptance. However, attempts to define HUS and TTP more precisely have been less successful. Gould (1) observed that scientific progress may result from an "interplay of theory and empirical observation. Theory can prod, suggest, integrate, and direct in fruitful ways; . . . But theory can also stifle, mislead and restrict" (1). We must also recognize "the ultimate sterility of a methodology without context and without aim beyond the noble, but unattainable, goal of piling pristine fact upon fact in the hope that generality would somehow mysteriously emerge at the end."

There is also the possibility that, once the definition of a syndrome is examined in detail, all of the king's horses and all the king's men may not be able to put it together again. However, an analysis of the relationship between HUS and TTP is required for practical rather than semantic reasons. These include interpretation of perturbations found in one with regard to their extrapolation to the other, questions about prognosis, and the application of specific and at times dangerous forms of treatment. We have noted that the more a case of HUS is perceived as atypical, the more it begins to resemble TTP. And we have also been criticized—fairly—that we have used "atypical" too loosely, especially in regard to the form of HUS encountered mainly in the subcontinent of India (5). We have also at different times thought of HUS and TTP as distinct entities, as part of a spectrum, as members of a community with overlapping features (15), and even as twin stars encircling each other in a far-off galaxy (8). We have never, however, suggested that they are a single entity.

Three approaches have been employed to unravel the overlapping syndromes of TTP and HUS: empirical documentation by evaluation of series of cases, theory, and the more objective method of cluster analysis (16).

COUNTING PEBBLES, DESCRIBING COLORS

"Correct" reading of the older literature confirms Wardle's contention that HUS and TTP may be different (17). But it does depend on which papers are read. Gautier et al. (Chapter 1) note candidly that at least three conditions were represented by their five original cases of HUS: acute cortical necrosis, HUS associated with bronchopneumonia, and a case of TTP. Mme. R. Habib (personal communication) believes that the illness in the patient described by Moschcowitz (18) more closely approximates what is now called HUS than Gasser's original cases of HUS. Symmers (19) defined the typical, fully developed case of thrombotic thrombocytopenic purpura (thrombotic microangiopathic haemolytic anemia or thrombotic microangiopathy), as a syndrome consisting of fever, hemolytic anemia, thrombocytopenic purpura, and fluctuating neurological disturbances. He emphasized the fact that the most characteristic component, the waxing and waning neurologic signs, often appeared in only the terminal stages; he also noted that disseminated lesions were seen only in vessels of microscopic caliber. Symmers' review of 31 "indisputable" cases yielded some important observations. The ages ranged from 9 years 6 months to 74 years, and there were no infants; there were slightly more females (19) than males (12); and six of the patients (20%) were black. He noted that "uremia has been a rare observation" and that the urine could also be completely normal, although proteinuria and microscopic hematuria were often detected and macroscopic hematuria was occasionally detected. Most cases had a leukocytosis with a left shift. Occult blood might sometimes be detected in stools. The juxtaglomerular portion of the afferent arteriole was most often affected; glomerular capillaries were often obliterated by hyaline material which was not clearly thrombotic in nature but appeared to represent a change in the capillary wall. A focal proliferative "glomerulitis" has been noted. Symmers discussed the fact that no familial cases had been reported.

It is interesting to observe, in retrospect, that, although Symmers' description was on the mark in so many aspects, he dismissed as unconvincing Jones and Loring's (20) argument that thrombotic microangiopathy was an unusually severe form of capillary thrombosis that could occur in glomeruli and occasionally elsewhere in some cases of bacterial infection or circulatory disturbance, possibly through toxic or anoxic damage to the endothelium.

CONCEPTUAL LOCKS

TTP is a syndrome and not a disease (21). Kwaan (22) has noted that the classical forms of TTP and HUS have their own characteristics that enable them to be classified as separate entities. In the atypical forms, the term HUS/TTP may be more appropriate.

Some authors have used the term thrombotic microangiopathy (TMA) to encompass the spectrum of TTP and HUS (22), but it may be advisable to restrict this appelation to those instances in which there is histologic evidence of thrombi in microvessels. It may be appropriate to introduce additional modifiers, such as idiopathic TMA and hereditary TMA. Or, it may be appropriate to restrict the term TMA to cases where there is no apparent cause, and where it is difficult to define the problem as unequivocally TTP or HUS (23). TMA is a very useful and descriptive term, but it is a pathologic observation and therefore can or should be used only when a tissue examination has confirmed its presence.

Nalbadian et al. (24) have regarded as pernicious the practice of lumping HUS and TTP together. There are two ironies in their criticism: They reproach us for advocating a syndromic approach to HUS and TTP although what we were attempting to do was in line with their approach; and they base their development of a TTP paradigm on the work of Kwaan, who now favors the TTP/HUS designation for some cases. These carpings aside, Nalbadian et al. (24) have written a review with many important observations. They deplore the fact that the diagnostic criteria for TTP have become so nonspecific that they include more than TTP. Unfortunately, their narrowly defined clinicopathological paradigm of TTP is also beset by problems. These are mainly apparent in the first table in their article in regard to the features ascribed to HUS. In contrast to what they have stated, HUS is not uncommon after 1 year of age; the pathology is not almost always limited to the kidneys; disseminated intravascular coagulation (DIC) is not commonly present; not all patients have thrombi, and if present, there is little evidence to support the notion that they are formed during the process of DIC; heparin is not effective in HUS.

BACK TO RICKETS AND OSTEOMALACIA

Rickets is childhood osteomalacia, and osteomalacia is adult rickets. Rickets and osteomalacia share many of the acquired causes of each, and there are no reasons to believe that each may not be caused by any of the exogenous factors that produce the other. Can the same line of reasoning be used for HUS and TTP? Is it the case that HUS is childhood TTP and that TTP is adult HUS? The answer seems to be yes—and no. Minimal-change nephrotic syndrome and membranous nephrotic syndrome have very similar clinical and laboratory features; however, the former is seen mainly in children, the latter mainly in adults. At one time some people believed that they were manifestations of the same disease. They are now known to be discrete entities. The same is probably true for most, but not all, cases of HUS and TTP.

In a small number of families, HUS and TTP *may be* variable expressions of the same disease (25); in other *they only seem* to be variable expressions (26). There are also patients with recurrent episodes of HUS who have HUS during some episodes and TTP during others (27, 28). Clearly, when the molecular defect responsible for these cases has been identified, a new name will be given to these subsets.

Although the first documented case of TTP was in a child (18), this syndrome is extremely uncommon in children. Berman and Finkelstein (29) found 13 cases of TTP in children when they reviewed the literature up to 1975. They excluded cases with acute renal failure and those with histopathologic changes that primarily affected the kidneys. They also added information on 12 cases from a survey of North America. A summary of Berman and Finkelstein's data is shown in Table 2. An important finding in their study is the relatively large number of affected black patients (30%). This figure is similar to that noted by others in adults. HUS is extremely uncommon in blacks. I have personally seen only one black child with HUS (in Montreal) among several hundred cases in South Africa, Montreal, London, and Philadelphia. There are few reports of HUS in black children in Africa.

CLUSTER ANALYSIS

A more objective method, cluster analysis, has been used in an attempt to separate them HUS from TTP (16). The main conclusion was that these two syndromes occupy

Table 2 TTP in Childhood

Number of patients	25
Sex (M:F)	9:16
Age (range)	20 mo –16 yr
Race (white/black)	15:5
Mortality	75%

Source: Ref. 29.

the opposite ends of a continuum with overlap in some cases. However, there is no doubt that the gestalt of a typical case of HUS is quite different from that of a typical case of TTP. A precise definition of each, and of the subsets of each, must reach beyond the clinical features. However, we must wait for the elucidation of the causes and/or of the mechanisms which produce HUS and TTP and their subsets or variant forms. HUS is a syndrome as well as a disease (3)—hence the need for a new iconography. HUS the syndrome can be classified into acquired and inherited forms

Table 3 Classification of the Putative Causes of the Hemolytic Uremic Syndrome and Thrombotic Thrombocytopenic Purpura

	HUS	TTP
A. Idiopathic	+	+
B. Acquired		
Infections		
Escherichia coli 0157:H7	+	
Shigella shigae	+	
Streptococcus pneumoniae	+	
Salmonella typhi	+	
Campylobacter jejuni	+	
Yersinia pseudotuberculosis	+	
Pseudomonas	+	
Bacteroides	+	
Portillo virus	+	
Coxsackie versuses	+	
Echo viruses	+	
Influenza viruses	+	
Epstein-Barr virus	+	
Rotoviruses	+	
Human immunodeficiency virus		+
Microtatabiote	+	+
Rickettsia		+
Inherited		
Autosomal recessive	+	+
Autosomal dominant	+	?
Cynanocobalamin-associated	+	
Treatment-associated		
Cyclosporin	+	
Mitomycin	+	
Oral contraceptives	+	+
Radiation	+	
Pregnancy-associated	+	+
Transplant-associated		
Renal	+	
Bone marrow	+	
Liver	+	
Glomerulopathy-associated	+	
Malignancy-associated	+	+
Kawasaki-associated	+	
Lupus-associated		+

(30). Many of the associations have not been proven beyond a reasonable doubt and are the subject of more in-depth analyses in some of the chapters that follow. A classification of HUS is shown in Table 3.

The most typical of the acquired forms could be called, for the sake of this argument, HUS the disease. HUS the disease occurs mainly, but not exclusively, in infants and children. Chances of surviving the acute phase are good, and the microvascular disease mainly affects the kidneys. HUS the disease is usually associated with a prodromal illness of bloody diarrhea (hemorrhagic colitis). Onset is usually very acute. The disease is associated with S-LT (verotoxin)–producing *E. coli*. These patients almost never have recurrences. Adults with a prodrome of bloody diarrhea, evidence of S-LT–producing *E. coli* infection, and a clinical syndrome affecting many organs seem to have HUS the disease rather than TTP. To think otherwise is to advocate forms of therapy that are more in vogue for the treatment of TTP but have not been proven to be of value in the treatment of HUS the disease.

A similar classification can be used for TTP (Table 3). TTP occurs mainly in adults, has a high mortality rate, and is characterized by a generalized vasculopathy. Onset is often insidious. In HUS the kidneys bear the brunt of the injury, whereas in TTP the brain injury is more prominent than the nephropathy. However, there is a lot of overlap when groups of cases are compared: Both syndromes occur at all ages; many organs may be damaged in HUS; renal disease may occur in TTP; HUS and TTP have occurred in the same patient at different times; and each has occurred in one of identical twins. Development of new types of treatment, such as plasma infusions and plasmapheresis, makes it imperative that HUS, TTP, and their subsets be defined more precisely because some patients may be at risk when a nondiscriminating approach to treatment is used.

> "HUS and TTP seem to rotate about each like the twin stars of U Cephei in a far-off galaxy each appearing intermittently brighter depending on their relationship to the observer, each in turn drawing energy from the other depending on the bias of the observer. From afar they seem to be one entity, closer up they seem to be discrete entities but their photospheres merge and confuse their separate identities. And yet it is of crucial importance that this problem be resolved because the treatment and outcome of HUS and TTP may be so different" (8).

The more carefully we look, the more clearly each star will begin to appear.

REFERENCES

1. Gould, S. J. Down on the farm. *NY. Rev. Books, 36:* 26–27 (1990).
2. *The Holy Bible. Genesis* 2:19 and 11:17. Oxford University Press, London.
3. Gasser, C., Gautier, C., Steck, A., Siebenmann, R. E., Oechslin, R. Hamolytisch-uramische syndrome: Bilaterale nierenindennekrosen bei akuten erworbenen hamolytischen anamien. *Schweiz. Med. Woschenschr., 85:* 905–909 (1955).
4. Walters, M. D. S., Matthei, I, U., Kay, R., Dillon, M. J., Barratt, T. M. The polymorphonuclear leukocyte count in childhood haemolytic uraemic syndrome. *Pediatr. Nephrol. 3:* 130–134 (1989).
5. Taylor, C. M., Milford, D. V., White, R. H. R. A plea for standardized terminology within the haemolytic-uraemic syndromes. *Pediatr. Nephrol, 5:* 97 (1991).
6. Byrnes, J. J., Similarities and differences between the hemolytic uremic syndrome and

thrombotic thrombocytopenic purpura. In *Acute Renal Disorders and Renal Emergencies*. (J. Strauss ed.) Martinus Nijhoff Publishing, Boston, pp. 51–68 (1984).
7. Remuzzi, G. HUS and TTP: Variable expression of a single entity. *Kidney Int.*, *32:* 292–308 (1987).
8. Kaplan, B. S., Remuzzi, G. The hemolytic uremic syndrome. In *Thrombosis and Hemostasis* (Remuzzi, G., Rossi, E., eds.) Butterworths, London, pp. 201–236 (1989).
9. Scriver, C. R. Nature, nurture, and human affairs. *Trans. R. Soc. Can.*, *19:* 211–232 (1981).
10. Neill, M. A., Agosti, J., Rosen, H. Hemorrhagic colitis with Escherichia coli 0157:H7 preceding adult hemolytic uremic syndrome. *Arch. Intern. Med.*, *145:* 2215–2217 (1985).
11. Griffin, P. M., Ostroff, S. M., Tauxe, R. V., Greene, K. D., Wells, J. G., Lewis, J. H., Blake, P. A. Illness associated with *E. coli* 0157:H7 infections. *Annu. Intern. Med.*, *109:* 705–712 (1988).
12. Kovacs, M. J., Cameron, W. Epidemiology of the hemolytic uremic syndrome. *N. Engl. J. Med.*, *324:* 1065 (1991).
13. Drummond, K. N. Hemolytic uremic syndrome—then and now. *N. Engl. J. Med.*, *312:* 116–118 (1985).
14. Kaplan, B. S., Proesmans, W. The hemolytic uremic syndrome of childhood and its variants. *Semin. Hematol.* *24:* 148–160 (1987).
15. Kaplan, B. S., de Chadarevian, J.-P. Hemolytic uremic syndrome. *Can. Med. Assoc. J.* *117:* 1246 (1977).
16. Vedaranayanan, V. V., Preus, M., Kaplan, B. S. An application of cluster analysis as an attempt to differentiate objectively between hemolytic-uremic syndrome (HUS) and thrombotic thrombocytopenic purpura (TTP). In *Recent Advances in Pediatric Nephrology* Murakami, K., Kitagawa, T., Yabuta, K., (eds.), Excerpta Medica, Amsterdam, pp. 573–576 (1987).
17. Wardle, N. What is HUS and what is TTP? *Nephron*, *50:* 389 (1988).
18. Moschcowitz, E. An acute febrile pleiochromic anemia with hyaline thrombosis of the terminal arterioles and capillaries. An undescribed disease. *Arch. Intern. Med.*, *36:* 89–93 (1925).
19. Symmers, W. St.C. Thrombotic microangiopathic haemolytic anaemia (thrombotic microangiopathy). *Br. Med. J.*, *2:* 897–903 (1952).
20. Jones, D. B., Loring, W. E. Glomerular thrombosis. *Am. J. Pathol.*, *27:* 841–852 (1951).
21. Umlas, J., Kaiser, J. Thrombohemolytic thrombocytopenic purpura (TTP). *Am. J. Med.*, *49:* 723–728 (1970).
22. Kwaan, H. C. Miscellaneous secondary thrombotic microangiopathy. *Semin. Hematol.*, *24:* 141–147 (1987).
23. Salant, D. J., Corwin, R. B. A 66-year-old woman with rapidly deteriorating renal function. *N. Engl. J. Med.*, *323:* 1050–1061 (1990).
24. Nalbadian, R. M., Henry, R. L., Bick, R. L. Thrombotic thrombocytopenic purpura. An extended editorial. *Semin. Thromb. Hemostas.*, *5:* 216–240 (1979).
25. Elias, M., Horowitz, J., Tal, I., Kohn, D., Flatau, E. Thrombotic thrombocytopenic purpura and haemolytic uraemic syndrome in three siblings. *Arch. Dis. Child.*, *63:* 644–646 (1988).
26. Hellman, R. M., Jackson, D. V., Buss, D. H. Thrombotic thrombocytopenic purpura and hemolytic-uremic syndrome in HLA-identical siblings. *Ann. Intern. Med.*, *93:* 283–284 (1980).
27. Mettler, N. E. Isolation of a microtatobiote from patients with hemolytic-uremic syndrome and thrombotic thrombocytopenic purpura and from mites in the United States. *N. Engl. J. Med.*, *281:* 1026–1027 (1969).
28. Ruggenenti, P., Remuzzi, G., Rossi, E. N. Epidemiology of the hemolytic uremic syndrome. *N. Engl. J. Med.*, *324:* 1064–1065 (1991).

29. Berman, N., Finkelstein, J. Z. Thrombotic thrombocytopenic purpura in childhood. Results of a survey and re-examination of the literature. *Scand. J. Haematol., 14:* 286–294 (1975).
30. Kaplan, B. S. Thrombotic thrombocytopenic purpura/ hemolytic uremic syndrome. In *The Principles and Practice of Nephrology* (Jacobson, H. R., Striker, G. E., Klahr, S., eds.), B. C. Decker Inc., p. 324 (1991).

II
Epidemiology of HUS

4
The Hemolytic Uremic Syndromes in the United Kingdom

David Milford *The Children's Hospital, Birmingham, England*

Interest in the hemolytic uremic syndromes (HUS) in the United Kingdom (UK) began in 1956 with the first case report of two children (1). These were sporadic cases and were followed by further case reports of HUS in children (2–5) and in adults (6). One of these reports (2) described cases presenting to a single pediatric unit over an 8-year period. The first report of an HUS epidemic came from a hospital serving a rural community (7), in which nine children from a small area developed HUS over a period of 8 weeks. No enteric pathogens were identified. Since then a further epidemic has been reported (8, 9); 11 children and two adults from the same locality within the West Midlands region presented over a period of 2 weeks in the summer of 1983. A dramatic and sustained rise in the incidence of HUS within the region had been noted to commence in the year preceding the epidemic. Significantly, verocytotoxin producing *Escherichia coli* (VTEC) were isolated from the stools of three of 10 children with HUS from this region, although not all these presented during the epidemic. These were among the first children found to have VTEC-associated HUS in the United Kingdom.

Despite the clear geographical boundary of an island nation, which favors a static population and is therefore an ideal setting in which to study the epidemiology of rare diseases and changing patterns of illness, there has only been one successful national study of HUS in UK children (10). However, although a large amount of valuable data was obtained during this study, changes in disease patterns with time could not be highlighted because of the lack of previous national studies for comparison. The analysis of data from HUS patients treated over a 17-year period at The Children's Hospital, Birmingham, permitted such comparisons and suggested that some features of the disease had changed (9), as outlined later.

It is now evident that children with the HUS can be subdivided into cases with a diarrheal prodrome (D+) and those without such a prodrome (D–) (10–16). In the

UK, Stuart et al. (11), and later Trompeter et al. (12), have shown that D-HUS carries a worse prognosis for renal outcome. This important distinction, which was not always made in previous studies, necessitated separate analysis of clinical and laboratory features for patients included in a collaborative national study of HUS conducted over a 3-year period. The findings of this study are outlined later in this chapter.

HUS IN THE WEST MIDLANDS REGION

Evidence of VTEC infection, especially *E. coli* 0157:H7, has been found in up to 75% of D+ HUS in North America and in more than 60% of cases in the UK (10, 17, 18). If this is a recent association, has this been reflected in changes in disease expression? Following an epidemic of D+ HUS in the West Midlands, it was suggested that there had been a change in the nature of the disease in the region (9), which appeared to coincide with an increase in referral rates. To examine this further, Coad et al. (9a) performed a retrospective analysis of clinical and laboratory data from 74 D+ children treated at The Children's Hospital, Birmingham, between 1970 and 1987. The cumulative sum (Cusum) technique (19), when applied to annual referral rates to detect the timing of any change from the previous norm, revealed a marked increase in annual referrals between 1981 and 1982 (Fig. 1). Therefore, the clinical features of children presenting between 1970 and 1981 were compared to those for the group presenting between 1982 and 1987 (Table 1a); this analysis provided further support for the notion that the expression of the disease had changed.

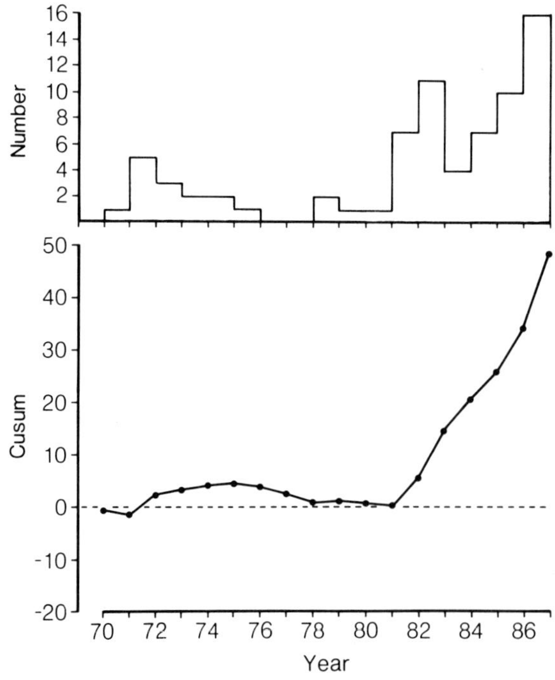

Figure 1 Annual HUS referral rates to The Children's Hospital, Birmingham, with Cusum analysis in the lower panel demonstrating the abrupt increase in the number of new cases presenting after 1981. (From Coad et al. 9a.)

Table 1a Comparison of Clinical Features in West Midlands Children Presenting to The Children's Hospital, Birmingham, Before and After 1981

	1970–81	1982–87	p
Number	19	55	<0.001
Mean Age (months)	23.8	48.3	<0.02
Male:female	11:8	22:33	ns
Bloody diarrhea	7 (37%)	39 (71%)	<0.02
Acute dialysis	17 (89%)	27 (49%)	<0.01
Seizures	5 (26%)	10 (18%)	ns
Residual CNS deficit	6 (32%)	5 (9%)	<0.05

Source: Coad et al. (9a).

Coad et al. demonstrated that children in the earlier period did well if they presented in the summer and were males, findings that were in agreement with Trompeter et al. (12); however, this did not apply to those presenting later. They also found that in the latter period neutrophilia was associated with a poor outcome (Table 1b), and that it explained half the variance of outcome in a logistic regression analysis of factors predictive of a good or poor outcome at presentation. In this group of closely followed up children, a good outcome was suggested by a neutrophil count less than 20,000 cmm (sensitivity 93%, specificity 66%, and positive predictive value 93%). A high initial hemoglobin concentration and male sex were also predictors of a poor outcome in this group, but it is notable that none of these factors (i.e., neutrophilia, high hemaglobin, male sex) contributed to outcome in the logistic regression analysis applied to the earlier group.

This regional study demonstrated an abrupt increase in the incidence of D+ HUS which was associated with a change in some clinical features of the disease and in clinical parameters predictive of outcome. A review of coliform isolates held in a UK reference center has shown that the commonest VTEC (0157:H7) has only emerged as a significant pathogen since the early 1980s (20). It remains to be shown that these changes in the nature of the disease, which corresponded with the

Table 1b Comparison of Laboratory Investigations at Presentation in Good and Poor Outcome Groups Before and After 1981

	1970–1981		p	1982–1987		p
Outcome	good	poor		good	poor	
Hemoglobin	6.4 (1.1)	7.8 (0.7)	ns	7.8 (0.3)	10.9 (0.9)	<0.01
Neutrophils	9.1 (1.6)	12.1 (2.4)	ns	10.6 (1.0)	24.9 (2.5)	<0.01
Lymphocytes	6.9 (1.2)	6.4 (1.6)	ns	5.5 (0.8)	5.4 (1.1)	ns
Monocytes	—	—		1.0 (0.2)	1.8 (0.2)	<0.01
Platelets	50.5 (8.2)	91.5 (20.4)	ns	89 (14)	133 (33.7)	ns

Source: Coad et al. (9a).

emergence of VTEC in mainland Britain, can be explained by this association, although the circumstantial evidence is compelling.

THE UK COLLABORATIVE STUDY, 1985–1988

This study, conducted between April 1, 1985, and March 31, 1988, was based on data from questionnaires completed by the attending physician, combined with a microbiological survey of stool specimens. It was made possible by collaboration among the British Association for Paediatric Nephrology (BAPN), the Communicable Diseases Surveillance Centre (CDSC), and the Division of Enteric Pathogens (DEP) of the Public Health Laboratory, London. The study was later aided by the establishment of the British Paediatric Surveillance Unit (BPSU), an epidemiological unit within the CDSC dedicated to the study of diseases in childhood (21).

Incidence of HUS

Annual Rates

Surveillance of HUS in Britain began in 1983 as a voluntary reporting scheme by the British Paediatric Association (BPA) and the CDSC (22). The combined BAPN/CDSC/DEP study began in April 1985; later, it was augmented by the establishment of the BPSU and the introduction of an active reporting scheme in which monthly requests were sent to all pediatricians within the BPA for notification of listed diseases. The incidence of the disease appeared to increase throughout the duration of the study; however, while the inception of the reporting scheme in July 1986 undoubtedly increased the number of cases reported, the increase in annual totals persisted until the end of BPSU surveillance in December 1989 (Table 2).

Sex

The overall male-to-female ratio was 141:157 (1:1.1). This slight female preponderance was not seen in D– cases, in whom there were 11 males and 5 females (2.2:1). If the D+ group was analyzed separately, the overall ratio was 130:152 (1:1.2). It is of interest that while the ratio for D+ children less than 10 years old was 1:1.1, that for the group aged 10 or more was 1:2.4. Thus, D– cases had an excess of males, and D+ cases had a female dominance most marked in those more than 10 years old. There is no explanation for the female preponderance in D+ cases; while

Table 2 Annual Reports of HUS in British Children

Year	No. of cases reported	Incidence/100,000/yr
1985	83	0.81
1986[a]	103	1.01
1987	116	1.14
1988	95	0.93
1989	193	1.89

[a]British Paediatric Surveillance Unit established in July.
Source: Dr. S. Hall of the BPSU (unpublished data).

other workers have reported similar findings (22–24), they have failed to comment on the excess of older females. It is perhaps relevant to these observations that Pai et al. (25) noted that the relative frequency of VTEC 0157:H7 infection in individuals over 15 years of age was 2.15 times greater in females, although the mechanisms underlying this finding were unexplained.

Age

The incidence by age and sex is diagrammatically shown in Figure 2. D+ HUS most commonly affected children under 5 years old, a finding that has been reported by other workers (9, 10, 12, 13, 22, 26, 27). The peak annual incidence was in the group aged 1–2 years (3.3 cases per 100,000 children), which was more than 10 times that for those aged 10 years or more (0.27 cases per 100,000 children). Nonetheless, the incidence in the under 5's is much lower than has been calculated for this age group in and around Buenos Aires, which has the highest reported incidence (21.7 cases per 100,000 children per year) (27). However, despite the predilection of D+ HUS for the young, only 7 (2.3%) children were less than 6 months of age. It may be pertinent that the dramatic rise in incidence of D+ HUS coincides with the age of weaning, a time when the immunologically "naive" individual is exposed to an increasing number of novel micro-organisms over a relatively short period of time. By contrast, the incidence of D– cases did not appear to alter with age (13).

Season

In keeping with other studies, the incidence of D+ HUS showed a marked seasonal variation (9, 10, 12, 13, 22, 26, 27), with most presenting between April and October (Fig. 3); these 7 months accounted for more than 80% of all cases reported to the study. No such seasonal distribution was found for the D– cases.

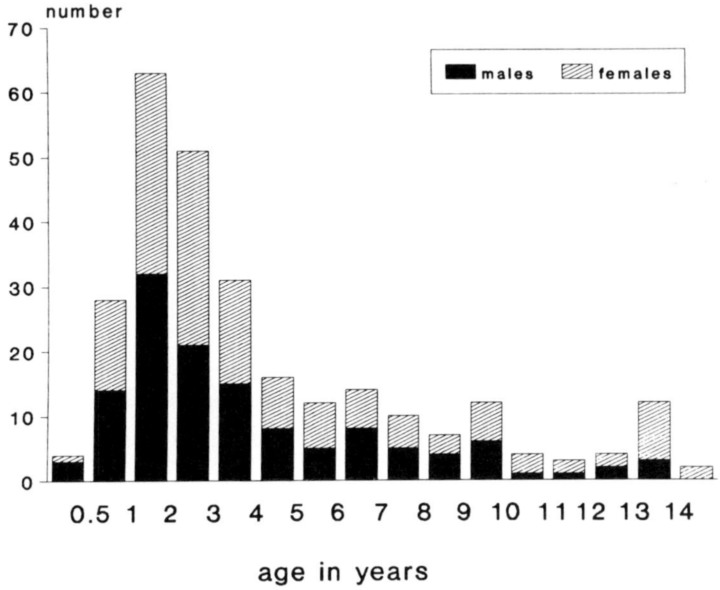

Figure 2 The age and sex distribution of children with D+ HUS reported to the UK collaborative study.

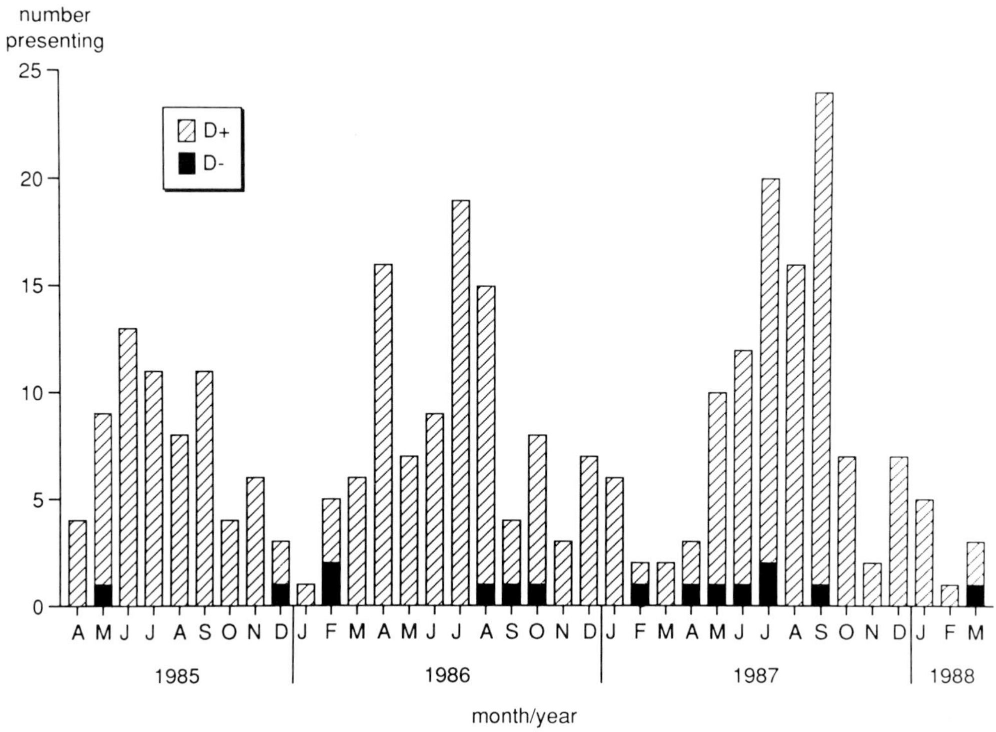

Figure 3 The monthly incidence of HUS in children reported to the UK collaborative study. Note the lack of a seasonal pattern for children with D− HUS (From Ref. 10.)

Ethnic Group

Studies from countries with mixed populations have previously reported that HUS appears to affect Caucasians particularly (28, 29). In this study, 277 (98.2%) children with D+ HUS were Caucasians, and five were Asians; while the precise populations of ethnic groups living in the United Kingdom are not known, it has been estimated that 92% of children less than 16 years of age are white (30), suggesting an under-representation of non-white children in the study. There were 15 Caucasians in the D– group (92%), the remaining child being Asian.

Clinical Findings in Nondiarrheal Cases

The difference between D+ and D– HUS was recently highlighted by finding evidence of VTEC infection only in D+ patients (18). In the tropics, HUS is associated with *Shigella dysenteriae* type 1 (31). In contrast, D– cases have numerous etiologies; while a minority are associated with other extrinsic toxins such as pneumococcal neuroaminidase (32), the majority are associated with intrinsic causes, including complement deficiencies (16, 33); however, most have an unknown etiology, may relapse, and may be inherited.

Of the 16 children who did not have a diarrheal prodrome, 13 had respiratory symptoms or vomiting preceding their illness. In contrast to D+ cases, none of the family contacts had concurrent illnesses, and although one boy came from a family with autosomal dominant inheritance of HUS (34), he did not have an obvious prodromal illness and none of the immediate family was reported to be unwell at the time. None of the 16 was reported to be pyrexial at the onset of the disease. Nine developed oliguria or anuria (56%) and required dialysis, a percentage similar to that for the D+ cases (Table 3); another had high-output renal failure.

Clinical Findings in Diarrheal Cases

Prodrome

Two hundred and eighty-two children developed HUS after a prodromal illness of diarrhea, and in 202 (71.6%) the stool was visibly blood-stained. The majority of these children (65.6%) had diarrhea on admission, but only 42.5% had diarrhea at the time of diagnosis—hence the difficulty encountered by workers seeking to identify VTEC using microbiological techniques alone. The interval between the onset of the prodrome to time of diagnosis varied from 1–34 days (the longest being in a child with *Shigella dysenteriae* type 1 infection), but the mean interval between onset of diarrhea and diagnosis was 8 days. Those with bloody diarrhea had a longer prodrome (median 7 days) when compared to those with diarrhea only (median 5 days, Mann-Whitney $p=0.0002$).

Severe abdominal pain can be associated with the enterocolitic prodrome, sometimes necessitating surgery and usually delaying diagnosis. Common misdiagnoses include inflammatory bowel disease, intussusception and appendicitis (26, 35–37). In the UK study, abdominal pain was reported in 40 children; of these, 11 underwent a laparotomy. Seven children had appendectomies performed prior to the diagnosis of HUS being made, and in all instances normal appendices were removed. Two

Table 3 Comparison of Clinical Features and Outcome Between Diarrhea Associated (D+) and Nondiarrheal (D−) HUS

	D+	D−
No. reported	282 (94.6%)	16 (5.4%)
Season	spring/summer	none
Age of onset	71% <5 years	any age
Males:females	1:1.2	2.2:1
Onset of prodrome	abrupt	vague
Dialyzed	175 (62%)	9 (56%)
VT/VTEC in stools	62% (early samples)	0
Outcome at >1 year from diagnosis:		
Followed up	182	11
Lone hypertension	1	1
Ht/Cr <1.5	18	1
ESRF	0	5
Died	15 (7.9%)	3 (27%)
mortality/morbidity	18%	91%

Ht/Cr = height/creatinine ratio
ESRF = end-stage renal failure

children had a laparotomy because intussusception had been diagnosed, and a further two required colonic resections for severe colitis (38), a situation akin to the toxic megacolon seen in inflammatory bowel disease.

The probability of an infective etiology in D+ HUS was suggested by a history of concurrent diarrheal symptoms in the contacts of 66 D+ children; 36 of the contacts were siblings and 27 were parents. Fourteen individuals developed D+ HUS within a few days of each other; eight of these children were included in the study, but the contacts of a further three were not reported. At least one of those not reported was known to be an adult.

Physical Signs at Presentation

Pallor was the commonest physical sign, and was noted in 92% of cases, while jaundice was reported in 35%. Forty-one children were pyrexial during their illness, but this did not correlate with the duration or severity of their prodrome or any other clinical or laboratory parameter. A clinical assessment of hydration was reported for 272 children, 50% of whom were assessed to be normally hydrated, 22% fluid overloaded, and 25% dehydrated. Nevertheless, only 60% of children had been diagnosed by the time oliguria was established, and in some instances the diagnosis was not made for 2 or more days after the onset of oliguria. The delay in diagnosis, coupled with subsequent failure to recognize the onset of oliguria, undoubtedly contributed to later electrolyte disturbances (37, 39).

Clinical Course

Not all children developing HUS require dialysis as oligoanuria is not invariable; indeed, a careful balance of fluids, base supplementation, and appropriate dietary management may maintain biochemical stability until renal function recovers. Of the 226 children reported to have had oliguria or anuria, 175 required dialysis, and of these 77% for less than 14 days. The initial neutrophil count was significantly higher in those patients developing oligoanuria, but there was no significant difference in the duration of thrombocytopenia for children with varying degrees of renal failure (Fig. 4).

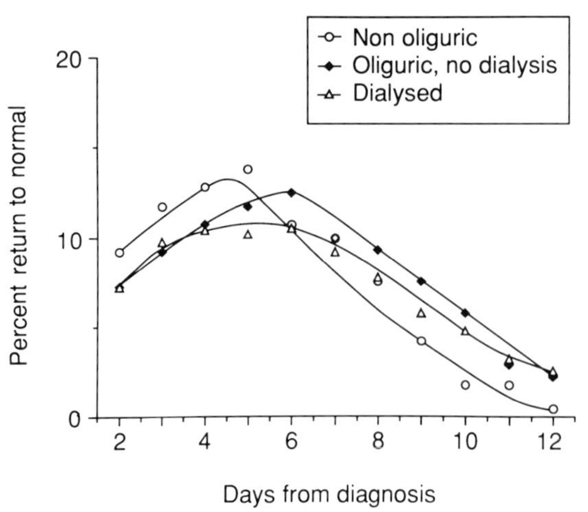

Figure 4 The time taken for the platelet count to return to normal in children with varying degrees of renal impairment (moving average smoothed curve).

Hypertension in the acute phase of the illness is well described, although the reported prevalence varies considerably (7, 26, 40). In this study, hypertension was reported in 79 (28%) children; however, while 29 of these also had seizures or neurological symptoms or signs, only in 11 did these disturbances occur within 2 days of the onset of hypertension. Furthermore, no temporal association was found between hypertension and intracranial hemorrhage in the 2 patients with this complication.

Hyponatremia (plasma sodium <130 mmol/L) was found in 203 children during the course of their illness; support for its importance in the pathogenesis of seizures (9, 39, 41, 42) comes from the finding that a greater proportion of children with seizures were hyponatremic (84%) compared to those who did not have seizures (50%). Furthermore, it was notable that in the 51 (17%) children with seizures, two thirds occurred within 24 hours of the lowest recorded plasma sodium concentrations. While it is recognized that widespread microvascular thromboses may be found in HUS (40, 43, 44), undue emphasis, in our opinion, continues to be placed on their significance in the etiology of neurological disturbances. Thrombotic lesions in the brain undoubtedly occur (40, 41, 43–46), but they usually cause severe CNS disturbances that are associated with either a fatal outcome in the acute phase or persisting neurological deficits. In contrast, the commonest neurological abnormality noted in this study was seizures, mostly confined to the first 3 days after admission, and without long-term sequelae. While all the children who died had neurological disturbances during the course of their illness, only one survivor was reported to have residual neurological symptoms, lending further support to the notion that, in recent D+ HUS, hyponatremia was responsible for the majority of symptoms, although others have suggested it may not be the sole cause (47).

Four children developed a cardiomyopathy (9, 46, 48), and another four developed diabetes mellitus (9, 46, 49, 50). It is not known if these complications persisted in these children.

Microbiological Findings in Controls and HUS

Konowalchuk et al. (51) first described a verocytotoxin produced by *E. coli* in 1977 (51), but it was not until 1983 that an association between HUS and VTEC was described (18), although its role in hemorrhagic colitis in adults had been noted previously (17, 52, 53). Microbiological studies have provided circumstantial evidence linking D+ HUS and VTEC infection (17, 18, 23, 54–56), but the duration of this association is less clear. In most studies, evidence for VTEC infection has been based on increasing titers of antibodies to verocytotoxin (VT) in the blood, the detection of neutralizable VT in stools, and the culture of VTEC from stool samples. The UK study did not include the detection of circulating antibodies, but used DNA probes for detection of VT1- and VT2-producing organisms, and the presence of free neturalizable VT in stools (56, 57). The latter required a Vero cell assay using specific antisera to VT1 and VT2 to quantify the level of VT present in the sample. Stool samples were obtained from four groups of children: healthy controls, those with diarrhea, those with bloody diarrhea, and HUS patients (58). Approximately two thirds of children with HUS reported to the study had stool samples or coliform isolates submitted to the DEP for culture and analysis, although 78% were obtained more than one week from the onset of diarrhea. Stool samples from eight contacts were also examined for the presence of VT or VTEC.

A total of 60 VTEC were isolated from the four patient groups studied; it is of note that 85% were obtained from children presenting between April and October. In a two-year population based survey of stools from diarrheal patients of all ages in the Calgary area, Pai et al. (25) noted a similar seasonal variation in the prevalence of VTEC, with 86% isolated from stool samples obtained between April and October. The results of DNA probe analysis and serotyping in the four patient groups are shown in Table 4 and clearly demonstrate an association between VTEC and D+ HUS in the United Kingdom. It was notable that 94% of these organisms produced VT2 either alone or with VT1, in keeping with findings from North America (59).

Eighty-five percent of children infected with *E. coli* 0157 had a prodrome of bloody diarrhea, but only 53% of non-0157 VTEC were associated with such a

Table 4 VTEC Serotypes and VT[a] Production in Patients With HUS, Bloody Diarrhea, Diarrhea Alone, and Healthy Controls

Study group	No. tested	VTEC serotype	VT type	No. of isolates
HUS	188	0157.H7	VT1 VT2	4
		0157.H7	VT2	32
		0157.H−	VT2	3
		05.H−	VT1 VT2	1
		026.H11	VT1	2
		026.H11	VT2	1
		055.H7	VT2	1
		055.H10	VT2	1
		0105ab.H18	VT1 VT2	1
		0115.H10	VT1	1
		0128ab.H25	VT2	1
		0145.H25	VT2	2
		0163.H19	VT2	1
		0165.H25	VT2	2
		0?.H−	VT2	1
		Total VTEC 54; VTEC + VT 31; VT alone 6		
Bloody diarrhea, no HUS	48	0157.H7	VT1 VT2	1
		0157.H7	VT2	2
		Total VTEC 3; VTEC + VT 0; VT alone 1		
Diarrhea, no HUS	54	0157.H7	VT2	1
		Total VTEC 1; VTEC + VT 0; VT alone 2		
Healthy controls	46	0 rough.H2	VT1 VT2	1
		0 rough.H10	VT1 VT2	1
		Total VTEC 2; VTEC + VT 0; VT alone 0		

[a]All VTEC/VT studies carried out by the Division of Enteric Pathogens, Public Health Laboratores, London, UK.
VTEC = verocytotoxin; VT = verotoxin
Source: Ref. 52.

prodrome ($p<0.025$, Fisher's exact test). Furthermore, 14 contacts of 35 children with 0157 VTEC had diarrhea or bloody diarrhea, compared to three contacts of 14 children with non-0157 VTEC. Despite the increased prevalence of bloody diarrhea in those with 0157 VTEC and the greater probability of diarrheal symptoms in contacts of patients with this organism, gene probe analysis revealed that 92% of 0157 VTEC and 80% of non-0157 VTEC produced VT2 alone or with VT1 (Table 4). It therefore appears unlikely from these data that a particular verocytotoxin was responsible for the frequent association of *E. coli* 0157 with bloody diarrhea or promoted its infectivity, as has been previously reported (25). This observation may be highly relevant to future studies of the role of VETC in HUS, indicating that other VETC components, such as 0157 lipopolysaccharide (LPS), may be informative; indeed, antibodies to *E. coli* 0157 LPS may be useful in future epidemiological studies (60, 61).

The isolation of VTEC was found to be dependent on the interval between the onset of diarrhea and the collection of stool specimens (Fig. 5) (18, 53), but this

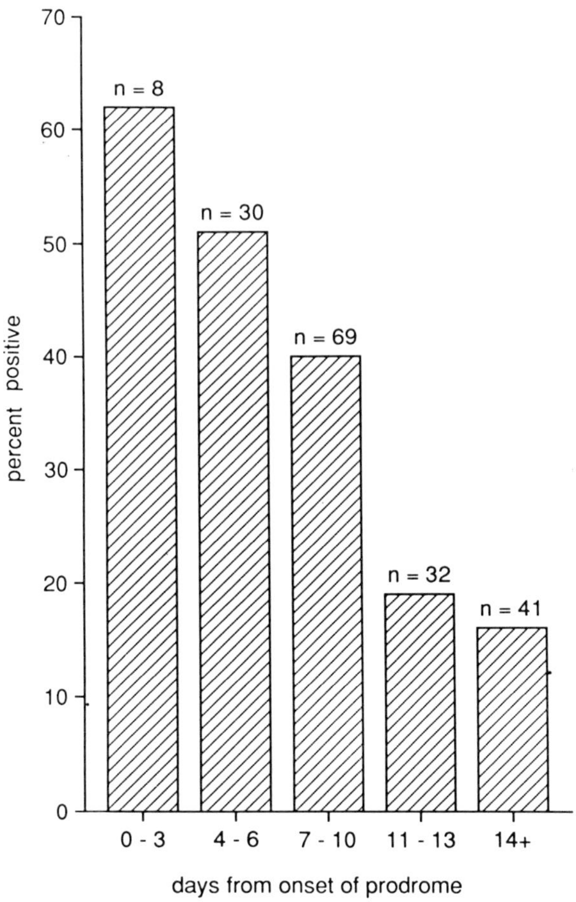

Figure 5 The relationship between time of stool sampling and successful demonstration of VTEC; the number of stool samples analysed is indicated above each bar (From Ref. 10.)

relationship only pertained to D+ cases as the 7 D– cases who had samples submitted were negative for VT and VTEC (18). Other fecal organisms were isolated by local laboratories and included five enteropathogenic *E. coli,* two *Campylobacter,* two *Salmonellae,* two *Clostridium difficile,* and single isolates of *Entameba histolytica, Candida albicans,* and *Shigella dysenteriae* type 1. The last organism was isolated from an Asian child who had returned from the Indian subcontinent.

Treatment of HUS

The high mortality and morbidity reported in early studies (7) has fallen markedly in D+ cases (10, 12, 40) following the introduction of peritoneal dialysis and better supportive care. Unfortunately, a similar improvement has not been noted in D– cases (10, 12, 13, 15), as can be seen from Table 3. In addition to dialysis, other therapies have been used in attempting to ameliorate the severity of HUS and so improve outcome. Steroids (7), heparin infusions (62, 63), streptokinase (11, 64), vitamin E (65), and antiplatelet drugs (62, 66) were used initially, but without proven benefit. Latterly, exchange transfusions, plasmapheresis (67), fresh frozen plasma infusion (68, 69), prostacyclin infusions (70), and immunoglobulin infusions (71) have been advocated, but none has been universally adopted. Such diversity of therapies reflects the inability to identify beneficial treatments, possibly because of the heterogenous nature of these diseases.

The present uncertainties regarding active treatment are reflected in the UK study, in which 87 children were reported to have received one or more of the aforementioned therapies (Table 5), with daily infusions of fresh frozen plasma the commonest adjunct. It was notable that the same treatments were used for both D+ and D– patients, despite the evident clinical and etiological differences between these two forms of HUS. It was not possible, however, to use the results from this study to determine whether any of the treatments used substantially altered the clinical course.

Table 5 "Active" Treatments Used in Children Reported to the National Study

Treatment	No. of cases D+ (good outcome)	No. of cases D–
FFP	62[a] (53)	3
Plasmapheresis	4 (3)	2
Exchange transfusion	3 (1)	2
Vitamin E alone	8 (7)	-
Prostacyclin	11[b] (8)	1[c]
Steroids	1 (1)	-

FFP = fresh frozen plasma
[a]Two patients also received vitamin E
[b]Three patients also received vitamin E; two others received FFP
[c]This patient was also plasmaphresed

Outcome

It was intended that follow-up data would be obtained in addition to details of the epidemiological, clinical, and microbiological findings reported during the acute phase. Questionnaires were sent to clinicians at 4 months and 1 year from diagnosis, requesting basic clinical and laboratory data. This was used to classify patients into outcome groups, enabling parameters recorded during the illness to be correlated with outcome. Unfortunately, although data were obtained from 280 children, they could not all be allocated to an outcome group because of inadequate information and in part because follow-up times varied considerably between centers.

Definition of Outcome

Patients were considered to have fully recovered, and therefore to have had a good outcome, if they were normotensive, if they had no significant proteinuria (clinic Albustix $<1+$), and if their body height : plasma creatinine ratio (Ht/Cr) was greater than 2.0 cm/μmol/L. Patients who were considered to have had a poor outcome were those with Ht/Cr less than 1.5, or with significant proteinuria or hypertension necessitating treatment, as were patients in end-stage renal failure and those who had died. As it is recognized that a Ht/Cr between 1.5 and 2.0 does not reliably identify patients with abnormal renal function (72), these patients were therefore considered as a intermediate group and were excluded from analyses of factors influencing outcome.

Timing

Nephrologists caring for children who have recovered from HUS know that an improvement in renal function may continue during the period of convalescence, although no consensus exists regarding how long it takes for renal function to return to normal. In the study, 50 children with D+ HUS could be allocated to an outcome group both at 4 months and again at 12–14 months from diagnosis. Although 20% were placed in the poor outcome category at initial follow-up, this was reduced to 10% by 1 year. The data suggest that it would be unwise to attempt to classify D+ patients until at least one year from diagnosis—a conclusion that is borne out by the results of earlier studies in which serial GFR estimations were performed on patients followed up at regional units (73, 74), and which demonstrated that the GFR may continue to rise until 1 year from the illness. Clearly, those planning future studies must take this period of continuing improvement in renal function into account and avoid the strategy of categorizing patients into outcome groups that are based either on events occurring during the illness (e.g., seizures, hypertension) or on renal status at discharge.

Clinical Features and Laboratory Parameters as Predictors of Outcome

In the D+ group, children with a poor outcome were more likely to have been dyalized than those with a good outcome ($p<0.02$ Fisher's exact test), and a greater proportion of these children were dialyzed for more than 14 days when compared with the good-outcome group. Similar findings have been previously reported, but in contrast to earlier studies (11), we found that younger children fared worse than older ones. A comparison between survivors less than two years of age and those greater than two at presentation revealed that 11.4% of the former and 5.3% of the latter than long-term renal impairment or hypertension. This difference remained when deaths in these age groups were included, 17.9% of the younger and 9.5% of the older children having had a poor outcome.

The presence of hypertension during D+ HUS did not necessarily mean that antihypertensive treatment would have to be continued (Fig. 6); 84% of these

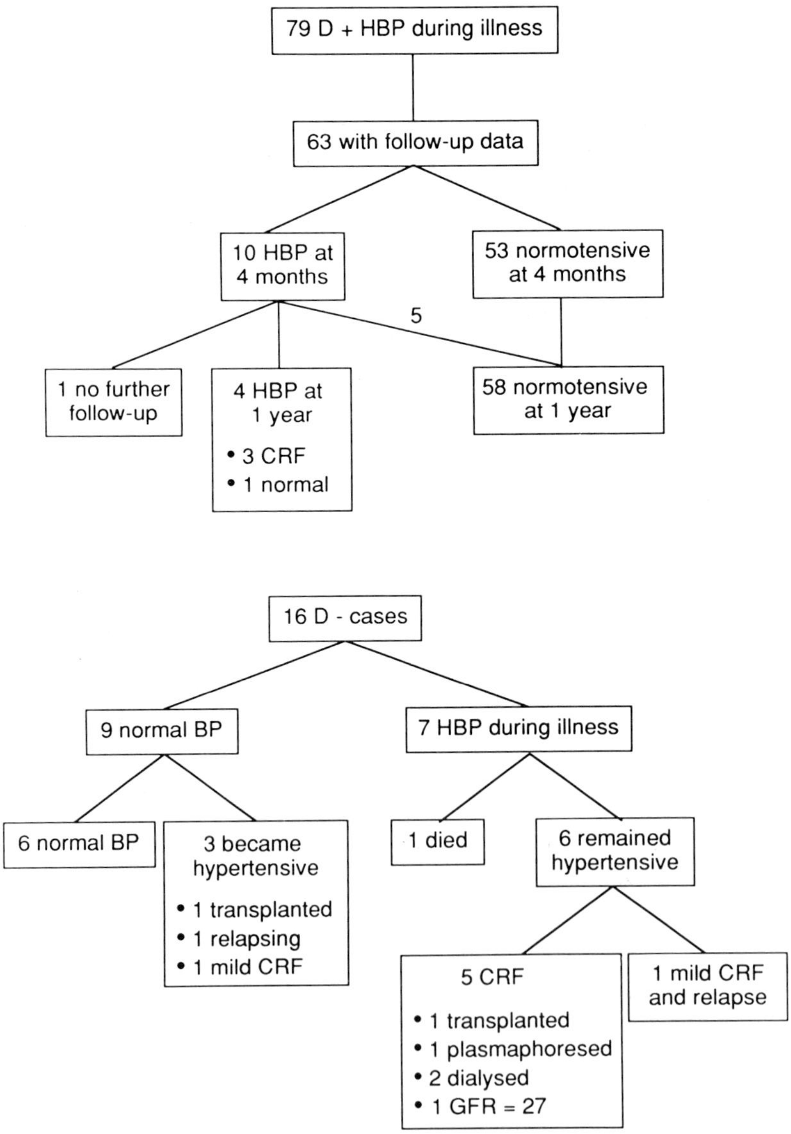

Figure 6 The outcome of children with D+ HUS who had hypertension during the acute phase of their illness (upper panel) compared with the progress of the D− cases. It is notable that three D− children developed hypertension after the acute illness, and all had residual renal impairment.

children who were followed up were normotensive at 4 months and 92% by one year from diagnosis. In contrast, not only was hypertension more common during the initial illness in D– cases (44%) than in D+ cases (27%), but treatment had to be continued in all survivors who had been hypertensive in the acute phase, all of whom also had impaired renal function later. Therefore, hypertension during the acute phase of D– HUS was strongly predictive of persisting renal impairment and hypertension. Four children became hypertensive after their initial illness; these included three children with D– HUS and one with D+ HUS. Although the three D– cases had abnormal renal function, the latter did not.

The initial neutrophil count was significantly higher in children with poor outcomes when compared to those with good outcomes (Fig. 7); this finding is in keeping with previous reports (75, 76). While 41% of the poor-outcome group had an initial neutrophil count greater than 20,000 only 15% of those with a good outcome had similarly high counts (Fisher's exact test p=0.025). A neutrophil count less than 20,000 was predictive of a good outcome with a sensitivity of 88%, a specificity of

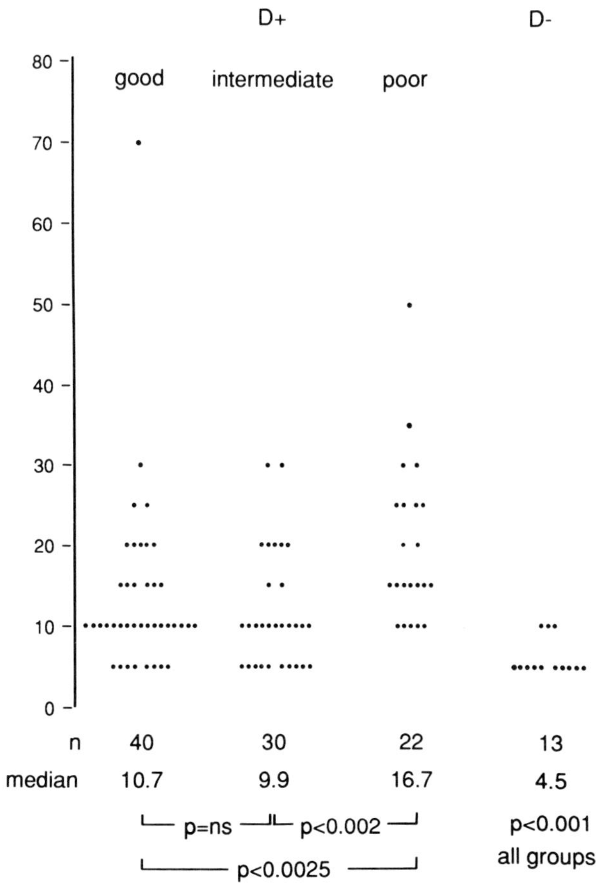

Figure 7 The initial neutrophil count as a predictor of outcome. Note that the children with D– HUS do not demonstrate a significant neutrophilia, despite their greater mortality and morbidity.

36%, and a positive predictive value of 78%. The disappointing specificity of this method was probably due to the difficulty of classifying patients into outcome groups using data provided by questionnaire. Further evidence of the fundamental difference between D+ and D– HUS is provided by the observation that this relationship between outcome and initial neutrophilia did not apply to D– patients, all of whom had low counts (Fig. 7) despite the very much greater risk of long-term renal impairment in this group (Table 3).

Relapses and Deaths

Four children, all D– cases, were reported to have had at least one relapse; all these had persisting hypertension, and three had renal impairment at follow-up. Eighteen children died; their clinical details are outlined in Table 6. It was notable that with one exception, all were less than 5 years of age. The remaining child had been oliguric and hypertensive, but he was not treated aggressively because of a spastic quadriplegia resulting in severe handicap from birth. Seizures or other neurological disturbances were present in 5 D– and 60 D+ cases; three of the former and 12 of the latter died. Thus the mortality in D– cases with CNS disturbances was 60%, and for D+ cases it was 20%. Central nervous system disorders in the acute phase have always been considered as clinical markers of poor outcome, and although this may

Table 6 Clinical Features and Reported Cause of Death

Age (yr)	Sex	Type of HUS	Days survived	Initial PMN count	Cause of death
0.11	F	D–	17	5.2	Intracranial hemorrhage
2.25	M	D–	30	12.0	Hypoxic brain damage
2.75	M	D–	12	3.0	Brain-stem death
1.25	M	D+	21	12.1	Seizures, CNS involvement
2.58	F	D+	3	29.3	Brain-stem death
3.50	F	D+	12	27.8	CNS involvement
1.75	M	D+	5	16.5	Renal cortical necrosis
0.17	M	D+	4	48.5	Septicemia, cardiac arrest
4.60	F	D+	17	50.2	Seizures, coma, CNS disease
1.83	F	D+	1	16.9	Intracranial hemorrhage
0.17	F	D+	1	—	Died within 8 hours
1.92	F	D+	38	—	Seizures, coma, CNS disease
4.5	M	D+	4	13.6	Cardiac arrest
2.08	M	D+	3	24.0	Cardiac arrest
2.83	F	D+	4	18.4	Brain-stem death
2.75	F	D+	15	15.0	Septicemia, raised ICP
0.58	M	D+	69	16.7	Septicemia 2° to colitis
13.58	M	D+	8	8.9	Untreated because of severe cerebral palsy

PMN = polymorphonuclear neutrophil leukocytes.

not be entirely justified (vide supra), these complications undoubtably occur more frequently in those children with more severe disease.

SUMMARY

Interest in HUS in the United Kingdom began in 1956, and since then there have been studies of sporadic and epidemic disease. A review of cases treated at a large pediatric nephrology center suggested that there had been a change in the nature of the disease which coincided with the emergence of VTEC in the early 1980s. This change was reflected in a dramatic increase in the incidence of HUS. It was also noted that clinical features previously thought to be prognostically significant were no longer useful after this point. However, in contrast to the earlier period, an initial neutrophilia was associated with a poor outcome.

Recently, a three-year national study of HUS was undertaken by British pediatric nephrologists in co-operation with the British Paediatric Surveillance Unit and the Division of Enteric Pathogens of the Public Health Laboratory. This study confirmed an association between D+ HUS and VTEC in the United Kingdom and demonstrated that patients without a diarrheal prodrome must be considered separately. The neutrophil count at presentation was the only clinical parameter of prognostic value.

REFERENCES

1. Fison, T. N. Acute glomerulonephritis in infancy. *Arch. Dis. Child., 31:* 101–109 (1956).
2. Brain, M. C., Dacie, J. V., Hourihane, D. O.'B. Microangiopathic haemolytic anaemia: the possible role of vascular leisions in pathogenesis. *Br. J. Haematol. 8:* 358–374 (1962).
3. Shinton, N. K., Galpine, J. F., Kendall, A. C., Williams, H. P. Haemolytic anaemia with acute renal failure. *Arch. Dis. Child, 39:* 455–464 (1964).
4. Moorhead, J. F., Edwards, E. C., Goldsmith, H. J. Haemodialysis of three children and one infant with a haemolytic-uraemic syndrome. *Lancet, 1:* 570–573 (1965).
5. Sharpstone, P., Evans, R. G., O'Shea, M., Alexander, L., Lee, H. A. Haemolytic-uraemic syndrome: Survival after prolonged oliguria. *Arch. Dis. Child., 43:* 711–716 (1968).
6. Linton, A. L., Gavras, H., Gleadle, R. I., Hutchison, H. E., Lawson, D. H., Lever, A. F., Macadam, R. F., McNicol, G. P., Robertson, J. I. Microangiopathic haemolytic anaemia and the pathogenesis of malignant hypertension. *Lancet, 1:* 1277–1282 (1969).
7. McLean, M. M., Jones, H. C., Sutherland, D. A. Haemolytic uraemic syndrome. *Arch. Dis. Child., 41:*76–89 (1966).
8. Gully, P. R. Haemolytic-uraemic syndrome: epidemiology and report of an outbreak. *R. Soc. Health, J., 104:* 214–217 (1984).
9. Taylor, C. M., White, R. H. R., Winterborn, M. H., Rowe, B. Haemolytic-uraemic syndrome: Clinical experience of an outbreak in the West Midlands. *Br. Med. J., 292:* 1513–1516 (1986).
9a. Coad, N. A. G., Marshall, T., Rowe, B., Taylor, C. M. Changes in the postenteropathic form of the hemolytic uremic syndrome in children. *Clin. Nephrol. 35*: 10–16 (1991).
10. Milford, D. V., Taylor, C. M., Gutteridge, B., Hall, S., Rowe, B., Kleanthous, H. Haemolytic uraemic syndromes in the British Isles 1985–1988; association with vero cytotoxin-producing *Escherichia coli*. Part 1, Clinical and epidemiological aspects. *Arch. Dis. Child. 65*: 716–721 (1990).
11. Stuart, J., Winterborn, M. H., White, R. H. R., Flinn, R. M. Thrombolytic therapy in haemolytic-uraemic syndrome. *Br. Med. J., 3*: 217–221 (1974).

12. Trompeter, R. S., Schwartz, R., Chantler, C., Dillon, M. J., Haycock, G. B., Kay, R., Barratt, T. M. Haemolytic uraemic syndrome: an analysis of prognostic features. *Arch. Dis. Child., 58:* 101–105 (1983).
13. Levin, M., Walters, M. D., Barratt, T. M. Hemolytic uremic syndrome. *Adv. Pediatr. Infect. Dis., 4:* 51–82 (1989).
14. Dollislager, D., Tune, B. The hemolytic-uremic syndrome. Spectrum of severity and significance of prodrome. *Am. J. Dis. Child., 132:* 55–58 (1978).
15. Kaplan, B. S. Hemolytic uremic syndrome with recurrent episodes: An important subset. *Clin. Nephrol., 8:* 495–498 (1977).
16. Kaplan, B. S., Proesmans, W. The hemolytic uremic syndrome of childhood and its variants. *Semin. Hematol., 24:* 148–160 (1987).
17. Karmali, M. A., Petric, M., Lim, C., Fleming, P. C., Arbus, G. S., Lior, H. The association between idiopathic hemolytic uremic syndrome and infection by verotoxin-producing *Escherichia coli. J. Infect. Dis., 151:* 775–781 (1985).
18. Karmali, M. A., Steele, B. T., Petric, M., Lim, C. Sporadic cases of hemolytic uremic syndrome associated with faecal cytotoxin-producing Escherichia coli in stools. *Lancet., 1:* 619 (1983).
19. Chapur de Saintonge, D. M., Vere, D. W. Why don't doctors use cusums? *Lancet., 1:* 120–121 (1974).
20. Day, N. P., Scotland, S. M., Cheasty, T., Rowe, B. *Escherichia coli* 0157:H7 associated with human infections in the United Kingdom. *Lancet., 1:* 825 (1983).
21. Hall, S., Glickman, M. The British Paediatric Surveillance Unit. *Arch. Dis. Child., 63:* 344–346 (1988).
22. British Paediatric Association—Communicable Disease Surveillance Centre surveillance of haemolytic uraemic syndrome 1983–4. *Br. Med. J., 292:* 115–117 (1986).
23. Neill, M. A., Tarr, P. I., Clausen, C. R., Christie, D. L., Hickman, R. O. *Escherichia coli* 0157:H7 as the predominent pathogen associated with the hemolytic uremic syndrome: A prospective study in the Pacific North West. *Pediatrics, 80:* 37–40 (1987).
24. Tarr, P. I., Hickman, R. O. Hemolytic uremic syndrome epidemiology: A population-based study in King County, Washington, 1971–1980. *Pediatrics, 80:* 41–45 (1987).
25. Pai, C. H., Ahmed, N., Lior, H., Johnson, W. M., Sims, H. V., Woods, D. E. Epidemiology of sporadic diarrhea due to verocytotoxin-producing *Escherichia coli:* A two-year prospective study. *J. Infect. Dis., 157:* 1054–1057 (1988).
26. Van Wieringen, P. M., Monnens, L. A., Schretlen, E. D. Haemolytic-uraemic syndrome. Epidemiological and clinical study. *Arch. Dis. Child., 49:* 432–437 (1974).
27. Lopez, E. L., Diaz, M., Grinstein, S., Devoto, S., Mendilaharzn, F., Murray, B. E., Ashkenazi, S., Rubeglio, E., Woloj, M., Vasquez, M., Turco, M., Pickering, L., Cleary, T. G. Hemolytic uremic syndrome and diarrhea in Argentine children: The role of shiga-like toxins. *J. Infect. Dis., 160:* 469–475 (1989).
28. Kibel, M., Barnard, P. J. The haemolytic uraemic syndrome—a survey in Southern Africa. *S. Afr. Med. J., 42:* 692–698 (1968).
29. Davies, P. The haemolytic uraemic syndrome. *E. Afr. Med. J. 48:* 136–139 (1968).
30. *Labour Force Survey 1985; Ethnic Group and Country of Birth. OPCS Monitor;* LFS 86/2. London, Office of Population Censuses and Surveys (1986).
31. Rhagupathy, P., Date, A., Shastry, J. C., Sudarsanam, A., Jodhar, M. Haemolytic-uraemic syndrome complicating shigella dysentery in South Indian children. *Br. Med. J., 1:* 1518–1521 (1978).
32. McGraw, M. E., Lendon, M., Stevens, R. F., Postlethwaite, R. J., Taylor, C. M. Haemolytic uraemic syndrome and the Thomsen Friedenreich antigen. *Pediatr. Nephrol., 3:* 135–139 (1989).
33. Thompson, R. A., Winterborn, M. H. Hypocomplementaemia due to a genetic deficiency in B1H globulin. *Clin. Exp. Immunol., 46:* 110–119 (1981).
34. Farr, M. J., Roberts, S., Morley, A. R., Dewar, P. J., Roberts, D. F., Uldall, P. R. The haemolytic uraemic syndrome—a family study. *Q. J. Med., 174:* 161–188 (1975).

35. Berman, W. The hemolytic-uremic syndrome: Initial presentation mimicking ulcerative colitis., *J. Pediatr., 81:* 275–278 (1972).
36. King, L. R., Wuslin, J. H., McAdams, A. J. Hemolytic-uremic syndrome in older children and adults. *J. Urol., 101:* 273–275 (1969).
37. Smith, C. D., Schuster, S. R., Gruppe, W. E., Vawter, G. F. Hemolytic-uremic syndrome: A diagnostic and theraputic dilemma for the surgeon. *J. Pediatr Surg., 13:* 597–604 (1978).
38. Kendall, P. A., Reid, I., Wright, J. E., Nanra, R. S. Gangrenous colitis in the haemolytic-uraemic syndrome. *Med. J. Aust., 140:* 543–544 (1984).
39. Milford, D. V., Taylor, C. M. Hyponatraemia and haemolytic uraemic syndrome. *Lancet, 1:* 439 (1989).
40. Gianantonio, C. A., Vitacco, M., Mendilaharzu, F., Gallo, G. E., Sojo, E. T. The hemolytic uremic syndrome. *Nephron, 11:* 174–192 (1973).
41. Bos, A. P., Donckerwolcke, R. A., von Vught, A. J. The hemolytic-uremic syndrome: prognostic significance of neurological abnormalities. *Helv. Paediatr. Acta., 40:* 381–389 (1985).
42. Bale, J. F., Brasher, C., Siegler, R. L. CNS manifestations of the hemolytic-uremic syndrome. *Am. J. Dis. Child., 134:* 869–782 (1980).
43. Upadhyaya, K., Barwick, K., Fishaut, M., Kashgarian, M., Siegel. N. The importance of nonrenal involvement in hemolytic-uremic syndrome. *Pediatrics, 65:* 115–120 (1980).
44. Argyle, J. C., Hogg, R. J., Pysher, T. J., Silva, F. G., Siegler, R. L. A clinicopathological study of 24 children with hemolytic uremic syndrome. A report of the Southwest Pediatric Nephrology Study Group. *Pediatr. Nephrol. 4:* 52–58 (1990).
45. Trevathan, E., Dooling, E. C. Large thrombotic strokes in hemolytic-uremic syndrome. *J. Pediatr., 111:* 863–865 (1987).
46. Gianantonio, C. A. Extra renal manifestations of the hemolytic uremic syndrome. In *Pediatric Nephrology Seminar 10. Acute renal disorders and renal emergencies. (Developments in Nephrology).* (J. Strauss, ed.), Martinus Nijhoff Publishing, Boston, pp. 43–50 (1984).
47. Sheth, K. J., Swick, H. M., Haworth, N. Neurological involvement in hemolytic-uremic syndrome. *Ann. Neurol., 19:* 90–93 (1986).
48. Poulton, J. S., Taylor, C. M., de Giovani, J. V. Dilated cardiomyopathy associated with haemolytic uraemic syndrome. *Br. Heart. J., 57:* 181–183 (1987).
49. Burns, J. C., Berman, E. R., Fagre, J. L., Shikes, R. H., Lum, G. M. Pancreatic islet cell necrosis: association with hemolytic-uremic syndrome. *J. Pediatrics, 100:* 582–584 (1982).
50. Primhak, R. A., Taitz, L. S., Variend, S., Webb, D. H., Cser, A. Necrosis of the pancreas in the haemolytic uraemic syndrome. *J. Clin. Pathol., 37:* 655–658 (1984).
51. Konowalchuk, J., Speirs, J. I., Stavric, S. Vero response to a cytotoxin of Escherichia coli. *Infect. Immun., 18:* 775–779 (1977).
52. Riley, L. W., Remis, R. S., Helgerson, S. D., McGee, H. B., Wells, J. G., Davis, B. R., Hebert, R. J., Olcott, E. S., Johnson, L. M., Hargrett, N. T., Blake, P. A., Cohen, M. C. Hemorrhagic colitis associated with a rare Escherichia coli serotype. *N. Engl. J. Med., 308:* 681–685 (1983).
53. Wells, J. G., Davis, B. R., Wachsmuth, I. K., Riley, L. W., Remis, R. S., Sokolow, R., Morris, G. K. Laboratory investigation of hemorrhagic colitis outbreaks associated with a rare *Escherichia coli* serotype. *J. Clin. Microbiol., 18:* 512–520 (1983).
54. Novillo, A. A., Voyer, L. E., Cravioto, R., Freine, M. C., Castano, G., Wainstein, R., Binzten, N. Haemolytic uraemic syndrome associated with faecal cytotoxin and verotoxin neutralizing antibodies. *Pediatr. Nephrol., 2:* 288–290 (1988).
55. Bitzan, M., Karch, H., Klemt, M., Buren, J., Atrogge, H. Relevance of verotoxin-mediated hemolytic-uremic syndrome in Germany. *Nieren-und Hochdruck Krankheiten., 17:* 246 (abstr.) (1988).

56. Scotland, S. M., Rowe, B., Smith, H., Willshaw, G., Gross, R. Verocytotoxin-producing strains of *Escherichia coli* from children with haemolytic uraemic syndrome and their detection by specific DNA probes. *J. Med. Microbiol., 25:* 237–243 (1988).
57. Willshaw, G. A., Smith, H. R., Scotland, S. M., Field, A. M., Rowe, B. Heterogeneity of Escherichia coli phages encoding Vero cytotoxins: comparison of cloned sequences determining VT1 and VT2 and development of specific gene probes. *J. Gen. Microbiol.*, 133: 1309–1317 (1987).
58. Kleanthous, H., Smith, H. R., Scotland, S. M., Gross, R. J., Rowe, B., Taylor, C. M., Milford, D. Haemolytic uraemic syndromes in the British Isles, 1985–1988: Association with verocytotoxin-producing *Escherichia coli*. Part 2, microbiological aspects. *Arch. Dis. Child. 65*: 722–727 (1990).
59. Ostroff, S. M., Tarr, P. I., Neill, M. A., Lewis, J. H., Hargrett-Bean, N., Kobayashi, J. M. Toxin genotypes and plasmid profiles as determinants of systemic sequelae in *Escherichia coli* 0157:H7 infections. *J. Infect. Dis., 160:* 994–998 (1989).
60. Chart, H., Scotland, S. M., Smith, H. R., Rowe, B. Antibodies to *Escherichia coli* 0157 in patients with haemorrhagic colitis and haemolytic uraemic syndrome. *J. Clin. Pathol., 42:* 973–976 (1989).
61. Chart, H., Scotland, S. M., Rowe, B. Serum antibodies to *Escherichia coli* serotype 0157:H7 in patients with haemolytic uraemic syndrome. *J. Clin. Microbiol., 27:* 285–290 (1989).
62. Moncrieff, M. W., Glasgow, E. F. Haemolytic-uraemic syndrome treated with heparin. *Br. Med. J., 3:* 188–191 (1970).
63. Damme-Lombaerts, R. van., Proesmans, W., van Damme, B., Eeckels, R., Ki Muaka, P. B., Mercieca, V., Vlietinck, R., Vermyeen, J. Heparin plus dipyridamole in childhood hemolytic-uremic syndrome: A prospective, randomized study. *J. Pediatr., 113:* 913–918 (1988).
64. Monnens, L., Kleynen, F., van Munster, P., Schretlen, E., Bonnerman, A. Coagulation studies and streptokinase therapy in the haemolytic-uraemic syndrome. *Helv. Paediatr. Acta., 27:* 45–54 (1972).
65. Powell, H. R., McCredie, D. A., Taylor, C. M., Burke, J. R., Walker, R. G. Vitamin E treatment of haemolytic uraemic syndrome. *Arch. Dis. Child., 59:* 401–404 (1984).
66. O'Regan, S., Chesney, R. W., Montear, J. G. Aspirin and dypyridamole therapy in the haemolytic-uraemic syndrome. *J. Pediatr., 97:* 473–476 (1980).
67. Camba, L., Al Hilah, M., Shulji, M. M. H., Joyner, M. V., Feest, T. G. Haemolytic uraemic syndrome with renal failure. The effect of plasmaphoresis. *Haematologica, 70:* 341–344 (1985).
68. Misiani, R., Appiani, A. C., Edefonti, A., Gotti, E., Bettinelli, A., Giani, M., Rossi, E., Rammuzi, G., Mecca, G. Haemolytic uraemic syndrome: theraputic effect of plasma infusion. *Br. Med. J., 285:* 1304–1306 (1982).
69. Loirat, C., Sensino, E., Hinglais, N., Pais, J. P., Landais, P., Fermanian, J. Treatment of the childhood haemolytic uraemic syndrome with plasma. *Pediatr. Nephrol., 2:* 279–285 (1988).
70. Beattie, T. J., Murphy, A. V., Willoughby, M. L., Belch, J. J. Prostacyclin infusion in haemolytic-uraemic syndrome of children. *Br. Med. J., 283:* 470 (1981).
71. Ashkenazi, S., Cleary, T. G., Lopez, E., Pickering, L. K. Anticytotoxin-neutralizing antibodies in immune globulin preparations: Potential use in hemolytic-uremic syndrome. *J. Pediatr., 113:* 1008–1014 (1988).
72. Haycock, G. B. Creatinine, body size and renal function *Pediatr. Nephrol., 3:* 22–24 (1989).
73. Ki Mauka, B. P., Proesmans, W., Eeckels, R. The haemolytic uraemic syndrome in childhood: a study of long-term prognosis. *Eur. J. Pediatr., 136:* 237–243 (1981).
74. Gusmano, R., Perfumo, F., Ciardi, M. R., Sarpen, M. Long-term prognosis of

haemolytic-uraemic syndrome in children. In *Acute Renal Failure. Advances in Experimental Medicine and Biology*, vol. 212. A. Amerio, P. Coratelli, V. M. Campese, S. G. Massry (eds.), Plenum Press, New York. pp. 199–204 (1987).

75. Walters, M. S., Matthei, I. U., Kay, R., Dillon, M. J., Barratt, T. M. (1989). The polymorphonuclear leucocyte count in childhood haemolytic uraemic syndrome. *Pediatr. Nephrol.*, *3:* 130–134.
76. Milford, D. V., Taylor, C. M., Rafaat, F., Halloran, E. Neutrophils elastase and haemolytic uraemic syndrome. *Lancet*, *2:* 1153 (1989).

5
Childhood Hemolytic Uremic Syndrome in Canada: a Multicenter Study

Peter N. McLaine *University of Ottawa and Children's Hospital of Eastern Ontario, Ottawa, Ontario, Canada* **Elaine Orrbine** *Children's Hospital of Eastern Ontario, Ottawa, Ontario, Canada* **Peter C. Rowe** *The Johns Hopkins Hospital, Baltimore, Maryland*

Canada, the second largest country in the world, has a population of 25 million people dispersed over an area of 3.8 million square miles. This fact presents a considerable geographic challenge to communication for the 23 pediatric nephrologists in the country. In 1985, the Pediatric Section of the Canadian Society of Nephrology established the Canadian Pediatric Kidney Disease Reference Centre (CPKDRC), with the intention of developing a communication network nationwide (1). The Reference Centre is located at the Children's Hospital of Eastern Ontario in Ottawa, under the direction and coordination of Dr. Peter N. McLaine and Mrs. Elaine Orrbine, respectively.

The objectives of the CPKDRC are:

1. to provide a unique opportunity to facilitate clinical research using a multicenter approach,
2. to study the epidemiology of renal disease in Canada to determine if regional differences exist,
3. to provide a patient population large enough to allow collaborative research to be efficiently conducted within a reasonable length of time, and
4. to co-ordinate the design, data collection, and statistical analyses of prospective and retrospective studies.

On January 1, 1986, pediatric nephrologists from across Canada (Fig. 1), began to submit basic descriptive data to the CPKDRC on all newly diagnosed pediatric nephrology patients seen in both in-hospital and ambulatory settings. At the end of

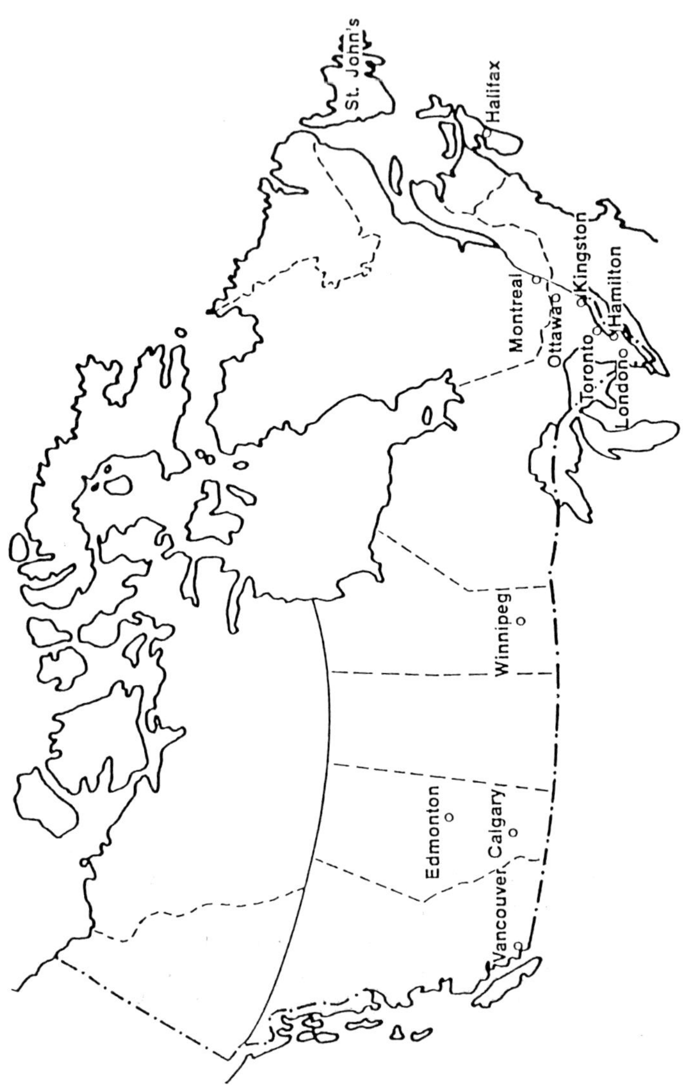

Figure 1 Participating Centers in the Canadian Pediatric Kidney Disease Reference Centre (CPKDRC).

June 1990, approximately 8,500 children were registered, with a wide variety of renal diseases.

This unique mechanism for data collection has facilitated the involvement of the CPKDRC in the initiation and completion of several research projects. These have included the identification of a non-nephrogenic marker for obligatory carriers of congenital nephrogenic diabetes insipidus (2); primary conditions associated with the development of acute renal failure in childhood; and a multicenter, 3-year cross-over study in the use of levamisole and prednisone alone in children with frequently relapsing nephrotic syndrome in childhood (3).

THE CPKDRC HUS STUDY

The CPKDRC also completed a 3-year descriptive study on hemolytic uremic syndrome (HUS), from January 1, 1986, to December 31, 1988 at 14 Canadian centers. With the exception of Quebec City, which joined the CPKDRC in 1989, these centers represent all 10 children's hospitals in Canada, as well as the children's wards in general hospitals of all Canadian cities with populations greater than 350,000. The results of the HUS study are summarized in this chapter; a more extensive report has been submitted for publication (4). The objective of this study was to examine the epidemiology of HUS in Canada, with particular emphasis on the proportion of HUS associated with *Escherichia coli* 0157:H7.

METHODS AND ASCERTAINMENT

From January 1, 1986, to December 31, 1988, all patients from each participating center were eligible for inclusion in the study if they had been diagnosed by a nephrologist as having HUS, or if they were identified, by a search of medical records, for discharge diagnoses for HUS in each institution. This search ensured a more complete ascertainment of hospitalized patients with HUS.

The same two investigators (P. N. McLaine and E. Orrbine) traveled to each participating institution to abstract pertinent data retrospectively from the medical records of eligible patients. Children were excluded after chart review if they had no evidence of acute renal injury, as indicated by hematuria or a urea greater than the 95% percentile. Children with recurrent or previously diagnosed HUS were not included in this study.

The denominator for calculating the incidence of HUS in Canada was the entire population of children less than 15 years of age obtained from the 1987 postcensal estimates (5), minus those from Quebec City. Since our numerator of HUS patients did not include those hospitalized in Quebec City or in some of the smaller hospitals in Canada, our estimate of the incidence of HUS in Canada should be regarded as the minimal annual incidence for the country.

The data were analyzed under the direction of Dr. George Wells at the Bureau of Biometrics, Laboratory Centre for Disease Control (LCDC), Health and Welfare Canada, Ottawa, Ontario, and the Department of Epidemiology and Community Medicine, University of Ottawa, Ontario, Canada.

RESULTS

A total of 228 children were either reported prospectively to the CPKDRC by the participating nephrologists or were identified through the medical records search for the discharge diagnosis of HUS (International Classification of Diseases, ICD-9-code 283.10). Two patients were excluded because their discharge diagnosis was "possible HUS" and they had no evidence of acute renal injury.

Of the 226 children, 126 (56%) were females and 100 (44%) were males. Although females outnumbered males, these data were not statistically significant when analyzed using the binomial test (p=0.10). Only six (3%) of the 226 had HUS associated with a point-source outbreak of *E. coli* 0157:H7 gastroenteritis.

The median age was 2.75 years, with a range of 1 month to 15 years. Twenty-five (11%) patients were under the age of 1 year (only three of whom were less than 6 months), and 163 (72%) of the children were less than 5 years of age. The peak prevalence of HUS was in the warmer months, with 185 (82%) occurring in the 6-month period from April to September (Fig. 2). Two hundred and fourteen (95%) children presented with diarrhea and 167 (74%) had evidence of bloody stools. In those cases where stools were cultured for *E. coli* 0157:H7, 51% (87/169), were positive for this organism (Fig. 3). Of the 226 children, 76% had stools screened for *Salmonella, Shigella,* or *Campylobacter* species; none of these organisms were identified. Prior to admission, vomiting was reported in 152 (67%) and hematemesis occurred in six.

On admission, 78 (35%) patients had documented CNS involvement with lethargy, irritability, or seizures. Twenty-three (10%) of the 226 children had documented seizures prior to admission.

By definition all patients had laboratory evidence of acute renal injury. This consisted of azotemia in 98%, and peak creatinine values greater than the 97.5th

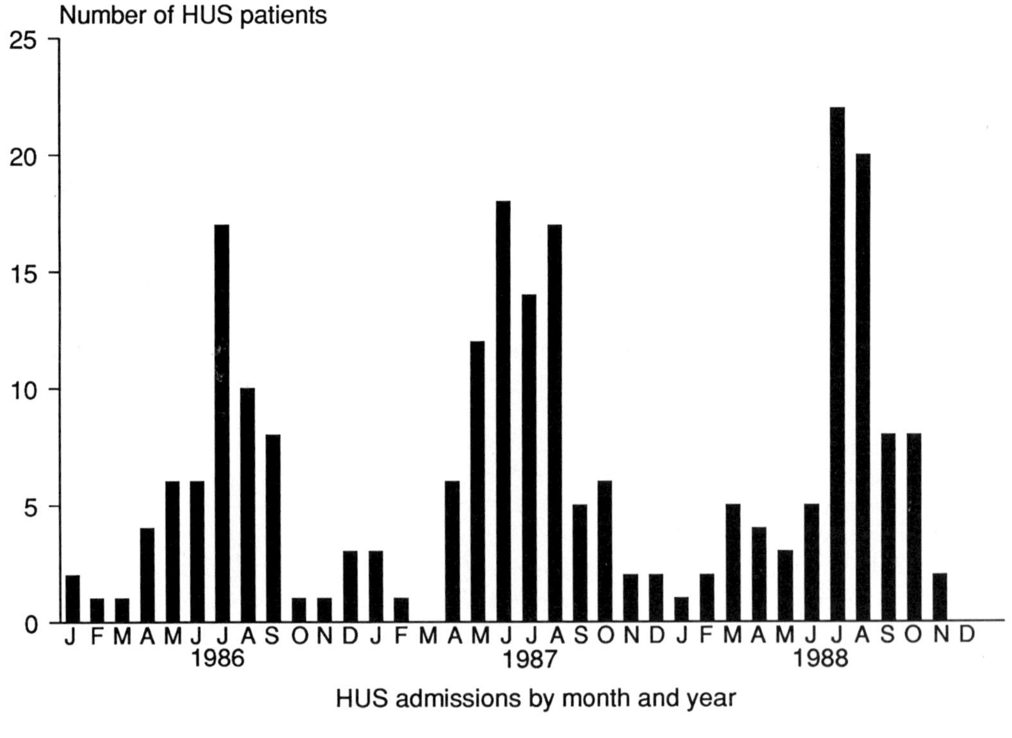

Figure 2 HUS admissions by month and year.

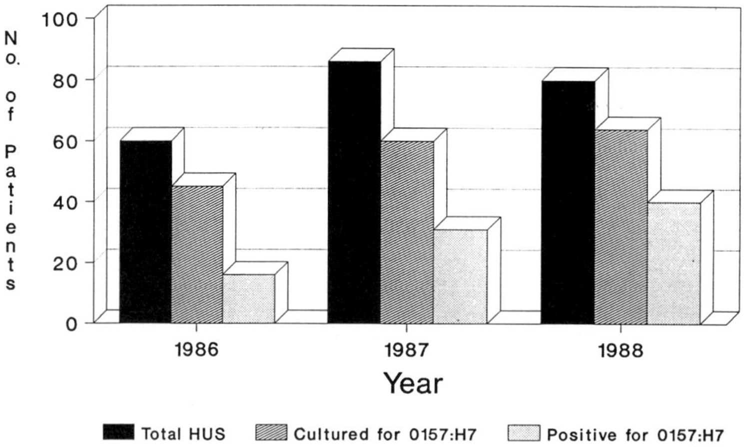

Figure 3 *E. coli* 0157:H7.

percentile for age (6) in 93%. The five children with peak urea values < 7 mmol/L all had evidence of creatinine elevation or hematuria, and their lowest hemoglobin values ranged from 43–83 g/L. Anemia was present in 99%; one of the remaining two patients had evidence of RBC fragments in association with an acute drop in hematocrit and the other was treated with a RBC transfusion before the hemoglobin fell below 105 g/L. Seventy-four percent had a white blood cell count greater than 15×10^9/L.

The minimal annual incidence of HUS in Canada during this study period was 1.44 per 100,000 children less than 15 years of age (Table 1). The minimal annual incidence for the province of Alberta was the highest at 2.8 per 100,000 children, which approaches three times the minimal annual incidence for the province of Ontario.

MORBIDITY AND MORTALITY

The morbidity and mortality of the 226 children are listed in Table 2. Anemia was severe enough to require at least one blood transfusion in 73% of the patients. One hundred and eight (48%) patients were treated with either hemo- or peritoneal dialysis. Of the 108 patients requiring dialysis, 64% were females and 36% were

Table 1 Minimal Annual Incidence[a] of HUS in Canada, 1986–1988

British Columbia	1.29
Alberta	2.78
Manitoba	2.09
Ontario	0.97
Quebec	1.42
Atlantic Provinces	1.48
Canada	1.44

[a]per 100,000 children <15 years of age.

Table 2 Morbidity and Mortality

>1 transfusion	73%
Dialysis	48%
Seizures	16%
Hypertension at discharge	3%
Chronic dialysis	1.8%
Renal transplant	0

males (Fig. 4), a statistically significant difference (p=0.019, or 1.89, 95% CI 1.07–3.35).

Seizures after admission developed in a further 6% of patients and 35 (15%) patients were reported to be hypertensive following admission. Only 3% were hypertensive at the time of discharge. Septicemia was reported in 11 (5%) children and pancreatitis in seven (3%).

Ten (4%) children had evidence of peritonitis; however, all were on peritoneal dialysis at the time of diagnosis. Six patients had a pleural effusion, but peritoneal dialysis was being performed in five of these children. Eight patients had significant pulmonary complications: four with adult respiratory distress syndrome, two with pulmonary edema, and two with pneumonia. Nineteen (8%) children had a documented urinary tract infection. Chronic dialysis was required in 1.8% of patients. In contrast to earlier reports which described a mortality rate of 4–7% (7–9), the mortality of this series was 2.7%. Of the six children who died, four were female and two were male. The mean age at death was 7.2 years. Three children were less than 5 years of age, and three were greater than 10 years of age. All six patients who died had evidence of CNS symptoms, four of whom had evidence of cerebral edema. Pathological findings on postmortem revealed evidence of vascular occlusion, typical of HUS; in the two oldest children (age 12 yr, 5 mo and 15 yr, 11 mo), a diagnosis of thrombotic thrombocytopenia purpura (TTP) was made on the basis of extensive organ involvement. The median length of stay in hospital was 11 days (range 1–107 days) and the median length of dialysis was 10 days (range 1–150 days).

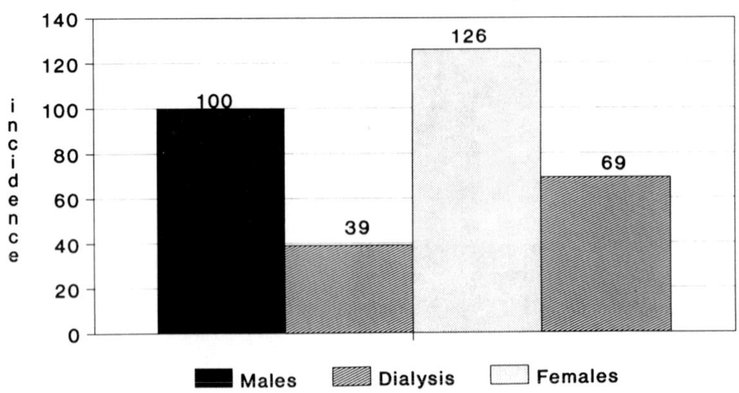

Figure 4 Gender distribution of patients requiring dialysis.

Conclusion

This study has confirmed that *E. coli* 0157:H7 is strongly associated with sporadic HUS in Canadian children, although the overall isolation rate of 51% for this organism likely underestimates the true proportion with infection by this and other verotoxin-producing *E. coli*. This work also confirms the wide regional variation in the annual incidence of HUS, as has been suspected in the past.

The apparent increase in the incidence of HUS in girls in our series has been reported in other population-based studies (10–12). However, we are unaware of other data suggesting an increased severity of renal involvement in females. These differences in the incidence and severity of HUS will be examined more closely in a 3-year prospective study now in progress.

EPIDEMIOLOGY AND THE DEFINITION OF HUS

As physicians increase their surveillance for hemolytic anemia, thrombocytopenia, and acute renal injury in patients with *E. coli* 0157:H7 gastroenteritis, dilemmas are bound to arise in the classification of HUS. The classic syndrome is defined by the laboratory triad of hemolytic anemia, thrombocytopenia, and evidence of acute renal injury, although thrombocytopenia may be an evanescent feature (13) and uremia is not always present (14). No one can argue with a diagnosis of HUS in a patient with a hemoglobin of 70 g/L with 10% schistocytes on the peripheral blood smear, a platelet count of 60 × 10^9/L, and a urea of 20 mmol/L. At the other end of the spectrum, however, there can be a considerable amount of disagreement in terms of whether or not to diagnose the patient as having had hemolytic uremic syndrome. Three case reports are presented in whom there was evidence of *E. coli* 0157:H7 infection as determined on stool cultures. These patients serve to illustrate this new dilemma:

Patient 1: A 1.3-year-old girl was admitted to hospital for investigation of fever, pallor, and lethargy after a two-week history of loose stools. Streaks of blood were present in the stools in the 4 days before admission. Her hemoglobin was 55 g/L and there were 101–250 fragmented cells per 1,000 RBCs in the peripheral blood smear. Her urea was 8.6 mmol/L, creatinine 76 μmol/L (> 97.5th percentile for age), and platelets 449 × 10^9/L. There were 3–5 RBCs per high-powered field on urine microscopy. She was treated with a single RBC transfusion and did not require dialysis. Her lowest platelet count during the 7-day hospitalization was 399.

Patient 2: A 2-year-old girl was admitted to hospital in June after a 4-day illness characterized by abdominal cramps and diarrhea mixed with blood. She developed rectal prolapse on the day of admission and was lethargic. Her lowest hemoglobin in hospital was 105 g/L; she had 6–50 fragmented RBCs per 1,000 on the blood film. Her platelet fell from 426 to 129 after three days. Her highest urea was 5.0 mmol/L, her highest creatinine 53 μmol/L, and her urine microscopy was normal.

Patient 3: A 14-month-old girl was seen in the outpatient department in 1985 because of diarrhea and vomiting for the preceding 5 days. The initial blood samples revealed a urea of 6.1 mmol/L, a hemoglobin of 101 g/L, and a platelet count of 153. She was sent home, but one week later she developed tea-colored urine, examination of which revealed 40–60 RBCs per microscopic field. Her platelet count was 279, her hemoglobin was 76 g/L, and the blood film showed evidence of 101–250 fragmented cells per 1,000 RBCs. Urea and creatinine were not measured at this visit. She recovered uneventfully without being admitted to hospital.

Patient 1 had a profound hemolytic anemia associated with mild, transient renal impairment but no evidence of thrombocytopenia. Patient 2 had borderline anemia. Definite schistocytes were seen on the blood smear and there was mild thrombocytopenia, but there was no laboratory confirmation of acute renal injury. Patient 3 was seen by a physician who was not aware of the association between the results of the stool culture and the hematologic abnormalities. She was not admitted to hospital, and was identified as having mild HUS only through a retrospective review as a result of the stool culture report. She had hemolytic anemia, borderline thrombocytopenia, and hematuria. Her BUN and serum creatinine were not measured.

Rahaman et al. (15) described the association of marked leukocytosis and erythrocyte fragmentation with *Shiga* bacillus dysentery in 1975. Although not included in the title, they mention that thrombocytopenia occurred during the period of hemolysis in most of the patients and that transient oliguric renal failure developed in

Table 3 Proposed Classification of Postinfectious Hematologic Abnormalities

1. *Postinfectious hemolytic anemia*
   a. No acute renal injury
   b. Hemolytic anemia ± thrombocytopenia

2. *Incomplete HUS*
   a. Acute renal injury *and either:*
   b. Hemolytic anemia *or*
   c. Thrombocytopenia

3. *HUS*
   a. Acute renal injury
   b. Hemolytic anemia
   c. Thrombocytopenia

4. Severe *HUS*
   a. HUS as defined above
   b. Creatinine ≥500 μmol/L *or*
   c. Death

Acute renal injury defined as at least one of:
- urea ≥7 mmol/L (≥2 SD above mean for all ages)
- creatinine ≥2 SD above mean for age *or* ≥ 50% increase in creatinine over baseline
- urine RBCs >5/HPF

Anemia defined as at least one of:
- Hgb ≤2 SD below mean for age
- >10% drop in Hct in first week
- RBC transfusion

Hemolysis defined as:
- schistocytes (≥6 fragmented RBCs/1000 RBCs on peripheral smear)

Thrombocytopenia defined as:
- platelets < 150 × 10^9/L

Creatinine value >2 SD above mean:

<5 yr:	62 umol/L
6–12 yr:	88 umol/L
12–15 yr:	88 umol/L [F]; 106 umol/L [M]

several. In 1978, Koster et al. (16) described the occurrence of hemolytic uremic syndrome in association with shigellosis. A cohort of 207 children and 34 adults were studied prospectively in Bangladesh. All had shigellosis. Nineteen of the children had evidence of acute hemolytic anemia, a leukomoid reaction, thrombocytopenia, and oliguria. In addition, nine other children also had a serum urea nitrogen level of greater than 100 mg/dL. Eight of these nine had pseudomembranous colitis and six of these died.

As a result of these studies and our own review, it has become abundantly clear that infection with shigella or *E. coli* 0157:H7 can produce a wide spectrum of clinical involvement. This may range from abdominal pain with cramps all the way to fulminant colitis, acute renal failure, seizures, and death. This observation raises many difficulties in the classification and indeed in the diagnosis of hemolytic uremic syndrome. In an attempt to circumvent some of these difficulties, and in order to provide a basis for more accurate comparisons among population groups, we have proposed four categories of postinfectious hematologic abnormalities (Table 3). The criterion of a creatinine value ≥500 μmol/L for severe HUS is based on the median creatinine value among the group of children who received ≥7 days of dialysis in the CPKDRC study. We realize that our approach is based primarily on laboratory values that include the serum creatinine and the severity of the anemia. This schema cannot entirely circumvent the problem posed by varying intensities of laboratory surveillance. However, if discrete laboratory values are required for the diagnosis of HUS, the use of this or a similar scheme will generate a more precise way of comparing the incidence of HUS and the spectrum of disease caused by *E. coli* from different centers.

ACKNOWLEDGMENTS

James Carter, M.D., FRCPC David Lirenman, M.D., FRCPC	Nephrology Service, British Columbia Children's Hospital, Vancouver, British Columbia
Lane Robson, M.D., FRCPC	Nephrology Service, Alberta Children's Hospital, Calgary, Alberta
Frances Harley, M.D., FRCPC Daniel Hasinoff, M.D., FRCPC	Nephrology Service, University of Alberta Hospital, Edmonton, Alberta
Robert Walker, M.D., FRCPC	Nephrology Service, Winnipeg Children's Hospital, Winnipeg, Manitoba
William Clark, M.D., FRCPC	Nephrology Service, Victoria Hospital, London, Ontario
Brian Steele, M.D., FRCPC	Nephrology Service, Children's Hospital at Chedoke-McMaster University Medical Centre, Hamilton, Ontario
Gerald Arbus, M.D., FRCPC Diane Hébèrt, M.D., FRCPC J. W. Balfe, M.D., FRCPC Allison Eddy, M.D., FRCPC Denis Geary, M.D., FRCPC	Division of Nephrology, Hospital for Sick Children, Toronto, Ontario

David Alexander, M.D., FRCPC	Department of Pediatrics, Hotel Dieu Hospital, Kingston, Ontario
Peter Morrin, M.D., FRCPC Moussa Cohanim, M.D., FRCPC Edwin Toffelmire, M.D., FRCPC Michael Singer, M.D., FRCPC Bryce Kiberd, M.D., FRCPC	Nephrology Service, Kingston General Hospital, Kingston, Ontario
Norman Wolfish, M.D., FRCPC	Nephrology Service, Children's Hospital of Eastern Ontario, Ottawa, Ontario
Lorraine Bell, M.D., FRCPC Keith Drummond, M.D., FRCPC Paul Goodyer, M.D., FRCPC	Nephrology Service, Montreal, Children's Hospital, Montreal, Quebec
Bernard Kaplan, M.D., FRCPC	Nephrology Service, Children's Hospital of Philadelphia, Philadelphia, Pennsylvania
Marie-Jose Clermont, M.D., FRCPC Jean Guy Mongeau, M.D., FRCPC Sean O'Regan, M.D., FRCPC Pierre Robitaille, M.D., FRCPC	Division of Nephrology, L'Hôpital Ste. Justine, Montreal, Quebec
John Crocker, M.D., FRCPC Malcolm Ogborne, M.D., FRCPC	Nephrology Service, Izaak Walton Killam Hospital for Children, Halifax, Nova Scotia
Henry Gault, M.D., FRCPC Patrick Parfrey, M.D., FRCPC Michael Paul, M.D., FRCPC	Health Sciences Centre, Memorial University, Charles A. Janeway Child Health Centre, St. John's, Newfoundland
George Wells, Ph.D.	Bureau of Biometrics, *LCDC, Ottawa, Ontario
Heba Ebied	Bureau of Biometrics, *LCDC, Ottawa, Ontario
Andrew MacKenzie, M.D., FRCPC	Department of Laboratory Medicine, Children's Hospital of Eastern Ontario, Ottawa, Ontario
Mohamed Karmali, MB, ChB, MRCP(UK), FRCPC	Department of Bacteriology, Hospital for Sick Children, Toronto, Ontario
Hermy Lior	National Laboratory for Enteric Pathogens, Bureau of Microbiology, *LCDC, Ottawa, Ontario
Nicole LeSaux, M.D., FRCPC	Bureau of Communicable Disease, *LCDC, Ottawa, Ontario.
Ed Ellis, M.D., FRCPC	Bureau of Communicable Disease, *LCDC, Ottawa, Ontario.

*LCDC = Laboratory Centre for Disease Control

Supported by grants from:

Kidney Foundation of Canada

Children's Hospital of Eastern Ontario Foundation

REFERENCES

1. McLaine, P. N., Orrbine, E., and members of the Pediatric Section, Canadian Society of Nephrology. Canadian Pediatric Kidney Disease Reference Centre. *Ann. RCPSC, 22*: 531–2 (1989).
2. Bichet, D. G., Razi, M., Lanergan, M., Arthus, M. F., Papukna, V., Kortas, C., Barjon, J-N. Hemodynamic and coagulation responses to 1-desamino (8-D-arginine) vasopressin in patients with congenital nephrogenic diabetes insipidus. *N. Engl. J. Med., 318*: 881–7 (1988).
3. Mongeau, J.-G., Robitaille, P. O., Roy, F. Clinical efficacy of Levamisole in the treatment of primary nephrosis in children. *Pediatr. Nephrol.,* 2(4): 398–401 (1988).
4. Rowe, P. C., Orrbine, E., Wells, G. A., McLaine, P. N. The Epidemiology of childhood hemolytic uremic syndrome in Canada; 1986–1988. *J. Peds., 119*: 218–224 (1991).
5. *Estimates of Population by Sex and Age, Canada, Provinces and Territories.* Statistics Canada, Demography Division, Ottawa, Ontario, Canada (1987).
6. Meites, S., ed. *Pediatric Clinical Chemistry,* 3rd ed. American Association of Clinical Chemistry Press, Washington, pp. 111–112 (1989).
7. Trompeter, R. S., Schwartz, R., Chantler, C., Dillon, M. J., Haycock, G. B., Kay, R., Barratt, T. M. Haemolytic-uraemic syndrome: An analysis of prognostic features. *Arch. Dis. Child, 58*: 101–105 (1983).
8. Van Dyck, M., Proesmans, W., Depraetere, M. Hemolytic Uremic Syndrome in Childhood: renal function ten years later. *Clin. Nephrol., 29*: 109–112 (1988).
9. Gianantonio, C., Vitacco, M., Mendilaharzu, F., Gallo, G. E., Sojo, E. T. The hemolytic uremic syndrome. *Nephron, 11*: 174–192 (1973).
10. Rogers, M. F., Rutherford, G. W., Alexander, S. R., DiLiberti, J. H., Foster, L., Schonberger, L. B., Hurwitz, E. S. A population-bases study of hemolytic uremic syndrome in Oregon, 1979–82. *Am. J. Epidemiol., 123*: 137–42. (1986).
11. Kinney, J. S., Gross, T. P., Porter, C. C., Rogers, M. F., Schonberger, L. B., Hurwitz, E. S. Hemolytic-uremic syndrome: A population-based study in Washington, DC and Baltimore, Maryland. Am. J. Public Health, *78*: 64–65 (1988).
12. Tarr, P. I., Neill, M. A., Allen, J., Siccardi, C. J., Watkins, S. L., Hickman, R. O. The increasing incidence of the hemolytic-uremic syndrome in King County, Washington: lack of evidence for ascertainment bias. *Am. J. Epidemiol. 129*: 582–586 (1989).
13. Milford, D. V., Taylor, C. M., Guttridge, B., Hall, S. M., Rowe, B., Kleanthous, H. Haemolytic uraemic syndromes in the British Isles 1985–8: association with Verocytotoxin producing *Escherichia coli.* Part 1: clinical and epidemiologic aspects. *Arch. Dis. Child, 65*: 716–721 (1990).
14. Dolislager, D., Tune, B. The hemolytic uremic syndrome: spectrum of severity and significance of prodrome. *Am. J. Dis. Child., 132*: 55–58 (1978).
15. Rahaman, M. M., Alam, A. K. M. J., Islam, M. R., Greenough, W. B. Shiga bacillus dysentery associated with marked leukocytosis and erythrocyte fragmentation. *Johns Hopkins Med. J., 136*: 65–70 (1975).
16. Koster, F., Levin, J., Walker, L., Tung, K. S., Gilman, R. H., Rahaman, M. M., Majid, M. A., Islam, S., Williams, R. C., Jr. Hemolytic-uremic syndrome after shigellosis. *N. Engl. J. Med., 298*: 927–933 (1978).

6
Hemolytic Uremic Syndrome in Asia

Rajendra N. Srivastava *All India Institute of Medical Sciences, New Delhi, India*

The first report of hemolytic uremic syndrome (HUS) in Asia was by Rahman et al. from Bangladesh in 1975 (1). The authors reviewed 560 cases of shigellosis presenting over a period of 14 months between 1972–1974, in whom *Shigella dysenteriae* 1 was the causative organism in 86% and *Shigella flexneri* in the remainder. They observed a marked leucocytosis and erythrocyte fragmentation in these patients; 51 (9.1%) had leucocyte counts greater than 50,000/cu mm at some stage of the illness. In 16 cases there was evidence of hemolytic anemia of a microangiopathic type; 11 had thrombocytopenia; and five had renal failure. The authors mentioned that this picture was "reminiscent" of HUS; however, renal failure was transient, lasting 3–10 days, and was considered secondary to dehydration. Despite the apparently mild renal involvement, it does appear that these cases were examples of HUS.

A second report from the same center appeared in 1978 (2). Of 207 children with *Shigella* dysentery seen between 1975 and 1976, 19 had HUS. Nine had severe renal insufficiency, and six died. Limulus lysate assay for endotoxemia was positive in nine of 18 patients. Four patients had evidence of consumptive coagulopathy, but none had generalized bleeding. The authors suggested that circulating endotoxin from the colon could produce a coagulopathy, renal microangiopathy, and hemolytic anemia.

From Vellore in South India, Raghupathy et al. in 1978 reported the occurrence of HUS in children with *Shigella* dysentery (3). Of 320 children admitted to hospital with acute dysentery, from January 1975 to September 1977, 40 had acute renal failure (ARF). The diagnosis was made on clinical assessment and microscopic examination of stools. These 40 patients comprised 65% of cases of ARF in children treated during the same period. All had features of HUS and were below the age of 5 years (mean age 16.5±14 months). Rectal swab cultures were obtained in 29 cases; *S. dysenteriae* 1 was isolated in 10 and *S. flexneri* in one. Most of those with negative results had already received antibiotics. In all cases a marked neutrophilic leucocytosis was present. Twenty-one patients died; 15 improved, but the degree of recovery of renal function and their subsequent course was not reported. Renal histology showed focal cortical necrosis in four of 12 cases. Necropsy examination was undertaken in five cases and showed features consistent with the diagnosis of bacillary dysentery in three and pseudomembrane formation in the colon in two. Fibrin deposits were not seen in other organs. The authors concluded that infection with *S. dysenteriae* 1 was an important cause of HUS. They noted that *Shigella* dysentery was endemic in their region, particularly in preschool children (4). The complication of HUS was not seen in an earlier study of shigellosis from the same center (5). In that report of 100 children under 5 years of age, *S. flexneri* was isolated in 73% and *Shigella sonnei* in 9%.

In a recent report from Vellore, South India, HUS was responsible for 66 of 166 cases of acute renal failure in infants over a 14-year period (1971–1984), with a mortality of 63% (6).

In Delhi, Northern India, HUS was rarely diagnosed until 1978 when isolated cases presented, their clinical and laboratory features being very similar to those reported from Bangladesh and South India. At the All India Institute of Medical Sciences, New Delhi, 73 cases were admitted between 1980–1988 (7). Ninety-two percent were below the age of 5 years. Eighty percent were associated with acute dysentery, which was usually severe with a poor response to different antibiotics. Stool cultures were positive for *Shigella* organisms in seven, *Escherichia coli* in 11, and nontyphoid *Salmonella* in nine. A neutrophilic leucocytosis was present in 85% and coagulation abnormalities suggestive of a consumptive coagulopathy in 24 of 30 cases. The condition was severe in most cases, with oligoanuria in 86%, and the mortality was 60%. Extensive or patchy renal cortical necrosis was seen in 40%.

During the last few years, reports of a large number of cases of HUS with a similar profile have appeared from different parts of India (8, 9).

The observation that HUS was rarely seen in the Indian subcontinent before the early 1970s has been the subject of much speculation. Epidemiological data suggested that appearance of a large number of cases of HUS followed epidemics of shigellosis due to *S. dysenteriae* 1, which occurred in Bangladesh and South India in 1972 and subsequently in several countries in South Asia (10). The dysenteric illness was usually severe with a high incidence, particularly in preschool children. Complications were frequent with a considerable mortality. The organisms were resistant to multiple antimicrobial drugs including ampicillin, chloramphenicol, and cotrimoxazole. In Bangladesh and India, *S. dysenteriae* 1 was rarely isolated before 1971 (10).

Shigella organisms have been isolated in 10–30% of patients with dysentery associated HUS in India, as also in hospital-based studies of dysentery (11). The low isolation rate could be partly due to previous administration of antibiotics. Even in epidemics of *Shigella* dysentery, the frequency of isolation has varied widely, being high when special media such xylose lysine desoxycholate and MacConkey agar were used (10). It is of interest that use of drugs to which the organisms were resistant could be a risk factor for the development of HUS (12).

Besides the Indian subcontinent, HUS in Asia has been observed recently in Thailand, where outbreaks of dysentery due to *S. dysenteriae* 1 appeared in 1986 (13). The organisms were resistant to several antimicrobials, including cotrimoxazole. Lertsukprasert et al. (14) examined 22 patients with HUS between April 1987 and June 1988. Eighteen were below the age of 2 years. Bloody diarrhea was present in all, with an average duration of 10 days. Blood transfusion and total blood exchange were used in 77% and 36% of the cases, respectively. The mortality was 9%. These authors noted that HUS was not a rare disease in Thailand—especially in their region, where shigellosis and invasive diarrhea were very common.

In some other Asian countries, HUS appears to be uncommon or rare, and there is little published information.

In Saudi Arabia, 14 patients with HUS were admitted to a children's hospital in Riyadh in 3.5 years, constituting 10% of all cases of acute renal failure (Mattoo, T. K., personal communication, 1990). Idiopathic, *Shigella* dysentery–related HUS as well as the familial autosomal recessive form (15) have been diagnosed in this center.

In Iraq HUS is uncommon; at a large medical center in Baghdad, only an occasional case has been reported (Al-dahhan, J., personal communication, 1989).

The prevalence of HUS is low in Indonesia, Singapore, and Malaysia. The Department of Child Health, Medical School, University of Indonesia, Jakarta, reported only one case of HUS out of 14,480 children admitted over a 3-year period (1986–1988); this patient developed chronic renal failure and died after 3 months (Tambunon, T., personal communication, 1989). Three cases were reported in 1987; all developed acute renal failure and required dialysis.

In Singapore, HUS has been observed occasionally in children between 3–5 years (Boon, W. H., personal communication, 1989); it is usually mild and full recovery ensues. Boon treated four patients with HUS in a family, all of whom died. The parents were consanguineous, and HUS was considered to have an autosomal recessive inheritance. In Malaysia, three cases of HUS were seen at one center in Kuala Lumpur over a period of 5 years.

In South Korea, HUS is uncommon; the first case was reported in 1972 (Choi, Y., personal communication, 1989). Choi's review of 41 cases showed that nine were infants below 2 years of age and the others between 2 and 6 years. Six each had a prodrome of either bloody diarrhea or an upper respiratory tract infection, three had jaundice, and another three had gross hematuria. Eight patients had leucocyte counts of over 10,000/cu mm, and nine had severe renal insufficiency. Nine patients recovered, two having persistent proteinuria, and five had end-stage renal disease.

From China, Weixum reported 38 cases of HUS in 1981. There were 31 boys and seven girls; 19 were below the age of 7 years and the others between 7 and 13 years. The prodromal illness included respiratory tract infection in 13, bloody diarrhea in six, and fever in some others. Oligoanuria was present in 36 cases, and 15 patients had convulsions. Twenty-one (55%) patients died of renal failure and other complications in the acute stage. On follow-up evaluation three of six patients had chronic renal failure and one had hypertension. Subsequently a total of 70 cases of HUS were presented by four different groups of workers at various national conferences in 1987 and 1989 (Yang, J.-Y., personal communication, 1990). These data indicate a profile of HUS characterized by a severe acute illness with a high mortality rate and a significant incidence of chronic renal damage among the survivors. The results of bacteriological studies in these cases were not avilable.

SUMMARY

It seems clear that on the Indian subcontinent and subsequently in Thailand, a large increase in the number of cases of HUS occurred following epidemics of dysentery caused by *S. dysenteriae* 1. However, in the absence of isolation of *Shigella* organisms, it cannot be assumed that *all* cases of dysentery-associated HUS were due to shigellosis. Other organisms, including nontyphoid *Salmonella* (7), have been isolated occasionally in such cases; their significance in the development of HUS needs to be examined. Comprehensive microbiological studies, particularly looking for verotoxin-producing *E. coli*, which have not been done in these cases, would be of particular importance in understanding the spread of the disease and the pathogenesis of HUS.

Epidemics of dystentery due to *S. dysenteriae* 1 have also occurred in Sri Lanka, Burma, Nepal, and Bhutan (10). There is no information as to whether cases of HUS were seen in these countries. Environmental and hygienic conditions that are not very different from those on the Indian subcontinent exist in other Asian countries. Whether HUS is truly rare in these countries or goes unreported needs to be ascertained.

REFERENCES

1. Rahman, M. M., Alam, A. K. M. J., Islam, M. R., Greenough, W. B. III, Lindebaum, J. Shiga bacillus dysentery associated with marked leukocytosis and erythrocyte fragmentation. *Johns Hopkins Med. J.*, *136*: 65–70 (1975).
2. Koster, F., Levin, J., Walker, L., Tung, K. S. K., Gilman, R. H., Rahman, M. M., Majid, M. A., Islam, S., Williams, R. C. Jr. Hemolytic-uremic syndrome after shigellosis: Relation to endotoxemia and circulating immune complexes. *N. Engl. J. Med. 298*: 927–933 (1978).
3. Raghupathy, P., Date, A., Shastry, J. C. M., Sudarsanam, A., Jadhav, M. Haemolytic-uraemic syndrome complicating shigella dysentery in south Indian children. *Br. Med. J.*, *1*: 1518–1521 (1978).
4. Feldman, R. A., Bhat, P., Kamath, K. R. Infection and disease in a group of South Indian families. IV: Bacteriologic methods and a report of the frequency of enteric bacterial infection in preschool children. *Am. J. Epidemiol.*, 92: 367–375 (1970).
5. Jadhav, M., Verghese, R., Bhat, P., Webb., J. K. G. Clinical and microbiological features of shigellosis in 100 South Indian infants and children under 5 years. *Ind. Pediatr.*, *3*: 393–400 (1966).
6. Unni, J. C., Date, A., Raghupathy, P., Shastry, J. C. M. Medical renal diseases in South Indian infants. *Acta. Paediatr. Scand.*, *75*: 1003–1031 (1986).
7. Srivastava, R. N., Moudigil, A., Bagga, A., Vasudev, A. Hemolytic uremic syndrome in children in northern India. *Pediatr. Nephrol.* 5: 284–288 (1991).
8. Nammalwar, B. R., Balasubramanian, N., Thangadurai, C., Santhanakrishnan, B. R. Hemolytic uremic syndrome. *Ind. J. Pediatr.*, *54*: 743–752 (1987).
9. Dedhia, N. M., Shah, B. V., Khanna, U. B., Almeida, A. F., Acharya, V. N. Hemolytic uremic syndrome. *J. Postgrad. Med.*, *32*: 4–8 (1986).
10. Pal, S. C., Sengupta, P. G., Sen, D., Bhattacharya, S. K., Deb, B. C. Epidemic shigellosis due to *Shigella dysenteriae* Type I in South Asia. *Ind. J. Med. Res.*, *89*: 57–64 (1989).
11. Santhanakrishan, B. R., Gang, N., Lakshminarayana, C. S. Shigellosis in children. *Ind. J. Pediatr.*, *54*: 739–742 (1987).
12. Butler, T., Islam, M. R., Azad, M. A. K., Jones, P. K. Risk factors for development of hemolytic uremic syndrome during shigellosis. *J. Pediatr.*, *110*: 894–897 (1987).
13. Taylor, D. N., Bodhidatta, L., Brown, J. E., Echeverria, P., Kunanusont, C., Naigowit, P., Hanchlay, S., Chatkaeomorakot, A., Lindberg, A. Introduction and spread of multiresistant *Shigella dysenteriae* 1 in Thailand. *Am. J. Trop. Med. Hyg.*, *40*: 77–85 (1989).

14. Lertsukprasert, S., Kowitangkul, K., Vasanawatana, S., "Hemolytic Uremic Syndrome in Khon Kaen," presented at 2nd Asian Symposium of Pediatric Nephrology Nagoya (1989).
15. Mattoo, T. K., Mahmood, M. A., Al-Harbi, M. S., Mikail, I. Familial, recurrent hemolytic-uremic syndrome. *J. Pediatr., 114:* 814–816 (1989).

7

HUS in Johannesburg, South Africa: Epidemiology and Long-term Follow-up

Peter D. Thomson *University of the Witwatersrand and Johannesburg Hospital, Johannesburg, South Africa*

HISTORICAL REVIEW

Bernard Kaplan and Peter Thomson saw their first cases of hemolytic uremic syndrome (HUS) at The Transvaal Memorial Hospital for Children (TMH), Johannesburg, in 1964 and 1965 when they were medical students. Both were Samuel Javett's senior house officers. In 1962 Javett and Boris Senior had reported six cases of HUS from Johannesburg (1). The previous year Joan Griffiths, also a pediatrician in Johannesburg, described cases with Irving, a hematologist (2). In addition, Utian, Fanaroff, and Plit included descriptions of HUS patients in their paper on glomerular diseases in 1964 (3). Another alumna, Joan Wagner, may have reported a case of HUS (Acute Tubular Necrosis with Anaemia) from The Hospital for Sick Children, Great Ormond Street, in 1954 (4). The first major epidemiological studies on HUS were reported from southern Africa by Kibel and Barnard (5, 6). There was a palpable sense of excitement in the air at TMH about this new syndrome. Sam Javett talked at length on ward rounds about HUS, Thrombotic thrombocytopenic purpura (TTP), disseminated intravascular coagulation, and the generalized Sanarelli-Shwartzman phenomenon. Something about the romance of those terms—the way they were talked about, or the stimulating way in which he taught, coupled with the sudden onset of a life-threatening illness in previously well babies and infants, and the high mortality rate of 30%—fired our imaginations. Thomson has treated and followed patients with HUS from the Transvaal Memorial Hospital for 23 years.

Many people have profound influences on a person's life yet do not know the extent of their input. Without Javett's approach to patient care and teaching and the input of many others, our involvement with HUS would never have occurred. James Gear, a renowned virologist, showed that enteroviruses were seldom associated with HUS. Gear also suggested in the 1960s that antibiotic treatment during the diarrheal prodrome may release a toxin. Avroy Fanaroff, Jack Katz, Aubrey Lurie, Solly Levin, and Piet Koornhof supported our efforts. Without the initial support of Boet Heese, the first Professor of Pediatrics in Johannesburg, nothing could have been accomplished. Thomson and Kaplan began a collaboration that has lasted for 20 years.

EPIDEMIOLOGY

The last comprehensive epidemiological survey of HUS in southern Africa was done in the late 1960s by Kibel and Barnard (6). Previous reports from this region noted that HUS occurred mainly in infants, that it usually followed a prodrome of diarrhea (2, 4, 5), and that it was unusual in blacks (5). This was also been noted in Uganda (7). Kibel and Barnard, in their survey of cases in southern Africa, found only eight black patients out of an estimated population of 15 million, but 96 white patients out of a population of 4 million. Earlier in 1968, Freiman et al. (8) reported the occurrence of atypical HUS in two of 15 black children with veno-occlusive disease of the liver. These were the first cases of HUS diagnosed at Baragwanath Hospital, which almost exclusively admits black patients. From the period 1962–1965, there were only three other patients with HUS at that hospital (S.E. Levin, unpublished information). In Johannesburg during the period of 1970–1981, Kaplan and Thomson documented 81 cases in whites but only three definite cases in blacks, plus seven other possible cases in blacks (9). The increased prevalence in whites was again found in the period 1982–1988, when children with pediatric renal diseases at Baragwanath hospital were compared with those at the Johannesburg Hospital (predominantly white admissions) (10). There were only two HUS black patients of 1,208 children admitted with renal diseases (one in 600) but there were 60 white patients out of 1137 admissions (one in 19 admissions). The numbers of the childhood populations from which the admissions were drawn were thought to be similar. HUS, therefore, seems to be 30 times more frequent in whites.

HLA typing of the A and B major histocompatibility antigens was studied in our HUS patients with a control group of white blood donors; there were no increases in any of the major histocompatibility antigens (11). This does not exclude the possibility that there may be an increased susceptibility among whites, but a more plausible explanation is presently being investigated. Our suggestion is that black children are more frequently exposed to diarrheal infections at earlier ages and may therefore produce antibodies able to deal with a significant "load" of verocytotoxin. It is possible that white infants lack the antibodies to counteract a verocytotoxin load because the diarrheal prodrome of HUS may often be their first significant illness. Our patients with HUS have not had measurable antibody titers to verocytotoxin when tested on presentation; two patients, however, had an increase in antibody titers when the test were repeated more than 2 weeks after admission for HUS (P.D. Thomson, unpublished data). We are now assessing HUS patients prospectively and are using age-matched black and white children with gastroenteritis as controls. If the postulate is correct, then the black children will have protective levels of verocytotoxin antibodies and the white children will not. The next step will be to compare cord blood levels from blacks and whites to see whether passive immunity plays a role in very young infants.

Kibel and Barnard (6) had also noted an increased prevalence of HUS "during the hot months" but thought that the disease was restricted to urban areas. They found no correlation with outbreaks of gastroenteritis. Utian et al. (3) noted that there were

23 admissions of HUS out of 150 cases of glomerular diseases at The Children's Hospital from August 1959 to January 1963. This high prevalence was sustained from 1982–1988 at the Johannesburg Hospital, where HUS accounted for 41.6% (60/144) of admissions for acute renal failure (10).

TREATMENT

In the latter part of 1969, the treatment of HUS was changed from a conservative approach in which dialysis was used infrequently and only late in the course of the illness to a more careful regimen in which dialysis was started when severely affected cases had been anuric for longer than 24 hours. (Patients without anuria were called mildly affected.) Hypertension was controlled more precisely in all patients. From 1959–1989, 231 patients with HUS were treated at TMH and the Johannesburg Hospital. These patients have been divided into two periods: pre-1970 (more conservative treatment) and post-1970 (more aggressive treatment).

The data from the 231 patients (121 females and 110 males) in the two periods have been compared (Table 1). Notable changes include an increase in the mean age at onset. Eight patients in the more recent period were older than age 4 years and all had an atypical prodrome. Six of eight of these patients required dialysis and transplantation. The increased prevalence of an upper respiratory tract infection prodrome in the older child is not evident in the total group, and the prevalence of a diarrheal prodrome has not changed pre- and post-1970.

The demographic distribution of the patients has changed from predominantly suburban to periurban and rural areas. Also, in the city, fewer patients came from the middle- to upper-class suburbs after 1970. This may be the result of changes in patterns of referral and hospitalization. Throughout the 30 years, 7.2% of the patients were immigrants or children of recent immigrants.

The seasonal distribution did not change pre- and post-1970 except for the month of April 2/76 pre and 17/149 post ($p < 0.034$). HUS occurs more often in spring and early summer in the southern hemisphere.

Table 1 Epidemiologic Features 1959–1989

	Pre-1970	Post-1970	p value
Number/Number per year	83/7.5	148/7.4	
Age at presentation (± SD years)	0.72 ± 0.37	1.15 ± 1.46	0.0009
Age range (years)	0.18-2.41 (2>2y)	0.25-11.08 (12>2y)	
Diarrheal prodrome (D+)	2/2 (0>4y)	3/12 (8>4y)	
D+ (total admissions)	58/77	118/138	NS
Acute and long-term mortality	24/83	8/148	0.001
Demographic Distribution			
Suburbs of major towns/cities	43/74	45/126	<0.005
Johannesburg suburbs	30/74	18/126	<0.0001
Johannesburg suburbs, middle-upper class	20/30	6/18	<0.05
Periurban and rural	31/74	81/126	<0.005
Seasonal (S Hemisphere)			
January-April	20	50*	0.001*
May-August	11	27	
September-December	45	72*	

*All nondiarrhoeal prodrome: 7 upper respiratory tract infection, 1 appendix abscess

ETIOLOGY

Over the total period, enteropathogenic E. coli was cultured from stool in only 15 patients; three were *E. coli* 011/B4 and two were *E. coli* 026/B6. An additional 26 patients had a profuse growth of *E. coli* which was not typed. Six stool cultures were positive for *Salmonella*, but none grew *Shigella*. A number of patients drank unpasteurized milk, and a few had been given dried meat (biltong) or herbal "rooi-bos" tea. Four patients had positive blood cultures: two were *E. coli*, one was *Enterococcus fecalis* and another was *S. typhi*.

An apparent association with viruses was noted in 10 cases: Coxsackie B was cultured from the blood of three patients and from stool of three others. Increasing blood titers were detected in one case; Coxsackie A type 8 was found in the stool of one patient; an unidentified enterovirus was noted in one patient, and corona viruses were seen on electron microscopy in the stool of another. One may speculate that enteroviruses, whether wild or postinoculation, blockade the reticuloendothelial system and render some infants more susceptible to the effects of bacterial toxins. In this regard it is of interest that the commencement of polio inoculation and the recognition of HUS in southern Africa occurred at the same time. Furthermore, from 1985–1989, polio virus isolation in the Johannesburg area was commoner in January–March and nonpolio enteroviral isolation was commonor in January–March and October–December (S. A. National Institute of Virology, unpublished data).

Six patients had significantly lower serum IgA levels. This may have made them more prone to intestinal-induced illnesses. Serum IgM levels were generally increased (12).

LONG-TERM FOLLOW-UP

We have evaluated the results of the long-term follow-up of 231 patients (121 females and 110 males) with HUS from Johannesburg who presented from 1959 to 1989. As noted above, patients had been treated differently prior to 1969 (1–3). After 1970 there was a reduction in the acute and long-term mortality compared with those who were treated from 1959–1969 (Table 2).

The survivors from the two periods were assessed. Ten of 59 patients treated prior to 1970 were traced. Many were lost to follow-up because they had been treated by private pediatricians and their records were no longer available. Forty of 140 patients treated after 1970 were excluded because they had been followed up for less than 5 years. Unfortunately, only 41 of 100 patients were available for assessment. No attempt has been made to determine whether the characteristics of these 41 patients differed from those of the 59 who could not be traced. In summary, 51

Table 2 Mortality (Acute and Long-term) Before and After 1970

Severity at presentation	1959 to end 1969	1970 to end 1989	p
Mild (no anuria)	6/52	2/71	n.s.
Severe (anuria >48 hours)	18/31	6/77	<0.0001
Total	24/83[a]	8/148[a]	0.001

[a]Includes acute and long-term deaths; also nonrenal (e.g., neurological, accidental).

patients (27 females and 24 males) were followed for 5 to 23 years. The mean period of follow-up was 10.9 ± 4.8 years for mildly affected cases and 13.5 ± 5.1 years for severely affected cases.

The mortality rate (acute and long-term) of the total group from 1959–1989 was 32/231 (17 females and 15 males). However, there has been a significant difference between the mortality rates of mildly affected cases (8 of 130) and severely affected patients (24 of 101) ($p<0.00025$). A significantly greater number of severely affected patients presented with hypertension, seizures, and leukocytosis (Table 3). More significant, however, is the observation that the mean calculated creatinine clearance after 10 years of follow-up was 58.7 for severely affected cases, compared with 93.3 ml/min/1.73 m^2 in the mildly affected cases.

The 51 patients followed for more than 5 years were divided into three categories:

Group A consisted of 17 mildly affected patients (nine females and eight males), who were not anuric.

Group B consisted of 13 severely affected patients who had been anuric for fewer than 7 days (seven females and six males).

Group C contained 17 severely affected patients who had been anuric for more than 7 days (11 females and 10 males).

Group D consisted of four severely affected patients who required ongoing dialysis and early renal transplantation. These patients have been excluded from this phase of the analysis but will be discussed in the section dealing with transplantation. Consequently, the long-term follow-up is based on 47 patients. More severely affected patients were more likely to have proteinuria (Table 4). Similarly, severely affected patients were more likely to require antihypertensive therapy (Table 5). None of the mildly affected patients required treatment. Despite treatment with antihypertensive agents, severely affected patients had significantly higher systolic and diastolic pressures than mildly affected patients.

The calculated creatinine clearances of mildly affected patients were much higher than those who were severely affected. Mildly affected patients had a mean of

Table 3 Acute Clinical Features and Long-Term Function and Growth

	Mild	Severe	p
At presentation			
Initial hypertension	43%	95%	<0.01
Initial seizures	12%	56%	<0.01
Initial neutrophil count (x 10^9/L)	6.209 ± 4.676	11.256 ± 5.649	<0.0001
Long-term Follow-up			
Calculated creatinine clearance[a] after >10 years' follow-up (ml/min./1.73 m^2)	93.3 ± 24.5	58.7 ± 26.5	<0.011
Age at >10 years' follow-up	13.29 ± 4.11	15.5 ± 4.76	n.s.
Mean percentiles after 5-23 years' follow-up	61%	52%	
	65%	55%	

[a]Calculated creatinine clearance = $\dfrac{\text{Ht(cm)} \times 40}{\text{Serum creatinine } \mu\text{mol/L}}$

Table 4 Proteinuria on Dipstick After Mean of 12 Years + Follow-up

	n	0 to trace	30 mg/dL or more	0–30 mg/dL	100 mg/dL or more
Group A (mild)	17	15	2	17	0
Group B (severe <7 days' anuria)	13	10	3	10	3
Group C (severe >7 days' anuria)	17	5	12	8	9

A vs. B	n.s.	A vs. B	n.s.
A vs. C	$p < 0.002$	A vs. C	$p < 0.003$
B vs. C	$p = 0.013$	B vs. C	n.s.
A vs. B&C	$p = 0.009$	A vs. B&C	$p = 0.002$

92.7 ± 13.2 ml/min/1.73 m^2 compared with Group B patients whose values were 77.6 ± 28.1 and Group C patients who had a mean value of 50.8 ± 26.4 (Table 6). There was no significant difference between Group A and Group B, but when Group A and Group C patients were compared, there was a significant difference at $p<0.001$. The difference was <0.013 when Group B and Group C patients were compared.

The 51 patients (including the four who required ongoing hemodialysis) were analyzed further in terms of their requirement for long-term antihypertensive therapy, and the presence of urine protein excretion in excess of 1 g/L, and a calculated creatinine clearance of less than 40 ml/min/1.73 M^2. After a mean follow-up period of more than 12 years, none of the 17 mildly affected patients had these unfavorable sequelae, as compared with two of 13 Group B patients and nine of 21 Group C+D patients (Table 7).

Seven of the patients have had a total of 13 renal allografts. Three of these

Table 5 Requiring Persistent Antihypertensive Therapy

		Systolic (mm Hg)	Diastolic (mm hg)
Group A (mild)	0/17	105 ± 11	66 ± 7
Group B (severe <7 days' anuria)	3/13	119 ± 16	72 ± 12
Group C (severe >7 days' anuria)	9/17	118 ± 13	75 ± 10

A vs. B+C	$p = 0.0017$	A vs. B	$p = 0.012$
A vs. C	$p < 0.003$	A vs. C	$p - 0.004$
A vs. C	$p = 0.005$		

Note: Systolic and diastolic measurements include those on therapy.

Table 6 Renal Function After Long-term Follow-up

	Calculated creatinine clearance (ml/min/1.73 m²)[a]	
Group A (mild)	92.7 ± 13.2	
Group B (severe <7 days' anuria)	77.6 ± 28.1	
Group C (severe >7 days' anuria)	50.8 ± 26.4	
	A vs B	n.s.
	A vs. C	$p < 0.0001$
	B vs. C	$p = 0.013$

[a]From the formula $\frac{\text{height (cm)} \times 40}{\text{serum creatinine } \mu\text{mol/L}}$

patients were older than 5 years at presentation, and one was between 2 and 3 years of age. The three who were older than 5 years required ongoing dialysis and early transplantation. The other patient recovered sufficient function to be off dialysis until age 5 years. The remaining three of seven patients presented in infancy with severe HUS but had ongoing proteinuria and hypertension. Hypertension was controlled in two of these, but this was not done in the third. The two with controlled hypertension were in Group C and the third was in Group B. The latter patient appeared to have a decrease in renal function as a result of uncontrolled hypertension. Six of the seven received kidneys from living related donors. With one exception, the second transplants were from cadavers. Graft survival from the first transplant has ranged from under 1 year to 13 years (Table 8). Graft survival from the second transplant has ranged from one month to more than 8 years.

DISCUSSION

Very little long-term follow-up data of HUS patients are available. A study from Argentina showed that in follow-up periods of 6 months to 13.6 years, only 5.6% of patients presenting without anuria had chronic renal failure, hypertension, or proteinuria, compared with 49% of those who presented with anuria (13). Studies from

Table 7 Persistent Antihypertension and Proteinuria >1 g/L and Calculated Creatinine Clearance <40 ml/min/1.73 M² After Follow-up of >12 Years

Group A (mild)	0/17
Group B (severe <7 days' anuria)	2[a]/13
Group C+D (severe >7 days' anuria)	9[b]/21
A vs C+D	$p = 0.0018$

[a]1 with arteriolar involvement on initial biopsy and the other transplanted (late) but did not have an initial biopsy

[b]7 with arteriolar involvement on initial biopsy, and 6 of these transplanted.

Table 8 HUS Patients Who Were Transplanted

		Sex	Age at first transplant (yr)	Graft	Graft survival	Age at second transplant (yr)	Graft	Graft survival	Outcome function
1	RB	M	10.06	RLD	<1 yr.	13.3	RLD	1 mo	Patient died on hemodialysis
2	CG	M	22.08	RLD	>1 yr.	—	—	—	Excellent
3	AL	F	14.75	CAD	1 yr	16.35	CAD	>8 yr	Excellent
4	JA	F	4.9	RLD	9 yr	14.83	CAD	Recent	Fair
5	YD	F	7.16	RLD	7 yr	13.4	CAD	>4 yr	Excellent
6	AdeV	F	7.09	RLD	5 yr	15.9	CAD	>5 yr	Excellent
7	AJ	M	6.75	RLD	13 yr	20.5	CAD	Recent	Fair
		Mean graft survival ± 6 yr (Patient 2 not included)				Mean graft survival >4 years to date (Patients 2, 4, and 7 not included)			

London, Paris, and Leuven (Belgium) showed that only 64% of 186 patients completely recovered (14). Additional data from Leuven showed that 10 years later, 30% of 46 patients had at least one abnormal finding indicative of renal disease; three adolescents had both hypertension and proteinuria (15). A 10-year follow-up study of 73 patients from Nijmegen (Netherlands) showed that all six patients with anuria that had lasted more than 7 days or oliguria of greater than 14 days duration had late sequelae (16). Two were started on hemodialysis more than 10 years after presentation, three had a decreased GFR, and concentrating ability, and one patient had a decreased concentrating ability. In another study (17), the GFR was measured by 99^{m}Tc DTPA plasma slope clearance, 6–11 years after presentation. Eleven of 37 patients (30%) had a GFR below 60 mL/min/1.73 m^2, and four had proteinuria.

In this Johannesburg study, 11 of 51 patients (21%) had a GFR of less than 40 mL/min/1.73 m^2 after a period of follow-up for a mean of more than 12 years. They also had proteinuria in excess of 1 g/L and required antihypertensive therapy.

John and Thoenes (18) have emphasized the relationship between arteriolar lesions and hypertension, and Habib et al. (19) have noted that both the severity of hypertension and a poorer prognosis occur in patients with arteriolar lesions. In this context, eight of our 11 patients with the triad of severe hypertension, proteinuria, and a reduced GFR had arteriolar lesions. Seven of these eight patients required renal transplantation.

The nonrenal long-term effects had not been critically analyzed, but at least three patients had severe mental retardation (one died), and another had bilateral sensorineural deafness. The majority have not had significant residual neurological problems (20), and many have done well both in the academic and sports arenas.

Careful treatment of hypertension and other complications as well as early dialysis in the severely affected cases have reduced the acute mortality rates (9, 12, 21). However, it is less certain whether or not the long-term prognosis has been favorably influenced. This could not be assessed because of the difficulties of providing adequate control groups. However, it seems that antihypertensive agents can be withdrawn in most severely affected cases if early control has been achieved. Fresh frozen plasma and allopurinol (to reduce hyperuricemia) have not made significant differences. Although a controlled trial of vitamin E therapy (22) was questioned because of the possibility of a type II (beta) error (23), vitamin E has no noteworthy effect in severely affected cases, when assessed in the acute stage and after a period of follow-up of at least 2 years. Mildly affected cases almost always recover and have an excellent long-term prognosis; therefore it is impossible to assess the effects of treatment in them. However, even in a mild case with acute anemia and hypertension, blood pressure control must still be meticulous because of the danger of cardiac failure and hypertensive encephalopathy.

We recommend that all severely affected cases of HUS should be followed for up to 20 years.

REFERENCES

1. Javett, S. N., Senior, B. Syndrome of hemolysis, thrombopenia and nephropathy in infancy. *Pediatrics, 29*: 209–223 (1962).
2. Griffiths, J., Irving, K. G. A haemolytic uraemic syndrome in infancy. *Arch. Dis. Child., 36*: 500–506 (1961).

3. Utian, H. L., Fanaroff, A. A., Plit, M. Glomerular disease in childhood: A review of 150 consecutive cases. *S. Afr. Med. J.*, *38*: 162–167 (1964).
4. Wagner, J. Acute tubular necrosis with anaemia. *Great Ormond St. J.*, *7*: 66–72 (1954).
5. Barnard, P. J., Kibel, M. The haemolytic-uraemic syndrome of infancy and childhood. A report of eleven cases. *Cent. Afr. J. Med.*, *11*: 4–11, 31–34 (1965).
6. Kibel, M., Barnard, P. J. The haemolytic-uraemic syndrome: A survey in southern Africa. *S. Afr. Med. J.*, *42*: 692–698 (1965).
7. Davies, P. The haemolytic-uraemic syndrome. *East. Afr. Med. J.*, *45*: 136–139 (1968).
8. Freiman, I., Schmaman, A., Zamit, R., Appleberg, M. Veno-occlusive disease of the liver—some new aspects. *S. Afr. Med. J.*, *42*: 126–129 (1968).
9. Kaplan, B. S., Thomson, P. D. Current approaches to the management of hemolytic uremic syndrome. In *Acute Renal Disorders and Renal Emergencies* (J. Strauss ed.), Marthinus Nijhoff Publishing, Boston, pp. 69–86 (1984).
10. Meyers, K. E. C., Thomson, P. D., Jacobs, D. W. C., Kala, U. K. "Paediatric Nephrology Experience. Johannesburg and Baragwanath Hospitals 1982–1988 Inclusive." Congress of the South African Renal Society, Johannesburg, August 9, 1990.
11. Thomson, P. D., Maier, G. "HLA Typing in the Haemolytic Uraemic Syndrome of Childhood." 11th Congress of the South African Renal Society, Port Elizabeth October 13–15, 1977.
12. Kaplan, B. S., Thomson, P. D., de Chadarevian, J. P. The hemolytic uremic syndrome. *Pediatr. Clin. N. Am.*, *23*: 761–777 (1976).
13. Biblioni, N. N. Nephrology around the world. In *Pediatric Nephrology*, ed. 2. (M. A. Holliday, T. M. Barratt, R. L. Vernier, eds.), Williams & Wilkins, Baltimore, p. 349 (1987).
14. Kaplan, B. S., Proesmans, W. The hemolytic-uremic syndrome of childhood and its variants. *Semin. Hematol.*, *24*: 148–160 (1987).
15. Van Dyck, M., Proesmans, W., Depraetere, M. Hemolytic uremic syndrome in childhood; renal function ten years later. *Clin. Nephrol.*, *29*: 109–112 (1988).
16. DeJong, M., Monnens, L. Haemolytic-uraemic syndrome: A 10 year follow-up study of 73 patients. *Nephrol. Dial. Transplant.*, *3*: 379–382 (1988).
17. O'Regan, S., Blais, N., Russo, P., Pison, C. F., Rousseau, E. Hemolytic uremic syndrome: Glomerular filtration rate, 6 to 11 years later measured by ^{99m}Tc DTPA plasma slope clearance. *Clin. Nephrol.*, *32*: 217–220 (1989).
18. John, H. D., and Thoenes, W. The glomerular lesions in endotheliotropic hemolytic nephroangiopathy. *Pathol. Res. Pract.*, *73*: 236–259 (1982).
19. Habib, R., Levy, M., Gagnadoux, M. F., Broyer, M. Prognosis of the Hemolytic Uremic Syndrome in Children. In: *Advances in Nephrology* (J. F. Bach et al., eds.), Yearbook Medical Publishers, Chicago, pp. 109–128 (1982).
20. Thomson, P. D., Kaplan, B. S., Marcus, J., Rothberg, A., Olinsky, A. Long term follow-up in children with the hemolytic-uremic syndrome South African Renal Society Congress, Bloemfontein. Oct. 6–8, 1976. (Abstract). *Kidney Int.*, *11*: 288 (1977).
21. Kaplan, B. S., Katz, J., Krawitz, S., Lurie, A. An analysis of the results of therapy in 67 cases of hemolytic uremic syndrome. *J. Pediatr.*, *78*: 420–425 (1971).
22. Thomson, P. D., Milner, L. S. A randomly selected trial of vitamin E in the haemolytic uraemic syndrome (Abstract). Tenth International Congress of Nephrology, London. 1987; 98.
23. Siegler, R. L. Management of hemolytic-uremic syndrome. *J. Pediatr.*, *91*: 1014–1012 (1988).

8
The Hemolytic Uremic Syndrome in Argentina

Eduardo L. Lopez *Hospital de Niños Ricardo Gutierrez, Buenos Aires, Argentina*
Carlos A. Gianantonio *Hospital Italiano, Buenos Aires, Argentina* **Thomas G. Cleary** *University of Texas Medical School, Houston, Texas*

HISTORY

Shortly after Gasser et al.'s description of HUS in 1955 (1), it became apparent that this rare disease was in fact extraordinarily common in a few locales. By the early 1960s, more cases of HUS were seen in Argentina than anywhere else. In a series of studies published from 1964 (2–7), Gianantonio and colleagues defined the spectrum of the illness, suggested possible causes, speculated about the pathophysiology, made observations on the pathology, and increased world-wide awareness and interest, in what was until then thought to be little more than a medical curiosity. While working at the Hospital de Niños Ricardo Gutierrez, the major municipal pediatric hospital in Buenos Aires, they were able to develop new insights into the natural history of HUS.

FEATURES OF HUS IN ARGENTINA

Epidemiology

Prevalence of HUS in Argentina

On the basis of census data, and cases diagnosed in Buenos Aires, the incidence of the disease appears to be 7–10 times greater than reported from "high-risk" areas such as the Pacific Northwest United States. Recent data (Table 1) would suggest that the current incidence may be decreasing. However, because not all cases are admitted to the Hospital de Niños, the decrease may reflect the fact that many pediatricians are now skilled in caring for these patients so that referral to this hospital is required less often.

Table 1 Hemolytic Uremic Syndrome Admissions to the Hospital de Niños Ricardo Gutierrez, Buenos Aires, Argentina

Period	No. of cases	Age (months) Mean	Age (months) Range	Cases admitted/yr
1957–61	32	12.8	4.5–36	6
1962–66	130	12.2	2–60	26
1967–72	516	13.2	2–180	86
1982–88	383	20.4	3–84	55

There are substantial differences between the HUS in Argentina and the disease in other countries, and there are also differences between the current pattern and that recognized between 1957–1973 in Buenos Aires. A simple explanation may be that socioeconomic and cultural factors may predispose to a more severe spectrum of disease in Argentina. However, although it is uncertain whether the HUS seen at the Hospital de Niños is representative of that seen nationally, the socioeconomic status of children with HUS at this hospital has usually been good. This suggests that referral to the municipal hospital has not resulted in a biased ascertainment with more poverty- or nutrition-related complications. Another simple explanation for the reported differences is that the spectrum of HUS reported from other countries may reflect the use of different diagnostic criteria because many series contain mild cases which may lack some elements of the complete syndrome. However, a likely explanation for the different features of the HUS in Argentina may relate to the frequency of infection with *Shiga*-like toxin (SLT)–producing *Escherichia coli*.

Seasonal Variation in HUS

Although HUS occurs throughout the year recently there has been a striking variation in seasonal onset with the numbers beginning to increase in spring and remaining high until the middle of fall. Although this summer peak is similar to that reported from many other places, it was not recognized in Argentina at the time of the initial studies. Whether this represents a true shift in the pattern is uncertain.

Age-Related Risk

The age of affected children varies geographically and changes over the years. In San Francisco, Piel et al. (8) have reported patients as young as one month of age, and about 20% of 152 cases were less than 6 months. This contrasts with the experience in Buenos Aires: onset of HUS occurred in only three of 383 patients (1982–1988) under age 6 months. The patients in Argentina have been between 6 and 48 months (average age of 12.5 months) as reported between 1957 and 1972. The contemporaneous South African experience was similar with a mean age of 8 months (9). Older children have been described as a population at risk with an average age at onset of 4.5 years (range 8 months to 9 years) (10). However, for reasons that are unclear, the average age of patients seen at the Hospital de Niños has increased in recent years, and is now an average of 20.4 months. Because the number of cases on which this estimate is based is so large, it probably reflects a real shift in the age-related frequency. This increase in age of affected patients now makes the

Argentine population similar to that reported from Wales (11) and the Netherlands (12, 13) both of which had a mean age at presentation of 26 months. In our experience, differences in severity of HUS do not appear to be related to the age of the patient.

Clinical Manifestations

Prodrome

The prodromal illness is characterized by abdominal complaints. Fever rarely or never exceeds 38.5°C. Colicky abdominal pain is noted in older children. Diarrhea was present in about 70%, was usually bloody, and typically lasted from 4–10 days; vomiting was common. In the series of Tune (10, 14), the prodromal diarrheal illness lasted longer (mean 7 days, range 3–16 days). The interval between prodromal symptoms and HUS in Argentina is 2–5 days but occasionally is as long as 2 weeks. Respiratory symptoms, noted in approximately one third of patients in the early Argentine studies, have occurred in only 8–10% of patients in recent years (Fig. 1).

Acute Manifestations of HUS

Coombs-negative hemolytic anemia with fragmented erythrocytes is present in every patient; there are often repeated hemolytic crises during which the hemoglobin level decreases by 3–5 g/dL within 24 hours. The nadir of the hemoglobin level averages 6.6 g/dL (range 3–12) while the reticulocyte count increases to a mean of 7.8% (range 2.6–20%). Not all patients have decreased platelet counts; 14% did not have thrombocytopenia. Bleeding is common, especially from the gastrointestinal tract. Anemia and thrombocytopenia resolve in 1–4 weeks. Leukocytosis is present early in the illness (mean 17,000/mm^3, range 4,600–62,000) but resolves within a few weeks.

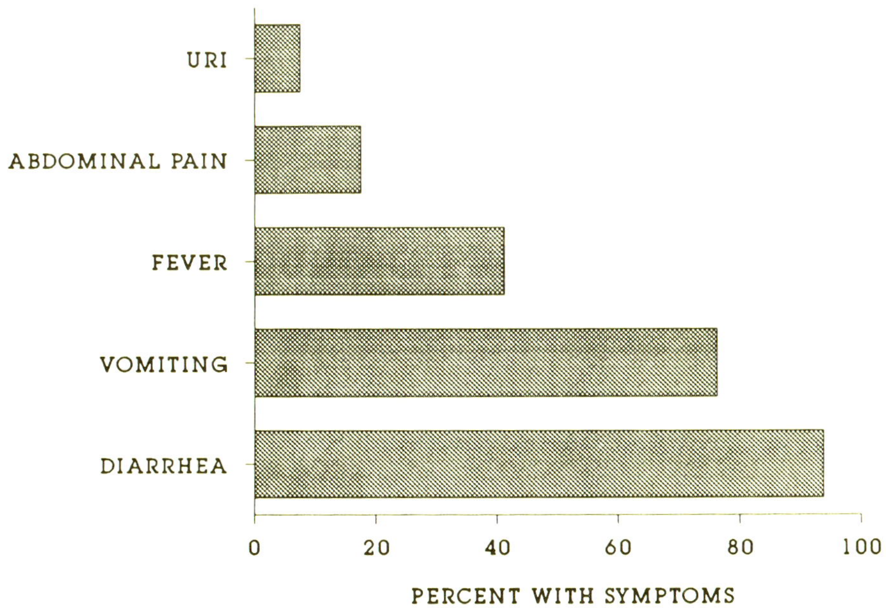

Figure 1 Symptoms during prodromal stage. Data based on 80 children.

Oliguria is present in nearly all patients. The duration of anuria is a mean of 8.5 days (maximum 28 days). In the 1974 report, oliguria averaged 14.2 days (range 2–72 days) and more than a third of patients were oliguric for more than 2 weeks. This degree of severity is in contrast with previous reports from North America. In California, 60% of affected children were oliguric or anuric but only 4% had oliguria/anuria that lasted for more than 21 days. Proteinuria and hematuria, usually microscopic, are present in all our patients. Azotemia is detected on admission (mean BUN 278± 103 mg/dl). Heart failure and hypertension commonly occur.

In contrast with other reports, central nervous system findings such as irritability, tremor, or ataxia are present in all our patients. Other important but less common findings include seizures (15–35%); stupor (20%); decerebrate rigidity, retinal hemorrhages, or coma (11%). We have not been able to relate the neurologic findings to metabolic abnormalities associated with renal failure.

Intussusception was suspected in 1–3% of cases on admission. Recently (15), we have cared for a child with intussusception proven by exploratory laparotomy in whom *E. coli* 0157:H7 was isolated. Eight of 383 patients evaluated between 1982–1988 (2.1%) had intussusception. HUS and intussusception may be part of the spectrum of complications associated with infection by toxin-producing enteropathogens. Intussusception may occur with *E. coli* 0157:H7 (and other toxin-producing *E. coli)* because edematous, hemorrhagic mucosa serves as a lead point for the invagination of a segment of intestine. Rectal prolapse was present on admission in 38 (9.9%), and acute myocardial infarction occurred in one (0.3%) patient.

Prognosis

The association of poor outcome with metabolic and hemodynamic complications, older age, leukocytosis, and severity of anemia have not been confirmed in our patient population. Mortality has decreased with each year since the HUS was first recognized (Fig. 2) because of improved management of renal failure and anemia. Renal failure, overwhelming infection and neurologic manifestations have tended to be poor prognostic features.

A poor prognosis has been associated with oliguria of more than 3 weeks' duration and/or anuria of more than 4 days' duration. This was usually secondary related to renal cortical necrosis. The prognosis is usually good if oliguria lasts for less than 2 weeks. Persistent or recurrent thrombocytopenia after the second week of illness also has been associated with a poorer prognosis.

Although duration of oliguria has prognostic value early in the course of the disease, evaluation of renal function months after the acute illness does not necessarily predict long-term outcome. Some patients who have had mild HUS, even with normal renal function 3–6 months after the acute stage, have then had markedly diminished GFR months or years later. Some degree of decreased renal function is common. In a group of 124 children followed for at least 5 years, renal function returned to normal in only 60. Ten (8.1%) had persistent arterial hypertension with no decrement in function. The remainder had progressive renal failure, stable renal dysfunction, or slowly improving function. Persistent hypertension was present in eight patients (6.4%) who also had evidence of chronic renal impairment. Nephrotic syndrome was never observed after recovery from the acute illness.

Neurological sequelae are not uncommon: 5% have permanent neurologic sequelae such as hemiparesis, involuntary movements, optic atrophy, seizures, or mental retardation.

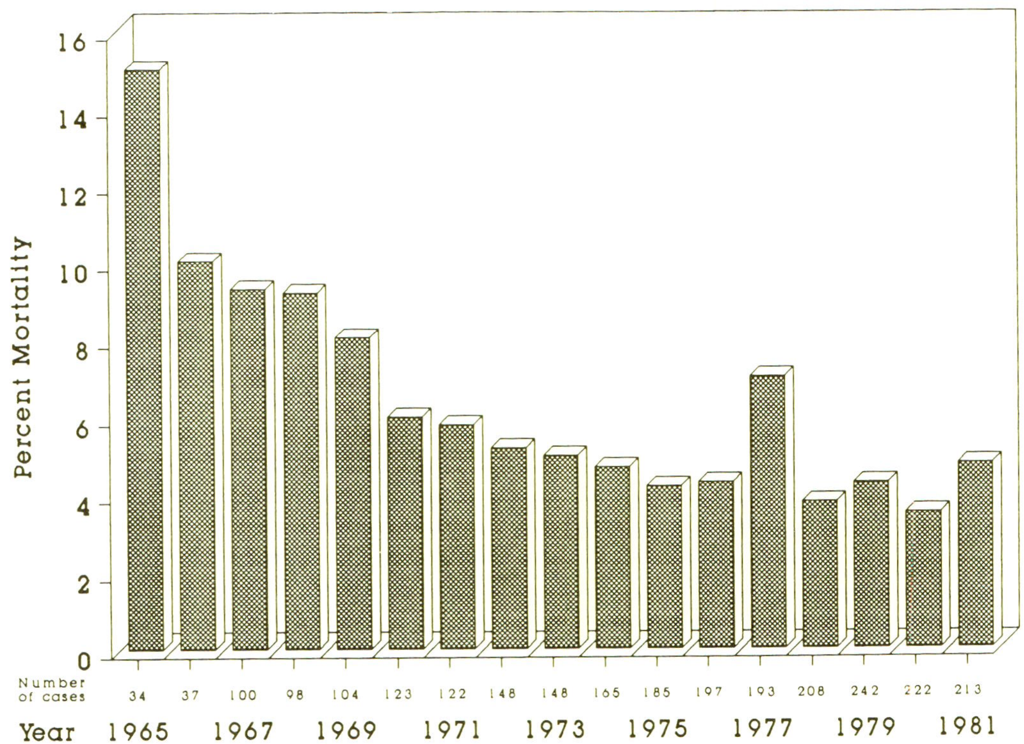

Figure 2 HUS mortality in Argentina between 1965–1981. Data based on 2,534 children compiled from eight (1965–1976) and 14 (1977–1981) pediatric nephrology services.

ETIOLOGY

Early Searches for Causative Agents

In the 1964 study, it was suggested that a virus related to Argentinian hemorrhagic fever might be an etiologic factor. A virus was isolated from the blood of five patients, but a definite causal link was not established. It was suggested that the Portillo virus of the Tacaribe group was responsible for HUS because of its isolation from the blood of eight patients during the acute stage, and because convalescent antibodies to the virus were detected in 36 of 55 cases. Subsequent demonstration of a number of other viral isolates from patients with HUS suggested these associations might be due to chance.

Recent Data on Etiology

Recent studies of etiology of HUS in Argentine (16–18) suggest that the usual cause of the syndrome is the toxin-producing *E. coli* as noted elsewhere (19).

De Cristofano et al. (16) found free fecal verotoxin in 8 of 18 (44%) stool specimens from patients with HUS. Novillo et al. (17) demonstrated free fecal cytotoxin in 15 of 49 (31%) patients. Lopez et al. (18) evaluated patients with HUS as well as healthy children in Buenos Aires. In those children with complete sample collections available (stool culture, DNA hybridization of isolated *E. coli* for toxin genes, stool for toxin neutralization assay, paired serologies for antibodies to SLT I and/or II), 96% of patients with HUS were associated with SLT-producing *E. coli*. Ninety-one percent had a prior episode of gastronenteritis which was usually bloody. No causes other than SLT-producing *E. coli* were found in these patients. The toxins were more frequently demonstrated in the feces of those whose diarrheal disease had recently ended; toxin-positive stools were obtained 4.5 ± 4.3 days after the end of diarrhea, and toxin-negative stools were obtained 10.4 ± 8.6 days after the end of diarrhea ($p<0.05$). No single test linking HUS to SLT was positive in all patients. Of interest, two of four patients who did not have the classic gastroenteritis prodrome had evidence of infection by SLT-producing *E. coli*. In comparison, none of the healthy children had free fecal toxin, cultures positive for *E. coli* 0157:H7, or DNA probe–positive organisms. However, 20% of healthy children had antibody titers to either SLT I or II. This unexpected finding was understood better when data from age-matched children with diarrhea occurring during the HUS season were evaluated. These studies showed that 32% of diarrheal disease was associated with SLT. This very high frequency of SLT enteritis is more than 10-fold greater than in other parts of the world where these organisms have been sought systematically. The diagnosis of toxin-associated diarrhea was based on free fecal cytotoxin, serum antibody, gene probe, and stool cultures. Only 33% of the children without HUS had bloody diarrhea, as compared to bloody diarrhea in 79% of children with HUS ($p<0.005$). Our most recent studies (unpublished observations) show that, over a 5-year period, the frequency of SLT-associated gasteroenteritis is about 23%. The majority of these infections are not complicated by HUS. We believe that the risk of HUS complicating SLT patients enteritis in this setting may be less than 5%. This low frequency may be due to interaction of complex phenomena including developing gut and endothelial receptors, developing serum and secretory immunity, passive immunity from breast feeding, transplacental antibodies, and exposure risk.

An additional finding from recent studies is that family members of the index case often have evidence of recent or current asymptomatic infection with SLT producing *E. coli* (unpublished observations). This was not unexpected, since person-to-person spread of these organisms has been demonstrated in a day-care center outbreak in North America (20). Studies of family contacts sometimes permits an episode of HUS to be ascribed to infection with SLT when the patient has been admitted too late in the illness to have detectable toxin or toxin-producing organisms in stool. In addition, we have found familial cases of HUS occurring years apart in which the second affected child had a toxin-related illness. This contrasts with that seen elsewhere in the world where the frequency of HUS is less common, so that familial cases of HUS which are not closely clustered in time often represent inherited variants of the syndrome (21).

The extraordinarily high frequency of SLT enteritis in Argentina explains the high prevalence of HUS. It further suggests that age-related risk may be due to risk of early infection. It is still unclear why patients are relatively spared from the ravages of these organisms in the first 6 months of life. Recent data in animal models suggest that the gut receptors for uptake of toxin (22) and adherence of organisms (23) are not present at birth but develop subsequently.

With the recent recognition that HUS is usually caused by SLT-producing *E. coli*, the whole subject of geographic differences in HUS must be re-examined. Whether differences will remain when cases of identical etiology are compared remains to be seen. In particular, the unusual frequency of severe disease in Argentina must be explained. We suspect that many geographic differences will persist. These will relate to differences in infection patterns and immunity. The high prevalence of SLT-producing *E. coli* as a cause of diarrhea in Argentina is likely to continue to cause frequent and early infection which will continue to be reflected in the occurrence of HUS at an early age. Transplacental and milk-related antibodies which may well be common in Argentina because of the frequency of exposure are likely to modify disease in ways as yet not understood.

ACKNOWLEDGMENT

The authors thank Dr. Susana Devoto for her critical review of the manuscript and Dr. Henry Gomez for preparation of the figures.

REFERENCES

1. Gasser, V. C., Gautier, E., Steck, A., Siebenmann, R. E., Oechslin, R. Hamolytische uramische Syndrome. *Schweiz. Med. Wochenschr.*, *85*: 905–909 (1955).
2. Gianantonio, C., Vitacco, M., Mendilaharzu, F., Rutty, A., Mendilaharzu, J. The hemolytic uremic syndrome. *J. Pediatr.*, *64*: 478–491 (1964).
3. Gianantonio, C. A., Vitacco, M., Mendilaharzu, F. The hemolytic uremic syndrome. *Proc. 3rd Int. Congr. Nephrol.*, *3*: 24–36 (1966).
4. Gianantonio, C., Vitacco, M., Mendilaharzu, F., Gallo, G. The hemolytic uremic syndrome: Renal status of 76 patients at long term follow up. *J. Pediatr.*, *72*: 757–765 (1968).
5. Avalos, J. S., Vitacco, M., Molinas, F., Peñalver, J., Gianantonio, C. Coagulation studies in the hemolytic uremic syndrome. *J. Pediatr.*, *76*: 538–548 (1970).

6. Gianantonio, C. A., Vitacco, M., Mendilaharzu, F., Gallo, G. E., Sojo, E. T. The hemolytic uremic syndrome. *Nephron, 11*: 174–192 (1973).
7. Gianantonio, C. The hemolytic uremic syndrome. *Kidney, 7*: 1–4 (1974).
8. Piel, C. F., Phibbs, R. H. The hemolytic uremic syndrome. *Pediatr. Clin. N. Am.*, 295–314 (1966).
9. Kibel, M. A., Barnard, P. J. The haemolytic uraemic syndrome: A survey of southern Africa. *S. Afr. Med. J., 42*: 692–698 (1968).
10. Tune, B. M., Leavitt, T. J., Gribble, T. J. The hemolytic uremic syndrome in California: A review of 28 nonheparinized cases with long term follow up. *J. Pediatr., 82*: 304–310 (1973).
11. McLean, M. M., Hilton-Jones, C., Sutherland, D. A. Haemolytic-uraemic syndrome: A report of an outbreak. *Arch. Dis. Child., 41*: 76–81 (1966).
12. Van Wieringen, P. M. V., Monnens, L. A. H., Schretlen, E. D. A. M. Haemolytic uraemic syndrome: Epidemiological and clinical study. *Arch. Dis. Child., 49*: 432–437 (1974).
13. Donckerwolcke, R. A., Kuyten, R. H., Tiddens, H. A. Haemolytic uraemic syndrome. *Paediatrician, 4*: 27–40 (1975).
14. Dolislager, D., Tune, B. The hemolytic uremic syndrome. *Am. J. Dis. Child., 132*: 55–58 (1978).
15. Lopez, E. L., Devoto, S., Woloj, M., Pickering, L. K., Cleary, T. G. Intussusception associated with Escherichia coli 0 157:H7. *Pediatr. Infect. Dis. J., 8*: 471–473 (1989).
16. De Cristofano, M. G., Fayad, A., Ferraris, J., Cortinez, C., Ramirez, J., Ascione, A., Gianantonio, C. Síndrome Urémico Hemolítico de la infancia. Su relación con la presencia de verotoxina libre fecal. *Arch. Arg. Pediatr., 84*: 339–342 (1986).
17. Lovillo, A., Voyer, L. E., Cravioto, R., Freire, M. C., Castaño, G., Wainstein, R., Binztein, N. Haemolytic uraemic syndrome associated with faecal cytotoxin and verotoxin neutralizing antibodies. *Pediatr. Nephrol., 2*: 288–290 (1988).
18. Lopez, E. L., Diaz, M., Grinstein, S., Devoto, S., Mendilaharzu, F., Murray, B. E., Ashkenazi, S., Rubeglio, E., Woloj, M., Vasquez, M., Turco, M., Pickering, L. K., Cleary, T. G. Hemolytic uremic syndrome and diarrhea in Argentine children: the role of shiga like toxins. *J. Infect. Dis., 160*: 469–475 (1989).
19. Karmali, M. A., Petric, M., Lim, C., Fleming, P. C., Arbus, G. S., Lior, H. The association between haemolytic uraemic syndrome and infection by verotoxin producing *E. coli*. *J. Infect. Dis., 151*: 619–620 (1985).
20. Spika, J. S., Parsons, J. E., Nordenberg, D., Wells, J. G., Gunn, R. A., Blake, P. A. Hemolytic uremic syndrome and diarrhea associated with *E. coli* 0157:H7 in a day care center. *J. Pediatr., 109*: 287–291 (1986).
21. Kaplan, B. S., Chesney, R. W., Drummond, K. N. Hemolytic uremic syndrome in families. *N. Engl. J. Med., 292*: 1090–1093 (1975).
22. Mobassaleh, M., Gross, S. K., McCluer, R. H., Donahue-Rolfe, A., Keusch, G. T. Quantitation of the rabbit intestinal glycolipid receptor of shiga toxin. *Gastroenterology*, 97: 384–391 (1989).
23. Ashkenazi, S., May, L., LaRocco, M., Lopez, E. L., Cleary, T. G. The effect of postnatal age on the adherence of enterohemorrhagic *E. coli* to rabbit intestinal cells. *Pediatr Res* 29: 14–19 (1991).

III
Clinical Manifestations of HUS

9
Gastrointestinal Features of the Hemolytic Uremic Syndrome

Russell W. Chesney *The University of Tennessee and Le Bonheur Children's Medical Center, Memphis, Tennessee* **Peter F. Whitington** *The University of Chicago, Chicago, Illinois*

Hemolytic uremic syndrome (HUS) frequently presents with gastrointestinal symptoms, including abdominal pain, vomiting, and diarrhea with blood and mucus (Table 1). These features appear to represent a prodrome, which is then followed by microangiopathic hemolytic anemia, thrombocytopenia, and renal impairment. This chapter focuses on the numerous gastrointestinal features of HUS and highlights other aspects of the syndrome that are pertinent to a better understanding of gastrointestinal disease. Specific topics that are discussed include: the clinical features, contributing etiologic agents, pathology, pathogenesis, radiology, treatment, and prognosis of gastrointestinal disease. A hypothesis will also be explored. It states that gastrointestinal disease is an important feature in HUS and an important component of the syndrome rather than a prodrome. The value of realizing HUS as having a gastrointestinal component as a major feature is that worrisome complications, including ischemia, stricture, perforation, and infarction, are not overlooked (1). Further, unnecessary therapy directed at diseases mimicked by HUS can be avoided.

CLINICAL FEATURES

The major gastrointestinal pathology in HUS occurs in the colon (2) (Table 2), usually initiated with bloody diarrhea, abdominal pain, and distention. In a study by van Wieringen, Monneus, and Schrethen, more than 90% of nearly 200 patients with HUS had diarrhea with blood and/or mucus (13). Numerous reports relate the difficulty in distinguishing the gastrointestinal lesion(s) of HUS from ulcerative colitis (3–8), appendicitis (3, 9, 10) and intussusception (11, 12). Other diagnostic possibilities include toxic megacolon (2, 6), suspected cecal polyp (2), and gastric hemorrhage (14). Other patients are diagnosed as having bacterial enteritis, diarrheal enteritis, or

Table 1 Gastrointestinal Components of the Hemolytic Uremic Syndrome

Abdominal pain
Acute pancreatitis
Bloody diarrhea
Diarrhea with mucus
Endocrine and exocrine pancreatic failure with calcinosis
Gangrenous colitis
Gastric hemorrhage
Hepatitis
Intestinal tract perforation
Intussusception
Ischemic colitis with stricture formation
Ischemic enterocolitis or hemolytic uremic syndrome colitis
Peritonitis, bacterial
Vomiting

gastroenteritis (2). The presence of leukocytosis heightens the illusion that the patient has acute bacterial enterocolitis (2). Finding diarrhea with blood (hematochezia) or mucus or both may further contribute to this illusion (13). Failure to recognize these features as early indicators of the HUS may result in diagnostic confusion and possibly lead to inappropriate intervention.

The notion that gastrointestinal disease represents a prodromal phase of HUS has been prevalent for years (3, 4, 15) and persists today (16). This is because abdominal pain, vomiting, and hematochezia usually disappear with the onset of pallor, anemia, thrombocytopenia, and azotemia, and the gastrointestinal features often presage the systemic disease. A typical observation is nonspecific gastroenteritis that manifests for 1–15 days followed by the triad of features that define HUS. Unfortunately for the clinician, the gastrointestinal features may be so dominant in the early stages to make it difficult, if not impossible, to establish the proper diagnosis without the passage of time and the development of systemic features.

In certain patients, although it is rare, florid colitic findings typical of ulcerative colitis are expressed (2, 4, 5, 7, 16). In such patients, sigmoidoscopy should be the first diagnostic examination. An interesting physical finding in the HUS that may be observed with sigmoidoscopy is a lax anal sphincter, which was evident in 2 of 12 subjects in one series (2). This observation has been of recent interest because it should alert the physician to possible child sexual abuse, sustained anal trauma, and

Table 2 Sites of Gastrointestinal Disease in the Hemolytic Uremic Syndrome

Colon
Liver
Pancreas
Peritoneum
Rectum
Small bowel (ileum and jejenum)
Stomach

constipation, but it is also a distinct finding in the HUS (17) and *Shigella* infection. Findings at sigmoidoscopy can also include mucosal friability, petechiae, and ulceration which are suggestive of ulcerative colitis. Edema, bowel wall thickening, and nodularity can also be noticed, but these are more suggestive of Crohn's colitis. Another finding, dirty gray pseudomembranes, can be confused with antibiotic-associated colitis (2, 4).

This acute colitis phase is usually self-limited, and recovery is almost always the rule (4). However, complications can develop, including rectal prolapse (18), toxic megacolon (2, 18), and necrosis of the bowel wall (1, 2). The colonic disease, which is considered to be a local vasculitis, may proceed to ischemic lesions with full-thickness necrosis requiring surgical intervention (1). Patients with features suggestive of intussusception that led to surgery are also reported (12, 19). Other clinical features include pseudomembranous enterocolitis (2, 18), colonic perforation (20), segmental colonic gangrene (19, 21), colonic infarction (1), ischemic colitis with stricture formation (22), and persistence of colonic symptoms well into the uremic phase (1, 2). Other reported features are: ischemic small bowel disease with necrosis of the ileum, jejunum, and colon (2, 23), as well as small bowel perforation and stricture formation (2).

Gastric hemorrhage has occurred in patients with the HUS (14; R. W. Chesney, unpublished observations). In a 2-year-old boy with the HUS, gastric hemorrhage followed a dosage of heparin (14). Similarly, gastric hemorrhage secondary to uremia or to heparin administration in preparation for hemodialysis has been described (14; R. W. Chesney, unpublished observations).

Acute and chronic pancreatitis have been described in HUS (25–27). Acute pancreatitis that releases into the circulation free trysinogen or trypsin complexed to α-2-macroglobulin. α-1-Protease inhibitor was reported in two patients with the HUS (26). A case of the HUS in a 3-year-old boy was complicated by hyperglycemia and a lack of circulating insulin (24), resulting in the child's death. Extensive necrosis of both the exocrine and endocrine pancreas was found at autopsy. An adolescent girl developed insulin-dependent diabetes mellitus and pancreatic calcinosis after having had acute pancreatic necrosis following HUS (25–27).

Liver function may be difficult to evaluate in HUS because the prothrombin time could be elevated due to consumptive coagulopathy, the serum albumin concentration may be reduced from intestinal losses, and the severe degree of microangiopathic hemolytic anemia often produces hyperbilirubinemia. Elevation of serum transaminases have been noted and appear to mark hepatocellular involvement in HUS (2, 29). In the series of Whitington et al. (2), all patients manifested elevations of serum transaminase concentrations. The SGOT varied from 58 to 468 IU/L and the SGPT from 89 to 149 IU/L. Though not proven, these hepatocellular lesions were ascribed to focal hepatic hypoxia. Hepatomegaly is a common physical finding in HUS (19), although cholestatic jaundice is an uncommon feature (30). Patients with more severe forms of HUS may also have liver function abnormalities as the result of peritonitis and portal sepsis. A liver biopsy specimen from one such patient exhibited acute portal inflammation, bile duct replication, bile plugs, and acute inflammatory cells within interlobular ducts (2).

To summarize, extensive gastrointestinal, hepatic, and pancreatic features of HUS may be found during any phase of the syndrome. However, the most important feature by far is hemorrhagic enterocolitis (2, 14).

RADIOLOGICAL FEATURES

The radiological features of the hemorrhagic colitis of HUS are well described (1, 2, 5–7, 19, 31). Abdominal flat plate often shows accumulation of gas in the colon with mild-to-severe colonic distention. The colon wall and, on occasion, the small bowel may be thickened. Although barium enema examination in HUS patients may prove normal, this same examination in HUS patients who present with bloody diarrhea, cramping, and vomiting usually shows thumbprinting, pseudotumor, and transverse ridging (5, 6, 19), which are related to submucosal hemorrhage and edema. These findings characterize ischemic bowel disease. In a series of seven patients, all showed "thumbprinting" and areas of narrowing alternating with distention (32). Often, fine serrations or spicules are noticed along the edges of the contrast column; these are indicative of mucosal ulceration (Fig. 1) (31). Bowel wall irritability has also been identified (5). The acute changes of narrowing and thumbprinting can progress in some patients to toxic megacolon (2, 18). Free intraperitoneal air can be evident if the patient has experienced intestinal perforation (2). Although nonspecific in them-

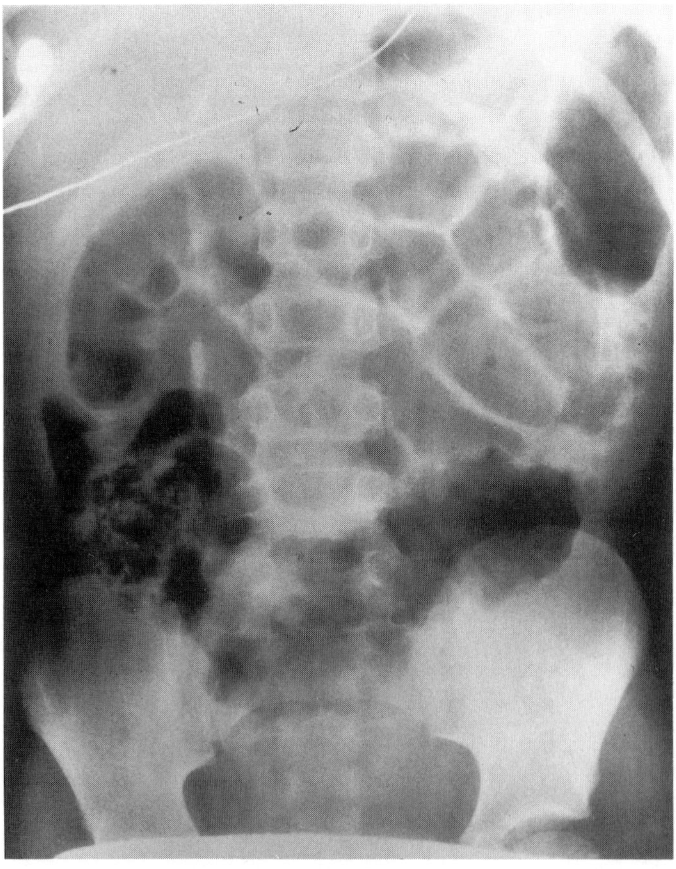

Figure 1 Supine abdominal x-ray of patient 11. This film demonstrates diffuse bowel wall edema most marked in the sigmoid colon. The sigmoid colon is dilated and has nodular mucosa. (From Ref. 2, with permission.)

selves, these findings associated with a history of bloody diarrhea may enable the radiologist to suggest the diagnosis of HUS (6). In two patients, colonic strictures developed 6 and 10 weeks after the onset of the HUS (Fig. 2) (6).

PATHOLOGICAL FINDINGS IN THE INTESTINE

Few detailed descriptions of colonic pathology have been reported (2, 4, 19, 21, 22); these involved only a few patients, but the pathological findings in the bowel wall appear to be the result of local ischemia (2). Abnormal findings include only edema and submucosal hemorrhage (4). In more severe disease, thrombosis of submucosal and intramural vessels has been identified, which is associated with focal, superficial ischemic necrosis involving the colonic mucosa. This, in turn, is associated with mucosal ulceration, hemorrhagic mucositis, and pseudomembrane formation (2). More widespread thrombosis results in transmural infarction (2, 21, 22) (Fig. 3) and even gangrene of the colon (19). Intramural hemorrhage of the small intestine has also been observed (2).

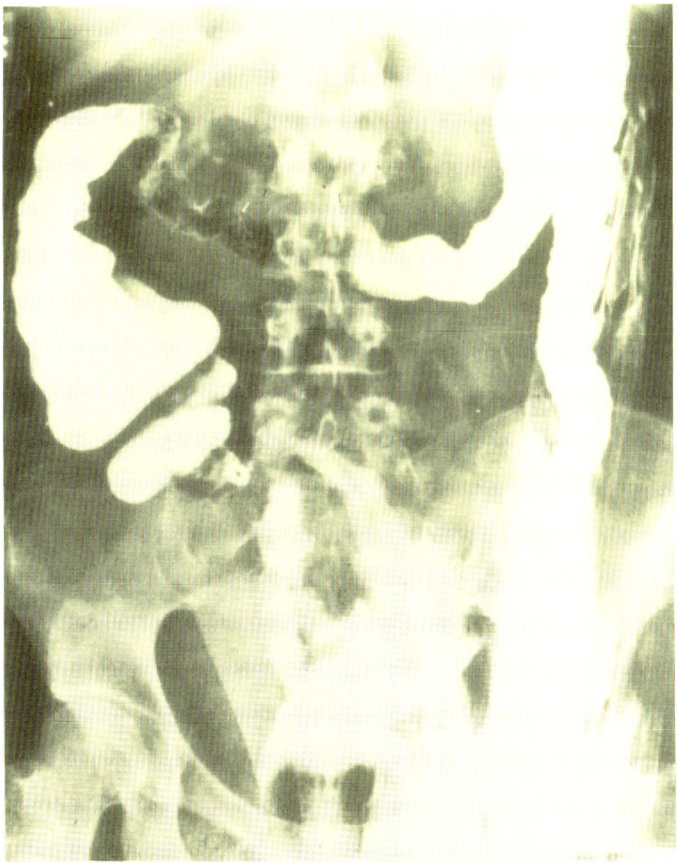

Figure 2 Barium enema of patient 2. There is diffuse superficial mucosal irregularity from the hepatic flexure through the sigmoid colon. This study was interpreted as being consistent with a clinical diagnosis of ulcerative colitis. (From Ref. 2, with permission.)

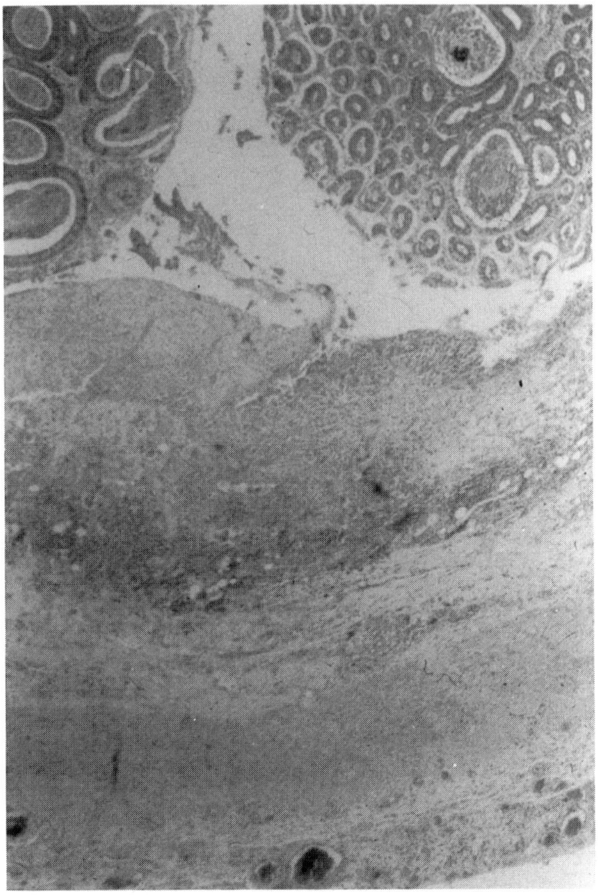

Figure 3 Light microscopic histology of a portion of resected colon of a patient with the severe form of hemolytic uremic syndrome. Acute mucosal necrosis with epithelial ulceration is evident (x100).

If sigmoidoscopy is performed, a biopsy specimen should be obtained to exclude other diagnoses. The distinct absence of findings such as crypt abscesses, loss of epithelial mucus, and any chronic inflammation clearly differentiates the bowel disease of HUS from either ulcerative colitis or Crohn's disease. In those patients with *Shigella*- or *Campylobacter*-associated HUS, there may be acute inflammation; but in most instances, the findings are also quite distinct from acute infectious enterocolitis.

ETIOLOGICAL AGENTS CONTRIBUTING TO GI DISEASE IN HUS

Numerous viral and bacterial agents which are associated with diarrhea are etiological agents implicated in leading to HUS. The list of infectious agents causing both gastrointestinal disease and full-blown HUS is long and includes *Mycoplasma pneumoniae* (13), *Yersinia enterocolitica* (33), *Yersinia* pseudotuberculosis (34), verocytotoxin-producing *Escherichia coli* (VTEC) (23), *Shigella dysenteriae* 1 (35), *Shigella flexneri* (35), *Campylobacter jejuni* (36), *Salmonella typhimurium* (37), *Salmonella typhi* (38), *Entamoeba histolytica* (39), *Clostridium septicum* (40) and, interestingly, *Streptococcus pyogenes* (41). Numerous viral agents have also been implicated: Echo 22 (42), Coxsackie B (43), Tacaribe group Portella virus (44), Coxsackie A4 (45), several enteroviruses including Coxsackie B1, B3, and B5, as well as A-4 (46), and other viruses not associated with gastrointestinal symptoms, including Epstein-Barr (47), influenza, and parainfluenza (14).

These agents were either directly cultured from the throat or stool or were found by serological evidence (42). The most consistently found agents are VTEC, related to *E. coli* O157:H7, 025:H11 (48), 011 (49), and *Shigella dysenteriae* type 1 (35). The contribution of these agents and the role of Shiga-like toxins 1 and 2 in the pathogenesis of HUS are discussed extensively in Chapter 28. We will focus on their role in bowel disease (vide infra).

PATHOGENESIS

This section will focus only on the pathogenesis of gastrointestinal disease in HUS, ignoring its development in other organs. Over 30 years ago, investigators showed that the results of the injection of Shiga toxin into laboratory animals were associated with ischemic lesions of the bowel, characterized by submucosal hemorrhage and edema (50, 51). The follow-up of these results occurred in the 1980s (52). Early in 1982, two outbreaks of bloody diarrhea were reported in Oregon and Michigan (49). Investigation of these outbreaks strongly suggested that the hitherto rare *E. coli* serotype O157:H7, a VTEC strain, was involved and had been transmitted by undercooked meat ingested at a fast food restaurant (50). Unpasteurized milk can be another source of this serotype of *E. coli* (53). Bloody diarrhea related to this strain has occurred in communities, in nursing homes, after banquets, in day-care centers, and in a kindergarten (54).

The careful analysis of an outbreak occurring in Walla Walla, Washington, between October 29 and November 24, 1986, provides extremely important information. In these 37 patients *E. coli* O157:H7 infection caused either bloody or nonbloody diarrhea, or HUS, or thrombotic thrombocytopenic purpura (TTP), representing the spectrum of possible diseases (54). Infection in some cases was asymptomatic, involved extraintestinal sites, or was fatal. Bloody diarrhea, severe abdominal cramps, and fever were common. Radiological and colonoscopic examinations showed inflammatory bowel disease or ischemic hemorrhagic colitis. Patients at extremes of age were at risk for hemorrhagic colitis, HUS, TTP, and death. In a separate study, three cases of HUS were reported in an outbreak of *E. coli* O157:H7 diarrhea in a day-care center (55). Thirty-four percent of 107 children at the center developed this diarrhea. Only 12% of the older children became ill, compared to 48% of children under age 4 who were sick. Eighteen percent of 56 family members of the ill children developed diarrhea, while only one of 45 of child-aged siblings of well children attending the center developed gastrointestinal complaints. The careful analysis of these two outbreaks indicates that this strain of *E. coli* can cause both diarrhea and HUS or TTP in an outbreak, that it can spread from person to person, and that young children are mostly affected.

By way of contrast, in another outbreak in Utah involving children in a residential treatment center for retarded children, older children and young adults were affected with bloody diarrhea and HUS, resulting in several deaths (56).

With these reports of HUS associated with *E. coli* O157:H7 enteric infections (57), several questions are raised: What is the nature of toxins in VTEC, and how do these toxins lead to ischemic or hemorrhagic colitis? There exist four major forms of diarrheagenic *E. coli:* enterotoxigenic (causing traveler's diarrhea and infant diarrhea in Third World countries); enteroinvasive (causing dysentery); enteropathogenic (causing infant diarrhea); and enterohemorrhagic (causing hemorrhagic diarrhea and HUS) (58). Aside from manifesting these distinct clinical patterns, these *E. coli* differ in their epidemiology, disease mechanism, and O:H serotypes. They have in common plasmid-encoded virulence properties, a characteristic proclivity for the intestinal mucosa, and elaboration of a variety of enterotoxins and/or cytotoxins. By convention, those VTEC *E. coli* that have been shown to produce a verotoxin (59) are now termed enterohemorrhagic *E. coli* (48). Thus, the term VTEC is replaced by enterohemorrhagic *E. coli* (EHEC). In addition to *E. coli* strain O157:H7 at least 26 different serotypes have been isolated from patients with hemorrhagic colitis and/or the HUS. Strains of these serotypes also produce cytotoxins to vero cells in culture (verocytotoxins or VT) (60). At least two cytoxotoxins are produced by *E. coli* O157:H7: VT1 and VT2 (61, 62). These two toxins are also termed Shiga-like toxin 1 and Shiga-like toxin 2, which are almost indistinguishable, both immunologically and genetically, from Shiga toxin (63). However, while the nucleotide sequence and deduced amino acid sequence of ST-1 is virtually identical to those of Shiga toxin produced by *Shigella dysenteriae* type 1, ST-2 is less closely related and is not universally neutralized by antiserum to Shiga toxin (63). ST-producing *E. coli* strains produce one or several closely related toxins (64). Each closely related toxin has a single copy of an enzymatically active 32.21 kD A subunit, but several copies of the receptor binding 7.69 kD B subunit are transcribed as an operon. Shiga toxin, produced by *Shigella dysenteriae* serotype 1, is almost completely identical to ST-1, the only difference being a single amino acid change at position 45 of the A subunit, threonine for serine. ST-2 and Shiga toxin have approximately 50–60% DNS homology (64). Cytotoxins produced by O157, O111:H, strain HUS 2 (Hamburg), and O26:H11 always have ST-1 properties (65).

The pathogenesis of disease associated with VTEC (EHEC) strains is related to their production of VT-1 and VT-2 (ST-1 and ST-2). These strains, when fed to infant rabbits, show intimate attachment and effacement binding to rabbit enterocytes and colonocytes in vivo (66). In addition to bacterial binding in the ceca and colon, these strains adhere to enterocytes in the distal small intestine after oral ingestion. Both Shiga toxin and *E. coli* ST act directly on the vascular endothelium of the intestinal villus in the rabbit model (67). Shiga toxin is also cytotoxic to cultured colonic epithelial cells (68). In addition, both ST-1 and 2 will cause fluid accumulation in rabbit ileal segments (69). Another model involving ST is the hemorrhagic colitis that develops when purified ST-2 is continuously infused into the peritoneal cavity of rabbits (70). Large doses of ST-2 result in paresis, azotemia, and elevated serum creatinine values as well as watery diarrhea. At 20% of that dose (200 ng) given continuously, rabbits develop diarrhea only after day 3, as manifested by cecal and colonic hemorrhage and leukocytosis. The appearance of the colonic mucosa is similar to that in human disease; namely, petechial and ecchymotic hemorrhages, submucosal edema, and hemorrhage of the lamina propria. The rabbit is a useful model for hemorrhagic colitis because its gut mucosa apparently has the purported functional receptor for ST-1 and 2, globotriaosyl ceramide, which is also found in human kidney (71). Thus, it appears that toxins may be elaborated from certain EHEC strains after they bind and adhere to the mucosal surface, that these Shiga-like toxins can cause enteric and colonic cell damage, and that the evolving histopathological appearance is similar to hemorrhagic colitis.

Recent developments concerning the pathogenesis of *Shigella*-induced disease are noticeable. In a rabbit model, exposure to Shiga toxin leads to accumulation of water in the jejunal lumen associated with reduced basal NaCl absorption. Glucose- and alanine-stimulated sodium absorption was also lower, but active anion secretion was unchanged (72). In this model selective targeting of Shiga toxin to villus cells was evident; villus cells had a greater content of the glycolipid Shiga toxin receptor Gb3 than did crypt cells. Villus cells were also much more sensitive to toxin-induced inhibition of protein synthesis. Shiga toxin, therefore, can account for the watery diarrhea seen in the gastrointestinal phase of *S. dysenteriae*-associated HUS.

Evidence is impressive that severe colitis with bloody diarrhea and the HUS can develop after *Campylobacter fetus* subspecies *jejuni* infection (73). These patients may demonstrate hypocomplementemia and bacteremia during their illness. It is unclear whether these are important in the pathogenesis of the hemorrhagic colitis. Finally, endotoxemia may be important in the development of more severe colitis and the complete development of HUS in patients with bacillary dysentery (74–76). These cases also may have overt evidence of disseminated intravascular coagulation.

It is evident that infection with EHEC, *Campylobacter*, or *Shigella dysenteriae* produce a spectrum of disease (54, 58, 74, 76), which includes asymptomatic infection or mild diarrhea, bloody diarrhea, diarrhea with hemorrhage and hemolysis (74), typical HUS, and TTP (54, 58). Perhaps as much as any piece of data, this finding of broad-spectrum disease indicates that hemorrhagic or ischemic colitis does not represent a prodromal phase but rather an integral component of the HUS. What still remains uncertain, however, is what will trigger the remainder of HUS features in that minority of patients who progress from hemorrhagic colitis to complete HUS or TTP.

TREATMENT

Regarding therapy of the gastrointestinal disease in the HUS, topics worthy of discussion include therapy of the hemorrhagic colitis phase, indications for surgical exploration (1), therapy of the patient who develops intestinal perforation, and avoidance of unnecessary treatment.

There is no specific therapy for the colitic phase of HUS. As with other acute enterocolitis, the patient should be placed at complete bowel rest. Fluid balance should be maintained assiduously. Infectious dehydration may be present in EHEC, shigellosis, and campylobacteriosis. It can generally be treated with oral rehydration solutions or intravenous fluid, with care not to overhydrate if oliguric renal failure supervenes. Intravenous fluids should be administered in amounts to maintain only a normal hydration status. Brisk hydration in response to diarrhea may lead to fluid overload before acute renal failure is appreciated. Blood can be administered to maintain an adequate hemoglobin concentration, but despite the hemorrhagic colitis, blood transfusions should rarely be needed until deemed necessary in the hemolytic phase of the disease. As the child or adult with the typical features of hemorrhagic or ischemic colitis will often have abdominal pain, colic, diarrhea, rectal bleeding, and rectal prolapse (2, 5, 6), it is tempting to use agents that retard peristalsis, such as atropine compounds, paregoric, or other antispasmotics. These medications are of no proven value (2) and could be potentially harmful.

There is no therapy of proven benefit in the patient with EHEC infection. While it might be tempting to use antibiotic agents, this mode is contraindicated, at least theoretically (77). Subinhibitory concentrations of antimicrobials affect the amount of toxin produced by *E. coli* O157:H7. Organisms exposed to sulfamethoxazole or trimethoprim in vitro increase toxin production, while ciprofloxacin exposure may reduce toxin production (77). Patients with HUS associated with EHEC O157:H7 or other EHEC serotypes develop a brisk serologic response to these organisms with a rise in ST-neutralizing antibody titers (49). Thus, at least in theory, it might be possible to administer intravenous immune globulin early in the course of disease to treat hemorrhagic colitis. Commercial immune globulin preparations appear to contain anticytotoxin-neutralizing antibodies (78). However, because EHEC are not invasive, this immune globulin may not be effective in eliminating organisms from the bowel per se. The use of immune globulin in HUS is controversial and is discussed further in Chapter 10.

The current chosen treatment for shigellosis is the administration of oral antibiotics (79). When organisms are sensitive, ampicillin is the current drug of choice; when they are resistant to this agent, trimethoprim-sulfamethoxazole should be used.

As has been frequently emphasized, the inaccurate diagnosis of these children often leads to improper therapeutic approaches. The administration of glucocorticoids for presumed idiopathic inflammatory bowel disease may actually be contraindicated in light of the thrombocytopenia often accompanying HUS (7) and is of no established value in the treatment of HUS. Several authors make the point that in the child presenting with acute ulcerative colitis, the diagnosis of HUS must be entertained (2, 4, 5, 7, 16, 31); blood smears should be examined daily in anticipation of later changes (7). Withholding corticosteroids until a proper diagnosis is established will seldom compromise the patient with ulcerative colitis, while administering them to the patient with HUS can do harm. It is most important to avoid unnecessary surgical intervention. This lesion in the child or adult presenting with colitis as part of HUS may have been diagnosed as appendicitis (3, 9, 10, 80), acute ulcerative colitis with toxic megacolon (2–7, 80), colonic polyp (2), intussusception (11), or other bowel pathology that can lead to a perceived need for emergency laparotomy (2, 9–11, 18). Unneeded surgery can obviously complicate the course of a patient with HUS (Table 3). Indeed, the mortality rate in this circumstance may be higher than usual for HUS because of the added burden of anesthesia, surgery, and recovery from a surgical procedure (1, 11, 18, 19). This contention is difficult to accurately assess because many of these reports come from an era when bowel disease in the HUS was recognized less efficiently and when the management of acute renal failure was not well established in young children.

It has been pointed out that on occasion the ischemic bowel lesion may progress to such an extent that surgical intervention may be required (1). Some individuals

Table 3 Gastrointestinal Conditions Possibly Mimicked by the Hemolytic Uremic Syndrome

Acute pancreatitis
Appendicitis
Bacterial enterocolitis
Bacterial peritonitis associated with bowel perforation
Intussusception
Necrotic polyp of cecum
Rectal prolapse
Segmental gangrene of colon
Ulcerative colitis

may even require a hemicolectomy for these ischemic lesions. Both cecal and ileal perforations which required surgical intervention have been described (2). Although the bowel disease of HUS is a diagnostic and therapeutic dilemma for the surgeon, in the absence of documented perforation, toxic megacolon, or intussusception, the decision to perform laparotomy must be individualized (81). The surgeon must decide which child will require a colostomy but is comforted by the fact that perforation is fairly infrequent and true intussusception quite rare (81). The therapy of the patient who develops perforation is made more difficult by the other components of the HUS and is a life-threatening complication.

PROGNOSIS

As has been repeatedly noted, the occurrence of hemorrhagic colitis in HUS is a favorable prognostic sign (82). Patients not presenting with gastrointestinal disease may actually have more severe forms of HUS including genetic forms, recurrent disease, and TTP (83). Using the prognostic features in 72 children from the south of England, the probability of a good outcome was analyzed by logistic regression (84). Children with a prolonged diarrheal phase did worse than those with diarrhea of short duration. The presence of diarrhea was a good prognostic sign among boys but not among girls.

In a series in which patients manifested severe colonic disease, including perforation and the requirement for extensive surgical removal of necrotic bowel, the prognosis was worse than those without severe colonic disease (1, 2, 11, 18–20, 81).

The prognosis in patients with shigellosis-associated HUS was not as good as in North American and English patients, who had an overall mortality rate of 38% or 16 of 42 cases (75, 76). These patients experienced a renal death with cortical necrosis after disseminated intravascular coagulation (DIC) was common.

Thus, regarding gastrointestinal manifestations of HUS, those children whose disease is associated with short-duration diarrhea or the epidemic form of the disease appear to have the best prognosis.

ACKNOWLEDGMENTS

We greatly appreciate the editorial assistance of Brenna Nichols and the secretarial assistance of Shirley Seymour in the preparation of this manuscript.

REFERENCES

1. Van Stiegmann, G., Lilly, J. R. Surgical lesions of the colon in the hemolytic uremic syndrome. *Surgery, 85*: 357–359 (1979).
2. Whitington, P. F., Friedman, A. L., Chesney, R. W. Gastrointestinal disease in the hemolytic uremic syndrome. *Gastroenterology, 76*: 728–733 (1979).
3. Lieberman, E. Hemolytic uremic syndrome. *J. Pediatr., 80*: 1–16 (1972).
4. Berman, W. The hemolytic uremic syndrome: initial clinical presentation mimicking ulcerative colitis. *J. Pediatr, 81*: 275–278 (1972).
5. Bar-Ziv, J., Ayoub, J.I.G., Fletcher, B. D. Hemolytic uremic syndrome: a case presenting with acute colitis. *Pediatr. Radiol., 2*: 203–206 (1974).
6. Peterson, R. B., Meseroll, W. P., Shargo, G. G., Goodling, O. Radiographic features of colitis associated with the hemolytic uremic syndrome. *Radiology, 118*: 667–671 (1976).
7. Craner, B. E., Burdick, G. E. Acute colitis resembling ulcerative colitis in the hemolytic uremic syndrome. *Digest Dis., 21*: 74–76 (1976).
8. Yates, R. S., Osterholm, R. K. Hemolytic-uremic syndrome colitis. *J. Clin. Gastroenterol., 2*: 359–363 (1980).
9. Edmonson, M. B., Chesney, R. W. Hemolytic-uremic syndrome confused with acute appendicitis. *Arch. Surg., 113*: 754–755 (1978).
10. Tune, B. M., Leavitt, T. J., Gribble, T. J. The hemolytic uremic syndrome in California: A review of 28 nonheparinized cases with long-term followup. *J. Pediatr., 82*: 304–310 (1973).
11. Maki, S., Miyata, H., Uda, H. Hemolytic-uremic syndrome: A fatal case after operation for intussusception as a complication of upper respiratory tract infection. *Med. J. Osaka U., 19*: 157–173 (1968).
12. Sun, C. C., Hill, J. L., Combs, J. W. Hemolytic-uremic syndrome: Initial presentation mimicking intestinal intussusception. *Pediatr. Pathol., 1*: 415–422 (1983).
13. Van Wieringen, P.M.V., Monneus, L.A.H., Schrethen, E.D.A.M. Hemolytic uremic syndrome: epidemiologic and clinical study. *Arch. Dis. Child, 49*:432–437 (1974).
14. Bugaier-Gleitman, H. E., Balzar, E., Lubec, G., May, L., Weissenbacher, G. The presence of cold agglutinins in the hemolytic uremic syndrome. *Pädiatrie und Rädologie, 11*: 245–253 (1976).
15. Gasser, C., Gautier, F., Steck, A., Siebermann, R. E., Oechslin, R. Hämolytisch-urämische syndrome: Bilaterale nierenrindennekrosen bei akuten erworbenen hamolytischen anämien. *Schweiz. Med. Wschr., 85*: 905–909 (1955).
16. Yates, R. S., Osterholin, R. K. Hemolytic-uremic syndrome colitis. *J. Clin. Gastroenterol., 2*: 359–363 (1980).
17. Vickers, D., Morris, K., Coulthard, M. G. and Eastham, E. J. Anal signs in hemolytic uremic syndrome (letter). *Lancet, 1*: 998 (1988).
18. Tochen, M. L. and Campbell, J. R. Colitis in children with the hemolytic uremic syndrome. *J. Pediatr. Surg., 12*: 213–219 (1977).
19. Kendall, P. A., Reid, I., Wright, J. E., Nanra, R. S. Gangrenous colitis in the hemolytic uremic syndrome. *Med. J. Aust., 140*: 543–544 (1984).
20. Liebharber, M. I., Parker, B. R., Morton, J. A., Tune, B. M. Abdominal mass and colonic perforation in a case of the hemolytic uremic syndrome. *Am. J. Dis. Child, 131*: 1168–1169 (1977).
21. Schwartz, D. L., Becker, J. M., So, H. B., Schneider, K. M. Segmental colonic gangrene: a surgical emergency in the hemolytic uremic syndrome. *Pediatrics, 62*: 54–56 (1972).
22. Swaf, H., Sharp, M. J., Youn, K. J. Ischemic colitis and stricture after hemolytic uremic syndrome. *Pediatrics, 61*: 315–317 (1978).
23. Richardson, S. E., Karmali, M. A., Becker, L. E., Smith, C. R. The histopathology of the hemolytic uremic syndrome associated with verocytotoxin-producing *Escherichia coli* infections. *Human Pathol., 19*: 1102–1108 (1988).

24. Primhak, R. A., Taitz, L. S., Variend, S., Webb, D. H., Cser, A. Necrosis of the pancreas in the haemolytic uremic syndrome. *J. Clin. Pathol.*, *37*: 655–658 (1984).
25. Taylor, C. M., White, R.H.R., Winterborn, M. H., Rowe, B. Haemolytic-uraemic syndrome: clinical experience of an outbreak in the West Midlands. *Br. Med. J.*, *292*: 1513–1516 (1986).
26. Burns, J. C., Berman, E. R., Fagre, J. L., Shikes, R. H., Lum, G. M. Pancreatic islet cell necrosis: association with hemolytic-uremic syndrome. *J. Pediatr*, *100*: 582–584 (1982).
27. Andreoli, S. P., Bergstein, J. M. Development of insulin-dependent diabetes mellitus during the hemolytic-uremic syndrome. *J. Pediatr.*, *100*: 541–545 (1982).
28. Durie, P. R., Gaskin, K. J., Ogilvie, J. E., Smith, C. R., Forstner, G. G., Largman, C. Serial alterations in the forms of immunoreactive pancreatic cationic trypsin in plasma from patients with acute pancreatitis. *J. Pediatr. Gastroenterol.*, *4*: 199–207 (1985).
29. Van Rhijn, A., Donckerwolcke, R. A., Kuijten, R. H., Van Der Heiden, C. Liver damage in the hemolytic uremic syndrome. *Helv. Paediatr. Acta.*, *32*: 77–81 (1977).
30. Jeffrey, G., Kibbler, C. C., Baillod, R., Farrington, K., Morgan, M. Y. Cholestatic jaundice in the hemolytic-uremic syndrome: a case report. *Gut*, *26*: 315–319 (1985).
31. Kawanami, T., Bowden, A'D., Girdany, B. R. Enterocolitis: prodrome of the hemolytic uremic syndrome. *Radiology*, *151*: 91–92 (1984).
32. Kirbs, D. R. The radiology of enteritis due to hemolytic-uremic syndrome. *Pediatr. Radiol.*, *12*: 179–183 (1982).
33. Kavi, J., Rose, P. E. Yersinia and hemolytic uremic syndrome. *Lancet*, *1*: 1224 (letter) (1988).
34. Davenport, A., Finn, R. Haemolytic uraemic syndrome induced by Yersinia pseudotuberculosis. *Lancet*, *1*: 358–359 (letter) (1988).
35. Rongnoparat, C., Panpanit, T. Hemolytic uremic syndrome associated with shigellosis: report of two cases. *S.E. Asian J. Trop. Med. Pub. Health*, *18*: 226–228 (1987).
36. San Joaquin, V. H., Welch, D. F. Campylobacter enteritis. A 3 year experience. *Clin. Pediatr.*, *23*: 311–316 (1984).
37. Maudgil, A., Bhan, M. K., Khoshoo, V. Hemolytic uremic syndrome associated with salmonella typhimurium. *Ind. Pediatr.*, *24*: 608–609 (letter) (1987).
38. Baker, N. M., Mills, A. E., Rachman, I., Thomas, J.P.E. Haemolytic uremic syndrome in typhoid fever. *Br. Med. J.*, *2*: 84–88 (1965).
39. McKnorey, R. E. Jr. Hemolytic uremic syndrome and Entamoeba histolytica infections. *J. Pediatr. Infect. Dis.*, *3*: 371 (letter) (1984).
40. Riccio, J. A., Oberkircher, O. R. Clostridium septicum sepsis and cerebrites: a rare complication of the hemolytic uremic syndrome. *Pediatr. Infect. Dis. J.*, *7*: 342–345 (1988).
41. Bollaert, P. E., Bauer, P., Judlin, P., Laprevote-Heully, M. C., Lambert, H., Larcan, A. Hemorrhagic colitis with streptococcus pyogenes preceding hemolytic uremic syndrome during early pregnancy. *Nephron*, *52*: 103–104 (letter) (1989).
42. O'Regan, S., Robitaille, P., Mongeau, J-G., McLaughlin, M. D. The hemolytic uremic syndrome associated with ECHO 22 infection. *Clin. Pediatr.*, *19*: 125–127 (1980).
43. Vecilla, M. C., Ruiz Moreno, M., Bernacer, M., Casado, Y., Rocandio, L. Coxsackie B-associated hemolytic uremic syndrome in two siblings. *An. Esp. Pediatr.*, *20*: 369–374 (1984).
44. Gianantonio, C. A., Vitacco, M., Mendilaharzu, F. The hemolytic uremic syndrome. *Nephron*, *11*: 174–189 (1973).
45. Glasgow, L. A., Baldizzi, P. Isolation of Coxsackie virus group A4 from a patient with hemolytic-uremic syndrome. *N. Engl. J. Med.*, *273*: 754–756 (1965).
46. Roy, C. G., Tucker, V. L., Harris, D., Cuppage, F. E., Chin, T.D.Y. Enterovirus associated with hemolytic uremic syndrome. *Pediatrics*, *46*: 378–388 (1970).
47. Shashaty, G. C., Atamer, M. A. Hemolytic uremic syndrome associated with infectious mononucleosis. *Am. J. Dis. Child.*, *127*: 720–722 (1974).

48. Levine, M. M., Xu, J. G., Kaper, J. B., Lior, H., Prado, V., Tall, B., Nataro, J., Karch, H., Wachsmuth, K. A DNA probe to identify enterohemorrhagic *Escherichia coli* of O157:H7 and other serotypes that cause hemorrhagic colitis and hemolytic uremic syndrome. *J. Infect. Dis. (USA), 156*: 175–182 (1987).
49. Karmali, M. A., Petric, M., Lim, C., Fleming, P. C., Arbus, G. S., Lior, H. The association between idiopathic hemolytic uremic syndrome and infection by verotoxin-producing *Escherichia coli*. *J. Infect. Dis. (USA), 151*: 775–782 (1985).
50. Cavanagh, J. B., Howard, J. G., Whitley, J. L. The neurotoxin of *Shigella shigae*: a comparative study of the effects produced in various laboratory animals. *Br. J. Exp. Pathol., 37*: 272–278 (1956).
51. Bridgewater, F.A.J., Morgan, R. S., Rowson, K.E.K., Payling Wright, G. The neurotoxin of *Shigella shigae*. Morphologic and functional lesions produced in the central nervous system. *Br. J. Exp. Pathol., 36*: 447–453 (1955).
52. Riley, L. W., Remis, R. S., Helgerson, S. D. Hemorrhagic colitis associated with a rare *Escherichia coli* serotype. *N. Engl. J. Med., 308*: 681–685 (1983).
53. Griffin, P. M., Ostroff, S. M., Tause, R. V., Greene, K. D., Wells, J. G., Lewis, J. H., Blake, P. A. Illnesses associated with *Escherichia coli* O157:H7 infections. A broad clinical spectrum. *Ann. Intern. Med., 109*: 705–712 (1988).
54. Anonymous. Outbreak of bloody diarrhea caused by *E. coli* O157:H7 *Wisc. Epidemiol. Bull., 10*: 1–2 (1988).
55. Spika, J. S., Parsons, J. E., Nordenberg, D., Wells, J. G., Gunn, R. A., Blake, P. A. Hemolytic uremic syndrome and diarrhea associated with *Escherichia coli* O157:H7 in a day care center. *J. Pediatr., 109*: 287–291 (1986).
56. Siegler, R. Hemolytic uremic syndrome during an outbreak of *Escherichia coli* O157:H7 infections in institutions for the mentally retarded: Clinical and epidemiologic observations. J. Pediatr. in press (1989).
57. Leads from MMWR: Hemolytic-uremic syndrome associated with *Escherichia coli* O157:H7 enteric infections—United States, 1984. *J.A.M.A., 253*: 1541 (1985).
58. Levine, M. M. *Escherichia coli* that cause diarrhea: enterotoxigenic, enteropathogenic, enteroinvasive, enterohemorrhagic and enteroadherent. *J. Infect. Dis., 155*: 377–389 (1987).
59. Johnson, W. M., Lior, H., Beganson, G. S. Cytotoxic *Escherichia coli* O157:H7 associated with haemorrhagic colitis in Canada. *Lancet, 1*: 76–79 (1983).
60. Dorn, C. R. Hemorrhagic colitis and hemolytic uremic syndrome caused by *Escherichia coli* in people consuming undercooked beef and unpasteurized milk. *J.A.V.M.A., 193*: 1360–1361 (1988).
61. Scotland, S., Smith, H. R., Rowe, B. Two distinct toxins active on vero cells from *Escherichia coli* O157. *Lancet, 2*: 885–886 (1985).
62. Scotland, S. M., Willshaw, G. A., Smith, H. R. Properties of strains of *Escherichia coli* belonging to serogroup O157 with special reference to production of vero cytotoxins VT1 and VT2 *Epidemiol. Infect., 99*: 613–624 (1987).
63. Strockbine, N. A., Jackson, M. P., Sung, L. M., Holmes, R. K., O'Brien, A. D. Cloning and sequencing of the genes for Shiga toxin from *Shigella dysenteriae* Type I. *J. Bacteriol., 170*: 1116–1122 (1988).
64. Cleary, T. G., Lopez, E. L. The Shiga-like toxin-producing *Escherichia coli* and hemolytic uremic syndrome. *Pediatr. Infect. Dis. J., 8*: 720–724 (1989).
65. Karch, H., Bitzan, M. Purification and characterization of a phage-encoded cytotoxin from an *Escherichia coli* O111 strain associated with the hemolytic uremic syndrome. *Zentralbl. Bakteriol. Mikrobiol. Hyg., [A] 270*: 41–51 (1988).
66. Sherman, P., Soni, R., Karmali, M. Attaching and effacing adherence of vero cytotoxin-producing *Escherichia coli* to rabbit intestinal epithelium in vivo. *Infect. Immun., 56*: 756–761 (1988).

67. Keenan, K. P., Sharpnack, D. D., Collins, H., Formal, S. B., O'Brien, A. D. Morphologic evaluation of the effect of Shiga toxin and *E. coli* Shiga-like toxin on the rabbit intestine. *Am. J. Pathol., 125*: 69–80 (1986).
68. Moyer, M. P., Dixon, P. S., Rothman, S. W., Brown, J. E. Cytotoxicity of Shiga-toxin for primary culture of human colonic and ileal epithelial cells. *Infect. Immun., 55*: 1533–1535 (1987).
69. Strockbine, N. A., Marques, L. R., Newland, J. W., Smith, H. W., Holmes, R. K., O'Brien, A. D. Two toxin converting phages from *Escherichia coli* O157:H7 strain 933 encode antigenically distinct toxins with similar biologic activities. *Infect. Immun., 53*: 135–140 (1987).
70. Barrett, T. J., Potter, M. E., Wachsmoth, I. K. Continuous peritoneal infusion of Shiga-like toxin II (SLT II) as a model for SLT II-induced diseases. *J. Infect. Dis., 159*: 774–777 (1989).
71. Boyd, B., Lingwood, C. Verotoxin receptor glycolipid in human renal tissue. *Nephron, 51*: 207–210 (1989).
72. Kandel, G., Donohue-Rolfe, A., Donowitz, M., Keusch, G. T. Pathogenesis of Shigella diarrhea XVI. Selective targetting of Shiga toxin to villus cells of rabbit jejunum explains the effect of the toxin on intestinal electrolyte transport. *J. Clin. Invest., 84*: 1509–1517 (1989).
73. Delans, R. J., Biuso, J. D., Saba, J. R., Ramirez, G. Hemolytic uremic syndrome after campylobacter-induced diarrhea in an adult. *Arch. Intern. Med., 144*: 1074–1076 (1984).
74. Koster, F., Levin, J., Walker, L. Hemolytic uremic syndrome after shigellosis. Relation to endotoxemia and circulating immune complexes. *N. Engl. J. Med., 298*: 927–933 (1978).
75. Date, A., Raghupathy, P., Jadhan, M., Pereira, S. M., Shastry, J.C.M. Outcome of the hemolytic-uremic syndrome complicating bacillary dysentery. *Ann. Trop. Paediatr., 2*: 1–6 (1982).
76. Badami, G., Srivastava, R. N., Kumar, R., Saraya, A. K. Disseminated intravascular coagulation in post-dysenteric haemolytic uremic syndrome. *Acta. Pediatr. Scand., 76*: 919–922 (1987).
77. Karch, H., Goroncy-Bermes, P., Operkuch, W., Kroll, H-P., O'Brien, A. Subinhibitory concentrations of antibiotics modulate amount of Shiga-like toxin produced by *Escherichia coli*. In *The Influence of Antibiotics on the Host-Parasite Relationship II*. (D. Adam, H. Halin, W. Opterkudi, eds.) Springer, Verlag, Berlin, pp. 239–245 (1985).
78. Ashkenazi, S., Cleary, T. G., Lopez, E., Pickering, L. K. Anticytotoxin-neutralizing antibodies in immune globulin preparations: potential use in hemolytic-uremic syndrome. *J. Pediatr., 113*: 1008–1014 (1988).
79. Keusch, G. T. Shigella infections. *Clin. Gastroenterol., 8*: 645–662 (1979).
80. Allan, A., Keighley, M. R., Thompson, H. Beware of hemolytic uremic syndrome presenting as colorectal disease in adults. Report of two cases. *Dis. Colon Rectum, 32*: 426–428 (1989).
81. Smith, C. D., Schuster, S. R., Gruppe, W. E., Vawter, G. F. Hemolytic-uremic syndrome: A diagnostic and therapeutic dilemma for the surgeon. *J. Pediatr. Surg., 13*: 597–604 (1978).
82. Dolislager, D., Tune, B. The hemolytic-uremic syndrome. *Am. J. Dis. Child, 132*: 55–58 (1978).
83. Kaplan, B. S., Thompson, P. D., de Chadarevian, J. P. The hemolytic-uremic syndrome. *Pediatr. Clin. N. Am., 23*: 761–777 (1977).
84. Trompeter, R. S., Schwartz, R., Chantler, C., Dillon, M. J., Haycock, G. B., Kay, R., Barratt, T. M. Haemolytic-uraemic syndrome: an analysis of prognostic features. *Arch. Dis. Child, 58*: 101–105 (1983).

10
Central Nervous System Involvement in the Hemolytic Uremic Syndrome

Richard L. Siegler *University of Utah School of Medicine, Salt Lake City, Utah*

The importance of central nervous system (CNS) involvement was recognized by Gasser et al. in their original description of the hemolytic uremic syndrome (HUS) in 1955 (1). It has subsequently been noted that the majority of children with HUS show evidence of minor CNS involvement such as irritability, somnolence, behavioral changes, restlessness, ataxia, dizziness, tremors, and twitching (2). Of greater concern is the fact that major CNS dysfunction (e.g., seizures) is also frequent, can be the most serious feature of the syndrome, and is an important determinant of outcome. Moreover, major CNS dysfunction may be the presenting feature of the illness, and late-onset major CNS involvement can occur when other aspects of the illness (e.g., renal failure, anemia, thrombocytopenia) are subsiding.

FREQUENCY AND PRESENTATION

Signs of major CNS dysfunction occur in approximately one third of HUS cases (Table 1). The most common signs are seizures (usually generalized) and severe alterations in consciousness such as stupor and coma. Less frequent signs include hemiparesis, decerebrate or dystonic posturing, cortical blindness, and brain stem involvement (e.g., respiratory dysrhythmia and apnea). Additional, but uncommon CNS findings include delirium, increased muscle tone, hypotonia, clonus, random eye movements, hyperreflexia, diplopia, hallucinations, and choreoathetoid movements.

In the world's largest reported series (2), 41% of 678 patients in Argentina experienced major dysfunction of the central nervous system, including stupor, coma, convulsions, and/or hemiparesis.

Rooney et al. (3) described major CNS disturbance in 13 (52%) of 25 patients from Australia. This included seizures, decerebrate spasms, and transient hemi-

Table 1 Major CNS Dysfunction in HUS

Feature and frequency (%)									
Seizures	Altered consciousness (e.g., coma, semicoma, stupor)	Hemi-paresis	Decerebrate posturing	Cortical blindness	Brain stem	Any major fea-tures	Report (Ref.)	Country	Size of HUS population
44	40	16	16	4	0	52	Rooney, 1971 (3)	Australia	25
35	11	3	0	0	10	41	Gianantonio, 1973 (2)	Argentinia	678
38	21	0	0	0	15	39	Donckerwolcke, 1979[a] (29)	Netherlands	72
40	10	2	3	0	0	49	Bale, 1980[b] (7)	USA	61
31	19	0	0	0	13	32	Bos, 1985 (4)	Netherlands	68
27	6.8	9	4.5	2.3	0	34	Sheth, 1986 (5)	USA	44
23	4.4	1.3	0	1.3	0.4	28	Siegler, 1987 (8)	USA	229
13	15	5.1	3.8	3.6	0	14	Hahn, 1989 (6)	USA	78
31	16	4.6	3.4	1.3	4.8	36			

[a]Some cases may by included in later article by Bos, et al.
[b]Some cases included in later article by Siegler.

plegia. Coma or semicoma occurred in 10; in one infant, coma persisted for 6 weeks.

In a series of 68 patients reported from the Netherlands by Bos et al. (4) 22 of 68 patients (32%) had major CNS involvement. A striking feature was the occurrence of dysregulation of breathing (periodic, atactic, apnea) in nine (13%) of their patients.

Ten (23%) of 44 American children described by Sheth et al. (5) experienced generalized seizures; in two, the seizures were focal. Moreover, seizures were the presenting feature in two patients (4.6%). Hemiparesis was seen in four (9%) children. Less frequent findings were decerebrate posturing, sixth nerve palsy and cortical blindness.

In a more recent report of 78 American children by Hahn et al. (6), CNS involvement was noted in 20%, and 14% were considered to have major CNS dysfunction. Their reported experience included coma, stupor, generalized or focal seizures, hemiplegia, decerebrate posturing, cortical blindness, hallucinations, and dystonic posturing.

Seizures occurred in 40% of 61 consecutive episodes of HUS in 60 patients seen by us from 1972 through 1978 (7). They were generalized in 33% of the cases and focal in 7%. Stupor or coma without seizure activity was seen in an additional 10% of the children. Decerebrate posturing occurred in 3% of the children, and transient hemiparesis in 2%.

In a recent collaborative review of 229 cases of classical childhood HUS seen in 11 medical centers that participate in the Southwest Pediatric Nephrology Study Group (SPNSG), seizures occurred prior to the diagnosis of HUS in 16% of the cases and occasionally were the first recognized feature of the syndrome (8). Coma was present on admission in 8% of the children. Seizures occurred sometime during hospitalization in 23% of the patients; they were seen more frequently in children less than 3 years of age (32%) than in older children (17%). In 83% of the cases they were generalized rather than focal. Additional neurological complications developed in 23 (10%) of the children. Coma occurred in ten. Three developed cortical blindness which persisted for at least one month, but eventually resolved. Three additional children experienced hemiparesis. Other miscellaneous CNS features included motor aphasia, delirium, increased lower extremity motor tone, hypotonia, clonus, random eye movements, hyperreflexia, respiratory dysrhythmia, and apnea. Thirteen of these 23 patients also experienced seizures.

It is curious that CNS involvement sometimes occurs late in the course of HUS after renal involvement and other signs of disease activity are subsiding. Rooney's (3) series included an 8-month-old who developed focal seizures and semicoma 2 months after the onset of HUS. One of the 78 children reported by Hahn et al. (6) was a 4-year-old girl who developed left hemiplegia, facial weakness, and blindness approximately 2 weeks after the onset of HUS. Steinberg et al. (9) reported the onset of focal seizures and expressive aphasia on the twelfth hospital day, about 6 days after the onset of HUS (9). DiMario et al. (10) observed basal ganglia infarction several weeks after the onset of HUS in a child who had recovered and had been discharged from the hospital. One of the patients reported by Trevathan and Dooling (11) developed a large-vessel stroke after renal involvement was subsiding. Rasoulpour et al. (12) described a 4-year-old boy who experienced a cerebrovascular accident during the beginning of the second hospital week, at a time when the child was no longer oliguric, had a serum creatinine of 1.6 mg/dL and had no signs of neurological involvement. Although the initial computerized axial tomography (CAT) scan was normal, a repeat scan 2 days later showed a large infarct in the right basal ganglia. One of the 16 patients with CNS manifestations described by Hahn and associates (6) developed neurological abnormalities secondary to a brain infarct about 2 weeks into her episode of HUS. We have also seen the sudden onset of structural CNS damage in patients who were in the recovery phase of HUS and who were otherwise doing well.

PATHOGENESIS OF CNS DYSFUNCTION

Metabolic Encephalopathy

There is an association between major neurological events and the patient's biochemical status. Bos et al. (4) noted that the average serum sodium concentration was lower in those with severe CNS involvement. They also noted, however, that serum urea values were lower in those with very severe neurological dysfunctions. They speculated that this might have been a reflection of the very rapid evolution of CNS involvement with death occurring before there had been time for advanced azotemia to develop.

In the series of 44 children reported by Sheth et al. (5), there were no significant differences in the admission laboratory values for serum sodium, total CO_2 content, serum calcium, plasma osmolality, or BUN between those with and without CNS dysfunction. However, the serum creatinine concentration was higher. When the most abnormal (i.e., extreme) laboratory values during hospitalization were compared, children with CNS dysfunction had significantly lower total CO_2 contents, lower serum calcium levels, and higher serum creatinine concentrations.

In an outbreak of HUS in the West Midlands of Great Britain, 12 of 35 children experienced seizures; in two cases; seizures occurred before admission to hospital (13). All but one child, who presumably had CNS vasculopathy, were severely hyponatremic (i.e., less than 126 mEq/L) at the time of the seizure. It was noted that hyponatremia resulted from intravenous rehydration with hypotonic saline solution (13).

Our experience (7) with our first 61 cases (1972–1978) revealed that potential immediate metabolic causes were present in more than half the children who developed severe CNS symptoms. Hyponatremia (serum sodium concentration less than 130 mEq/L) and/or aggressive hydration with hypotonic fluids were associated temporally with seizures or altered consciousness in 17 children. An additional 10 children had hypocalcemia (calcium less than 8 mg/dL). Moreover, children with seizures and/or coma were more likely to have a BUN above 100 mg/dL; 80% of children with severe CNS findings required dialysis in contrast to only 29% of those without CNS involvement. None of our patients had hypertensive encephalopathy or hypoglycemia. We therefore concluded that a combination of metabolic abnormalities was probably responsible for the encephalopathy in most of our patients.

CNS Thrombotic Microangiopathy

While the thrombotic microangiopathy (TMA) of HUS always involves the microvasculature of the kidney, extrarenal TMA can also occur. It has become easier to recognize CNS structural damage with the introduction of CAT scans and magnetic resonance imaging (MRI). With perhaps even more sensitive instrumentation such as positron emission tomography (PET) (14) and single positron emission computed tomography (SPECT) (15), it might be possible to detect abnormalities in regional blood flow or metabolism that occur in the absence of structural changes. Functional abnormalities of this nature would offer an explanation for severe encephalopathy that occurs in the absence of severe hypertension, metabolic derangement, or structural damage as detected by CAT or MRI.

In 1981, we described two children (16) who developed ischemic (pale) cerebral infarctions with delayed hemorrhage (Fig. 1, a & b). There have subsequently been several other reports of CNS structural damage documented by CAT (5, 6, 9, 11, 12, 17) or MRI (10). Areas of involvement have included the frontal-parietal cortex, sylvian area, visual cortex, basal ganglia (e.g., caudate and lentiform nuclei), and cerebellum. Since then, we have seen seven additional patients who experienced cerebral infarctions documented by CAT scan or MRI. This represents an overall frequency of 3.9% (nine out of 230 cases of HUS).

Infarction may initially be undetectable if the CAT scan is obtained soon after the onset of dysfunction (e.g., hemiparesis). This may be particularly true of small lacunar infarcts resulting from the occlusion of small penetrating branches of large cerebral vessels (10). It has been our experience that MRI is more sensitive than CAT scan in identifying small lesions.

While the CNS vasculopathy usually involves the microcirculation (TMA), Trevathan et al. (11) focused attention on large-vessel thrombosis—that is, stroke in the distribution of the large branches of the anterior and middle cerebral arteries. Similar examples are probably contained in the reports of Mendelsohn et al. (17) and Hahn et al. (6).

Children experiencing infarction generally exhibit one or more of a combination of paresis, seizures, decorticate or decerebrate posturing, extensor plantar responses, blindness, coma, or evidence of brain stem involvement (e.g., breathing abnormalities).

When cerebral infarction occurs, it presumably results from the same type of TMA that involves the renal vasculature. In this context, it is interesting that the administration of exotoxin-producing *Shigella shigae* to rabbits causes neurotoxicity by damaging the endothelium of the small blood vessels in the neuraxis, rather than by attacking the nerve cells (19). Tzipori et al. (20) administered *Escherichia coli* O157:H7 (an organism that produces Shiga-like toxin), isolated from a 20-month-old infant who had succumbed to HUS, to piglets. It was administered orally to six and intraperitoneally to four. Three of the six piglets who received the inoculant orally developed neurological abnormalities including incoordination, staggering gate leading to complete ataxia, paralysis, and recumbency. Once the neurological symptoms occurred, the piglets experienced rapid deterioration. Similar CNS complications developed in the four piglets who were inoculated intraperitoneally with bacterial lysates (i.e., following treatment of *E. coli* O157:H7 with polymyxin B). When the brains were examined, they were diffusely edematous and had areas of cerebellar hemorrhagic infarction. A few of the capillaries were occluded with fibrin. It is therefore tempting to theorize that, in classical, postdiarrhea childhood HUS, absorption of enteric bacterial toxin (e.g., Shiga-like toxin) is responsible for the TMA, irrespective of whether it occurs in the kidney or elsewhere (e.g., CNS). It is difficult, however, to reconcile this hypothesis with late-onset CNS involvement in patients who have already recovered from hemorrhagic colitis.

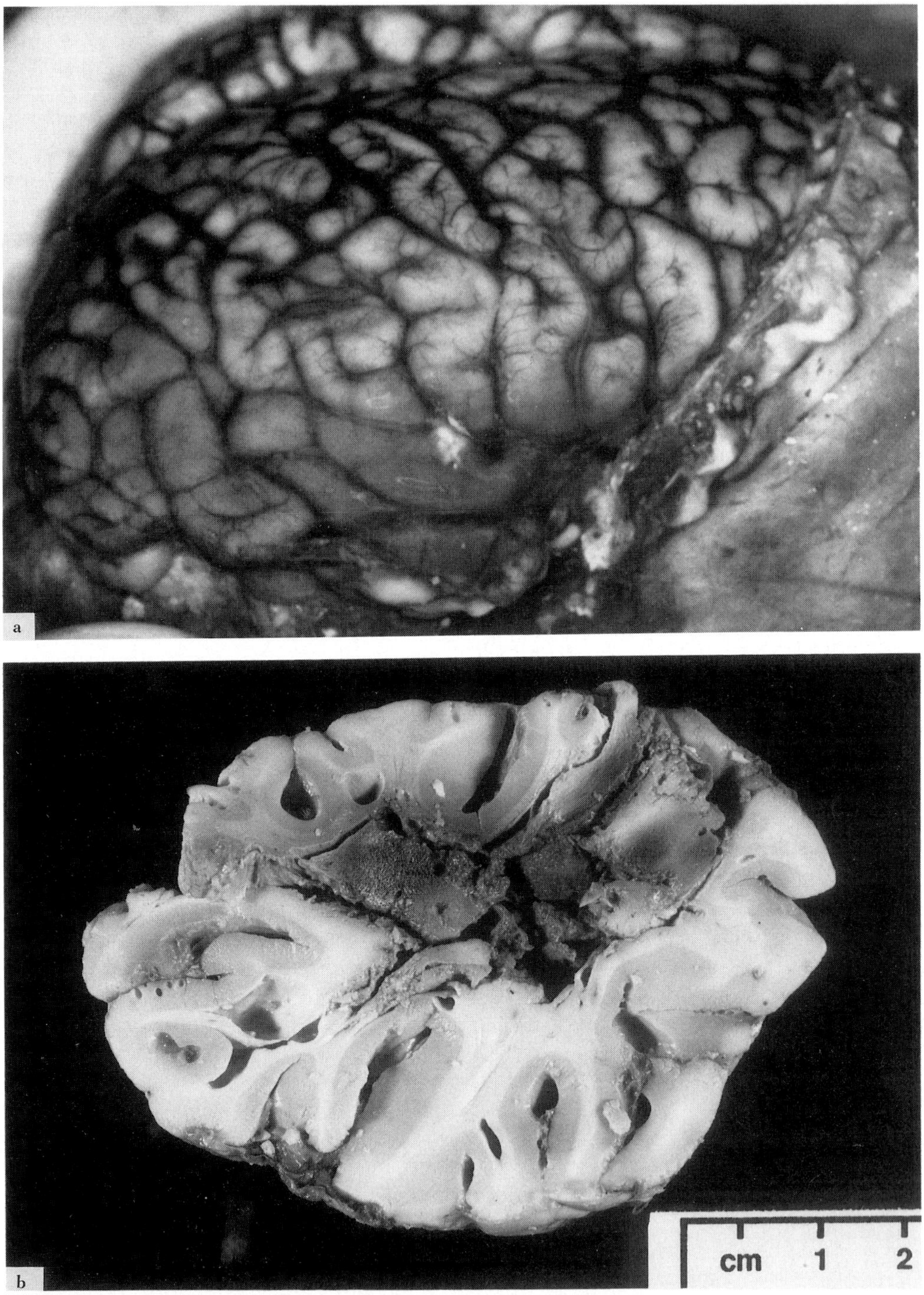

Figure 1 (a) Gross photograph showing marked cerebral edema evidenced by hemispheric gyral flattening, deepened sulci and meningeal congestion (Brain wt = 1,340 g (970–1,059 g expected for age). **Figure 1 (b)** Gross photograph of formalin fixed brain section demonstrating acute parenchymal hemorrhage and necrosis of right parieto-occipital cortex, and internal capsule. Microangiopathy with intra-ateriolar and capillary fibrin microthrombi were found on light and immunofluorescence microscopy. (Courtesy of O. M. Faye-Petersen, M.D., Salt Lake City, Utah.)

NEUROPATHOLOGY

Upadhyaya et al. (21) focused attention on the importance of nonrenal involvement by describing the histopathology of tissue from three fatal cases of HUS. While all three children had clinical signs of severe CNS involvement, CNS microthrombi were found in only two. All three however, showed focal areas of cerebral cortex infarction surrounded by edema. Similar findings were found in the basal ganglia of one patient. Rooney et al. (3) usually found no evidence of brain vessel thrombi in a series of seven fatal cases. Their experience included two children who died within 24 and 72 hours. Thrombi were present in the renal vasculature. They did find areas of anoxic damage, hemorrhage, and infarcts in a variety of CNS regions including the parietal, temporal, and occipital cortex, internal capsule, basal ganglia, and cerebellum.

In a recent clinicopathological study of 24 children conducted by the Southwest Pediatric Nephrology Study Group (SPNSG), the brain was examined in nine children who came to autopsy (22). Cerebral thrombi were found in three; each of the three had experienced seizures.

Bos et al. (4) examined the brains of five patients who came to autopsy. One patient had microthrombi in the medulla oblongata, putamen, internal capsule, and cerebral cortex. Brain stem microthrombi were found in another patient. There was no mention of microthrombi in the brain tissue of the other three patients, but cerebral edema was found in all specimens.

Examination of the brain in three of five patients who died in the series reported by Hahn et al. (6) showed extensive cerebral edema with cerebellar tonsillar and tentorial herniations. They also found a combination of anoxic damage, hemorrhagic infarction, and necrosis involving the basal ganglia, internal capsule, pons, anterior thalamus, amygdala, hippocampus, insular cortex, and forebrain. No small- or large-vessel thrombi were noted in any of the cases.

Therefore, while it is tempting to assume that all CNS structural damage in HUS is the result of TMA, histopathological studies have often failed to show evidence of TMA in cases of histologically abnormal brain tissue.

Figure 1 illustrates severe cerebral edema (A), and hemorrhage and necrosis (B) in a 2-year-old with HUS who died suddenly on the third day of hospitalization.

DIAGNOSTIC TESTS

With the widespread availability of modern CNS imaging techniques (e.g., CAT, MRI) there are few reasons to rely on less sensitive and nonspecific tests like the lumbar puncture (LP) and electroencephalogram (EEG) to diagnose structural brain damage.

Lumbar Puncture (LP)

Both pleocytosis and elevated cerebrospinal fluid (CSF) protein concentrations have been described. In Rooney's 1971 report (3) of 13 patients who had severe CNS dysfunction, the CSF was examined in three. One patient had increased numbers of cells but normal protein and sugar concentrations. Subsequent examination of the brain revealed a cerebral infarct. Another patient had an elevated CSF protein concentration.

Sheth et al. (5) desccribed the CSF findings of 11 patients who experienced major CNS dysfunction. Four had increased protein levels and one showed evidence of hemorrhage. The cell counts and glucose levels were normal in all cases.

In our 1980 report (7), the cerebrospinal fluid was examined in 19 of 30 children who had severe CNS findings. The glucose concentrations were normal and there was no pleocytosis. Two of the 19 children had elevated CSF protein concentrations (i.e., >50 mg/dL). One of these two died and the other was left with cortical blindness.

Since generalized cerebral edema and, occasionally, herniation are seen in fatal cases that come to autopsy, it may no longer be prudent to perform a LP without first excluding cerebral edema with a CAT scan or MRI. Moreover, lack of sensitivity and specificity in identifying structural damage also limits the usefulness of a LP. We therefore no longer do a LP, except on rare occasions when it is necessary to exclude an infectious cause of the CNS manifestations.

Electroencephalogram (EEG)

EEGs generally show slow wave and/or epileptiform activity. Rooney described EEG findings in eight of 13 patients who had severe CNS dysfunction (3). Excess slow wave activity was noted in five.

The EEGs were abnormal in all nine patients studied by Sheth et al. (5). Seven had diffuse slowing suggestive of metabolic encephalopathy, whereas two had focal or multifocal seizure spikes.

We obtained EEGs in 11 of 30 children with severe encephalopathy (7). There was diffuse slowing in nine, and three showed epileptiform or sharp wave discharges. One child, who died within 48 hours from the onset of HUS, had an isoelectric tracing.

CAT Scan

CAT scan has become the usual method of looking for evidence of structural damage in patients who show signs of severe neurological dysfunction, especially with focal findings such as hemiparesis. It is also a reasonable study in patients who become comatose with or without decerebrate or decorticate posturing. We described two young children (16) who initially showed hypodense areas of infarction that later progressed to hemorrhagic infarction (Fig. 2). Quinet et al. (18) reported infarction in the sylvian area of an 8-month-old female. Mendelsohn et al. (17) described extensive bilateral frontal and parietal hypodensities. A follow-up study showed dilation of the ventricles and eventually cerebral atrophy with subcortical white matter demyelination. A report of Rasoulpour et al. (12) described a large area of infarction in the right basal ganglia of a 4-year-old boy. Steinberg et al. (9) detailed CAT scan evidence of moderate cortical atrophy associated with two areas of infarction in the left parietal and frontal areas of a female aged 2.5 years. Sheth et al. (5) described cerebral vascular abnormalities in four of 14 patients (5). Trevathan and Dooling (11) focused attention on CAT evidence of large-vessel stroke in three patients. Hahn et al. (6) included a detailed report of three children who developed severe CNS involvement with CAT evidence of multiple CNS infarcts.

It is noteworthy that CAT scans initially may be normal in patients who exhibit severe focal neurological findings (6, 10, 12). Moreover, scans that first show

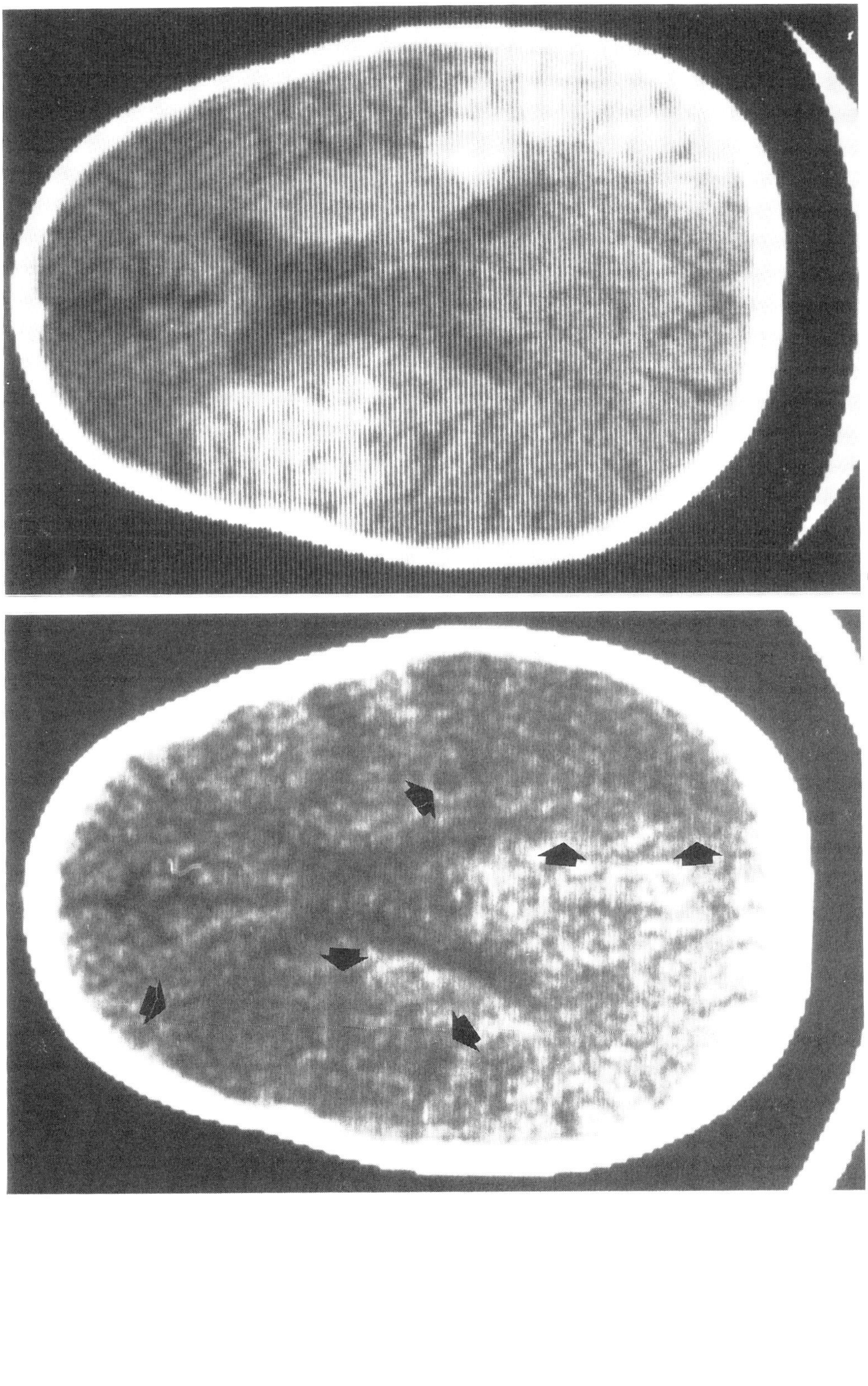

A B

Figure 2 CAT scans (unenhanced), Patient 1. *A*, The initial study showed hypodense areas of infarction in the left frontal and right parietal-occipital areas (arrows). *B*, Scan two weeks later showed hemorrhage in these areas. (Courtesy of Journal of Pediatrics, The C. V. Mosby Company.)

hypodense areas (i.e., pale infarction), may later demonstrate hemorrhage into the same areas (16).

Additional findings occasionally seen on CAT scan include cerebral atrophy, dilated ventricles, subcortical white matter demyelination, and diffuse leukomalacia (17).

While we have usually used unenhanced scans in oliguric patients, enhanced studies have been performed in oliguric patients who are undergoing peritoneal dialysis (17).

Magnetic Resonance Imaging (MRI)

MRI is a sensitive procedure for detecting structural CNS damage. While we have not systematically compared the sensitivity and specificity of CAT scans with MRI, and while reports of MRI in HUS encephalopathy are limited (10), it has been our impression that MRI is more sensitive for the early detection of structural lesions. DiMario et al. (10) described a lacunar infarct resulting from occlusion of small penetrating branches of the middle cerebral, basilar, and upper vertebral arteries. They stressed that small lacunar infarcts, which may not be demonstrable by CAT scan for weeks after onset, may be detectable by MRI. Figure 3 illustrates MRI findings in one of our patients who sustained severe CNS damage.

Miscellaneous Studies

While we have had no experience with radionuclide brain scans in HUS patients, Sheth et al. (5) described patchy abnormal nuclide accumulation in two of five patients who exhibited severe neurological involvement.

Sheth et al. (5) also described decreased amplitude and increase latency in four patients studied with flashed visual evoked potentials and slow conduction in two of four patients studied by brain stem auditory evoked potentials.

The only report of transcranial doppler study in HUS is by Trevathan and Dooling (11). They found it helpful in a patient who had CAT evidence of large-vessel stroke by showing no flow in the left middle and anterior cerebral arteries, as well as low peak velocities and blunted wave form in the same vessels on the contralateral side. On autopsy, large-vessel thrombi with associated infarctions were found in the cerebral vasculature. Doppler studies may therefore be useful in children who are developing large-vessel strokes.

Even though there have not yet been reports of positron emission tomography (PET) or single position emission computed tomography (SPECT) in HUS patients, it should be useful in detecting functional impairment (decreases in regional flow or metabolism) that might precede, or even occur in the absence of detectable structural abnormalities as seen by CAT or MRI (14, 15). In adult patients with classical stroke, for example, there is a reduction in oxygen metabolism, as detectable with PET, that precedes low attenuation (i.e., infarction) on CAT scan (14).

TREATMENT

Preventive and Prophylactic Measures

Given the strong association between hyponatremia and seizures in HUS patients (4, 5, 7, 13), it is important to refrain from the routine use of hyponatremic intravenous

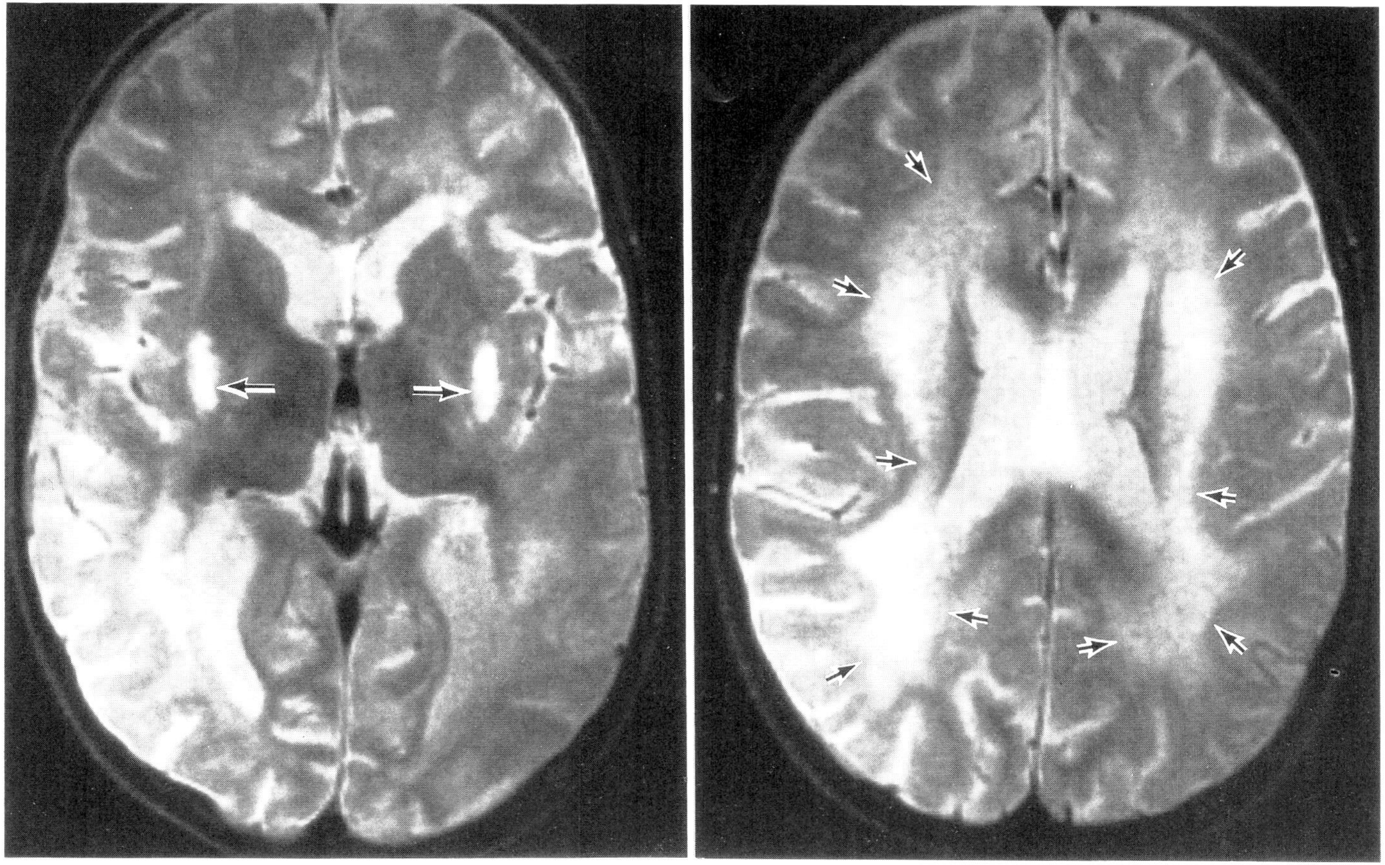

(A) (B)

Figure 3 Axial heavily T2-weighted brain MR scan images at the level of the basal ganglia (A) and the upper ventricle-centrum semiovale region (B). The scan images show focal areas of increased signal symmetrically in the lateral basal ganglia region, probably the putamina (arrows - image A) and in the periventricular and centrum semiovale white matter (arrows - image B). The findings indicate increased water content at these sites indicative of gliosis, edema and/or demyelination, secondary to previous vascular insult. No evidence of hemorrhage is seen. Also noted is mild enlargement of the ventricles and extraaxial CSF spaces, most likely secondary to brain shrinkage related to the patient's primary disease. (Courtesy of Richard S. Boyer, M.D., Pediatric Medical Imaging Department, Primary Children's Medical Center, Salt Lake City, Utah.)

repletion fluids in children who might be in the prodromal phase of HUS. This admonition is particularly relevant in treating dehydrated children with hemorrhagic colitis. Infusing hyponatremic repletion fluids (e.g., 0.2%–0.5% normal saline) to children developing oliguric renal failure may cause a fall in the serum sodium concentration. Furthermore, administering "boluses" of hyponatremic fluids, as "fluid challenges" to oliguric children experiencing early HUS renal failure, will also cause hyponatremia. Once dehydration has been appropriately treated, meticulous attention must be paid to salt and water balance. Care must be taken to replace ongoing losses with fluid of similar volume and composition. This approach should decrease the likelihood of a metabolic encephalopathy.

Early initiation of dialysis (e.g., before the BUN exceeds 100–150 mg/dL) and prompt control of severe hypertension may also decrease the likelihood of encephalopathy and seizures. It has been our practice to administer intravenous (IV) Dilantin® (phenytoin) prophylactically to children exhibiting frequent muscular twitching. In our experience, this sign of increased neuromuscular irritability often precedes seizures. We customarily treat hypertension with sublingual or oral nifedipine if the patient is alert. IV Hyperstat ® (diazoxide) is used in children with altered consciousness.

Seizure Control

For immediate control of seizures, we usually administer IV Valium® (diazepam) in a loading dosage of 0.1–0.2 mg/kg or IV Ativan® (lorazepam) in a dose of 0.05–0.25 mg/kg. If seizures persist or recur, we give IV Dilantin® (phenytoin) in a loading dose of 10–20 mg/kg. It is necessary to measure "free" phenytoin concentrations when using the drug in azotemic children, as decreased protein binding in azotemia increases the percentage of total phenytoin that is "free" (i.e., metabolically active). We initially give a dose of 10 mg/kg of body weight, followed by one, or occasionally two additional infusions of 5 mg/kg as needed. Since a total dose of 20 mg/kg may cause toxicity in these children, it is advisable to measure the "free" phenytoin concentration before administering a total of more than 10 mg/kg, or at the most 15 mg/kg. A normal maintenance dose can usually be used.

Intravenous phenobarbital (15–25 mg/kg loading dose) is also effective. Because of the risk of respiratory depression, it should not be given in conjunction with IV benzodiazepams (e.g., diazepam) unless one is prepared to support ventilation mechanically.

While the seizures usually occur early in the disease and generally are brief and easy to control, children may, on rare occasions, develop status epilepticus and require high doses of anticonvulsants (e.g., continuous IV infusion of pentobarbital with concurrent mechanical ventilatory support). In the absence of recurrent seizures or structural CNS damage (e.g., infarction) we generally discontinue anticonvulsants prior to discharge from the hospital.

Breathing Abnormalities

Children with brain stem involvement often experience dysrhythmic breathing (e.g., periodic breathing or apneic attacks). Bos et al. (4) reported that nine of 22 patients with major neurological symptoms developed dysregulation of breathing. Eight were also comatose and had generalized seizures that were difficult to control. Eight of the nine patients died, even though all had been intubated, placed on mechanical ventilation, and had frequent analysis of arterial blood gases. Therefore, even though this subset of patients has a high mortality rate with the best of care, prompt intubation and mechanical ventilation offer the best chance for survival.

Miscellaneous and Innovative Treatments

When treating children exhibiting life-threatening CNS involvement, one is tempted to utilize unproven treatments. There is no convincing evidence, however, that anticoagulant, antiplatelet, or fibrinolytic therapy is useful in treating any of the features of HUS. Given our experience with pale CNS infarction progressing to hemorrhagic stroke (7), the use of any of these drugs might be risky in patients with cerebral infarction. A possible exception might be children with evolving large-vessel stroke. There is some suggestion, based on experience with cerebrovascular accidents in adults without HUS, that short-term anticoagulation with heparin might be beneficial early in evolving large-vessel stroke if the neurological deficit is still small and is fluctuating or progressing (23). At the present time, however, except perhaps as part of approved controlled trials, it seems prudent to avoid using drugs that impair coagulation or platelet function, or increase fibrinolysis.

Although there were initially a number of anecdotal reports suggesting benefit from fresh frozen plasma (FFP) infusions, more recent controlled prospective studies have been unable to confirm a long-term benefit (24, 25). The same can be said of other innovative treatments such as antioxidants and intravenous immune globulin. Therefore, if one elects to use these, it must be done with the understanding that they are of unproven value and are not without risk (26–28).

If future technological advances (e.g., SPECT, PET) are able to demonstrate that brain tissue is ischemic but still viable, then decreasing metabolic needs by administering anesthetics or drugs that block CNS receptors might someday be helpful (14).

NATURAL HISTORY

There is no evidence that minor CNS dysfunction, which is present to some extent in almost all patients, predicts outcome. There is compelling evidence, however, that major CNS involvement, at least when secondary to structural CNS damage, is a major predictor of outcome. It is noteworthy (3–7) that severe CNS involvement is a feature of almost all fatal cases (Table 2), and that a substantial percentage of survivors (2, 4–7, 30) are left with neurological sequelae (Table 3).

In the report by Rooney et al. (3), nine of 13 patients (69%) with severe CNS dysfunction died. This contrasted to a death rate of 17% in those who did not have severe CNS involvement. Death occurred in nine of the 10 children who had coma, hemiplegia, or decerebrate spasms, while the three who had convulsions as the only manifestation of neurological dysfunction recovered.

Donckerwolcke et al. (29), in a series of 72 patients treated in the Netherlands, reported a mortality of only 4% in those without CNS involvement. The mortality rate rose to 36%, however, in those with seizures and/or coma. A very high mortality rate (73%) was found in those with brain stem involvement.

Bos and Donckerwolcke (4), who detailed their experience with 22 of 68 HUS patients who had CNS involvement, focused on a subset of nine (13%) who ex-

Table 2 Acute Mortality (%)

With severe CNS involvement	Without severe CNS involvement	Report (Ref.)
69[a]	17	Rooney, 1971 (3)
74[b]	—	Gianantonio, 1973 (2)
36[c]	4	Dockerwolke, 1979 (29)
15	0	Bale, 1980 (7)
14[d]	0	Bos, 1985 (4)
20	0	Sheth, 1986 (5)
29	0	Siegler, 1987 (8)
45	0	Hahn, 1989 (6)
38		

[a]Mortality was 90% (9/10) in those with very severe CNS involvement (hemiparesis, coma, decerebrate spasms).
[b]Very severe CNS damage. Acute mortality in those free of CNS involvement not mentioned.
[c]Mortality 73% with brain stem involvement. Some of these patients may be included in later article by Bos, Donckerwolke, et al.
[d]Mortality 89% with bran stem involvement.

perienced dysregulation of breathing (4). Eight (89%) expired despite aggressive ventilatory support.

In a report of 15 consecutive cases of HUS by Upadhyaya et al. (21), all three of the fatal cases had severe CNS involvement, and two of the three deaths were directly due to brain damage (i.e., cessation of brain function).

Sheth et al. (5) reported severe neurological involvement in 15 of 44 patients. Three of the 15 expired, and neurological sequelae were noted in half of the survivors. Therefore, nine of 15 (60%) with severe CNS dysfunction either died or had chronic neurological sequelae. Survival was 100% in those who escaped CNS involvement.

In the report of Hahn et al. (6), death occurred in five of 78 children (6.4%) treated for HUS at Boston Children's Hospital from 1976–1986. All five who died had major CNS involvement. These five deaths occurred among a group of 11 patients

Table 3 Neurological Sequelae (%)

In survivors with major CNS involvement during acute phase of HUS	In total HUS population	Report (Ref.)
5.8	2.4	Gianantonio, 1973 (2)
10	5	Bale, 1980 (7)
23	7.4	Bos, 1985 (4)
40	14	Sheth, 1986 (5)
55	7.7	Hahn, 1989 (6)
27	7.3	

who had major CNS dysfunction. The surviving six children had persistent neurological dysfunction at discharge that included hemiparesis, altered consciousness, cortical blindness, or dystonic posturing.

One half of the 60 patients seen by us from 1972–1978 (7) had major CNS dysfunction. Although seizures occurred in 40% of the children during the acute phase of the disease, they were not by themselves predictive of death or CNS sequelae. All of the children, however, who died or sustained permanent CNS damage experienced severe CNS dysfunction during the acute phase of the illness. In addition, coma on admission in five patients predicted a poor outcome. There were two deaths in this group, and the remaining three were left with severe CNS sequelae. Moreover, an elevated CSF protein concentration (greater than 50 mg/dL) was also a predictor of poor outcome, as one of the two with elevated CSF protein died and the other was left cortically blind.

In a recent review of the collective experience (229 cases) of the Southwest Pediatric Nephrology Study Group (8), CNS involvement and hypertension were present in each of the eight patients who died. The CNS disturbances included seizures, coma, and hemiparesis. At least two of these three neurological signs were present in five of the eight fatal cases.

The presence of CNS involvement during the acute phase of HUS also predicts nonneurological sequelae. Sheth et al. (5) noted that those with neurological involvement had a higher prevalence of residual hypertension (49% versus 11%) and chronic renal damage (40% vs. 3.5%). In a recent long-term follow-up study of 61 patients conducted by us (30), the presence of seizures during the acute phase of HUS increased the chances that proteinuria or impaired creatinine clearance would be found at follow-up (average interval since HUS 9.6 years) from 17%–71%, and 17%–64%, respectively (relative risk 4.2 and 3.8, respectively).

Although children who sustain structural CNS damage during the acute phase of HUS may certainly be left with severe and persistent neurological impairment (5–7, 17), there is tremendous potential for improvement and recovery. Quinet et al. (18) reported the case of a 9-month-old girl who showed substantial improvement 3 years after a large brain infarction that resulted in hemiplegia and coma that had lasted for 3 months (18). Steinberg et al. (9) described the case of a 2.5-year-old who had two large infarctions in the parietal and frontal areas which resulted in hemiplegia, expressive aphasia, and moderate cortical atrophy. One year later she had only mild residual hemiparesis. Our personal experience with eight children who survived structural CNS damage (i.e., stroke) is also encouraging. All improved, and five of the eight (63%) had complete or nearly complete recoveries.

REFERENCES

1. Gasser, V. C., Gautier, E., Steck, A., Siebenmann, R. E., Oechslin, R. Hamolytisch-uramische syndrome: Bilaterale nierenrindennekrosen bei akuten erworbenen hamolytischen anamien. *Schweiz. Med. Wochenschr.*, *85*: 905–909 (1955).
2. Gianantonio, C. A., Vitacco, M., Mendilaharzu, F., Gallo, G. E., Sojo, E. T. The hemolytic-uremic syndrome. *Nephron.*, *11*: 174–192 (1973).
3. Rooney, J. C., Anderson, R. McD., and Hopkins, I. J. Clinical and pathologic aspects of central nervous system involvement in the haemolytic uraemic syndrome. *Proc. Aust. Assoc. Neurol.*, *8*: 67–75 (1971).
4. Bos, A. P., Donckerwolcke, R. A., van Vught, A. J. The hemolytic-uremic syndrome:

prognostic significance of neurological abnormalities. *Helv. Paediatr. Acta., 40*: 381–389 (1985).

5. Sheth, K. J., Swick, H. M., Haworth, N. Neurological involvement in hemolytic-uremic syndrome. *Ann. Neurol., 19*: 90–93 (1986).
6. Hahn, J. S., Havens, P. L., Higgins, J. J., O'Rourke, P. P., Estroff, J. A., Strand, R. Neurological complications of hemolytic-uremic syndrome. *J. Child Neurol., 4*: 108–113 (1989).
7. Bale J. F. Jr., Brasher, C., Siegler, R. L. CNS manifestations of the hemolytic-uremic syndrome. *Am. J. Dis. Child, 134*: 869–872 (1980).
8. Siegler, R. L., Wenzel, J., Berry, P., Argyle, C., Silva, G., Hogg, R. A review of 229 children with hemolytic uremic syndrome comparing cases from high and low incidence regions. (unpublished observations).
9. Steinberg, A., Ish-Horowitcz, M., El-Peleg, O., Mor, J., Branski, D. Stroke in a patient with hemolytic-uremic syndrome with a good outcome. *Brain Dev., 8*: 70–72 (1986).
10. DiMario, F. J. Jr., Bronte-Stewart, H., Sherbotie, J., Turner, M. E. Lacunar infarction of the basal ganglia as a complication of hemolytic-uremic syndrome. *Clin. Pediatr., 26*: 586–590 (1987).
11. Trevathan, E., Dooling, E. C. Large thrombotic strokes in hemolytic-uremic syndrome. *J. Pediatr., 3*: 863–866 (1987).
12. Rasoulpour, A., Leichtner, A., San Jorge, M., Hyams, J. Cerebral vascular accident during the recovery phase of hemolytic uremic syndrome. *Int. J. Pediatr. Nephrol., 6*: 287–288 (1985).
13. Taylor, C. M., White, R.H.R., Winterborn, M. H., Rowe, R. Haemolytic-uraemic syndrome: clinical experience of an outbreak in the west midlands. *Br. Med. J., 292*: 1513–1516 (1986).
14. Council on Scientific Affairs. Jacobson, H. G. (section editor). Positron emission tomography—A new approach to brain chemistry. *J.A.M.A., 260*: 2704–2710 (1988).
15. Podreka, I., Suess, E., Goldenberg, G., Steiner, M., Brucke, T., Muller, Ch., Lang, W., Neirinckx, R. D., Deecke, L. Initial experience with technetium-99m HM-PAO brain SPECT. *J. Nucl. Med., 28*: 1657–1666 (1987).
16. Crisp, D. E., Siegler, R. L., Bale, J. F., Thompson, J. A. Hemorrhagic cerebral infarction in the hemolytic-uremic syndrome. *J. Pediatr., 99*: 273–276 (1981).
17. Mendelsohn D. B., Hertzanu, Y., Chaitowitz, B., Cartwright, J. D. Cranial CT in the haemolytic uraemic syndrome. *J. Neurol. Neurosurg. Psychiatri., 47*: 876–878 (1984).
18. Quinet, B., Bensman, A., Mathe, J. C., Berger, J. P., Costil, J. Ramollissement cerebral etendu au cours d'un syndrome hemolytique et uremique. *Arch. Fr. Pediatr., 41*: 55–56 (1984).
19. Cavanagh, J. B., Howard, J. G., Whitby, J. L. The neurotoxin of shigella shigae. The comparative study of the effects produced in various laboratory animals. *Br. J. Exp. Pathol., 37*: 272–278 (1956).
20. Tzipori, S., Chow, C. W., Powell, H. R. Cerebral infection with *Escherichia coli* O157:H7 in humans and gnotobiotic piglets. *J. Clin. Pathol., 41*: 1099–1103 (1988).
21. Upadhyaya, K., Barwick, K., Fishaut, M., Kashgarian, M., Siegel, N. J. The importance of nonrenal involvement in hemolytic-uremic syndrome. *Pediatrics, 65*: 115–120 (1980).
22. Argyle, J. C., Hogg, R. J., Pysher, T. J., Silva, F. G., Siegler, R. L. *Pediatr. Nephrol., 4*: 52–58 (1990).
23. Kistler, J. P., Ropper, A. H., Heros, R. C. Therapy of ischemic cerebral vascular disease due to atherothrombosis. *N. Engl. J. Med., 311*: 27–34 (1984).
24. Rizzoni, G., Claris-Appiani, A., Edefonti, A., Facchin, P., Franchini, F., Gusmano, R., Imbasciati, E., Pavanello, L., Perfumo, F., Remuzzi, G. Plasma infusion for hemolytic-uremic syndrome in children: Results of a multicenter controlled trial. *J. Pediatr., 112*: 284–290 (1988).

25. Loirat, C., Sonsino, E., Hinglais, N., Jais, J. P., Landais, P., Fermanian, J. Treatment of the childhood haemolytic uraemic syndrome with plasma. *Pediatr. Nephrol.*, *2*: 279–285 (1988).
26. Eddy, A. A., Geary, D. F., Balfe, J. W., Clark, W. F., Baumal, R. Prolongation of acute renal failure in two patients with haemolytic-uremic syndrome due to excessive plasma infusion therapy. *Pediatr. Nephrol.*, *3*: 420–423 (1989).
27. Cole, B. R. Plasma infusion therapy in hemolytic uremic syndrome: is it warranted? *Pediatr. Nephrol.*, *2*: 286–287 (1988).
28. Siegler, R. L. Management of hemolytic-uremic syndrome. *J. Pediatr.*, *112*: 1014–1020 (1988).
29. Donckerwolcke, R. A., Kuijten, R. H., Tiddens, H. A., van Gool, J. D. Haemolytic uraemic syndrome. *Paediatrician*, *8*: 378–393 (1979).
30. Siegler, R. L., Milligan, M. K., Burningham, T. H., Christofferson, R. D., Chang, S-Y., Jorde, L. B. Long-term outcome and prognostic indicators in the hemolytic uremic syndrome. *J. Pediatr.* *118*: 195–200 (1991).

11
Pancreatic Involvement in the Hemolytic Uremic Syndrome

Sharon Phillips Andreoli *Indiana University Medical Center, Indianapolis, Indiana*

Although the kidney is the organ most commonly affected in the hemolytic uremic syndrome (HUS), evidence of gastrointestinal, central nervous system, pancreatic, skeletal, and myocardial involvement may also be present (1–9). Technical advances in dialysis therapy and better supportive care have resulted in a dramatic reduction in the acute mortality of HUS so that multiple nonrenal manifestations are now recognized. The pancreas, in particular the pancreatic islets, may be involved in the microangiopathic process, resulting in transient or permanent insulin dependent diabetes mellitus (6, 10–13). In some cases, severe pancreatic disease results in pancreatic endocrine and exocrine necrosis (14).

INCIDENCE

Although the precise incidence of pancreatic involvement is unknown, studies of larger series suggest that fewer than ten percent of patients with HUS develop clinically recognizable pancreatic involvement as manifested by glucose intolerance (6, 8). Of 61 children with HUS seen at our hospital over a 12-year interval, four demonstrated pancreatic islet cell involvement as manifested by insulin-dependent diabetes mellitus during the acute phase (Table 1). When carbohydrate intolerance was first recognized as a complication of HUS, we then noted an incidence of three out of 20 children (6). However, of 41 children with HUS seen since our original report, only one has developed glucose intolerance suggesting that the incidence of pancreatic involvement is variable. A similar trend was seen in the West Midlands; during an epidemic in 1982–1983, two of 35 children developed insulin-dependent diabetes mellitus (8). The incidence of extrarenal disease in that epidemic was higher than had been seen in the previous 13 years. In a recent study of 24 children with severe HUS, hyperglycemia was noted in two of nine children who died;

Table 1 Clinical, Biochemical, and Pathological Features of Children with Insulin-Dependent Diabetes Mellitus as a Result of HUS

	Incidence	CNS disease	Insulin levels	Amylase	Pathology	Outcome
Loo, 1977	1/?	?	Low	ND	ND	Off insulin, nomoglycemic
Adelman, 1980	1/?	+	ND	ND	ND	Permanent diabetic
Andreoli, 1982	3/20	3/3	Low	Slightly increased	Normal islets in one	1 died 1 permanent diabetic late exocrine insufficiency 1 off insulin, normoglycemic for 9 years, then permanent diabetic
Andreoli, since 1982	1/41	+	Low	Normal	ND	1 off insulin, normoglycemic
Burns, 1982	1/?	+	ND	Normal	Islet cell necrosis exocrine pancreas essentially normal	Died
Primak, 1984	1/?	+	Low	Slightly increased, then normal	Islet cell necrosis exocrine necrosis	Died
Taylor, 1986	2/35	2/2	ND	ND	ND	1 died 1 permanent diabetic later exocrine insufficiency
before 1986	0/32					
Zeidan, 1987	1/?	No	Low	Slightly increased	ND	Off insulin, normoglycemic normal glucose tolerance test
Argyle, 1990	2/24	+	ND	ND	Islet cell necrosis	2 died

ND = not done.

pancreatic microthrombi and pancreatic islet necrosis were found at autopsy in these two, as well as in an additional child who died during the acute phase (15). Several isolated case reports (12–14) have reported insulin-dependent diabetes mellitus during the acute phase of HUS. These reports do not detail the total number of patients with HUS, but the fact that glucose intolerance was observed in only one child suggested that pancreatic involvement is not a common complication. The incidence of pancreatic exocrine involvement is even more difficult to evaluate. Since amylase and lipase are cleared by renal mechanisms, these pancreatic enzymes are frequently elevated in patients who have renal insufficiency but who do not have pancreatic disease (16, 17). However, even a normal serum amylase concentration does not exclude pancreatic exocrine disease, as pancreatic necrosis was seen at autopsy in a case whose amylase was normal prior to death (14).

Although glucose intolerance with insulin deficiency seems to occur in less than 10% of cases, microscopic evidence of pancreatic involvement is more common (5, 18–21). In a study of 26 autopsies with sufficient material for evaluation of extrarenal disease, the pancreas was the third most common organ in which microthrombi were found (the kidneys and colon were most frequently affected) (18). Microthrombi in the pancreatic vasculature have been noted at autopsy in many other reports of HUS (5, 19–21). Necrosis of the islets of Langerhans has also been described in some reports (15, 21). Therefore, microscopic evidence of pancreatic damage may be more common than the clinical evidence of glucose intolerance seems to indicate.

CLINICAL MANIFESTATIONS

The development of insulin-dependent diabetes mellitus during the acute phase of hemolytic uremic syndrome nearly always occurs in children *with severe renal disease and additional extrarenal manifestations*. Each of our four patients who developed insulin-dependent diabetes mellitus had severe renal and CNS involvement. One girl never recovered renal function; one girl died two months after onset of HUS from an intracranial hemorrhage when her serum creatinine was 2.0 mg/dL one girl currently has a creatinine of 2.6 mg/dL, and one has residual hypertension requiring antihypertensive therapy. Each had seizures during the acute episode; two had prolonged coma and one died of an intracranial hemorrhage. In the Midlands epidemic, each of the two patients who developed insulin-dependent diabetes mellitus had severe CNS involvement. The majority of the additional reported cases also had severe CNS involvement (Table 1). The morbidity and mortality of HUS complicated by insulin-dependent diabetes mellitus is substantially higher than the overall mortality in the syndrome. Of the first 12 cases with glucose intolerance caused by HUS, six died during the acute phase; many of the survivors have long-term morbidity due to chronic renal failure, neurological impairment, and/or permanent insulin-dependent diabetes mellitus (Table 1).

Hyperglycemia is usually the first manifestation of pancreatic islet cell involvement in HUS. Glucose intolerance is frequently noted within the first few days of hospitalization but has also been observed on admission when HUS is first diagnosed (10). Hyperglycemia may be severe; values have ranged from 230–1400 mg/dL. Death was attributed to hyperosmolar coma in one case (15). Because most patients are anuric, the typical signs of diabetes mellitus that include polyuria and polydipsia are not seen. Insulin levels have been undectable or inappropriately low for the level of hyperglycemia (Table 1). The insulin deficiency may lead to the acidosis as a result of accumulation of ketone bodies.

Simultaneous glucose and insulin levels in a patient with HUS are shown in Figure 1. The serum glucose concentration increased to 200 mg/dL during peritoneal dialysis with a 1.5% glucose solution; after dialysis was discontinued, the glucose level declined. During the second peritoneal dialysis, the glucose increased to 360 mg/dL in association with a slight but inadequate rise of the insulin level to 15 μU/mL. However, on the following day, pancreatic endocrine failure became complete, as demonstrated by the increase of the serum glucose level to 972 mg/dL while the insulin level declined to 6 μU/mL. The patient required insulin therapy for nearly 2 weeks and then recovered pancreatic endocrine function and has remained normoglycemic for 9 years. At the time of admission of another patient, serum glucose was 136 mg/dL while the insulin level was 10 μU/mL (Fig. 2). On the third hospital day, the serum glucose increased to 762 mg/dL while the insulin level declined to 8 μU/mL. Each time insulin therapy was discontinued, hyperglycemia recurred while the insulin level remained inappropriately low. She has become an insulin-dependent diabetic. In other reports insulin levels were either nondetectable or inappropriately low for the severity of hyperglycemia. Interestingly, the serum

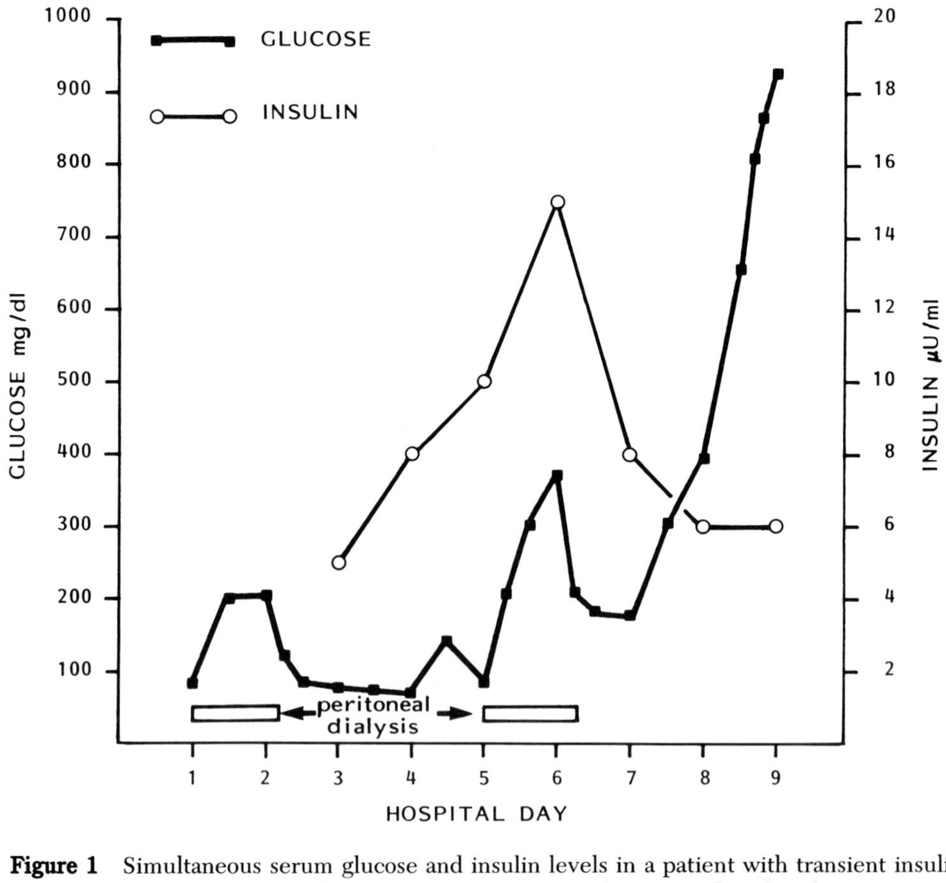

Figure 1 Simultaneous serum glucose and insulin levels in a patient with transient insulin-dependent diabetes mellitus during the HUS (From Ref. 6; reproduced with permission.)

insulin concentration was undetectable or was less than 1% of normal in the pancreas of one fatal case (14). Curiously, the serum amylase level has been either normal or mildly elevated, even when extensive pancreatic exocrine necrosis has been noted at autopsy (14).

Hyperglycemia, ketonemia, and acidosis should be treated with insulin therapy. Because of absorption of glucose from the peritoneal dialysate, insulin requirements typically increase during the peritoneal dialysis with high concentrations of glucose. Regular insulin may be given as an intravenous drip (0.05–0.10 U/kg/1hr) depending on the blood glucose. As with idiopathic insulin-dependent diabetes mellitus, the serum glucose should not be lowered rapidly. Once the glucose has declined, insulin may be given subcutaneously according to a sliding scale. The insulin deficiency may be transient or permanent. Among the six patients who survived the acute episode, three remain permanent insulin-dependent diabetics while three recovered pancreatic function. When the insulin-dependent diabetes mellitus is transient, recovery usually occurs after a few weeks to months. The three patients who recovered

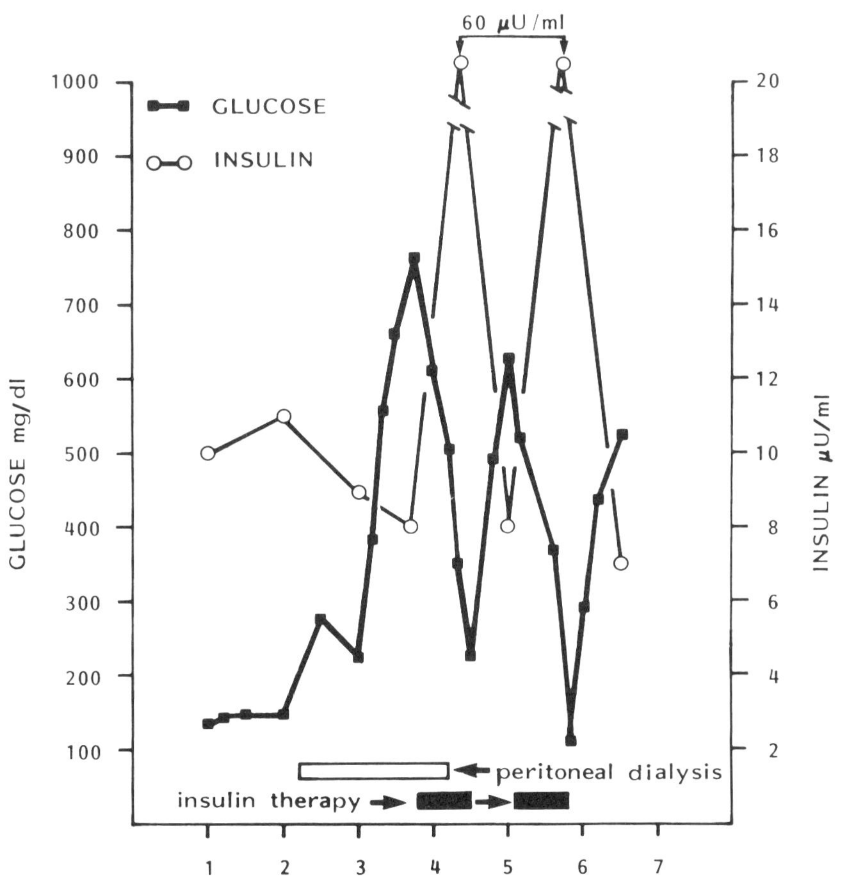

Figure 2 Simultaneous serum and insulin levels in a patient who remained a permanent insulin-dependent diabetic as a result of HUS (From Ref. 6; reproduced with permission.)

pancreatic endocrine function had normal glucose tolerance tests 5 months, 4 years, and 6 years later. However, as detailed later, patients who apparently recover pancreatic function are at risk for late complications and need long-term follow-up.

PATHOLOGY AND PATHOGENESIS

The pathogenesis of the hyperglycemia and insulin deficiency is probably due to thrombotic occlusion of the pancreatic microvasculature with resultant ischemia and islet cell dysfunction. In severe cases, the thrombotic occlusion leads to necrosis and permanent insulin deficiency. Examination of the pancreas from five patients with glucose intolerance and HUS who died during the acute episode demonstrated islet cell necrosis in four and normal islets in one (6, 11, 14–15). It is likely that our findings of normal islets was the result of a sampling error, as only one microscopic section of the pancreas was obtained at autopsy (6). In the case of Burns et al. (11), nearly all the islets were obliterated and replaced by fibrin and hemorrhage (Fig. 3). Indirect immunoperoxidase staining for beta cells did not show preferential destruc-

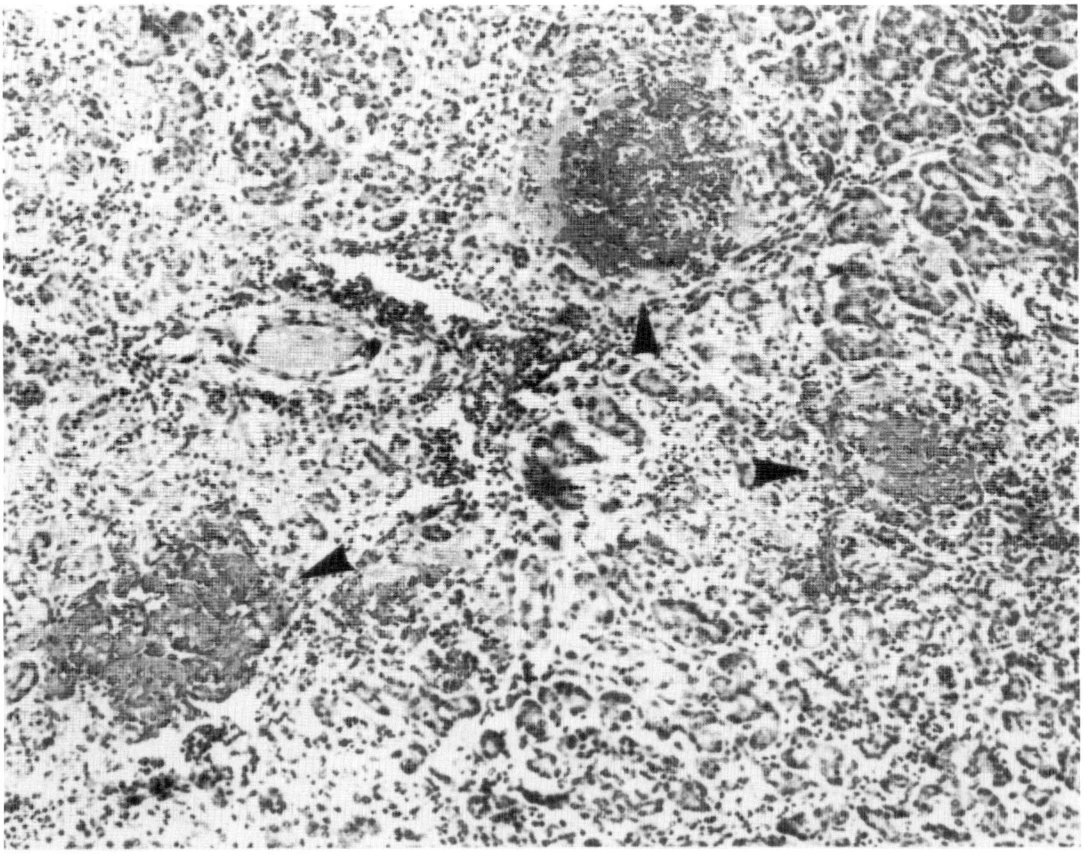

Figure 3 Pancreatic islets (arrows) are obliterated and replaced by fibrin and hemorrhage; intervening exocrine glands are intact (From Ref. 11; reproduced with permission.)

tion. A few islets were not destroyed and appeared unremarkable. The exocrine pancreas was intact except for occasional focal areas of acute and chronic inflammation and hemorrhage. Thrombi were not identified in the pancreatic vessels. In the case of Primack et al. (14), necrosis was not confined to the pancreatic islets but involved almost the entire pancreas (Fig. 4). Necrotic areas were heavily infiltrated by polymorphonuclear leukocytes. Fibrin thrombi were observed in the vasculature. Pancreatic microthrombi and islet cell necrosis have been reported in three of nine children who died of HUS (15). Before the reports of clinically apparent pancreatic involvement, microthrombi in the pancreatic vessels had been described in many reports (5, 18–21).

The pathogenesis of the pancreatic microvascular thrombi is unknown. The endothelium of both the glomerulus and the pancreatic islets may be particularly vulnerable to the microvascular insult that occurs in HUS. If the microvascular injury

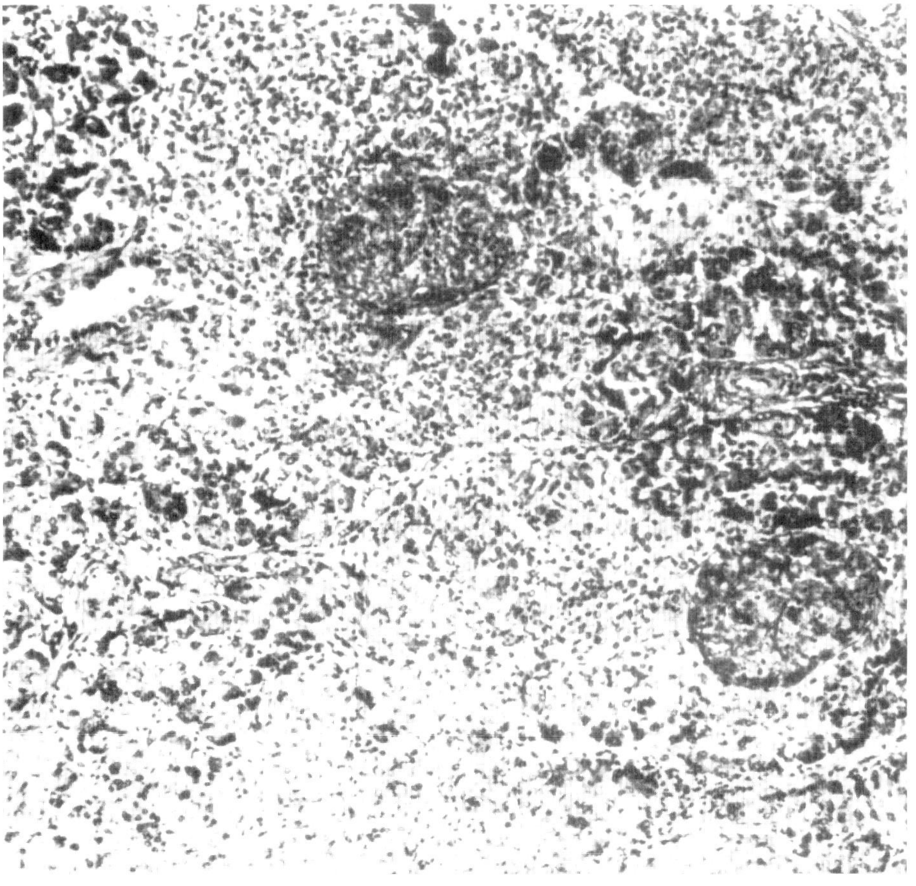

Figure 4 Extensive necrosis of the endocrine and exocrine pancreas with prominent polymorphonuclear leukocyte infiltration. The two round structures devoid of cellur detail are probably islets of Langerhans that have undergone necrosis. (From Ref. 14; reproduced with permission.)

that occurs in HUS is a result of reactive oxygen molecules (22), then a propensity to pancreatic involvement can be explained by an enhanced susceptibility of the pancreatic beta cells to oxidant injury (23, 24). Both alloxan and streptozotocin induce beta cell injury and diabetes in animals, in part by the generation of reactive oxygen molecules (23). In addition, pancreatic beta cells contain low levels of enzymes such as glutathione peroxidase which are important in detoxifying reactive oxygen molecules (23). Endothelial cells are also more susceptible to oxidant injury than renal tubular epithelial cells; the mechanism for this response is probably related to reduced levels of catalase in endothelial cells, allowing for enhanced oxidant injury (25). A role for verotoxin in the pathogenesis of the pancreatic injury has not been determined to date. It is possible that verotoxin directly injures islet cells, as has been shown for subconfluent endothelial cells in an in vitro cell culture system (26).

A role for viral infections or immunological mechanisms in the pathogenesis of islet cell injury during HUS has been investigated but not found. Viral particles were not found by electron microscopic studies in one case (11). Insulin and islet cell antibodies have not been detected (6, 14). This is in contrast to the majority of patients with idiopathic insulin-dependent diabetes mellitus who have anti-islet cell antibodies (27). A primary role of diazoxide in the pathogenesis of the insulin deficiency is unlikely. Diazoxide may alter carbohydrate metabolism by direct inhibition of insulin secretion by pancreatic beta cells causing transient hyperglycemia and ketoacidosis (28, 29). Only a few of the children with HUS and glucose intolerance received intravenous diazoxide for treatment of hypertension. Although a potentiating effect is possible the timing of the administration of diazoxide and the onset of hyperglycemia did not suggest a causal association.

LATE COMPLICATIONS

Patients who develop pancreatic involvement during the acute phase of HUS are also at risk for late complications. One of our original patients became an insulin-dependent diabetic 9 years after the acute episode of HUS, during which she had transient insulin deficiency (patient 1 in the previous report) (6). Although she had normal blood glucose and glycosolated hemoglobin levels for several years, polyuria, polydipsia, weight loss, enuresis, headaches, and abdominal pain developed when she was 11 years old. The blood glucose was 706 mg/dL, serum creatinine was 1.1 mg/dL, the insulin level was 6.7 IU/mL, the glycosolated hemoglobin was 17.6% (normal 5–12%) and ketonemia was not detected. Neither insulin nor islet cell antibodies were detected. Pancreatic exocrine function was normal as demonstrated by a normal carotene concentration and a normal 72-hour fecal fat value. A computerized tomography (CT) scan of the pancreas was normal. In addition, one of our other original patients who never recovered pancreatic endocrine function developed pancreatic exocrine insufficiency 6 years after the acute phase of HUS (30). Malabsorption was documented by a low serum carotene level, elevated 72-hour fecal fat excretion, and absent stool chymotrypsin. A CT scan of the pancreas demonstrated extensive calcification (Fig. 5). Similarly, one patient with permanent insulin-dependent diabetes mellitus from HUS in the Midlands epidemic also had a reduced fecal chymotrypsin 6 months after the acute onset (8). Therefore, pancreatic exocrine and endocrine insufficiency can occur as late sequelae in patients who

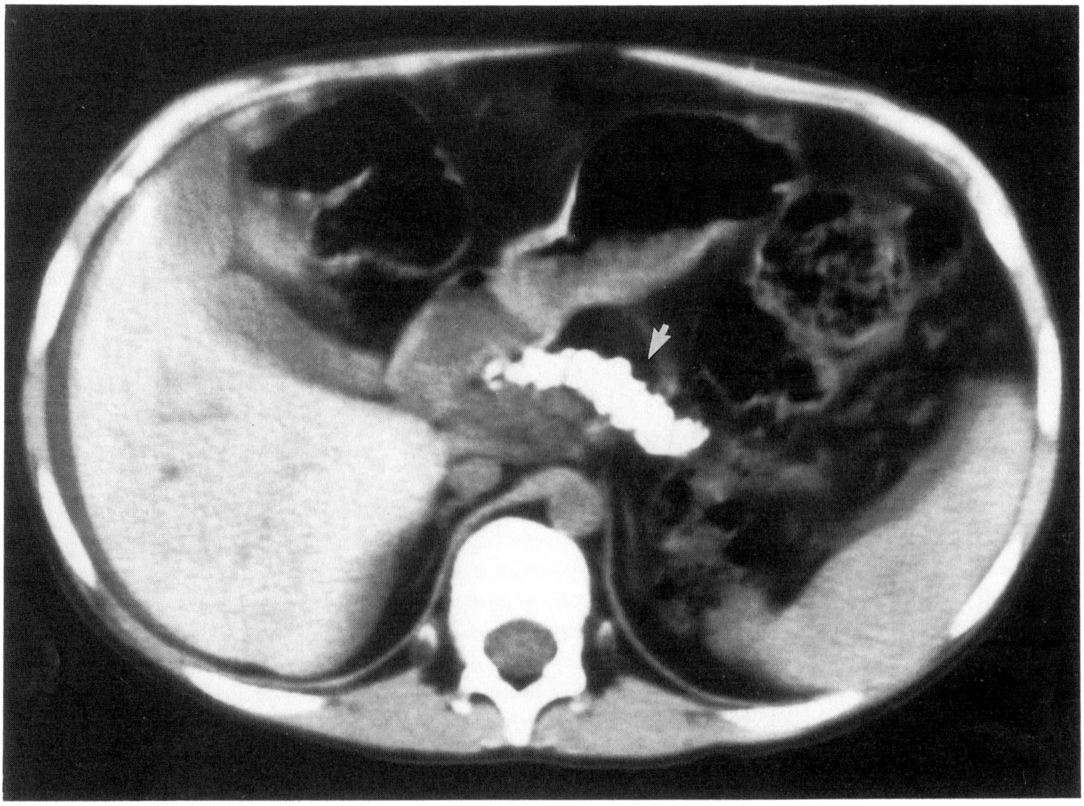

Figure 5 Computerized tomography of the abdomen of the patient depicted in Figure 2, 6 years after the acute phase of HUS when she developed pancreatic exocrine insufficiency. Arrowhead demonstrates extensive pancreatic calcifications.

seemed to have had complete or partial recovery of pancreatic function following the acute phase.

The pathogenesis of the delayed pancreatic insufficiency following HUS is also unknown. The absence of insulin and islet cell antibodies during the acute or late phase suggests that autoimmune mechanisms are unlikely. Because ischemic necrosis of the pancreas has been observed during the acute phase of the HUS, it seems likely that ischemic necrosis and subsequent scar formation can lead to endocrine and exocrine insufficiency long after the initial insult.

SUMMARY

Pancreatic microthrombi are a common occurrence in HUS. In some cases, microthrombi lead to ischemia and dysfunction of the pancreatic islets with insulin deficiency, hyperglycemia, and ketoacidosis. The insulin-dependent diabetes mellitus may be transient or permanent. In severe cases, pancreatic exocrine necrosis may also occur during the acute phase. Studies of the pancreas at autopsy demonstrate necrosis of the islets of Langerhans with a normal exocrine pancreas and occasionally exocrine necrosis. Late complications of pancreatic endocrine and exocrine insufficiency may occur in patients who have had complete or partial recovery of pancreatic function following the acute episode of HUS.

REFERENCES

1. Ray, C. G., Portman, J. N., Stamn, S. J., Hickman, R. O. Hemolytic-uremic syndrome and myocarditis. *Am. J. Dis. Child.*, *122*: 418–420 (1971).
2. Rooney, J. C., Anderson, R. M., Hopkins, I. J. Clinical and pathological aspects of central nervous system involvement in the haemolytic uraemic syndrome. *Aust. Paediatr. J.*, *7*: 28–33 (1971).
3. Berman, W. The hemolytic-uremic syndrome: Initial presentation mimicking ulcerative colitis. *J. Pediatr.*, *81*: 275–278 (1972).
4. Schwartz, D. L., Becker, J. M., So, H. B., Schneider, K. M. Segmental colonic gangrene: A surgical emergency in the hemolytic-uremic syndrome. *Pediatrics*, *62*: 54–56 (1978).
5. Upadhyaya, K., Barwick, K., Fishaut, M., Kashgarian, M., Siegel, N.J. The importance of nonrenal involvement in hemolytic-uremic syndrome. *Pediatrics*, *65*: 115–120 (1980).
6. Andreoli, S. P., Bergstein, J. M. Development of insulin-dependent diabetes mellitus during the hemolytic-uremic syndrome. *J. Pediatr.*, *100*: 541–545 (1982).
7. Kendall, P. A., Reid, I., Wright, J. E., Nanra, R. S. Gangrenous colitis in the haemolytic-uraemic syndrome. *Med. J. Aust.*, *140*: 543–544 (1984).
8. Taylor, G. M., White, R.H.R., Winterborn, M. H., Rowe, B. Haemolytic-uraemic syndrome: clinical experience of an outbreak in the West Midlands. *Br. Med. J.*, *292*: 1513–1516 (1986).
9. Andreoli, S. P., Bergstein, J. M. Acute rhabdomyolysis associated with hemolytic-uremic syndrome. *J. Pediatr.*, *103*: 78–80 (1983).
10. Adelman, R. D., Halsted, C. C., Sheikholishlam, B. M. Hemolytic uremic syndrome: associated conditions. *J. Pediatr.*, *96*: 161–162 (1980).
11. Burns, J. C., Berman, E. R., Fagre, J. L., Shikes, R. H., Lum, G. M. Pancreatic islet cell necrosis: Association with hemolytic-uremic syndrome. *J. Pediatr.*, *100*: 582–584 (1982).
12. Loo, S., Harmon, W., Gabbay, K. H. Hyperglycemia associated with the hemolytic uremic syndrome. *Pediatr. Res.*, *11*: 518 (1977).
13. Zeidan, S. F., Coulthard, M. G. Transient glucose intolerance associated with the haemolytic-uraemic syndrome. *Pediatr. Nephrol.*, *1*: 605–607 (1987).
14. Primhak, R. A., Taitz, L. S., Variend, S., Webb, D.H.K., Cser, A. Necrosis of the pancreas in the haemolytic uraemic syndrome. *J. Clin. Pathol.*, *37*: 655–658 (1984).
15. Argyle, J. C., Hogg, R. J., Pysher, T. J., Silva, F. G., Siegler, R. L. A clinicopathological study of 24 children with hemolytic uremic syndrome. *Pediatr. Nephrol.*, *4*: 52–58 (1990).
16. Zachee, P., Lins, R. L., DeBroe, M. E. Serum amylase and lipase values in acute renal failure. *Clin. Chem.*, *31*: 1237 (1985).
17. Vaziri, N. D., Chang, D., Malekpour, A., Radaht, S. Pancreatic enzymes in patients with end-stage renal disease maintained on hemodialysis. *Am. J. Gastroenterol.* *83*: 410–412 (1988).
18. Gianantonio, C. A., Vitacco, M., Mendilaharzu, F., Gallo, G. E., Sojo, E. T. The hemolytic-uremic syndrome. *Nephron*, *11*: 174–192 (1973).
19. Hammond, D., Lieberman, E. The hemolytic uremic syndrome. *Arch. Intern. Med.*, *126*: 816–822 (1970).
20. Lieberman, E., Heuser, E., Donnell, G. N., Landing, B. H., Hammond, G. D.

Hemolytic-uremic syndrome; clinical and pathological considerations. *N. Engl. J. Med.*, *275*: 227–235 (1966).
21. Shumway, C. N., Terplan, K. L. Hemolytic anemia, thrombocytopenia and renal disease in childhood: the hemolytic-uremic syndrome. *Pediatr. Clin. N. Am.*, *11*: 577–591 (1964).
22. Fong, J.S.C., de Chadarevian, J. P., Kaplan, B. S. Hemolytic-uremic syndrome. *Pediatr. Clin. N. Am.*, *29*: 835–856 (1982).
23. Malaisse, W. J., Malaisse-Lagae, F., Sener, A., Pipeleers, D. G. Determinants of the selective toxicity of alloxan to the pancreatic B cell. *Proc. Natl. Acad. Sci.*, *79*: 927–930 (1982).
24. Oberley, L. W. Free radicals and diabetes. *Free Radical Biol. & Med.*, *5*: 113–124 (1988).
25. Andreoli, S. P., McAteer, J. M. Reactive oxygen molecule-mediated injury in endothelial and renal tubular epithelial cells. *Kidney Int.* *38*: 785–794 (1990).
26. Obrig, T. G., DelVecchio, P. J., Karmali, M. A., Petric, M., Moran, T. P., Judge, T. K. Pathogenesis of haemolytic uraemic syndrome. *Lancet*, *2*: 687 (1987).
27. Dobersen, M. J., Scharff, J. E., Ginsberg-Fellner, F., Notkins, A. L. Cytotoxic autoantibodies to beta cells in the serum of patients with insulin-dependent diabetes mellitus. *N. Engl. J. Med.*, *303*: 1493–1498 (1980).
28. Updike, S. J., Harrington, A. R. Acute diabetic ketoacidosis—a complication of intravenous diazoxide treatment for refractory hypertension. *N. Engl. J. Med.*, *280*: 768 (1969).
29. Koch-Weser, J. Drug therapy: diazoxide. *N. Engl. J. Med.*, *294*: 1271–1274 (1976).
30. Andreoli, S. P., Bergstein, J. M. Exocrine and endocrine pancreatic insufficiency and calcinosis after hemolytic uremic syndrome. *J. Pediatr.*, *110*: 816–817 (1987).

12
Cardiovascular Involvement in the Hemolytic Uremic Syndrome

Richard L. Siegler *University of Utah School of Medicine, Salt Lake City, Utah*

Cardiovascular involvement in the form of salt and water retention (peripheral edema, pulmonary venous congestion), and hypertension occurs frequently in the hemolytic uremic syndrome (HUS). Occasionally, heart failure occurs as a result of persistent severe hypertension, and rarely, cardiomyopathy from thrombotic microangiopathy (TMA) of the heart muscle.

SECONDARY CARDIOVASCULAR INVOLVEMENT

Fluid Overload

Peripheral edema and pulmonary venous congestion occur frequently in patients with oliguric renal failure. This often results from the injudicious administration of intravenous fluids; patients who present with dehydration secondary to diarrhea are often given generous volumes of fluids before the oliguria is appreciated and the diagnosis of HUS established. Moreover, intravenous "fluid challenges" are often given to oliguric patients in the hope that the renal failure is prerenal and due to volume depletion. Excessive fluid administration usually results in peripheral edema and mild pulmonary venous congestion. Occasionally, however, it causes pulmonary edema. In a 1972 report of 39 children seen at Children's Hospital of Los Angeles between 1954 and 1970, two of eight deaths (25%) were secondary to pulmonary edema (1). In the 1964 report of 58 children from the Buenos Aires region of Argentina, 21 (36%) patients presented with signs of circulatory congestion or failure (2). It was noted that many had cardiomegaly, hepatomegaly, venous engorgement, generalized edema, and severe respiratory distress. Electrocardiograms were performed in 30 of the patients, and changes secondary to hyperkalemia or hypocalcemia were frequent. Excessive volumes of transfused blood or overhydration with intravenous fluids were the cause in some cases. While 32 (55%) patients initially had hypertension, this resolved in 13 once urine volume increased and the excess salt and water were excreted.

Fluid overload and pulmonary edema can be avoided if, as soon as dehydration has been corrected, administration of fluids is limited to ongoing losses only (insensible, gastrointestinal, and urine).

Mineral and Electrolyte Abnormalities

Although severe hypocalcemia and uremia can impair cardiac function, it is uncommon for either to cause clinically detectable heart failure. Hyperkalemia, on the other hand, occurs in almost 50% of cases (3) and occasionally can cause life-threatening cardiac arrhythmias. Patients with HUS who have oliguric renal failure are at risk for hyperkalemia for several reasons in addition to diminished renal excretory capability. Large amounts of potassium are released from red blood cells secondary to the hemolytic anemia. Most have hemorrhagic colitis with absorption of red blood cell potassium from the intestine. Many are catabolic. Metabolic acidosis of diarrhea and renal failure shifts intracellular potassium to the extracellular space. For every 0.1 unit fall in serum pH, a 0.6 mEq rise in serum potassium concentration can be anticipated (4).

Hypertensive Heart Disease

Left ventricular hypertrophy and occasionally, left ventricular failure can occur as a result of persistent severe hypertension. Gianantonio et al. (2) reported that hypertension occurred in 32 (55%) of their 58 patients and in 13 (22%) occurred early in the course and was transient. In 19, it was delayed in onset and/or was persistent. Six (10%) of this group eventually died because of severe persistent hypertension and refractory heart failure.

We have seen hypertensive heart failure in two of our 230 (0.87%) patients. One of these was a child who developed uncontrollable hypertension following an episode of recurrent HUS. A kidney biopsy showed severe arteriolar changes characterized by extensive intimal proliferation. She subsequently developed congestive heart failure (Fig. 1) and required treatment with digoxin. The second case was a 10-month-old infant who was left with persistent proteinuria, mild azotemia, and severe hypertension following an episode of classical childhood postdiarrheal HUS. He developed congestive heart failure 2 weeks following discharge from the hospital and required treatment with digoxin. He was eventually able to discontinue the digoxin, although he had persistent hypertension and slowly progressive azotemia. He recently received a renal allograft.

MYOCARDITIS

In 1971 Ray and associates (5) described two patients who had severe heart disease during the acute phase of HUS. Both had a significant rise in neutralizing antibody titers to the Coxsackie B_4 antigen. In addition, one was found to have immunofluorescent evidence of coxsackie B_4 in renal tissue, and Coxsackie B_4 virus was isolated from the blood and throat in the other patient. One had a cardiac gallop rhythm, hepatomegaly and distended neck veins, radiographic evidence of pulmo-

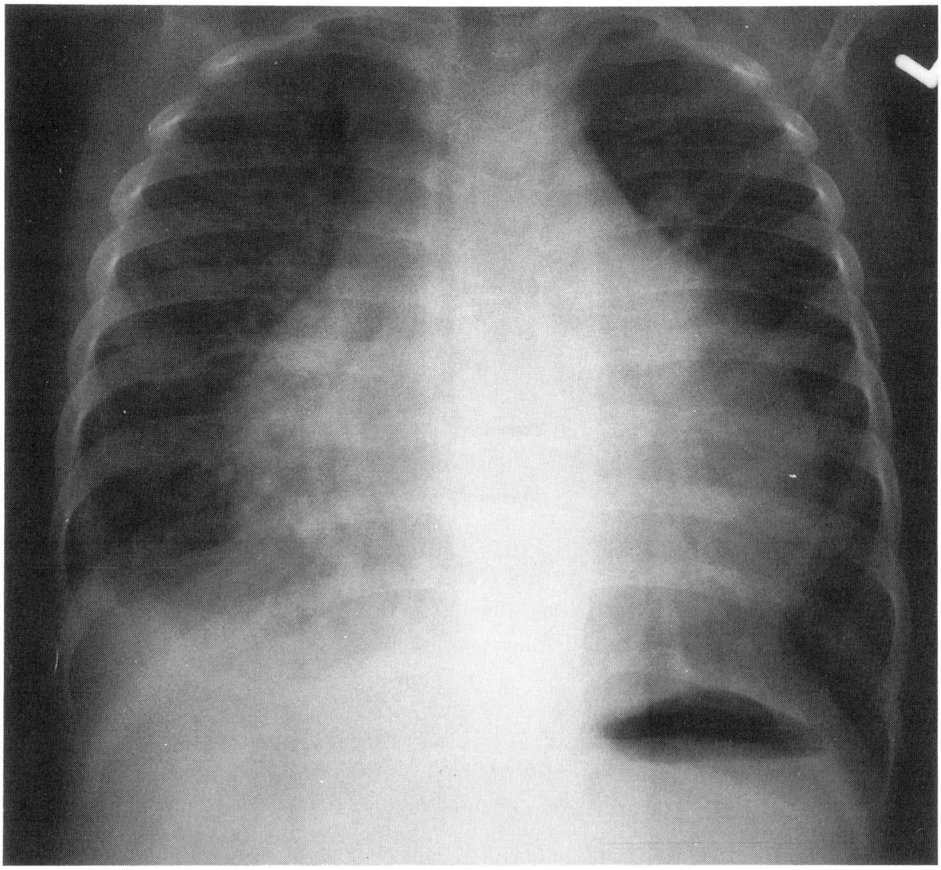

Figure 1 Cardiomegaly, interstitial pulmonary edema, pulmonary venous congestion, and pleural effusions in a HUS patient with severe hypertension.

nary edema, and cardiac enlargement; the ECG showed first-degree atrioventricular (AV) block with flattened T-waves. The other patient had an enlarged globular heart, first-degree heart block, and decreased voltage with flat T-waves that suggested pericarditis with a pericardial effusion. A pericardiocentesis yielded modest amounts of sterile blood–tinged fluid. Persistent cardiac dysfunction led to cardiac catheterization which revealed poor left ventricular contractility and dilatation. This patient, in contrast to the other patient, did not have the classical HUS diarrhea prodrome, and had coagulation studies which were more suggestive of disseminated intravascular coagulation (DIC) than classical childhood HUS. In addition, because no cardiac tissue was available for examination in either of the patients, it is possible that they had TMA of the heart rather than viral inflammation. Bugajer-Gteitman et al. (6) also described the case of a 2-year-old in whom HUS was complicated by myocarditis. Although the patient had a cold agglutinin titer of 1:256, suggesting mycoplasma myocarditis, the patient survived and no tissue was available to enable exclusion of TMA of the cardiac microcirculation. In another report (1), one of 39 patients had findings consistent with myocarditis and experienced an episode of congestive heart failure 2 months after onset of HUS, at a time when she had normal blood pressure and kidney function. There was no mention of viral cultures or serological studies in the report.

TMA OF HEART MUSCLE

When the TMA of HUS occurs in extrarenal organs, it most often involves the central nervous system (CNS). TMA of the heart muscle is uncommon but life threatening.

In a report (2) of 58 infants and children, five of 30 electrocardiogram had (ECG) findings suggestive of myocardial injury. None had signs of congestive heart failure. In a later report (7) of 678 patients which included autopsy findings in 52, the importance of ischemic cardiac injury was mentioned, but no histopathological details were given.

Upadhyaya and associates (8) called attention to the importance of extrarenal involvement by describing 15 consecutive patients admitted over a 6-year period. Three died, and one of the deaths was caused by refractory hypotension that probably was secondary to cardiogenic shock. The patient had persistent tachycardia, ST-T wave abnormalities on ECG, and an elevated SGOT level. At autopsy, fibrin microthrombi were found within the microvasculature of the heart.

Taylor and associates (9) saw evidence of a cardiomyopathy in one of 35 patients who developed HUS during an epidemic in the West Midlands of Great Britain. The patient developed left ventricular (LV) failure 2 months after the onset of HUS. The ECG showed only transient nonspecific T-wave and ST segment abnormalities, but the echocardiogram demonstrated LV dilatation with poor contractility. The patient had been normotensive, and had negative antibody titers to Coxsackie B viruses, sero types 1–6. Although heart returned to normal size, LV function, as assessed by an echocardiogram, was still abnormal a year later. In a more detailed report, Poulton et al. (10) described this patient and an 8-year-old whose HUS was preceded by headaches, lethargy, and vomiting, but no diarrhea. This patient also had transient left hemiparesis and had two focal seizures. Although blood pressure was initially normal, it became intermittently elevated about 2 weeks later. An ECG demonstrated LV hypertrophy; pulmonary edema developed 5 days later. An echocardiographic study demonstrated mild dilatation and poor function of the left ventricle. LV contractility returned to normal within 4 months. There was no serological evidence of infection for 11 common viruses, including six types of Coxsackie B. It might be argued that the features and course of this case were more typical of thrombotic thrombocytopenic purpura (TTP) than HUS.

A patient is included in a report of neurological complications, who developed, in addition to multiple brain infarcts, ECG evidence of left lateral wall ischemia and echocardiographic findings of LV dysfunction (11). She survived, and no cardiac tissue was available for histopathological studies.

We recently took care of a 2-year-old boy with postdiarrheal HUS who was admitted with tachycardia, tachypnea, severe pallor, irritability, occasional respiratory grunting, and a gallop rhythm. Shortly thereafter, the patient suddenly became profoundly hypotensive. He died from cardiogenic shock a few hours later. An autopsy examination revealed biventricular chamber enlargement, apicle erythematus mottling of the left ventricular free wall, and diffuse myocardial capillary microthrombi, particularly in the areas that were mottled (Fig. 2a). There was marked

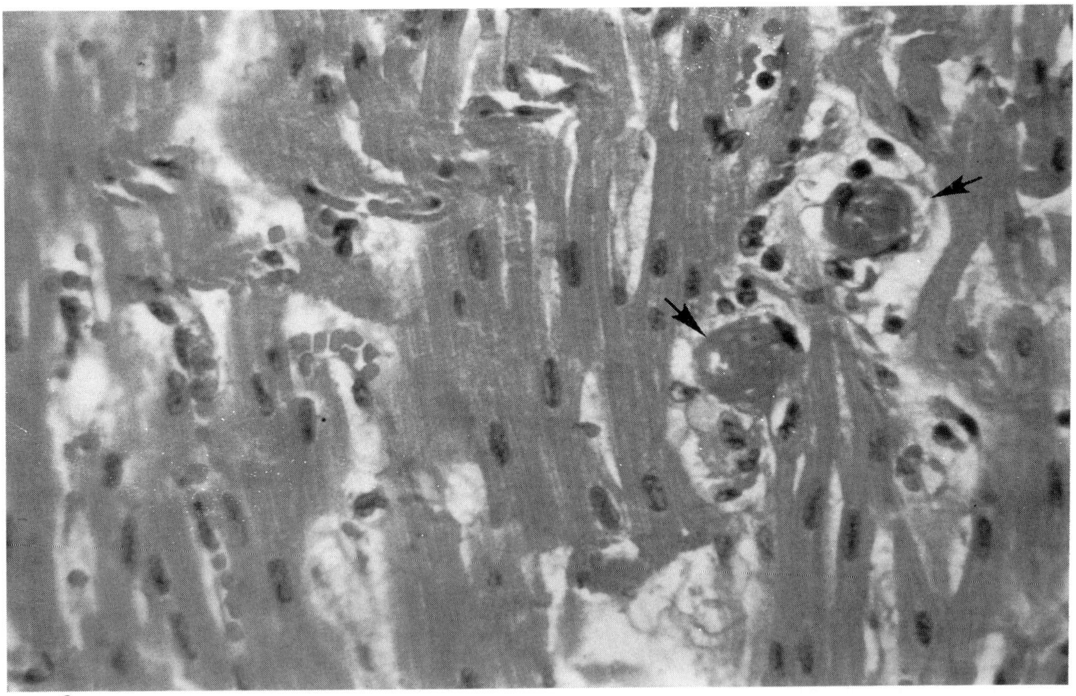

a

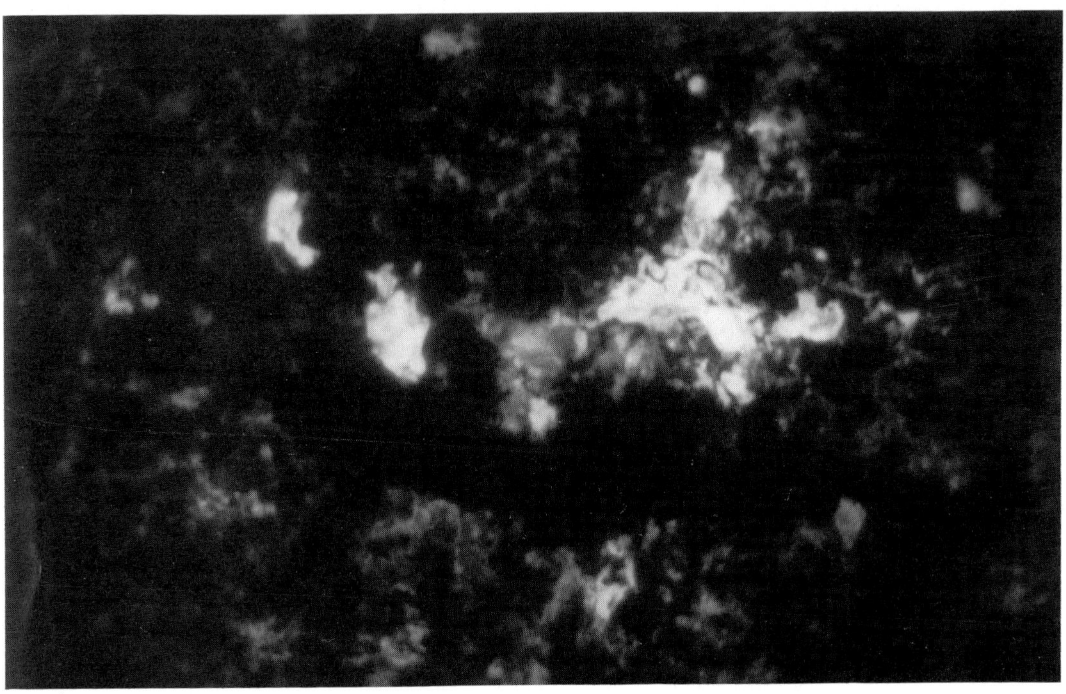

b

Figure 2 (a) Hematoxylin-eosin–stained section of myocardial tissue showing intracapillary fibrin and features of acute myocardial ischemia including interstitial edema, wavy fiber change, and myofiber hypereosinophilia (×400). (Courtesy of O. M. Faye-Petersen, M.D., and M. E. Hammond, M.D., Salt Lake City, Utah.) **Figure 2 (b)** Immunofluorescence photograph of myocardial tissue demonstrating fibrinogen within small arterioles and capillaries (×250). (Courtesy of O. M. Faye-Petersen, M.D., and M. E. Hammond, M.D., Salt Lake City, Utah.)

interstitial edema, but no fibrosis or inflammation. Immunofluorescent studies confirmed the presence of microthrombi (Fig. 2b), and electronmicroscopy showed capillary subendothelial lucent zones, similar to those seen in the kidney. Although there were a few microthrombi in the capillaries of the lung and colon, there were no signs of TMA of the brain as might be expected in TTP. Moreover, there was no evidence of DIC, as the PT, PTT, and fibrinogen concentrations were normal. This is the only case of clinically apparent primary myocardial involvement that we have seen in 230 cases of HUS.

TREATMENT

Fluid Overload

Most patients with HUS who have peripheral and/or pulmonary edema have normal-to-high cardiac output. Correction of the hypervolemic state is all that is needed. While potent loop diuretics may be tried, fluid removal is visually indicated by means of peritoneal dialysis using 2.5% or 4.25% dextrose, or hemodialysis combined with ultrafiltration, or pure ultrafiltration. If the patient is not severely azotemic or hyperkalemic, continuous arterial venous hemofiltration (CAVH) can also be used, but establishing arterial access might be risky in a child with thrombocytopenia and azotemia. Pump-assisted venous-to-venous hemofiltration poses less of a risk of bleeding; the addition of hemodiafiltration (12) increases the efficiency of solute removal.

Hyperkalemia

It is impossible to equate serum potassium concentration with the risk of cardiac arrest. Severity of toxicity appears to be related also to the magnitude of other concurrent mineral or electrolyte abnormalities (e.g., hyponatremia, hypocalcemia), and the presence of any concurrent TMA of the coronary circulation. We generally treat hyperkalemia if the potassium levels are greater than 6 mEq/L, or if the serum potassium concentration is rising rapidly. For lesser levels of hyperkalemia, with little if any peaking of T-waves and no other ECG abnormalities, cation exchange resins—e.g., Kayexalate® (sodium polystyrene sulfonate, USP)—may suffice. We usually administer Kayexalate® orally (1 g/kg body weight with 1 mL of 70% sorbitol/g Kayexalate®) if the patient does not have severe enteritis or ileus and is not vomiting. It can also be given by retention enema, although it needs to be retained for 20–40 minutes for effective potassium exchange. In the presence of severe enteritis with ileus or bloody diarrhea, it is safer not to administer Kayexalate®. For severe hyperkalemia, intravenous (IV) drugs can be given to facilitate the movement of potassium into cells while arrangements are being made for emergency dialysis. These include IV sodium bicarbonate (1 mEq/kg of body weight), and/or IV glucose with or without small amounts of insulin (50% dextrose, 1 mL/kg/body weight, with regular insulin, 1 unit/3–10 g/glucose). In the advent of immediate life-threatening hyperkalemia (i.e., severe ECG abnormalities), the slow intravenous administration of 10% calcium gluconate (0.25–0.5 mL/kg/body weight) with careful monitoring of cardiac activity can be life saving. Its effects are short-lived, however, and this should be used only while emergency dialysis is being arranged.

If there is evidence of poor LV function associated with severe systemic hypertension, afterload reduction with medications such as selective $alpha_1$ adrenergic receptor blocking agents (e.g., prazosin) or sodium nitroprusside (which also decreases preload) should be initiated promptly.

Primary LV failure resulting from TMA of the heart muscle is an indication for $beta_1$ agonists (e.g., dolbutamine) coupled with the cautious use of digoxin. A Swan-Ganz catheter to measure pulmonary wedge pressure and cardiac output will facilitate selective manipulation of both preload and afterload to maximize cardiac output and oxygen tissue delivery. If the patient's cardiovascular status fails to improve following utilization of these conventional forms of treatment, consideration might be given to the use of an intraaortic balloon pump (13) to temporarily support cardiac output while waiting for LV function to improve.

REFERENCES

1. Lieberman, E. Hemolytic-uremic syndrome. *J. Pediatr., 80*: 1–16 (1972).
2. Gianantonio, C., Vitacco, M., Mendilaharzu, F., Rutty, A., Mendilaharzu, J. The hemolytic-uremic syndrome. *J. Pediatr., 64*: 478–491 (1964).
3. Brasher, C., Siegler, R. L. The hemolytic-uremic syndrome. *West. J. Med., 134*: 193–197 (1981).
4. Rose, B. D. *Clinical Physiology of Acid-Base and Electrolyte Disorders*. McGraw-Hill Book Company, New York, pp. 213–214 (1977).
5. Ray, C. G., Portman, J. N., Stamm, S. J., Hickman, R. O. Hemolytic-uremic syndrome and myocarditis. *Am. J. Dis. Child, 122*: 418–420 (1971).
6. Bugajer-Gleitman, H. E., Balzar, E., Lubec, G., May, L., Weissenbacher, G. The presence of cold agglutinins in hemolytic uremic syndrome. *Pediatr. Padol., 11*: 245–253 (1976).
7. Gianantonio, C. A., Vitacco, M., Mendilaharzu, F., Gallo, G. E., Sojo, E. T. The hemolytic-uremic syndrome. *Nephron, 11*: 174–192 (1973).
8. Upadhyaya, K., Barwick, K., Fishaut, M., Kashgarian, M., Siegel, N. J. The importance of nonrenal involvement in hemolytic-uremic syndrome. *Pediatrics, 65*: 115–120 (1980).
9. Taylor, C. M., White, R.H.R., Winterborn, M. H., Rowe, R. Haemolytic-uraemic syndrome: Clinical experience of an outbreak in the west midlands. *Br. Med. J., 292*: 1513–1516 (1986).
10. Poulton, J., Taylor, C. M., DeGiovanni, J. V. Dilated cardiomyopathy associated with haemolytic uraemic syndrome. *Br. Heart J., 57*: 181–183 (1987).
11. Hahn, J. S., Havens, P. L., Higgins, J. J., O'Rourke, P. P., Estroff, J. A., Strand, R. Neurological complications of hemolytic-uremic syndrome. *J. Child Neurol., 4*: 108–113 (1989).
12. Bishof, N. A., Welch, T. R., Strife, C. F., Ryckman, F. C. *Pediatrics, 85*: 819–823 (1990).
13. Veasy, L. G., Blalock, R. C., Orth, J. L., Boucek, M. M. Intra-aortic balloon pumping in infants and children. *Circulation, 68*: 1095–1100 (1983).

13
Recurrent Hemolytic Uremic Syndrome

Bernard S. Kaplan *Children's Hospital of Philadelphia and University of Pennsylvania, Philadelphia, Pennsylvania*

In a seminal review of the hemolytic uremic syndrome (HUS), Brain (1) noted that "very occasionally, recurrent episodes of the haemolytic-uraemic syndrome have been associated with a seemingly wide variety of infective episodes." This was based on a few reports of recurrent HUS (2–5) that included one case with insufficient information to determine whether she had HUS (case 12) (2). Gasser (6) also described the recurrence of HUS in a patient, Franz J., several years after complete recovery. Despite these reports, the subject was largely ignored in reviews of HUS until 1977 (7).

This chapter provides an up-to-date review of more than twice the number of cases that were analysed in 1977 and a re-evaluation of the problem of recurrent HUS. An attempt has been made to group apparently similar phenotypes (Table 1), but it is a fact that some cases fit into more than one category. For example, there are patients with recurrences of HUS in association with oral contraception whose serum complement levels were low and who had other affected family members. One inference is that several factors may trigger the illness. Another possibility is that some or all of the apparent provocations have no etiologic roles.

Table 1 Recurrent Hemolytic Uremic Syndrome: Associations

1. Nonspecific prodromal illnesses
2. Hereditary HUS
3. Renal transplantation
4. Hypocomplementemia
5. Prostacyclin deficiency
6. Pregnancy
7. Oral contraception
8. Malignancy

DEFINITIONS

A recurrent episode of HUS is defined as a second (or subsequent) well-documented episode of HUS that occurs after recovery from previous HUS. We have found it useful to differentiate between a recurrence and a relapse. The latter can be defined as worsening of a patient's condition after a period of improvement. This subtle and perhaps even unnecessary distinction pertains to some reported cases (8–10) and unpublished observations (Kaplan).

Problems can arise in the assignment of some patients to the category of either HUS or thrombotic thrombocytopenic purpura (TTP). Precise assignment may be impossible because of insufficient information (11). Assignment may be difficult because one episode is confidently diagnosed as HUS (severe renal involvement, no neurologic symptoms) and another is equally confidently diagnosed as TTP (severe neurologic involvement, mild renal insufficiency) (12). The difficulties that have been experienced in defining HUS and TTP are discussed in more detail in Chapter 3.

ASSOCIATIONS

Recurrences With Nonspecific Prodromal Illnesses

Recurrences of HUS are uncommon (13) and rarely occur in patients with the typical form of HUS who have bloody stools. In general, the first episode and recurrences follows nonspecific symptoms (Table 2). In some patients recurrences have occurred after exanthemata or inoculations. Fever, an uncommon symptom in typical cases, is often prominent in patients with recurrences. Similar nonspecific prodromata can occur whether or not there is a family history of HUS. There may be no obvious prodrome at all. Prodromal illnesses and possible provocations that have been reported include bloody diarrhea (in one case; 10), watery diarrhea, gastroenteritis, upper respiratory tract infection, *Escherichia coli* urinary tract infection, streptococcal infection, exanthemata, inoculations. Symptoms prior to onset of the first episode or a recurrence have included fever, headache, vomiting, lassitude, malaise, myalgia, jaundice, and abdominal pain.

Table 2 Prodromal Illnesses

Case #	Author (Ref.)	
1.	Shumway and Miller (3)	
	McWhinney et al. (44)	URTIs
2.	Case Records (45)	
3.	Gasser (6)	
4.	Dacie (46)	
5.	Schubothe et al. (5)	Fever
6.	Hagge et al. (11)	Fever
7.	Wehinger et al. (47)	Fever
8.	Egli et al. (48)	
9.	Belobradkova and Nozicka (49)	
10.	Mettler (34)	Fever, lethargy
		Wk 14 pregnancy, headache, vomiting, garbled speech

Table 2 Prodromal Illnesses (*continued*)

Case #	Author (Ref.)	
11.	Markiewicz (50)	Small pox vaccination
12.	Willoughby et al. (51)	URTI, vomiting
13.	Westra (52)	URTI, abdominal pain
14.	Bergstein et al. (21)	
15.	Janssen et al. (53)	Gastroenteritis
16.	Olgaard et al. (54)	Fatigue, nausea, vomiting, jaundice each episode
17.	Courtecuisse et al. (15)	Fever, jaundice
18.		Fever
19.		Fever
20.		Fever
21.		
22.	Drukker et al. (16)	Fever, vomiting
23.	Barre et al. (17)	Nausea, diarrhea, fever, ?varicella
24.	Shigematsu et al. (55)	
25.		
26.	de Jong et al. (10)	Vomiting, bloody diarrhea
		Gastroenteritis
27.		DPT before each recurrence
28.	Spirer et al. (56)	Fever, jaundice
29.		Headache, fever, chills, epistaxis
30.	Rao et al. (57)	*E. coli* UTIs × many
31.	Rifle et al. (36)	ENT infection
		Measles
		Varicella
		ENT infection
		Angine bactrerienne; oral contraceptives
32.	Larbre et al. (43)	Vomiting, fever
33.		Vomiting, fever
34.		Vomiting, fever
35.		URTI, fever, vomiting
36.		Fever, vomiting
37.		Vomiting, jaundice
38.	Coulthard (58)	Lethargy, anorexia, fever
39.	Carreras et al. (14)	Anorexia, headaches, vomiting, myalgias
		E. coli UTI
40.		URTI
41.	Brasher and Siegler (59)	
42.	Hoornje et al. (60)	Oral contraceptives
43.	Kreisinger and Janda et al. (61)	Vomiting, fever
44.	Habib et al. (13)	
45.	Wyatt et al. (24)	Malaise, fever, diarrhea, URTI
46.	Strom (20)	Fever, lethargy, headache, vomiting
47.	Meroni et al. (12)	Bloody diarrhea each episode
48.	Elias et al. (62)	Fever, anorexia, lethargy, jaundice
49.	Bogdanovic et al. (23)	Fever, cough, vomiting, diarrhea
		Vomiting, diarrhea
		Fever, vomiting, diarrhea
50.	Mattoo et al. (63)	URTI

Recurrent HUS in Families

Recurrences most frequently occur in the autosomal recessive forms of HUS. Recurrences may occasionally occur in patients with autosomal dominant HUS (14). When the subject was reviewed in 1977, eight of 30 patients with recurrent episodes (27%) had an affected sibling or cousin (7). In the present review, 23 of 70 patients had an affected family member (30%). Recurrences of HUS occurred in more than one family member in five kindreds (14, 15; W. Balfe and F. Harley; J. Katz, personal communications). If it is accepted that some patients seem to have an inherited predisposition toward HUS, and, because many of these have recurrent episodes, may one infer that patients with hereditary HUS are more likely to have recurrent episodes? A more important inference may be that patients who have had recurrent episodes, but whose family histories are negative, may have an inherited form of HUS. Perturbations in the functions of serum complement are the only underlying inherited defects thus far identified that may predispose an individual toward recurrent HUS (14, 16, 17).

HUS has occurred in several family members at the same time, usually in association with the typical post–bloody diarrheal form of the syndrome (18, 19; Kaplan, unpublished observations). Recurrent episodes have not been reported in any of these cases.

Recurrent HUS Before and After Renal Transplantation

Recurrence of HUS in renal allografts is discussed in detail in Chapter 15. A few points are stressed in this chapter for completeness. Some patients who have had recurrences in their allografts have had several episodes of HUS prior to transplantation (20), whereas others have had a single episode (21). Some have had an inherited form of HUS (21); others have occurred sporadically. The prodromal illnesses have usually been atypical. Recurrences have occurred with and without administration of cyclosporine (22).

Recurrent HUS with Abnormalities of Complement

Several patients with recurrent HUS have had abnormalities in serum complement, recurrent episodes, and in some cases, affected family members. Of interest is a report (14) describing a familial, relapsing, autosomal dominant form of HUS associated with recurrences, persistent hypocomplementemia, and the HLA haplotype A3,B7. C3 nephritic factor has been detected in some patients with recurrent episodes (17). Reduced levels of serum C3, but not Clq, C4, C5, or CH50, have been found during recurrences and in four of five intervening periods in one patient (23). Decreased levels of factor B during two episodes in this patient suggested activation of the alternate pathway of complement (23). Both persistent and intermittent depression of C3 have been reported; it is possible that an underlying defect of depression of serum C3 concentration may predispose some individuals toward HUS or recurrences of HUS (24). Abnormalities of complement have been demonstrated in otherwise unaffected individuals in some kindreds (14, 24, 25). One posita had a persistently low C3 concentration and the C3fS phenotype; her unaffected father and paternal grandmother had the same phenotype (24). Another patient, whose parents were first cousins, had recurrent HUS, a very low level of C3 which persisted after recovery, and no demonstrable C3Nef. A healthy brother and both parents had very low levels of B1H globulin; C3b inactivator was normal (25).

The significance of these associations is difficult to determine because low levels of C3, C4, and CH50 have been described in patients with typical HUS (26–29). On the other hand, persistently low levels of serum C3 with evidence of intravascular activation have been detected pre- and postnephrectomy in patients with atypical forms of HUS (30, 31); none of these patients is known to have recurrent HUS. It is noteworthy that many patients with recurrent episodes have never had low levels of any of the components of complement.

Recurrences with Reduced Production of Prostacyclin

Levin et al. (32) found an inhibitor of prostacyclin production in six patients with atypical HUS. This was not found in seven patients with the typical syndrome. Two of the six patients with reduced prostacyclin production had recurrences.

Recurrent of HUS Associated with Pregnancy

HUS and pregnancy is discussed in detail in Chapter 20. An 18-year-old had HUS a few days after delivery following an uneventful pregnancy; urine culture grew *Staphylococcus pyogenes*. More than 5 years after her first illness, she had a second episode of HUS a few days after the delivery of a normal child. She recovered completely (33). In some patients HUS has followed febrile illnesses on several occasions and TTP (or HUS) has then occurred in association with pregnancy (34).

Recurrent HUS and Oral Contraception

The possible association of HUS and the use of oral contraception is reviewed in detail in Chapter 19. There are a number of reports of recurrent HUS in which one or more episodes, but rarely every recurrence, were associated with use of oral contraceptives. Bonsib et al. (35) described recurrent thrombotic microangiopathy in a renal allograft of a 20-year-old female who presented with HUS after a week of nausea, vomiting, diarrhea, mental confusion, and obtundation. She had been taking oral contraceptives for 2 years after an abortion. Thrombotic microangiopathy developed in the allograft 19 days after transplantation. The authors concluded that several factors may have been responsible for the recurrence but favored a role played by donor-specific antimonocyte antibody (35).

A report by Carreras et al. (14) described a case of HUS in a woman taking oral contraceptives. However, the occurrence of HUS in her daughter and nephew, and the recurrence of HUS in the subject when she was not using oral contraceptives, might suggest that her HUS was not related to use of oral contraceptives.

A girl aged 3 years had an upper respiratory tract infection followed by HUS. A second episode of HUS was associated with measles, a third with varicella, and a fourth with an ENT infection (36). At age 17 years, she had another episode of HUS, 15 days after a bacterial infection (angine bactrerienne). This occurred after she had been using oral contraceptives for 4 months. She also had a low serum C3 concentration, a reduced factor B level, and a positive C3NeF. Despite the occurrence of HUS with a variety of infections, the title of the paper is "Irreversible Cortical Necrosis While on Oestro-progestifs."

A 17-year-old girl complained of headaches, had oliguria, and then became anuric and developed malignant hypertension. She had been taking an oral contraceptive (Microgynon®) for 14 months. Two years later she had what was called a relapse of HUS on the basis of a mild microangiopathic hemolytic anemia and consumption coagulopathy (there are no details; renal function had not recovered completely after the initial episode). Despite these caveats, it is interesting that the recurrence happened after she had surreptitiously started taking Microgynon® again (37).

Five months before admission, a 23-year-old woman had a normal delivery of her second child, after which she was treated with ergotamine, estrogen, and then the oral contraceptive Sequens®. Four months prior to admission she had weakness and vomiting (38). In December 1972 she had a cadaveric transplant and was kept on progestogen. In April 1977 she was given estroprogestogen. In February 1978, she experienced feverishness and weakness and had a recurrence of HUS. Viral antibody titers revealed a 4-fold rise for influenza A, herpes simplex, and cytomegalovirus. A repeat biopsy showed similar changes to the first biopsy with thrombi in the tufts, interlobular and afferent arterioles, subintimal bleeding, and mucinous thickening of the intima. She had a second transplant and was well 2 years later. This patient had a recurrence of HUS associated with oral contraception and well-documented viral infections.

Recurrent HUS and Cancer

Two episodes of HUS occurred 8 months apart in a male aged 64 years with an adenocarcinoma of the prostate (39). The first occurred before the cancer was diagnosed, and neither were associated with anticancer treatment. The patient recovered completely after each episode.

HUS AND IDIOPATHIC THROMBOCYTOPENIC PURPURA

Idiopathic thrombocytopenic purpura (ITP) has been reported 1 year (40) and 3 months (41) after recovery from HUS. In neither patient was there evidence of hemolysis or renal failure during the episode of ITP. Varicella occurred during the episode of ITP in one of the patients (40). The same phenomenon has occurred in patients with TTP (42). Two patients presented with HUS and then had recurrent episodes of acute hemolytic anemia with fragmented erythrocytes and thrombocytopenia, but without any evidence whatsoever of renal injury over periods of several years. (Kaplan, unpublished observations, Cases 68 and 70 Table 3). These cases are uncommon, puzzling problems. Their outcomes seem to have been good in that none is known to have died. Treatment has included prednisone, infusions of fresh frozen plasma, plasmapheresis, and splenectomy.

PATHOLOGY OF RECURRENT HUS

The characteristic histological changes of the HUS are seen in the glomeruli of some (16) but not all (15) patients with recurrent episodes. In some of these cases the histologic changes are "exaggerations" of those seen in typical HUS and may be similar to those seen in membranoproliferative glomerulonephritis (17). Large deposits of C3 have been observed in the glomeruli of occasional cases (8, 17).

Table 3 Outcome of Patients with Recurrent HUS

Reference & Case #	Age Onset	(y)	Rec* #	Period	Affected family	Outcome**
1. Shumway and Miller (3) McWhinney et al. (44)	21m	F	++	12 y	—	Died, 13.5 y
2. Case Records of N. Engl. J. Med. (45)	6	F	4	15 y	—	Died
3. Gasser (6)	12	M	1	4 y	—	Alive
4. Dacie (46)	7m	F	6	6 y	?	Died, 7 y
5. Schubothe et al. (5)	17	M	4	10 y	—	Alive
6. Hagge et al. (11)	8m	F	++	?	Sib	ESRF 9 y, died
7. Wehinger et al. (47)	7m	?	1	2 m	—	Alive
8. Egli et al. (48)	5.5	F	1	2 m	—	Died, 6 y
9. Belobradkova and Nozicka (49)	6	F	1	2 y	Sib	Alive
10. Mettler (34)	2	F	?	20 y	—	Died
11. Markiewicz (50)	49	F	2	4 y	—	Alive
12. Willoughby et al. (51)	9	F	1	1 y	—	Died
13. Westra (52)	4	F	1	3 y	—	Alive
14. Bergstein et al. (21)	3	M	1	1 y	Sib	Alive
15. Janssen et al. (53)	3.6	?	1	4 y	—	Alive
16. Olgaard et al. (54)	3	M	6	?	—	Alive
Courtecuisse et al. (15)						
17.	6	M	1	4 y	Sib	Alive, 21 y
18.	8	M	1		Sib	Alive
19.	5.5	M	1	4 y	Cousin	Alive
20.	2	F	2	4 y	—	Alive
21.	6	M	1		Cousin	Alive
22. Drukker et al. (16)	2	F	4	2.5 y	—	Alive
23. Barre et al. (17)	4.5	M	1	3 m	—	Allograft, died
Shigematsu et al. (55)						
24.	1.5	F	2	1.5 y	—	Alive
25.	22	F	1	1.5 y	—	ESRF
de Jong et al. (10)						
26.	4	M	2	1 y	—	Alive
27.	3 m	M	3	3 m	—	Died
Spirer et al. (56)						
28.	1	M	2	9 y	—	Alive, adult
29.	12	M	1	4 y	—	Alive, adult
30. Rao et al. (57)	2d	F	++	5 y	—	Died, "TTP"
31. Rifle et al. (36)	3	F	5	14 y	—	ESRF
Larbre et al. (43)						
32.	3	F	4	9 y	—	Alive
33.	8	M	1	6.5 y	—	Alive
34.	4	M	1	14 m	—	Alive
35.	5	M	3	7 y	—	Alive
36.	4	F	1	2 y	—	Alive
37.	6	F	4	5 y	—	Alive
38. Coulthard (58)	3.3	F	1	1 y	—	Alive

Table 3 Outcome of Patients with Recurrent HUS (*continued*)

Reference & Case #	Age Onset	(y)	Rec #	Period	Affected Family	Outcome**
Carreras et al. (14)						
39.	34	F	1	2 y	daughter	ESRF
	3	M	3		Nephew	
40.	2	M	?	?	Aunt	Alive
41. Brasher and Siegler (59)	7m	F	1	3.5 y	—	CRF, Hypertension
42. Hoornje et al. (60)	17	F	1	2 y	—	
43. Kreisinger and Janda (61)	8	F	1	13 m	—	Alive, 11 y
44. Habib et al. (13)	6.5	F	1	3 m	—	ESRF
45. Wyatt et al. (24)	9.5	F	2	+2 y	—	Mild CRF
46. Strom (20)	8.5	F	1	31 m	—	ESRF Recurred in allograft
47. Thompson and Winterborn (25)	8m	M	1	1 m	—	Alive
Levin et al. (32)						
48.	5					
49.	13.5					
50. Meroni et al. (12)	?42	F	?5	12 y	—	Died
51. Elias et al. (62)	1.5	M			Sibs	TTP alive
52. Bogdanovic et al. (23)	8.5	M	4	3 y	—	Alive, 14 y
53. Mattoo et al. (63)	6 m	M	2	2.5 y	5 sibs	Alive
Personal Communications						
54. Kunzer	8.5	M	1	2 y	—	Died
Balfe and Harley						
55.	3	M	+++		3 sibs	Alive, 26 y
56.		M	+		3 sibs	Alive, 22 y
57.		M	+		3 sibs	Alive, 21 y
58.		M	+		3 sibs	Alive, 15 y
59. Tune	8	M	1	1 y	—	Alive
60. Gautier	6m	M	1	6 m	3 sibs	Hypertension
61. Swee	?	F	1	?	3 sibs	Hypertension
Deboukelear						
62.	9	M	2	?	Sib	Alive, 32 y
63.	?	M	3	?	Sib	Alive
64. Honda	12	F	1	?	Sib	ESRF
Katz						
65.	>1	M	3	17 y	Twin	Alive
66.	3 m	M	2	17 y	Twin	Alive
67. Mongeau	1	F	2	3 m	Sib	Died
Kaplan						
68.	2 d	M	3	13 y	—	Alive
69.	9	M	5	2 y	—	?TTP
70. Weiss, Sagel	8	M	3	5 y	—	Alive

*Rec # is the number of recurrences: + one, ++ some, +++ many.
**Outcome at time of report or last communication.

ADDITIONAL COMMENTS

With one exception, patients with recurrences have not originated from a particular geographic region. The exception was the report of six patients from the Rhône-Alpes region who had a total of 20 recurrent episodes over a period of 22 years. None of these patients had a family history of HUS (43).

In our original analysis of information from 30 cases, the mortality rate was 30% compared with 19% in the present survey of 71 cases. Six patients (8%) have progressed to end-stage renal failure. Several factors may have accounted for this apparent reduction in mortality. These include infusions of fresh frozen plasma, vigorous plasmapheresis, and better control of hypertension. Although no controlled trials have been done, it has been our practice to offer a trial of therapy with fresh frozen plasma for several days. If the patient has failed to respond, we have used plasmapheresis. We do not use plasmapheresis for the treatment of typical cases of HUS. The treatment of recurrent episodes of HUS with plasmapheresis is discussed in Chapter 30.

REFERENCES

1. Brain, M. C. The haemolytic-uraemic syndrome. *Semin. Hematol., 6*: 162–180 (1969).
2. Dacie, J. V., Mollison, P. L., Richardson, N., Selwyn, J. G., Shapiro, L. Atypical congenital haemolytic anaemia. *Quart. J. Med., 22*: 79–98 (1953).
3. Shumway, C. N., Miller, G. Hemolytic anemia, thrombocytopenic purpura and renal disease. *Blood, 12*: 1045–1060 (1957).
4. MacFarlane, P. S. Haemolytic anaemia associated with acute renal damage in infancy. *Arch. Dis. Child, 33*: 181 (1958).
5. Von Schubothe, H., Kerp, L., Klemm, D. Hamolytisch-uramisches syndrom im erwachsenenalter. *Blut, 15*: 65–70 (1967).
6. Gasser, C. Hamolyticsh-Uramisches Syndrom. In: *Handbuch Der Kinderheilkunde* (H. Opitz, F. S. Schmid, eds.) Springer-Verlag, Berlin, pp. 951–963 (1967).
7. Kaplan, B. S. Hemolytic uremic syndrome with recurrent episodes: an important subset. *Clin. Nephrol., 8*: 495–498 (1977).
8. Gervais, M., Richardson, J. B., Chiu, J., Drummond, K. N. Immunofluorescent and histologic findings in the hemolytic uremic syndrome. *Pediatrics, 47*: 352–359 (1971).
9. Seiler, G., Tietze, H. U. Hamolytisch-uramisches syndrom. Bericht uber 3 falle. Z. *Kinderheilk., 106*: 249–259 (1969).
10. De Jong, M.C.J.W., Monnens, L. A. Recurrent haemolytic uraemic syndrome. *Padiatr. Padologie, 11*: 521–527 (1976).
11. Hagge, W. F., Holley, K. E., Burke, E. G., Stickler, G. B. Hemolytic-uremic syndrome in two siblings. *N. Engl. J. Med., 277*: 138–139 (1967).
12. Meroni, M., Volpi, A., Battini, G., Conte, F., Ferrario, G., Giordano, F., Tarelli, L. T., Tommasi, A., Sessa, A. Recurrent hemolytic uremic syndrome: Case report. *Nephron, 44*: 263–264 (1986).
13. Habib, R., Levy, M., Gagnadoux, M-F., Broyer, M. Prognosis of the hemolytic uremic syndrome in children. *Adv. Nephrol., 11*: 109–128 (1982).
14. Carreras, L., Romero, R., Requesens, C., Oliver, A. J., Carrera, M., Clavo, M., Alsina, J. Familial hypocomplementemic hemolytic uremic syndrome with HLA-A3,B7 haplotype. *J.A.M.A., 245*: 602–604 (1981).
15. Courtecuisse, V., Dommergues, J-P., Rivron, J., Chaon, P. Syndrome hemolytique et uremique familial avec biopsie renale normale. *Arch. Fr. Pediatr., 32*: 749–755 (1975).

16. Drukker, A., Winterborn, M., Bennett, B., Churg, J., Spitzer, A., Greifer, I. Recurrent hemolytic-uremic syndrome: A case report. *Clin. Nephrol., 4*: 68–72 (1975).
17. Barre, P., Kaplan, B. S., de Chadarevian, J-P., Drummond, K. N. Hemolytic uremic syndrome with hypocomplementemia, serum C3Nef, and glomerular deposits of C3. *Arch. Pathol. Lab. Med., 101*: 357–361 (1977).
18. Tune, B. M., Groshong, T., Plumer, L. B., Mendoza, S. A. The hemolytic-uremic syndrome in siblings: A prospective survey. *J. Pediatr., 85*: 682–683 (1974).
19. Karmali, M. A., Arbus, G. S., Ish-Shalom, N., Fleming, P. C., Malkin, D., Petric, M., Cheung, R., Louie, S., Humphreys, G. R., Srachan, M. A familial outbreak of hemolytic-uremic syndrome associated with verotoxin-producing *Escherichia coli* serotype O157:H7. *Pediatr. Nephrol., 2*: 409–414 (1987).
20. Strom, T. B. Hemolytic uremic syndrome recurrent in renal allograft. Case Records of New England Journal of medicine. *N. Engl. J. Med., 314*: 1032–1040 (1986).
21. Bergstein, J., Michael, A. Jr., Kjellstrand, C., Simmons, R., Najarian, J. Hemolytic-uremic syndrome in adult sisters. *Transplantation, 17*: 487–489 (1974).
22. Goodman, D. J., Walker, R. G., Birchall, I. E., d'Apice, A.J.F., Powell, H. R., Kincaid-Smith, P. (1991). Recurrent haemolytic uraemic syndrome in a transplant recipient on Orthoclone (OKT3). *Pediatr. Nephrol. 5*: 240–1.
23. Bogdanovic, R., Cvoric, A., Nikolic, V., Sindjic, M. Recurrent haemolytic-uraemic syndrome with hypocomplementaemia: A case report. *Pediatr. Nephrol., 2*: 236–238 (1988).
24. Wyatt, R. J., Jones, D., Stapleton, F. B., Roy III, S., Odom, T. W., McLean, R. H. Recurrent hemolytic-uremic syndrome with the hypomorphic fast allele of the third component of complement. *J. Pediatr., 107*: 564–566 (1985).
25. Thompson, R. A., Winterborn, M H. Hypocomplementemia due to a genetic deficiency of b1H globulin. *Clin. Exp. Immunol., 46*: 119–119 (1981).
26. Cameron, J. S., Vick, R. Plasma C3 in haemolytic uraemic syndrome and thrombotic thrombocytopenic purpura. *Lancet, 2*: 975 (1973).
27. Kaplan, B. S., Thompson, P. D., McNab, G. N. Serum complement levels in haemolytic-uraemic syndrome. *Lancet, 2*: 1505–1506 (1973).
28. Kim, Y., Miller, K., Michael, A. F. Breakdown products of C3 and Factor B in hemolytic-uremic syndrome. *J. Lab. Clin. Med. 80*: 845–850 (1977).
29. Olavarria, F., Mezzano, S., Ardiles, L., Lopez, M. Presence of circulating immune complexes in the classic form of hemolytic syndrome: a constant finding. *Nephron, 52*: 313–316. (1989).
30. Kourilsky, O., Vandewalle, A., Smith, M. D., Stuhlinger, W., Verroust, P. J., Neuilly, G., Kanfer, A., Sraer, J. D., Morel-Moroger, L. Persistent intravascular C3 activation after bilateral nephrectomy in patients with thrombotic microangiopathy. *Clin. Nephrol., 6*: 417–419 (1976).
31. Teisberg, P., Grottum, K. A., Myhre, E., Flatmark, A. In-vivo activation of complement in hereditary nephropathy. *Lancet, 2*: 356–358 (1973).
32. Levin, M., Elkon, K. B., Noakes, T.J.C., Buckle, A. M., Dillom, M. J., Hardisty, R. M., Barratt, T. M. Inhibitor of prostacyclin production in sporadic haemolytic uraemic syndrome. *Arch. Dis. Child, 58*: 703–708 (1983).
33. Gomperts, E. D., Sessel, L., du Plessis, V., Hersch, C. Recurrent post-partum haemolytic uraemic syndrome. *Lancet, 1*: 48 (1978).
34. Mettler, N. E. Isolation of a microtatobiote from patients with hemolytic-uremic syndrome and thrombotic thrombocytopenic purpura and from mites in the United States. *N. Engl. J. Med., 281*: 1026–1027 (1969).
35. Bonsib, S. M., Ercolani, L., Ngheim, D., Hamilton, H. E. Recurrent thrombotic microangiopathy in a renal allograft. Case report and review of the literature. *Am. J. Med., 79*: 520–527 (1985).

36. Rifle, G., Chalopin, J. M., Genin, R., Justrabo, E., Severac, J., Balte, F. Syndrome hemolytique et uremique recidivant. Necrose cortical irreversible sous oestro-progestatifs. *J. Urol. Nephrol. (Paris), 85*: 331 (1979).
37. Hoorntje, S. J., Prins, E.J.L., Smith, A. J., Donker, AB., J. M. Reversal of long-standing renal insufficiency by captopril in a patient with relapsing hemolytic uremic syndrome due to an oral contraceptive. *Ann. Intern. Med., 94*: 355–357 (1981).
38. Hauglustaine, D., van Damme, B., Vanrenterghem, Y., Michielsen, P. Recurrent hemolytic uremic syndrome during oral contraception. *Clin. Nephrol., 15*: 148–153 (1981).
39. Sennesael, J. J., Vanden Houte, K. M., Spapen, H. D., de Bruyne, R.M.G., Verbeelen, D. L. Recurrent hemolytic uremic syndrome and metastatic malignancy. *Am. J. Nephrol., 7*: 60–64 (1987).
40. Mendoza, S. A., Sellers, B. B. Jr., Griswold, W. R. Hemolytic uremic syndrome and idiopathic thrombocytopenic purpura in a single patient. *J. Pediatr., 91*: 851–852 (1977).
41. Kaplan, B. S. Hemolytic-uremic syndrome followed by idiopathic thrombocytopenic purpura. *Int. J. Pediatr. Nephrol., 2*: 97–98 (1981).
42. Stein, C. S., Flexner, J. M. Idiopathic thrombocytopenic purpura during remission of thrombotic thrombocytopenic purpura. *South. Med. J., 77*: 1599–1601 (1984).
43. Larbre, F., Dechelette, E., Sellem, C., Parchoux, B., Marchal, A. Le syndrome hémolytique et uremique recidivant. A propos de 6 observations recueillies dans la région Rhône-Alpes. *Pediatrie, 34*: 433–441 (1979).
44. MacWhinney, J. B., Packer, J. T., Miller, G., Greendyke, R. M. Thrombotic thrombocytopenic purpura in childhood. *Blood 19*: 181–199 (1962).
45. Case Records of the Massachusetts General Hospital. *N. Engl. J. Med., 269*: 1195–1203 (1963).
46. Dacie, J. V. Haemolytic-uraemic syndrome. In: *The Hemolytic Anemias*, ed. 2. J. & A. Churchill, Ltd., London, pp. 841–907 (1967).
47. Wehinger, H., Zollinger, H. U., Schenck, W., Kunzer, W. Hamolytisch-uramisches syndrom (Gasser). Bericht uber zwei kinder mit ungewohnlichem verlauf. *Klin. Wschr.*, 874–881 (1968).
48. Egli, F., Stalder, G., Gloor, F., Duckert, F., Keller, F., Hottinger, A. Heparintherapie des hamolytisch-uramischen syndroms. *Helv. Paediatr. Acta., 24*: 13–37 (1969).
49. Belobradkova, J., Nozicka, Z. Hemolytico-uremicky syndrom. *Cas. Lek. Cesk., 111*: 85–90 (1972).
50. Markiewicz, K. Nawracajaca ostra niewydolnose nerek. *Polski Tygodnik Lekarski, 27*: 272–273 (1972).
51. Willoughby, M.L.N., Murphy, A. V., McMorris, S., Jewell, F. G. Coagulation studies in haemolytic uraemic syndrome. *Arch. Dis. Child, 47*: 766–771 (1972).
52. Westra, B. Recurrent haemolytic-uraemic syndrome treatment with and without heparin. *N.Z. Med. J., 80*: 209–210 (1974).
53. Janssen, F., Potvliege, P. R., Vainsel, M., Vis, H-L. Le prognostic a court et a long terme du syndrome hemolytique et uremique. *Arch. Fr. Pediatr., 31*: 59–69.
54. Olgaard, K., Madsen, S., Jacobsen, S. V. Recurrent attacks of hemolytic anemia, thrombocytopenia, and uremia—hemolytic uremic syndrome? *Acta. Med. Scand., 196*: 541–543 (1974).
55. Shigematsu, H., Dikman, S. H., Churg, J., Grishman, E., Duffy. Mesangial involvement in hemolytic-uremic syndrome. A light and electron microscopic study. *Am. J. Pathol., 85*: 349–362 (1976).
56. Spirer, Z., Knobel, B., Earon, J., Heyman, I., Bogair, N. Recurrent hemolytic-uremic syndrome. A report of two cases. *Helv. Paediatr. Acta., 32*: 165–172 (1977).
57. Rao, S. P., Sutton, A. L., Falter, M. L., Robinson, M. G. Chronic microangiopathic

hemolytic anemia. Association with Escherichia coli infections. *N.Y. State J. Med.*, *79*: 1763–1765 (1979).

58. Coulthard, M. G. An evaluation of treatment with heparin in the haemolytic-uraemic syndrome successfully treated by peritoneal dialysis. *Arch. Dis. Child*, *55*: 393–397 (1980).
59. Brasher, C., Siegler, R. L. The hemolytic-uremic syndrome. *West. J. Med.*, *134*: 193–197 (1981).
60. Hoorntje, S. J., Prins, E.J.L., Smith, A. J., Donker, AB. J. M. Reversal of long-standing renal insufficiency by captopril in a patient with relapsing hemolytic uremic syndrome due to an oral contraceptive. *Ann. Intern. Med.*, *94*: 355–357 (1981).
61. Kreisinger, J., Janda, J. Zweiterkrankung eines hamolytisch-uramischen syndroms bei einem 8 jarhrigen madchen. *Monatsschr. Kinderheilkd.*, *128*: 435–437 (1980).
62. Elias, M., Horowitz, J., Tal, I., Kohn, D., Flatau, E. Thrombotic thrombocytopenic purpura and haemolytic uraemic syndrome in three siblings. *Arch. Dis. Child*, *63*: 644–646 (1988).
63. Mattoo, T. J., Mahmood, M. A., Al-Harbi, M. S., Mikail, I. Familial, recurrent hemolytic-uremic syndrome. *J. Pediatr.*, *114*: 814– (1989).

14
Atypical Hemolytic Uremic Syndrome

Margaret M. Fitzpatrick, Michael J. Dillon, and T. Martin Barratt *Institute of Child Health, London, England* **Richard S. Trompeter** *Hospitals for Sick Children, London, England*

The concept of heterogeneity of the hemolytic uremic syndrome (HUS) is well established (1–7). Variability in outcome has long been recognized, and follow-up studies indicated that the absence of prodromal diarrhea was the most powerful predictor of relapse and/or residual renal dysfunction in children with HUS (5). Other studies pointed to recurrence of HUS as identifying an important subset with a poor prognosis (2). These two phenomena are highly but not exclusively correlated. This chapter assumes the primary subdivision of HUS to be those cases with prodromal diarrhea (D+ HUS) and those without (D– HUS) (8); it is based on the 21 cases of D– HUS referred to the Hospital for Sick Children (HSC), London, from 1968–1990. The clinical features of the 10 patients who relapsed are given in Table 1; those of the 11 who died during their initial illness or did not relapse are given in Table 2.

D+ HUS is synonymous with typical, epidemic, or enteropathic HUS. It characteristically affects infants and young children, usually in the summer months. Microangiopathic hemolytic anemia, thrombocytopenia, and renal failure develop suddenly about 1 week after the onset of the diarrhea. The majority of affected children recover completely, and relapses do not occur. A strain of *Escherichia coli* (*E. coli* O157:H7) was isolated from cases of hemorrhagic colitis, and subsequently from children with D+ HUS which produced a toxin cytopathic to Vero cells: verocytotoxin-producing *E. coli* (VTEC) are now thought to be responsible for most cases of D+ HUS.

In contrast, D– HUS, also referred to as atypical or sporadic HUS, affects children of all ages. It develops insidiously, often without a prodromal illness (6, 7). This form of HUS may be familial (1) and frequently follows a relapsing or progressive course (2, 5). Severe hypertension, end-stage renal failure (ESRF), and multisystem involvement, especially neurological, may occur; the ultimate prognosis is poor (1, 2,

Table 1 Patients with Relapsing D− HUS

Pt	Sex	Age	FH	PMNL count	CNS involvement	Dial	Relapses	PEx	Outcome
1	F	13.5	−	3.2	+	+	3	22	Died
2	F	4.9	−	3.7	−	+	4	67	P/BP
3	M	0.2	+	10.3	+	+	2	14	ESRF
4	M	0.15	−	14.1	+	+	1	NIL	Died
5	F	0.75	+	5.9	−	+	4	52	P/BP
6	M	5.9	−	4.8	−	+	8	227	P/BP
7	M	3.3	−	4.5	−	−	2	15	P/BP
8	M	0.3	−	5.4	−	+	3	233	ESRF
9	F	10.5	−	5.9	−	−	2	58	P/BP
10	F	0.9	−	13.6	−	+	1	4	N

N = normal
P/BP = proteinuria/hypertensive
ESRF = end-stage renal failure
Dial = dialysis
PEx = plasma exchange
FH = family history

5, 10). Many cases of D– HUS are indeed indistinguishable from thrombotic thrombocytopenic purpura (TTP) as described in adults, and the literature on the two conditions overlaps (3, 11, 12). The major features associated with D– HUS are listed in Table 3.

EPIDEMIOLOGY

D– HUS is a rare disorder. From 1968–1990 inclusive, 176 children with HUS, defined as the simultaneous occurrence of a microangiopathic hemolytic anemia,

Table 2 Patients Who Died During Initial Illness or Did Not Relapse

Pt	Sex	Age	Dialysis	PMNL count	CNS involvement	Outcome
1	M	0.7	+	4.6	+	Died
2	M	4.5	+	5.7	+	Died
3	F	4.5	+	7.8	+	Died
4	F	2.1	−	8.9	−	N
5	M	6.5	+	2.9	−	ESRF
6	M	0.5	−	8.4	+	P/BP
7	M	5.6	+	3.9	−	P/BP
8	F	9.5	+	4.6	−	ESRF
9	F	2.5	+	7.8	+	P/BP
10	M	12.0	+	14.4	−	BP
11	F	9.0	+	5.5	−	P/BP

N = normal
P/BP = proteinuria/hypertensive
ESRF = end-stage renal failure

Table 3 Features Associated with D− HUS

Genetic factors	Consanguinity/FH
Age	Infants/older children
Season	No seasonal variation
Prodrome	Nonspecific/respiratory
Onset	Insidious
CNS involvement	Common
Hypertension	Severe
Polymorphonuclear leukocyte count	Normal
Complement abnormalities	Present
Platelet-derived growth factor	High
Prostacyclin	Deficiency/inhibitor
Renal pathology	Arteriolar
Relapse	Common
Plasma exchange	Therapeutic role
End-stage renal failure	Common
Death	Common

thrombocytopenia, and acute renal failure, were treated at the HSC. Of these, 155 had prodromal diarrhea (D+ HUS) and 21 (12.4%) did not (D– HUS). The proportion of D– cases is probably an overestimate of the true situation because of a referral bias. We have excluded cases in which disseminated intravascular coagulation with an HUS-like picture has complicated *E. coli* septicemia, and HUS complicating pneumococcal infection—a well-defined entity mediated by neuraminidase.

Eleven of the 21 D– HUS children were male and 10 were female. Their age at presentation ranged from 0.1–13.5 years (median 4.6) (Fig. 1); in contrast, age at presentation of D+ HUS was grouped more tightly around a median of 2.3 years.

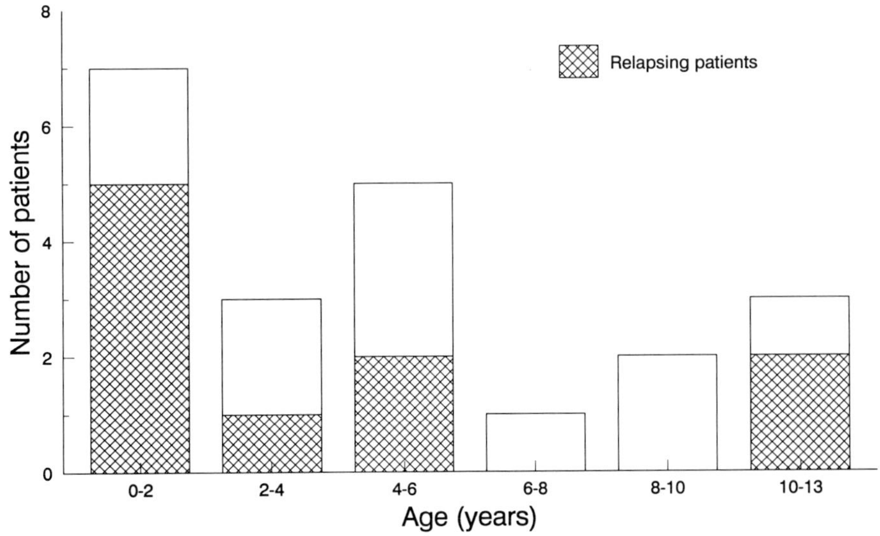

Figure 1 Age distribution of 21 children with atypical (non-diarrhea-associated) hemolytic uremic syndrome (D− HUS).

D+ HUS occurs more often in the summer months, with 103 (66%) of the 155 children presenting between May and September inclusive, whereas D– HUS does not have a seasonal variation in incidence, with only nine (43%) presenting in the summer months.

GENETIC AND RACIAL FACTORS

Both recessive and dominant inheritance of HUS has been reported (1, 12, 14). Kaplan et al. (1) analyzed familial HUS and reported two distinct patterns. There were families in whom siblings were affected more or less simultaneously (within 1 month of each other); these tended to occur in regions where HUS was common, to be associated with diarrhea, and to have a good outcome. In other families, often reported from nonendemic areas, siblings were affected sequentially and tended to follow a relapsing course with a poor outcome. The former familial pattern is now interpreted as D+ HUS resulting from common exposure to a causative infectious agent, the latter as D– HUS resulting from a genetically determined predisposition.

Four (19%) of the 21 HSC children were from African or Asian families, all but one of whom were resident in the United Kingdom at the time of onset of the illness. This contrasts with our experience of children with D+ HUS, of whom only seven (4.5%) of the 155 were from immigrant families. Only one of the D– HUS children had affected siblings (Fig. 2); in none was there history of the disorder in preceding generations, but two (9%) had consanguinous parents.

It is not clear whether the greater incidence of D– HUS in immigrant families represents a true difference in racial susceptibility or reflects the practice of consanguinous marriage in those communities.

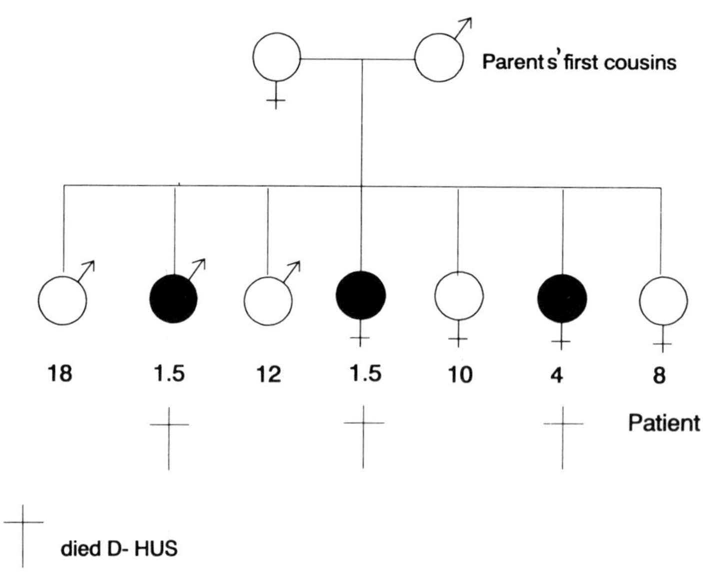

Figure 2 Family tree of a child with D– HUS, currently under our care, undergoing a program of intermittent plasma exchange.

CLINICAL FEATURES

The prodromal symptoms in the 21 D– HUS children included vomiting (n = 16), fever (n = 7), maculopapular rash (n = 7), upper respiratory tract infection (n = 7), malaise (n = 4), and jaundice (n = 4). One child had tuberculous adenitis and was being treated with rifampicin. Three others had documented infections: an *E. coli* urinary tract infection, a group B β-hemolytic streptococcal septicemia, and a *Mycoplasma pneumoniae* infection complicated by an anti-p autoimmune hemolytic anaemia.

Fifteen of the 21 D– HUS children required dialysis for treatment of renal failure. In many of these, however, the progression of the renal failure was slow, and dialysis was not initiated until several days after admission to hospital. Of these 15, three died during the acute phase of their illness while still being dialyzed and two progressed to ESRF and remained dialysis dependent. In the remaining 10 children, the mean duration of dialysis was 21 days (range 4–46).

Hypertension is characteristically severe and resistant to treatment. Seventeen of the D– HUS patients were hypertensive at presentation, and 14 of these were resistant to volume depletion. The hypertension is believed to be renin-mediated, a consequence of the afferent arteriolar narrowing characteristic of the condition. Central nervous system (CNS) involvement unrelated to the complications of renal failure is one of the principal features taken to differentiate TTP from HUS. Two of our relapsing cases of D– HUS had CNS involvement at presentation and subsequently died from them—one following an intracranial hemorrhage and the other after a cerebral infarct. Three of four others who had CNS involvement with fits died during the acute illness as a result of septicemia and peritonitis.

LABORATORY INVESTIGATIONS

Microangiopathic Hemolytic Anemia

The pattern of erythrocyte fragmentation is similar in D+ and D– HUS. There are, however, a few D– HUS cases in which the anemia is a marked feature but there is little evidence of renal involvement.

Polymorphoneutrophil Leukocytes (PMNL)

A raised peripheral blood PMNL count is typical of D+ HUS, with a high count heralding a poor outcome (15). There is evidence of PMNL activation, with marked elevation of circulating α_1-antitrypsin–bound elastase indicating release of granule contents (Fig. 3) (16). In D– HUS, however, the circulating PMNL count is usually normal or only slightly elevated (and this is a very helpful diagnostic feature). In the present series the median PMNL count was 5.7 (range 2.9–14.4). Oddly, there are a few cases of D– HUS with marked elevation of circulating α_1-antitrypsin–bound elastase but normal PMNL counts; this feature is unexplained (16).

Complement

Complement activation with low plasma concentrations of C3 and C4 has been observed in both D+ and D– HUS. The presence of increased breakdown products of C3 and factor B suggest activation of the alternate pathway.

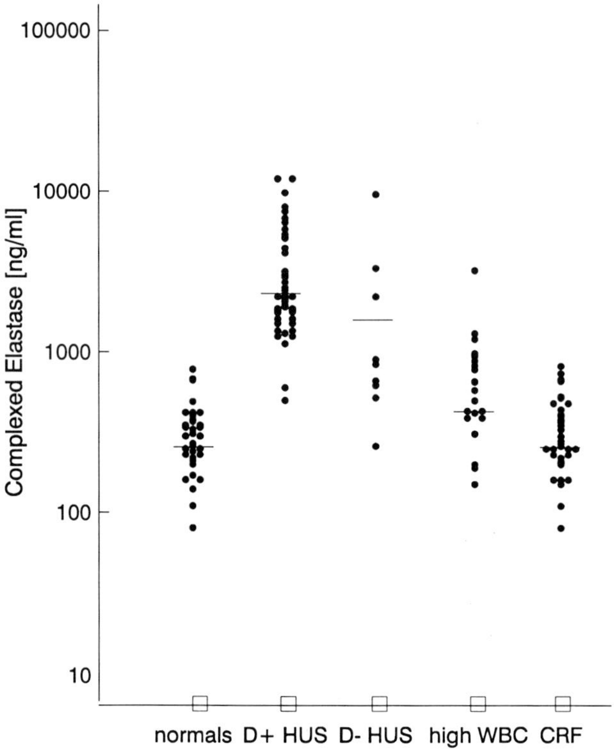

Figure 3 Alpha-1-antitrypsin complexed elastase levels in the plasma of children with D+ HUS, D− HUS, chronic renal failure, high white blood cell counts secondary to other febrile illnesses, and normal controls.

A number of different complement abnormalities have been observed in families with familial or recurrent D– HUS; a low C3 with C3 nephritic factor, a hypomorphic fast allele of C3, and a deficiency of β_1h-globulin. These observations indicate that D– HUS is itself a heterogeneous disorder, possibly with many different genetically determined defects leading to similar disease patterns.

Platelets

Intravascular platelet activation and increased platelet destruction occur in both forms of HUS (20). Platelet survival is shortened, and platelets circulate in a degranulated form (20–23). Such "exhausted" platelets do not aggregate in response to ADP, and are associated with prolonged bleeding times and occasionally severe hemorrhage (21). Plasma levels of platelet factors such as serotonin and platelet-derived growth factor (PDGF) are increased and their intraplatelet concentrations diminished. Raised plasma levels of PDGF are characteristic of D– HUS, and it has been postulated that they are responsible for the characteristic proliferative lesion (24).

Intravascular platelet activation persists for several weeks after the platelet count has returned to normal in both D+ and D– HUS (20). In relapsing D– HUS, platelet activation eventually returns to normal during remission. A fall in platelet serotonin content is a sensitive marker of relapse, and may be present even though the peripheral blood platelet count is within the normal range (Fig. 4).

Endothelium

The recognition of prostacyclin (PGI_2) as a powerful inhibitor of platelet aggregation led Remuzzi et al. (25) to postulate that the intravascular platelet activation seen in HUS resulted from a failure of the vessel wall to produce PGI_2. This was considered to be due either to a lack of a normal plasma factor stimulating PGI_2 production or to an inhibitor of PGI_2 synthesis (4, 26). Subsequent studies confirmed reduction in PGI_2 production in vitro after incubation of endothelial cells with HUS plasma. This abnormality is generally only found in children with D– HUS or adults with TTP, and plasma from children with D+ HUS usually supports PGI_2 production normally (4, 26, 27). Using cultured human umbilical endothelial cells and a bioassay for PGI_2, Walters et al. (21) found reduced support of PGI_2 by plasma from 7 of 9 (77%) D– HUS children but only 9 of 33 (27%) D+ HUS children.

The detection of abnormalities of PGI_2 production during relapse of D– HUS and in unaffected individuals from families with D– HUS suggests that inherited or acquired defects of PGI_2 synthesis may be of pathogenetic importance in the disorder (28–30). These data also emphasize the need to consider the heterogeneity of HUS when investigating its pathogenesis.

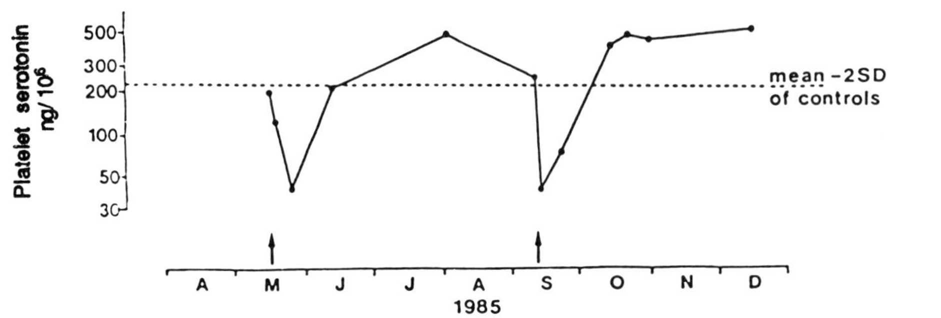

Figure 4 Platelet serotonin concentrations and platelet/plasma serotonin ratios in a child with D– HUS showing a rapid fall during two successive relapses. Relapses are marked by an arrow and show a simultaneous fall in the platelet count and a rise in plasma creatinine.

RENAL PATHOLOGY

The two clinically and epidemiologically distinct subgroups of HUS have different renal histology (31, 32). D+ HUS is associated predominantly with glomerular pathology characterized by endothelial cell swelling, separation of the endothelial cells from the basement membrane, narrowing of the glomerular capillary lumen, and capillary thrombosis. In contrast, the pathological changes of D– HUS are primarily vascular, with proliferation of endothelial and smooth muscle cells to produce changes resembling the "onion skin" proliferative lesions of malignant hypertension (31–33) (Fig. 5).

NATURAL HISTORY AND OUTCOME

The outcome of D+ HUS has improved considerably over the past 3 decades with better management of acute renal failure (34–36). Of the 155 cases of D+ HUS treated at HSC between 1968 and 1990, 10 (6.5%) died; 46 (29.6%) had some degree of residual renal impairment with reduced glomerular filtration rate, proteinuria, or hypertension; and 99 (63.9%) recovered (Fig. 6). However, a closer scrutiny of cases that have apparently recovered completely shows a significant degree of residual occult nephropathy (37). Children with D+ HUS do not relapse with further episodes of acute renal failure or recurrence of the haematological abnormalities.

In contrast, D– HUS has a much worse outlook. Three of the 21 cases died in the acute phase and a further two never recovered renal function; of the remaining 16, 10

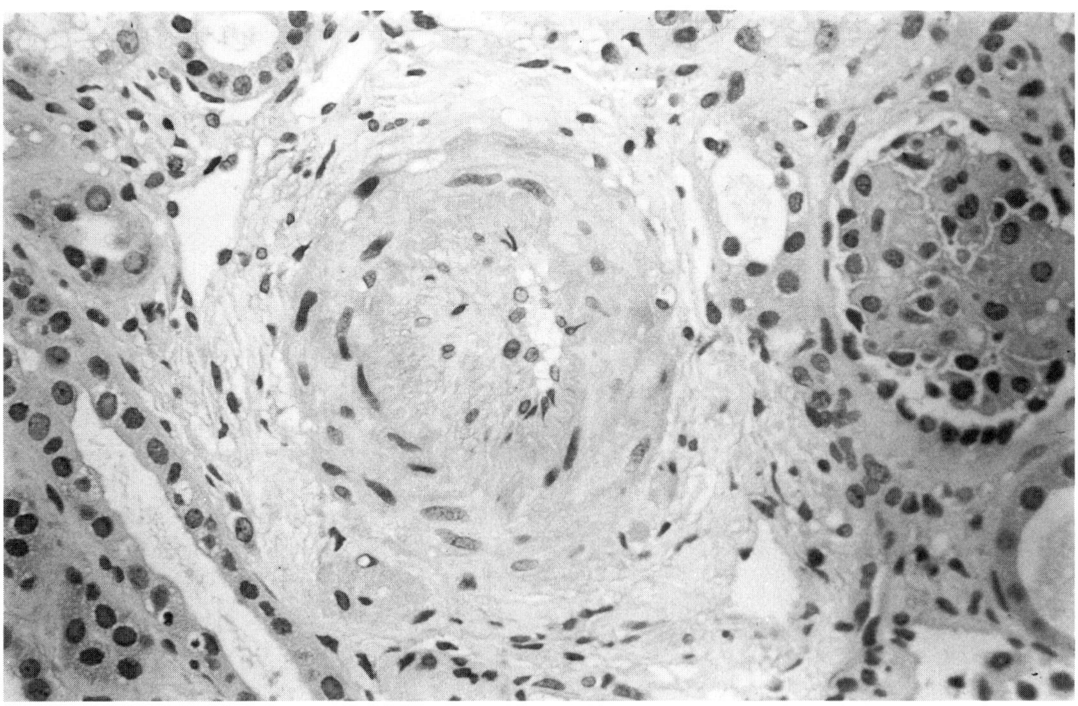

Figure 5 Characteristic histological features associated with D– HUS.

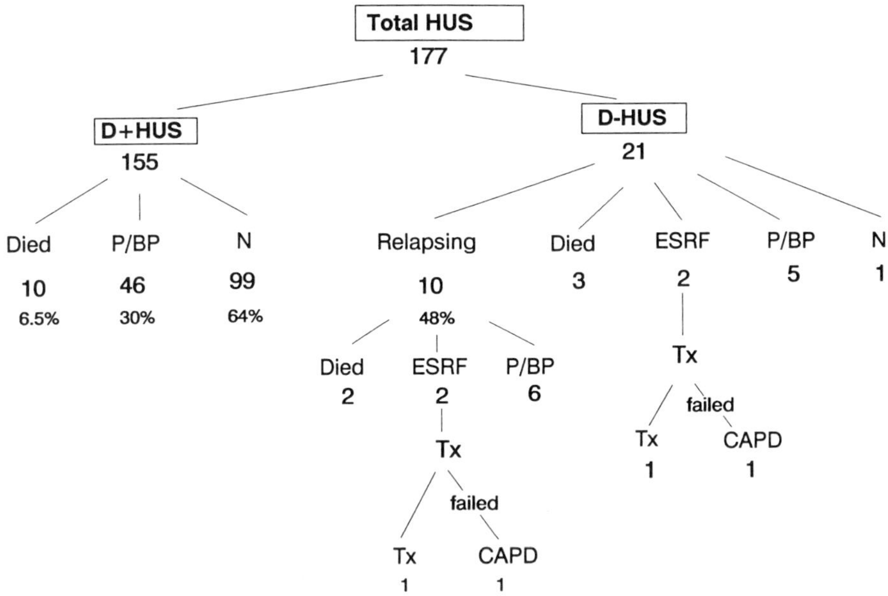

Figure 6 Diagrammatic representation of the renal outcome of 177 children presenting to the HSC between 1970 and 1990 with HUS. N: Normal, P/BP: proteinuria/hypertension, ESRF: end-stage renal failure, Tx: transplanted, CAPD: continuous peritoneal dialysis.

had one or more relapses with episodes of acute deterioration of renal function associated with a dip in the platelet count. Both relapsing and nonrelapsing D– HUS fare badly (Fig. 6); five are dead, four are on ESRF programs, 11 have proteinuria and/or hypertension, and only one has apparently recovered completely.

No differences were observed at presentation between the clinical features of those who relapsed and those who did not (Tables 1 and 2). Eight of the 10 patients with recurrent HUS had more than one relapse, the maximum number being eight spread over a period of several years. Relapses were sometimes associated with infection and were often heralded by a deterioration in control of hypertension.

Five (23.9%) children died: three in the acute phase with infection, coagulopathy and neurological involvement in addition to renal failure, and two during a relapse with neurological complications. The four children with ESRF have all been transplanted. Of the two who had nonrelapsing disease, one has a functioning graft, but the other lost her graft with recurrence of HUS after 4 years. One of the two relapsing cases has a functioning graft, but the other lost two grafts within 2 weeks of transplantation from recurrent HUS: on the second occasion there was glomerular capillary thrombosis with a flare-up of microangiopathic hemolytic anaemia and thrombocytopenia after a quiescent period of more than 1 year.

TREATMENT

The cornerstone of treatment for all cases of HUS is early control of renal failure and hypertension with careful correction of electrolyte imbalance and anaemia. Dialysis should be initiated promptly. Vigorous control of hypertension, often a striking feature of D– HUS, is essential, the objective being to maintain the blood pressure at or below the mean normal for age. In most instances volume depletion alone is insufficient to control the blood pressure, and angiotensin-converting inhibition is appropriate as the hypertension appears to be mediated by the renin angiotensin system.

A number of therapeutic measures directed at the underlying pathogenesis of the disorder have been used in D– HUS, but none have been substantiated by controlled clinical trial—in part because of the complexity and heterogeneity of the individual clinical situations, and in part because of the lack of suitable short-term outcome parameters.

Prostacyclin

In view of the evidence pointing to a deficiency of PGI_2 in patients with HUS (4, 26–28), it has seemed logical to combat acute crises, essentially those associated with severe hypertension and CNS involvement, with PGI_2 infusion. PGI_2 is a powerful vasodilator and inhibitor of platelet aggregation with a very short half-life. It has to be administered by constant intravenous infusion, and it is very expensive. The usual starting dose is 2 ng/kg/min; infusion rates up to 20 ng/kg/min have been used. The most troublesome complications are hypotension and diarrhea.

Although there are a number of reports of prostacyclin being used in D– HUS and TTP, and we ourselves used it in four of the 21 cases, the heterogeneity and lack of structure of this data preclude formulation of a view on its efficacy.

Plasma Infusion

Infusions of fresh plasma have been observed to have a beneficial effect in some adults with TTP (38). This has been attributed to supply of a deficient plasma factor essential to prostacyclin synthesis. Infusions of fresh plasma have been used quite extensively in D+ HUS. In one prospective controlled study undertaken on behalf of the French Society of Pediatric Nephrology (39) of the treatment of childhood HUS with plasma, infusions of 10 mL/kg of fresh plasma for 3 days resulted in a better outcome of renal function and a reduction in residual histological damage.

The experience of fresh plasma infusions in D– HUS is less clearly defined, and there are no reports which substantiate a beneficial effect.

Plasma Exchange

In view of reports of occasional cases of TTP and HUS which failed to respond to infusions of fresh plasma but responded to plasma exchange (40, 41), as well as the possibility that deficient PGI_2 production is a consequence of a circulating inhibitor, a number of centers, including our own, have used plasma exchange extensively in the management of relapsing D– HUS (42–45). Again it must be emphasised that there are no controlled therapeutic studies, and there are reports of spontaneous recovery from relapsing episodes of HUS in individual patients which make assessment of case reports of plasma exchange in D– HUS difficult to evaluate.

Plasma exchange can be effected by either of two different methods—plasma filtration or centrifugation. The choice of method selected is influenced by body size and cardiovascular stability of the patient, from which the maximum safe extracorporeal volume is determined, usually 8–10% of total blood volume (taken as 100 mL/kg in infants <10 kg, and 80 mL/kg in children >10 kg). Plasma filtration entails pumping the patient's blood through a hollow-fiber plasma filter which has pores with a maximum size of 0.5–0.6 μ, allowing water and plasma to pass through. The filtered plasma is replaced by the same volume of plasma protein fraction (PPF), followed finally by fresh frozen plasma (FFP). The total extracorporeal volume of the plasma filtration circuit is less than 100 mL, making this the most suitable method for use in small patients or in those whose circulation is unstable.

The system of centrifugal plasma exchange involves pumping blood into a centrifuge in which whole blood is separated into red blood cells and plasma. The plasma and red cells are pumped separately out of the centrifuge, the plasma to waste and the red blood cells to be reconstituted as whole blood with PPF and reinfused. In both methods of exchange, the patient's circulating volume is maintained but the plasma replaced. The total extracorporeal circuit volume in the centrifugal system is usually about 250 mL; this method is therefore only suitable for the larger more stable patients. We are currently using the COBE Spectra Apheresis System (COBE Laboratories Inc) for the centrifugal technique. This system individualizes the procedure for each patient and allows rapid removal of plasma without the loss of cellular components. The extracorporeal blood volume of this circuit is only 170 mL, making it safer for use in small children.

Both types of treatment require anticoagulation. Acid citrate dextrose solution is used and infused throughout the procedure. The replacement plasma should be diluted with normal saline or half normal saline/dextrose mixture to produce a replacement fluid with a sodium and albumin content similar to that of the patient. This is done to avoid sudden shifts in extra cellular fluid volume, particularly the intravascular expansion which may result from a sudden increase in the plasma albumin concentration. We have found that the incidence of hypertension, fluid overload, and pulmonary edema occurring after exchange has been reduced with this modification. The plasma exchange is completed using 10 ml/kg of FFP to replace the intrinsic clotting factors which are not present in PPF and are lost by either filtration or centrifugation. All patients are given hydrocortisone and piriton prior to plasma exchange to reduce the risk of anaphylaxis. Patients with D– HUS in our hospital are currently treated with 2-volume plasma exchange; the volume of plasma exchanged being calculated as 2 × ⅔ total blood volume. The procedure is initially performed daily for 5 days if tolerated. Only one of the nonrelapsing children in this review was managed by plasma exchange, as the other patients presented before this treatment was available. This child presented in 1981 and had five plasma exchanges. She made a good recovery from the acute episode and now has a glomerular filtration rate of 98 mL/min/1.73m^2SA but is hypertensive and has significant proteinuria. The children with relapsing disease are now managed by a program of intermittent plasma exchange at increasing intervals for several months after the last relapse. Nine of the 10 relapsing cases were managed in this way, the remaining child having died at first relapse prior to the initiation of this treatment. These nine patients had a median of 2.5 relapses (range 1–8) and received a median of 37 plasma exchanges (range 4–233). These cases are too few in number and too heterogeneous for firm conclusions to be drawn. However, the episodes of acute renal failure were reversed but the former baseline renal function was seldom achieved. In all but one case, a gradual decline in renal function occurred. In the two children who had frequent relapses it was observed that as the frequency of exchanges declined there was a tendency to relapse 6–8 weeks following the last exchange (Fig. 7).

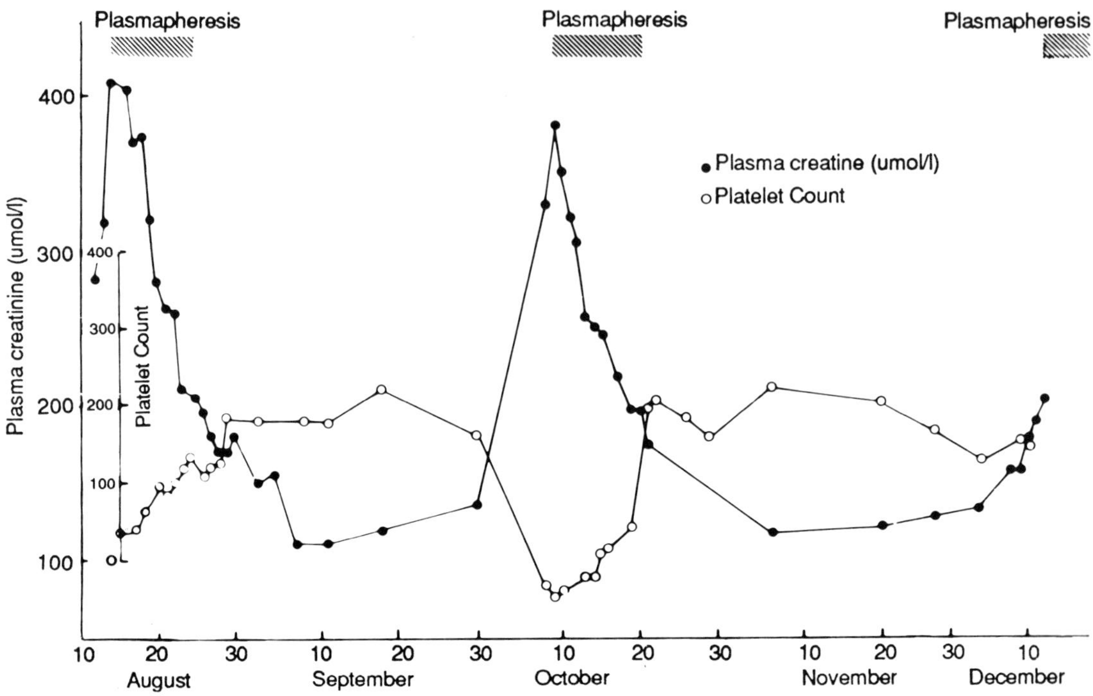

Figure 7 Case of D− HUS treated with a program of plasma exchange. A relapse is shown by a simultaneous rise in plasma creatinine and fall in platelet count. The number of plasma exchanges are shown at the top of the figure.

There are problems and complications associated with plasma exchange. The procedure requires appropriate vascular access in the form of a double-lumen catheter inserted either centrally or peripherally into a major vessel. There may be electrolyte and fluid disturbances resulting in hypervolemia and pulmonary edema or hypovolemia and shock. Anaphylactic reactions are relatively common despite appropriate cover and may be accompanied by cyanosis, bronchospasm, soft-tissue edema, and stridor. There is a risk of infection and of bleeding. It is also an expensive treatment both in terms of the hardware used and plasma required and the specialist medical and nursing time involved.

RECURRENCE FOLLOWING TRANSPLANTATION

In renal transplant recipients, de novo HUS is rare (46) but recurrence of HUS is more common (47); both have assumed greater importance since the introduction of cyclosporin A (CyA) to immunosuppressive regimens. Folman et al. (48) first reported a child with recurrent HUS 1 month following transplantation, and Hauglustine et al. (49) observed recurrent HUS in woman whose two episodes were triggered by oral contraceptives. Interpretation of reports of the outcome of transplantation in HUS is difficult, as it is not always clear whether the initial illness was D+ HUS complicated by acute cortical necrosis or D– HUS, but as these are different disease processes they should be considered separately, with recurrence of HUS being more likely in D– HUS than in D+ cases with cortical necrosis.

A particular problem exists in relation to CyA, which is known to cause a nephropathy that has many features in common with D– HUS and is probably best avoided in these cases. Recurrence of HUS has certainly been documented in both CyA and non-CyA-treated patients (46, 47, 50–52). The onset of allograft rejection (53) and hypertension (54) may trigger HUS. It has also been reported in association with antilymphocyte globulin (ALG) (55) and Orthoclone OKT®3 Sterile Solution (56). It is, however, very difficult to distinguish recurrence of HUS from severe acute vascular or chronic rejection on histological examination of kidney tissue: in all cases, glomerular and arteriolar fibrin thrombi, double contours and necrosis of glomeruli and tubuli may occur.

Four of the 21 children in our series have been transplanted. One child has received two grafts. Two children currently have a functioning transplant, and neither received CyA as immunosuppression. The three graft losses were attributed to recurrence of HUS, and in two of these instances CyA was used. Currently, two patients are on dialysis and a further two have declining renal function with glomerular filtration rates of less than 30 mL/min/m^2SA.

It is clear that there is a significant risk of recurrence of HUS post renal transplantation (43, 48) which may occur in patients receiving a wide range of immunosuppressive agents and how recurrence of HUS can best be predicted or avoided following transplantation remains an important clinical problem.

REFERENCES

1. Kaplan, B. S., Chesney, R. W., Drummond, R. N. Hemolytic uremic syndrome in families. *N. Engl. J. Med., 292*: 1090–1093 (1975).
2. Kaplan, B. S. Hemolytic uremic syndrome with recurrent episodes: An important subset. *Clin. Nephrol., 8*: 495–498 (1977).
3. Fong, J.S.C., de Chadaverian, J. P., Kaplan, B. S. Hemolytic uremic syndrome: Current concepts and management. *Pediatr. Clin. N. Am., 4*: 835–856 (1982).
4. Levin, M., Elkon, K. B., Nokes, T.J.C., Buchle, A. M., Dillon, M. J., Hardisty, R. M., Barratt, T. M. Inhibitor of prostacylin production in sporadic haemolytic uraemic syndrome. *Arch. Dis. Child, 58*: 703–708 (1983).
5. Trompeter, R. S., Schwartz, R., Chantler, C., Dillon, M. J., Haycock, G. B., Kay, R., Barratt, T. M. Haemolytic uraemic syndrome in childhood: Analysis of prognostic features. *Arch. Dis. Child, 58*: 101–105 (1983).
6. Levin, M., Barratt, T. M. Haemolytic uraemic syndrome. *Arch. Dis. Child, 59*: 397–400 (1984).
7. Drummond, K. N. Hemolytic uremic syndrome—then and now. *N. Engl. J. Med. 312*: 116–118 (1985).
8. Barratt, T. M., Dillon, M. J., Hardisty, R. M., Nokes, T.J.C., Smith, C., Stroobant, P., Walters, M.D.S. The role of platelets and platelet derived growth factors in the pathogenesis of haemolytic uraemic syndrome. In: *Recent Advances in Pediatric Nephrology*. (K. Murakami et al., eds.). Elsevier Science Publishers, New York. pp. 577–580 (1987).
9. Karmali, M. A., Petric, M., Lim, C., Fleming, P. C., Arbus, G. S., Lior, H. The association between idiopathic hemolytic-uremic syndrome and infection by verotoxin-producing *Escherichia coli J. Infect. Dis., 151*: 775–782 (1985).
10. Levin, M., Walters, M.D.S., Barratt, T. M. Hemolytic uremic syndrome. *Adv. Pediatr. Infect. Dis., 4*: 51–82 (1989).

11. Remuzzi, G. HUS and TTP: Variable expression of a single entity. *Kidney Int.*, *32*: 292–308 (1987).
12. Kaplan, B. S., Levin, M., de Chadaverian, J. P. The hemolytic uremic syndrome. In: *Pediatric Nephrology*, ed 2. (C. E. Edelman ed). Boston, Little, Brown & Co. (In press).
13. Gasser, C., Gautier, E., Steck, A., Siebermann, R. E., Oeschslin, R. L. Hamolytisch uramische syndrome: Bilaterale nierenrindennekrosen bei akuten erwobenen hamolytischen anamien. *Schweiz. Med. Wochenschr.*, *38*: 905–909 (1955).
14. Farr, M. J., Roberts, S., Morley, A. R., Dewar, D. F., Uldall, P. R. The haemolytic uraemic syndrome—A family study. *Q. J. Med.*, *174*: 161–168 (1975).
15. Walters, M.D.S., Matthei, U., Kay, R., Dillon, M. J., Barratt, T. M. The polymorphonuclear leucocyte count in childhood haemolytic uraemic syndrome. *Pediatr. Nephrol.*, *3*: 130–134 (1989).
16. Fitzpatrick, M. M., Shah, V., Filler, G., Dillon, M. J., Barratt, T. M. Neutrophil activation in the haemolytic: Free and complexed elastase in plasma. *Pediatr. Nephrol.* (in press).
17. Cameron, J. S., Vick, R. Plasma C3 in haemolytic uraemic syndrome and thrombotic thrombocytopaenic purpura. *Lancet*, *2*: 975 (1973).
18. Gonzalo, A., Mampaso, F., Gallego, N., Bellas, C., Segui, J., Ortuno, J. Hemolytic uremic syndrome with hypocomplementemia and deposits of IgM and C3 in the involved renal tissue. *Clin. Nephrol.*, *16*: 193–199 (1981).
19. Bogdanovic, R., Cvoric, A., Nikolic, V., Sindjic, M. Recurrent haemolytic-uraemic syndrome with hypocomplementemia: A case report. *Pediatr. Nephrol.* *2*: 236–238 (1988).
20. Monnens, L., Molenaar, J., Lambert, P. H., Proesmans, W., Van Munster, P. The complement system in haemolytic uraemic syndrome in childhood. *Clin. Nephrol.* *13*: 168–171 (1980).
21. Walters, M.D.S., Levin, M., Smith, C., Nohes, T. J. C., Hardisty, R. M., Dillon, M. J., Barratt, T. M. Intravascular platelet activation in the hemolytic uremic syndrome: Studies on the typical (epidemic) and atypical (sporadic) sub-groups. *Kidney Int.*, *33*: 107–115 (1988).
22. Fong, J.S.C., Kaplan, B. S. Impairment of platelet aggregation in hemolytic uremic syndrome: Evidence for platelet 'exhaustion.' *Blood*, *60*: 564–569 (1982).
23. Pareti, F. I., Capitano, A., Mannucci, L., Ponticelli, C., Manucci, P. M. Acquired dysfunction due to the circulation of 'exhausted' platelets. *Am. J. Med.*, *69*: 235–239 (1980).
24. Edefonti, A., Bettinelli, A., Mondonico, P., Clans Appiani, A., Picca, M., Cossu, M. M., Tenton, F., Giani, M., Rossi, E. Intraplatelet serotonin in children with the haemolytic uraemic syndrome. *Clin. Nephrol.*, *23*: 207–211 (1985).
25. Remuzzi, G., Marchesi, D., Mecca, G., Misiani, R., Maucheri, D., Livio, M., Mecca, G. Haemolytic-uraemic syndrome: Deficiency of plasma factor(s) regulating prostacyclin activity? *Lancet*, *2*: 871–872 (1978).
26. Levin, M., Stroobant, P., Walters, M.D.S., Cheng, D. J., Watefield, M. D., Barratt, T. M. Platelet-derived growth factors are possible mediators of vascular proliferation in the sporadic haemolytic uraemic syndrome. *Lancet*, *2*: 830–833 (1986).
27. Stuart, M. J., Spitzer, R. E., Walenga, R. W., Boone, S. Prostanoids in the hemolytic uremic syndrome. *J. Pediatr.*, *106*: 936–939 (1985).
28. Stuart, M. J., Spitzer, R. E., Coppe, D., de Gaetano, G., Donati, M. B. Abnormal platelet and vascular prostaglandin synthesis in an infant with the hemolytic uremic syndrome. *Pediatrics*, *71*: 120–124 (1983).
29. Jorgenson, K. A., Petersen, R. S. Familial deficiency of prostacyclin production stimulating factor in the hemolytic uremic syndrome of childhood. *Thromb. Res.*, *21*: 311–315 (1981).

30. Wiles, P. G., Soloman, L. R., Lawler, W., Mallick, N. P., Johnson, M. Inherited plasma factor deficiency in haemolytic uraemic syndrome. *Lancet, 1*: 1105–1106 (1981).
31. Habib, R., Levy, M., Gagnadoux, M. F., Broyer, M. Prognosis of the haemolytic uraemic syndrome in children. In: *Advances in Nephrology*, vol II. (J. Hamburger et al., eds.) Year Book Medical Publishers, Chicago, London. pp. 99–128 (1982).
32. Theones, W., John, H. D. Endotheliotropic (hemolytic) nephroangiopathy and its various manifestation forms (thrombotic microangiopathy, primary malignant nephrosclerosis, hemolytic uraemic syndrome) *Klin. Wochenschr., 58*: 173–184 (1980).
33. Heptinstall, R. H. Hypertension. II: Essential hypertension. In: *Pathology of the Kidney*. (R. H. Heptinstall, ed.) Little, Brown, & Co., Boston. pp. 181–246 (1983).
34. Gianantonio, C. A., Vitacco, M., Mendilharzu, F., Gallo, G. E., Sojo, E. T. The hemolytic-uremic syndrome. *Nephron, 11*: 174–192 (1973).
35. Lieberman, E. Hemolytic uremic syndrome. *J. Pediatr., 80*: 1–35 (1972).
36. Kaplan, B. S., Katz, J., Krawitz, S., Line, A. An analysis of the results of therapy in 67 cases of the hemolytic uremic syndrome. *J. Pediatr., 78*: 420–425 (1971).
37. Fitzpatrick, M. M., Shah, V., Trompeter, R. S., Dillon, M. J., Barratt, T. M. Long term renal outcome of childhood haemolytic uraemic syndrome. *Br. Med. J., 303*: 489–492 (1991).
38. Aster, R. H. Plasma therapy for thrombotic thrombocytopenic purpura. *N. Engl. J. Med., 312*: 985–987 (1985).
39. Loirat, C., Sonsino, E., Hinglais, N., Jais, J. P., Fermanian, J. Treatment of the childhood haemolytic uraemic syndrome with plasma. A multicentre randomized controlled trial. *Pediatr. Nephrology, 2*: 279–285 (1988).
40. Camba, L., Al Hilali, M., Schulji, M.M.H., Joyne, M. V., Feest, I. G. Haemolytic uraemic syndrome with renal failure. The effect of plasmapheresis. *Haematologica, 70*: 341–344 (1985).
41. Bukowski, R. M., King, J. W., Hewlett, J. S. Plasmapheresis in the treatment of thrombotic thrombocytopenic purpura. *Blood, 50*: 413–417 (1977).
42. Dillon, M. J., Barratt, T. M., Sabbagh, P. A., Urquhart, I. A., Ryall, M. A., Deal, J. E., Walters, M.D.S. Plasma exchange in children: results in vasculitis and haemolytic uraemic syndrome. In: Recent Advances in Pediatric Nephrology. Eds Murakami K, Kitigawa T, Yabuta K, Sakai T. Amsterdam: Elsevier Science Publishers, 1987; 447–452.
43. Beattie, T. J., Murphy, A. V., Willoughby, M.L.N., Machin, S. J., Defreyn, G. Plasmapheresis in the haemolytic-uraemic syndrome children. *Br. Med. J., 282*: 1667–1668 (1981).
44. Gillor, A., Bulla, M., Rith, B., Bubmann, K., Schor, K., Tekook, A., Gladtke, E. Plasmapheresis as a theraputic measure in hemolytic-uremic syndrome in children. *Klin. Wochenschr., 61*: 363–367 (1983).
45. Tizard, E. J., Dillon, M. J. Plasmapheresis in childhood. Care of the Critically Ill 1991 (in press).
46. Van Buren, D., Van Buren, C. T., Flechner, S. M., Maddox, A. M., Verani, R., Kahan, B. D. De novo hemolytic uremic syndrome in renal transplant recipients immunosuppressed with cyclosporine. *Surgery, 98*: 54–62 (1985).
47. Herbert, D., Sibley, R. K., Mauer, S. M. Recurrence of hemolytic uremic syndrome in renal transplant recipients. *Kidney Int. 19*: s51–s58 (1986).
48. Folman, R., Arbus, G. S., Churchill, B., Gaum, L., Huber, J. Recurrence of hemolytic uremic syndrome in a 3 year old child, 4 months after second renal transplant. *Clin. Nephrol., 10*: 121–127 (1978).
49. Hauglustaine, D., van Damme, B., Vanrenterghem, Y., Michielsen, P. Recurrent hemolytic syndrome during oral contraception. *Clin. Nephrol., 15*: 148–153 (1981).
50. Grino, G. M., Caralps, A., Carreras, L., Nogués, R., Casletao, A. M., Ramero Ranón

Cameras, M., Alsina, J. Apparent recurrence of haemolytic uraemic syndrome in azathioprine-treated allograft recipients. *Nephron 49*: 301–304 (1988).
51. Springate, J., Fildes, R., Anthone, C., Anthone, R., Brentjens, J., O'Shea, M., Feld, L. Recurrent haemolytic uraemic syndrome after renal transplantation. *Transplant 20*: 559–561 (1988).
52. Eijgenraam, F. J., Donckerwolcke, R. A., Monnens, L.A.H., Proesman, W., Wolff, E. D., van Damme, B. Renal transplantation in 20 children with hemolytic-uremic syndrome. *Clin. Nephrol., 33*: 87–93 (1990).
53. Pillay, V.K.J., Kurtzman, N. A., Manaligod, J. R., Jonasson, O. Selective thrombocytopaenia due to localized microangiopathy of renal allografts. *Lancet, 2*: 988–991 (1973).
54. Magalhaes, R. L., Braun, W. E., Straffon, R. A., Hoffman, G. C., Shainoff, J. R., Osborne, G., Deodhar, S. D. Microangiopathic hemolytic anaemia in allotransplantation: Report of a successfully treated case and a review of the literature. *Am. J. Med., 58*: 862–868 (1975).
55. Van den Berg-Wolf, M. G., Koote, A.M.M., Weening, J. J., Paul, L. C. Recurrent haemolytic uraemic syndrome in a renal transplant recipient and review of the Leiden experience. *Surgery, 98*: 54–62 (1985).
56. Goodman, D. J., Walker, R. G., Birchall, I. E., d'Apice, A.J.F., Powell, H. R. Recurrent haemolytic uraemic syndrome in a transplant recipient on Orthoclone (OKT 3). *Pediatr. Nephrol., 5*: 240–241 (1991).

15
Hemolytic Uremic Syndrome and Transplantation

Diane Hébert *University of Toronto, Toronto, Ontario, Canada* **S. Michael Mauer** *University of Minnesota, Minneapolis, Minnesota*

The actual risk of recurrence of the hemolytic uremic syndrome (HUS) in the renal allograft of a patient whose primary glomerulopathy was HUS cannot be calculated. The risk is probably influenced by factors that include the variance in geographical incidence of the disease, immunosuppressive therapies used postengraftment, and a fundamental difficulty in distinguishing the histology of recurrent nephropathy from that of allograft rejection. In this chapter, recurrent disease and "de novo" HUS occurring in the renal transplant of patients whose original disease was not HUS, will be discussed.

Howard et al. (1) in 1976 probably reported the first case of recurrent HUS, in a 51-year-old male who received a living-related renal allograft from his son 5 months following the onset of end-stage renal failure. Primary allograft function was good until the third postoperative day when the patient developed hemolytic anemia, thrombocytopenia, and oligoanuria. A renal transplant biopsy revealed extensive glomerular and arteriolar thrombus formation with no evidence of interstitial or perivascular cellular infiltrate. These findings were considered to be consistent with a histologic diagnosis of HUS. Renal function improved spontaneously and there were no further recurrences of HUS. The patient died 11 years post–renal transplant following a septicemic episode.

Until Hébert et al. (2, 3) reported a definite recurrence of HUS in renal allografts in children, the problem was restricted to occasional case reports. Folman et al. (4) described a 2-year-old male who developed HUS following a respiratory prodrome. The patient then received four cadaver renal transplants over a period of 2 years. The first was rejected within 3 weeks of engraftment. Four months after the second transplant, he developed hemolytic anemia, thrombocytopenia, hypertension, and renal failure. A transplant renal biopsy contained glomerular thrombi, mesangial hypercellularity with increased mesangial matrix, and only a mild interstitial infiltrate of mononuclear cells. These findings were consistent with a diagnosis of HUS plus acute allograft rejection. The hematological changes returned to normal and renal function temporarily improved. Transplant nephrectomy was performed after 11 months. Cortical necrosis resulted in the loss of the third renal transplant. The patient died from a cerebral hemorrhage following a fourth transplant. Histopathological changes in the graft were again consistent with a recurrence of HUS.

In 1986 Hébert et al. (2) reported on a series of adults and children whose primary disease was HUS. Their review was updated in 1991 (3). Over a 20-year period (1969–1989), 17 patients whose primary diagnosis was HUS received a renal transplant. Seven patients suffered a definite recurrence, diagnosed on the basis of both the typical clinical features of HUS and histopathological changes on renal transplant biopsy. Fourteen allografts were transplanted into the seven patients; 11 (nine living related, two cadaver) were lost as a result of recurrent disease, three in one patient alone. Three patients recovered renal function. In 10 of 17 there was either no recurrence (7) or a combination of biopsy-proven chronic vascular rejection and changes consistent with recurrent HUS (3). Immunosuppression consisted of antilymphocyte globulin in all patients except for one patient. Four patients received cyclosporin A (CyA). In this group there was one graft loss with recurrent disease and no recurrence in three. A monoclonal antibody was used in a patient with a history of two previous graft losses, but recurrent disease occurred within one week of the third engraftment. One patient had familial HUS because of the occurrence of HUS in her donor sister postnephrectomy.

With the exception of three adults reported by Grino et al. (5), these poor results generally have not been confirmed by others (6–9). Van der Berg et al. (7) reported five adults and three children, of whom two adults presented with recurrent disease. One of these patients, whose recurrence was associated with estrogen therapy, was left with poor graft function; in the second, the graft was lost. Eijgenraam et al. (8) reported 24 grafts of mostly cadaver kidneys (n = 22), that were transplanted into 20 children. All patients except for one were considered to have had the classical or epidemic type of primary disease, and none had sustained a recurrence prior to transplantation. Recurrence was suspected but not proven to be the cause of graft failure in two patients. A short interval between renal failure due to HUS and kidney transplantation seemed to affect graft function adversely.

Gagnadoux et al. (10) reported that the risk of recurrence in 31 children was exceptionally low, even in living-related donor organs. However, graft loss secondary to chronic vascular rejection was seen more frequently in HUS patients compared with children whose original disease was different. Actuarial graft survival for cadaver grafts (n = 28) in HUS compared to all other recipients was 66% at 1 year, versus 80%; and 37% at 5 years, versus 69%. Currently only 12 of 28 (45%) cadaveric grafts are functioning. Four grafts were lost within the first 10 days as a result of acute rejection in one and vascular thrombosis in three. Ten grafts were lost secondary to chronic rejection between 4 and 8 years posttransplantation. In only one patient was recurrent HUS diagnosed 3 weeks postengraftment, 6 months after the onset of the original illness. Retransplantation was successful for 12 years. Seventeen patients were transplanted using cyclosporin A (CyA) as immunosuppression, and no patient experienced a recurrence of HUS. Repetto et al. (9) described only one child with recurrent HUS in a series of 14 transplant recipients. This patient probably had a familial form of the disease.

Additional case reports are listed in Table 1 (11–20). In the majority of cases, graft loss occurred secondary to a recurrence of HUS. Post-transplant disease has been documented in association with the use of estrogen-based oral contraceptives (7, 12), and individual observers remain concerned about the role of CyA in the pathogenesis of the syndrome (13, 19, 20). Thrombotic thrombocytopenic purpura and recurrence post-transplant have also been reported (21, 22).

The diagnosis of post–renal transplant recurrent HUS is difficult and demands the presence of both clinical and histopathological features. It is of course important to recognize that the constellation of hemolytic anemia, thrombocytopenia, and acute renal failure is not pathognomonic and may also be associated with acute allograft rejection and malignant hypertension, conditions that in their own right are likely to complicate the postoperative transplant period. In the former, physical signs such as fever and/or graft tenderness are likely to be absent. It is usual for the onset of the recurrence to occur early in the posttransplant period, usually within days or weeks. The extrarenal manifestations of HUS frequently encountered with the original disease are infrequent in the post-transplant period. However, central nervous system involvement has been described in both adults and children and has presented with spontaneous cerebral hemorrhage (5, 20).

The histopathological changes seen in the kidney that are in keeping with the clinical spectrum of the disease, are not pathognomonic of HUS; similar changes are seen in acute allograft rejection, malignant hypertension, and autoimmune hemolytic anemia (23–28). The pathologic changes in the graft are generally similar to those seen in the native kidneys affected by the same disease process.

There is no direct evidence to suggest that polyclonal antilymphocyte globulins (ALG) induce HUS postrenal transplant. However, an HUS-like illness affecting the

Table 1 Case Reports of Recurrent HUS Post-Transplantation

Lead author	Ref.	Number patients	Outcome	Comment
Cerilli, 1972	11	1	Recovery	
Hauglustaine, 1981	12	1	Graft loss	Association with oral contraceptives
Leithner, 1982	13	1	Graft loss	CyA used
Cameron, 1983	14	2	Graft loss	
Strom, 1986	15	2	Graft loss, hypertension	
Remuzzi, 1987	16	1	Poor function, graft loss	Plasmapheresis, plasma infusions
Granato, 1988	17	1	Graft loss	
Springate, 1988	18	1	Recovery	Plasma infusions
Matthew, 1988	19	1	?	CyA used
Mochon, 1990	20	1	Function	CyA used

CyA = cyclosporin A

allograft may occur as a result of release of cytokines, such as tumor necrosis factor and α interferon, which are damaging to the endothelial cell (29). Here, there is evidence to suggest that cytokine release can adversely affect the vascular endothelium and perhaps play an important role in the pathogenesis of HUS.

CyA has been implicated as a possible cause of HUS in renal allograft recipients, either as recurrent disease or as de novo HUS in liver (30, 31) and bone marrow recipients (32–48). In the majority of cases, this complication was related to the use of CyA to prevent graft versus host disease (32–37). In the two reports in which histopathological information is given, HUS occurred early postengraftment and the renal involvement was characterized by the presence of few glomerular and arteriolar thrombi (33, 34). In contrast, 10 of 66 allogeneic bone marrow graft recipients suffered a severe microangiopathy resembling thrombotic thrombocytopenic purpura (TTP) (37). Nephrotoxicity was considered to be secondary to generalized endothelial damage; it is difficult to implicate CyA specifically from their data. Similarly, the thrombotic microangiopathy reported in bone marrow transplant recipients by Nizze et al. (38) was considered to be specific for CyA and may well have been the result of other causes. Antignac et al. (39) reported seven patients who developed acute renal failure several months after bone marrow transplantation and total body irradiation. In four of seven there was an associated hemolytic anemia and thrombocytopenia. In all patients the histology was that of a severe glomerulopathy with extensive mesangiolysis and arteriolar necrosis. The similarity to radiation nephritis suggests that chemotherapy alone may not have been the causative agent (see Chapter 16).

The precise mechanism of CyA nephrotoxicity is uncertain, but in experimental studies CyA has been linked with increased production of thromboxane A_2, decreased production of prostacyclin, reduction in the vasodilator response to acetylcholine, and decreased endothelium-dependent relaxation in arteries (33, 49, 50). CyA enhances platelet aggregation induced by ADP, adrenaline, and collagen, and it enhances thromboxane A_2 production in humans (51). Furthermore, CyA enhances in vitro hemostasis and reduces thrombolysis in renal transplant recipients (52). The enhanced platelet aggregation in the context of reduced vascular production of endothelium-derived relaxing factor and that of prostacyclin could be associated with an increased platelet–vessel wall interaction which might enhance vasoconstriction, and intravascular thrombosis, in the renal vasculature (53).

The treatment of recurrent and de novo HUS remains controversial (54–57). Plasma infusions and/or plasma exchange, and antiplatelet agents such as dipyridamole have been tried in individual patients with variable outcomes (58, 59). Early recognition of the syndrome and discontinuation of CyA occasionally has led to reversal of the disease (58, 60, 61). Substitution of CyA by newer immunosuppressive agents derived from fungal peptides, such as FK506, does not appear to suppress recurrence of the syndrome (62).

The risk of recurrence of HUS post–renal transplant is linked to the heterogeneity of the syndrome itself. There are no data defining the risk, but it would appear that: 1. recurrent disease is less common in children than in adults; and 2. children affected with the typical or epidemic form of the original disease are less likely to suffer recurrence postengraftment. If the endothelial cell of the kidney is the target for injury in HUS, it is tantalizing to speculate that cytokine release occurrs during the immunoregulatory response to organ transplantation and leads to endothelial cell damage. This might be the trigger for HUS in a susceptible individual. Perhaps prevention of allograft rejection could therefore theoretically reduce the small but significant incidence of this recurrent syndrome.

REFERENCES

1. Howard, R. J., Mauer, S. M., Miller, K., Simmons, R. L., Najarian, J. S. Biopsy proven recurrence of hemolytic uremic syndrome early after kidney transplantation with a favorable outcome. *Kidney Int.* (abstract), *10*: 544 (1976).
2. Hébert, D., Sibley, R. K., Mauer, S. M. Recurrence of hemolytic uremic syndrome in renal transplant recipients. *Kidney Int., 30*: S51–S58 (1986).
3. Hébert, D., Kim, E. M., Sibley, R. K., Mauer, S. M. Post-transplantation outcome of patients with hemolytic-uremic syndrome: Update. *Pediatr. Nephrol.*, *5*: 162–167 (1991).
4. Folman, R., Arbus, G. S., Churchill, B., Gaum, L., Huber, J. Recurrence of the hemolytic uremic syndrome in a 3½ year old child, 4 months after second renal transplantation. *Clin. Nephrol., 10*: 121–127 (1978).
5. Griñó, J. M., Caralps, A., Carreras, L., et al. Apparent recurrence of hemolytic uremic syndrome in azathioprine-treated allograft recipients. *Nephron 49*: 301–304 (1988).
6. Pirson, Y., Leclerq, B., Squifflet, J. P., Alexandre, G.P.J., van Ypersele de Strihou, C. Good prognosis of the hemolytic uremic syndrome after renal transplantation. *Nephrol. Dial Trans.* (abstract), *1*: 134 (1986).
7. Van den Berg-Wolf, M. G., Kootte, A., Weening, J. J., Paul, L. C. Recurrent hemolytic uremic syndrome in a renal transplant recipient and review of the Leiden experience. *Transplantation, 45*: 248–251 (1988).
8. Eijgenraam, F. J., Donckerwolcke, R. A., Monnens, L.A.H., Proesmans, W., Wolff, E. D., van Damme, B. Renal transplantation in 20 children with hemolytic-uremic syndrome. *Clin. Nephrol., 33*: 87–93 (1990).
9. Repetto, H. A., Vazquez, L. A., Calvo, P., Palti, G. Renal transplantation in children with idiopathic 'classic' hemolytic uremic syndrome. *Pediatr. Nephrol.* (abstract), *3*: C185 (1989).
10. Gagnadoux, M. F., Broyer, M., Habib, R. Renal transplantation in hemolytic-uremic syndrome. *Pediatr. Nephrol.* (abstract), *3*: C184 (1989).
11. Cerilli, G. S., Nelsen, C., Dorfmann, L. Homotransplantation in infants and children with the hemolytic-uremic syndrome. *Surgery, 71*: 66–71 (1972).
12. Hauglustaine, D., van Damme, B., Vanrenterghem, Y., Michielsen, P. Recurrent hemolytic uremic syndrome during oral contraception. *Clin. Nephrol., 15*: 148–153 (1981).
13. Leithner, C., Sinzinger, H., Pohanka, E., Schwarz, M., Kretschmer, G., Syre, G. Recurrence of haemolytic uraemic syndrome triggered by Cylosporin A after renal transplantation. *Lancet, 1*: 1470. (1982).
14. Cameron, J. S. Effect of the recipient's disease on the results of transplantation (other than diabetes mellitus). *Kidney Int., 23*: S42–S43 (1983).
15. Strom, T. B., McCluskey, R. T. Case records of the Massachusetts General Hospital. Case 15-1986. *N. Engl. J. Med. 314*: 1032–1040 (1986).
16. Remuzzi, G. HUS and TTP: variable expression of a single entity. *Kidney Int., 32*: 292–308 (1987).
17. Granato, D. B., Salimi, Z., George, E. A., Salinas-Madrigal, L., Garvin, P. J. Hemolytic uremic syndrome in renal transplant recipient. *Clin. Nucl. Med., 13*: 171–174 (1988).
18. Springate, J., Fildes, R., Anthone, S., et al. Recurrent hemolytic syndrome after renal transplantation. *Transplant Proc., 20*: 559–561 (1988).
19. Mathew T. H. Recurrence of disease following renal transplantation. *Am. J. Kidney Dis., 12*: 85–96 (1988).

20. Mochon, M., Kaiser, B., Dunn, S., Shulman, S., Baluarte, H. J. Cerebral infarct with recurrence of hemolytic uremic syndrome in a child following renal allograft. *J. Am. Soc. Nephrol.*, *1*: 765 (1990).
21. Stevenson, J. A., Dumke, A., Glassock, R. J., Raifer, J., Cohen, A. H. Thrombotic microangiopathy: recurrence following renal transplant and response to plasma infusion. *Am. J. Nephrol.*, *2*: 227–231 (1981).
22. Bonsib, S. M., Ercolani, L., Ngheim, D., Hamilton, H. E. Recurrent thrombotic microangiopathy in a renal allograft. Case report and review of the literature. *Am. J. Med.*, *79*: 520–527 (1985).
23. Kohler, T. R., Tilney, N. L. Microangiopathic hemolytic anemia associated with hyperacute rejection of kidney allograft. *Transplant Proc. 14*: 444–446 (1982).
24. Pillay, V.K.G., Kurtzman, N. A., Manaligod, J. R., Jonasson, O. Selective thrombocytopenia due to localised microangiopathy of renal allografts. *Lancet 2*: 988–991 (1973).
25. Magalhaes, R. L., Brown, W. E., Straffon, R. A., et al. Microangiopathic hemolytic anaemia in renal allotransplantation: report of a successfully treated case and review of the literature. *Am. J. Med.*, *58*: 862–868 (1975).
26. Croker, B. P., Salomon, D. S. Pathology of the renal allograft. In: (C. C. Tisher, B. M. Brenner, eds.) *Renal Pathology with Clinical and Functional Correlations*. J. B. Lippincott, Philadelphia, pp 1518–1554 (1989).
27. Goldblatt, P. J., Gohara, A. F., Khan, N. H., Hampton, J. H. Benign and malignant nephrosclerosis and renovascular hypertension. In: (C. C. Tisher, B. M. Brenner eds.) *Renal Pathology with Clinical and Functional Correlations*. Philadelphia, J. B. Lippincott, pp. 1131–1162 (1989).
28. Nyberg, G., Sandberd, L., Rydberg, L., et al. ABO autoimmune hemolytic anemia in a renal transplant patient treated with cyclosporin. A case report. *Transplantation 37*: 529–530 (1984).
29. Cotran, R. S., Pober, J. S. Cytokine-endothelial interactions in inflammation, immunity and vascular injury. *J. Am. Soc. Nephrol.*, *1*: 225–235 (1990).
30. Bonser, R. S., Adu, D., Franklin, I., McMaster, P. Cyclosporin-induced hemolytic uremic syndrome in liver allograft recipient. *Lancet 2*: 1337 (letter) (1984).
31. Dzik, W. H., Georgi, B. A., Khettry, U., Jenkins, R. L. Cyclosporine-associated thrombotic thrombocytopenic purpura following liver transplantation. Successful treatment with plasma exchange. *Transplantation*, *44*: 570–572 (1987).
32. Powles, R. L., Clink, H. M., Spence, D., Morgenstern, G., Watson, J. C., Selby, P. J., Woods, M., Barret, A., Jameson, B., Sloane, J., Lawler, S. D., Kay, H.E.M., Lawson, D., McElwain, T. J., Alexander, P. Cyclosporin A to prevent graft-versus host disease in man after allogeneic bone-marrow transplantation. *Lancet 1*: 327–329 (1980).
33. Shulman, H., Striker, G., Deeg, H. J., Kennedy, M., Storb, R., Thomas, E. D. Nephrotoxicity of cyclosporin A after allogeneic marrow transplantation. Glomerular thromboses and tubular injury. *N. Engl. J. Med.*, *305*: 1392–1395 (1981).
34. Atkinson, K., Briggs, J. C., Hayes, H., Ralston, M., Dodds, A. J., Concannon, A. J., Naidoo, D. Cyclosporin A associated nephrotoxicity in the first 100 days after allogeneic bone marrow transplantation: 3 distinct syndromes. *Br. J. Hematol.*, *54*: 59–67 (1983).
35. Hows, J. M., Smith, J. M., Baughan, A., Gordon Smith, E. C. Nephrotoxicity in marrow graft recipients treated with cyclosporine. *Transpl. Proc.*, *15* (suppl. 1): 2708–2711 (1983).
36. Textor, S. C., Forman, S. J., Bravo, E. L., Carlson, J. De novo accelerated hypertension during sequential cyclosporine and prednisone therapy in normotensive bone marrow transplant recipients. *Transpl. Proc.*, *20*: 480–486 (1988).
37. Holler, E., Kolb, H. J., Hiller, E., Mraz, W., Lehmacher, B., Gleixner, C., Seeber, U., Jehn, H. H., Gerhatz, G., Brehm, G., Wilmanns, N. Microangiopathy in patients on cyclosporine prophylaxis who developed acute graft-versus-host disease after HLA identical bone marrow transplantation. *Blood 73*: 2018–2024 (1989).

38. Nizze, H., Mihatsch, M. J., Zollinger, H. U., Brocheriou, C., Gokel, J. M., Henry, K., Sloane, J. P., Stovin, P. G. Cyclosporine associated nephropathy in patients with heart and bone marrow transplants. *Clin. Nephrol., 30*: 248–260 (1988).
39. Antignac, C., Gubler, M. C., Leverger, G., Broyer, M., Habib, R. Delayed renal failure with extensive mesangiolysis following bone marrow transplantation. *Kidney Int., 35*: 1336–1344 (1989).
40. Spruce, W. E., Forman, S. J., Blume, K. G., Bearman, R. M., Bixby, H., Ching, A., Drinkard, J., San Marco, A. Hemolytic uraemic syndrome after bone marrow transplantation. *Acta. Haematol.* (Basel), *67*: 206–210 (1982).
41. Rozenbaum, A., Colin, J. P., Flesh, M., Hory B., Saint-Hillier, Y., Leconte des Floris R., Pérol, C. Syndrome hémolytique et urémique (SHU) après chimiothérapie et greffe autologue de moelle osseuse: à propos de 2 observations. *Néphrologie* (abstract), *5*: 48 (1984).
42. Bergstein, J., Andreoli, S. P., Provisor, A. J., Yum, M. Radiation nephritis following total-body irradiation and cyclosphosphamide in preparation for bone marrow transplantation. *Transplantation, 41*: 63–66 (1986).
43. Craig, J.I.O., Sheehan, T., Bell, K. The haemolytic uraemic syndrome and bone marrow transplantation. *Br. Med. J.* (letter), *295*: 887 (1987).
44. Marshall, R. J., Sweny, P. HUS in recipients of bone marrow transplants not treated with CSA. *Histopathology, 10*: 953–962 (1986).
45. Guinan, E., Tarbell, N., Niemeyer, C., Sallan, S., Weinstein, H. Intravascular hemolysis and renal insufficiency after bone marrow transplantation. *Blood, 72*: 451–455 (1988).
46. Chappell, M. E., Keeling, D. M., Prentice, H. G., Sweny, P. Haemolytic uraemic syndrome after bone marrow transplantation: an adverse effect of total body irradiation? *Bone Marrow Transpl. 3*: 339–347 (1988).
47. Loomis, L. J., Aronson, A. J., Rudinsky, R., Spargo, B. H. Hemolytic uremic syndrome following bone marrow transplantation: a case report and review of the literature. *Am. J. Kidney Dis., 14*: 324–328 (1989).
48. Tschuchnigg, M., Bradstock, K. F., Koutts, J., Stewart, J., Enno, A., Seldon, M. A case of thrombotic thrombocytopenic purpura following allogeneic bone marrow transplantation. *Bone Marrow Transpl., 5*: 61–63 (1990).
49. Voss, B. L., Hamilton, K. K., Samara, E.N.S., McKee, P. A. Cyclosporine suppression of endothelial prostacyclin generation. A possible mechanism for nephrotoxicity. *Transplantation 45*: 793–796 (1988).
50. Bossaler, C., Förstermann, U., Hertel, R., Olbricht, C., Reschke, V., Fleck, E. Cyclosporine A inhibits endothelin-dependent vasodilatation and vascular prostacyclproduction. *Eur. J. Pharmacol. 165*: 165–169 (1989).
51. Grace, A. A., Barradas, A. A., Mikhailidis, D., et al. Cyclosporine A enchances platelet aggregation. *Kidney Int. 32*: 889–895 (1987).
52. Baker, L. R., Tucker, B., Kovacs, I. B. Enhanced in vitro hemostasis and reduced thrombolysis in cyclosporine-treated renal transplant recipients. *Transplantation 49*: 905–909 (1990).
53. Lüscher, T. F., Bock, H. A., Yang, Z., Diederich, D. Endothelium-derived relaxing and contracting factors: Perspectives in nephrology. *Kidney Int., 39*: 575–590 (1991).
54. O'Regan, S., Chesney, R. W., Mongeau, J. G., Robitaille, P. Aspirin and dipyridamole therapy in the hemolytic-uremic syndrome. *J. Pediatr. 97*: 473–476 (1980).
55. Van Damme-Lombaerts, R., Proesmans, W., van Damme, B., et al. Heparin plus dypiridamole in childhood hemolytic-uremic syndrome: A prospective, randomized study. *J. Pediatr., 113*: 913–918 (1988).
56. Sheth, K. J., Gill, J. C., Leitchter, H. E. High-dose intravenous gamma globulin infusions in hemolytic-uremic syndrome: A preliminary report. *A.J.D.C. 144*: 268–270 (1990).
57. Rizzoni, G., Claris-Appiani, A., Edefonti, A., et al. Plasma infusion for hemolytic-uremic

syndrome in children: Results of a multicenter controlled trial. *J. Pediatr.*, *112*: 284–290 (1988).
58. Dyck, R. F., Kappell, J. E., Sheridan, D., Card, R. T. Reversible Cyclosporine-associated hemolytic uremic syndrome in a renal transplant recipient: a role for a platelet aggregating factor? *Transplant Proc.*, *18*: 228–229 (1986).
59. Venkat, K., Kupin, W., Oh, H., Mozes, M., Tkach, D. Reversal of Cyclosporine-associated hemolytic-uremic syndrome by plasma exchange with fresh-frozen plasma replacement in renal transplant recipients. In: XIII International Congress of the Transplantation Society, San Francisco (1990).
60. Bonser, R. S., Adu, D., Franklin, L., McMaster, P. Cyclosporin-induced haemolytic uraemic syndrome in liver allograft recipient. *Lancet*, *2*: 1337 (1984).
61. Wolfe, J. A., McCann, R. L., Sanfilippo, F. Cyclosporine-associated microangiopathy in renal transplantation: A severe but potentially reversible form of early graft injury. *Transplantation*, *41*: 514–544 (1986).
62. McCauley, J., Bronsther, O., Fung, J., Todo, S., Starzl, T. E. Treatment of cyclosporin-induced haemolytic uraemic syndrome with FK506. *Lancet*, *2*: 1516 (1989).

16
Bone Marrow Transplantation-Associated Thrombotic Microangiopathy

Yaacov Frishberg and Bernard S. Kaplan *Children's Hospital of Philadelphia and University of Pennsylvania, Philadelphia, Pennsylvania*

Over the past 2 decades there have been improvements in the success rates of allogeneic and autologous bone marrow transplantation (BMT) for the treatment of several malignant and nonmalignant hematological diseases and nonbone marrow-derived solid tumors (1). As a result, the number of long-term survivors has increased, and physicians who take care of these patients are faced with diagnosing and treating new and often fatal complications in this unique population. The clinicopathological presentations of the renal complications in BMT recipients vary from thrombotic microangiopathy (TM) to glomerular mesangiolysis. The term *thrombotic microangiopathy* was introduced by Symmers (2) as an abbreviation for *thrombotic microangiopathic hemolytic anemia*. It encompasses the typical and atypical forms of hemolytic uremic syndrome (HUS) and thrombotic thrombocytopenic purpura (TTP).

The clinical findings and pathological characteristics of this association are reviewed in this chapter. An attempt has been made to evaluate potential factors involved in the pathogenesis of TM following BMT. Unfortunately, this review suffers from inadequate descriptions of the clinical findings, laboratory studies, and patients' courses, in the literature that has been surveyed.

CLINICAL MANIFESTATIONS

There are 59 reported cases of patients who developed TM following BMT (3–16). Over 60% were aged less than 18 years. It is impossible to comment on gender differences or on the incidence of this complication.

Seven reported cases with TM had a BMT for stage IV neuroblastoma (8). The remainder had bone marrow-derived malignancies or severe aplastic anemia. Seventeen of the 59 patients had autologous bone marrow transplantations, and the rest had an allogeneic BMT.

In contrast with patients with typical HUS who are usually diagnosed by the acute onset of pallor, purpura, and oliguria, following prodromal symptoms (17), many of the patients with BMT-associated TM were not ill at presentation, in that they had no prodromal disease, but were diagnosed as a result of abnormal laboratory results. Signs and symptoms, when present, were usually secondary to acute renal failure and were often related to volume overload. They included dyspnea on exertion (more pronounced in anemic patients), increasing peripheral edema and body weight, congestive heart failure, and pulmonary edema. The most common finding was hypertension, which was detected in over 60% of the patients and, at times, was severe enough to cause a hypertensive encephalopathy (5,8). Nonspecific symptoms of malaise and low-grade fever were reported in only one patient (10).

Loomis et al. (5) reported on a patient who developed seizures with a cerebrospinal fluid pleocytosis during the course of the disease. Because the patient was hypertensive, it is possible that this was a form of hypertensive encephalopathy, rather than a central nervous system manifestation of TM. Atkinson et al. (11) described two patients who succumbed to a rapidly progressive disease complicated by acute renal failure, grand mal seizures, and hemorrhagic pulmonary edema. Both had microscopic disseminated cytomegalovirus infection, which may have caused their devastating illnesses. Therefore, it is unclear whether TM, in this context, has any extrarenal manifestations.

LABORATORY FINDINGS

The urinary sediment was abnormal with microscopic hematuria and hyaline, granular and, occasionally, red blood cell casts. In most cases, there was slight proteinuria, whereas, in a few instances, protein excretion was massive (5,6,10). Renal insufficiency was manifested universally by increased serum blood urea nitrogen (BUN) and creatinine concentrations. Urine output was normal, with the exception of patients who progressed rapidly to end-stage renal failure and who required replacement therapy. Whereas there was evidence of renal dysfunction in every patient, hematological abnormalities were detected in a smaller number of cases. Microangiopathic hemolytic anemia was diagnosed in 80% of the patients. The main findings were a significant fall in the hemoglobin concentration and the presence of fragmented red blood cells in peripheral blood smears. Elevated serum lactate dehydrogenase (LDH) levels and low plasma haptoglobin concentrations were found in the patients in whom they were measured. In some cases, the hemolysis was severe and rendered the patient transfusion-dependent.

About 50% of the patients had thrombocytopenia. This was considered to be the result of the microangiopathic process, but this still requires confirmation. It is of interest that one patient had an autoimmune thrombocytopenia that required treatment by splenectomy (13).

One should be particularly cautious when interpreting the hematological findings. Some patients may have been transfusion-dependent at presentation because of delayed engraftment or because of hemolysis that was secondary to ABO-incompatible marrow. The latter group may have continued to produce host-type isoagglutinins against the donor ABO blood for as long as 330 days after transplantation (19). Furthermore, reticulocyte counts may be difficult to interpret in the context of the patient's ongoing posttransplant erythroid reconstitution (8). Therefore, all the hematological findings must be assessed in reference to the period before the onset of TM.

PATHOLOGY

Some patients developed a more prominent glomerular disease, whereas others had mainly vascular lesions. In addition, patients differed in the severity of the kidney involvement. This reflected, at least in part, the timing of the clinical presentation in reference to the BMT as well as the stage of the disease.

Light Microscopy

The most prominent glomerular abnormality was ballooning of the lobules of the tufts of variable portions of the glomeruli. The expanded lobules were filled with a spongy material that was the result of peripheral extension of the mesangial matrix along the inner aspect of the glomerular basement membrane. The subendothelial space was considerably widened. The overall appearance was that of disintegration of the mesangial matrix. This has been referred to as *mesangiolysis* (18). Unaffected lobules had the typical features of thrombotic microangiopathy, with an increase in mesangial matrix and a widened subendothelial space (7). Arteriolar changes consisted of marked narrowing of the lumina, with widening of the subendothelial space from mucoid thickening of the intima. Occasionally, the lumina were occluded by fibrinoid material. The myocytes of the muscular layer were swollen and were occasionally necrotic. Overall, the changes were consistent with a picture of diffuse arteriolar necrosis (7). There were also variable degrees of interstitial edema and fibrosis.

A repeat renal biopsy was done a year after the presentation in two patients. One had regained normal kidney function, and the other had mild renal insufficiency. The mesangiolytic changes had almost completely disappeared (7). About a third of the glomeruli revealed mesangial hypercellularity with an increase in mesangial matrix, a third showed global glomerulosclerosis, and the remaining glomeruli had ischemic changes that were manifested by wrinkling of the glomerular basement membrane. There was only minimal intimal thickening of the arterioles. It seems that these changes demonstrate both extremes of the pathological process: repair, on the one hand, and progression to end-stage disease on the other. Thromboses in the arterioles and capillary tufts seemed to occur more frequently in patients who had been treated with cyclosporine as prophylaxis against graft-versus-host disease (GVHD) (6).

Electron Microscopy

The glomerular changes consisted of uneven thickening of the capillary walls, which led to variable degrees of obstruction of the capillary lumina and focal loosening of the mesangial stalks. Both changes were related to the accumulation of a clear heterogeneous material in the subendothelial zone as well as in the mesangium (7). Flocculent deposits occasionally formed on the internal side of the normal lamina densa and were separated from the endothelial cell by a thin layer of newly formed basement membrane. Most of the endothelial cells were enlarged and had abundant perinuclear cytoplasm. Mesangial lesions were characterized by a massive edematous infiltration of the mesangial stalks and disruption of the mesangial matrix. Arteriolar changes consisted of various types of degenerative changes in smooth-muscle cells, massive electron-dense deposits at the site of necrotic smooth-muscle cells, heterogeneous deposits in the subendothelial space, and enlargement of the endothelial cells.

Immunofluorescence Microscopy

Deposits of fibrin and IgM were found in most of the glomeruli. The arteriolar changes consisted of coarse granular deposits of C3 arranged in a pearl-like pattern on the muscular layer of the arterioles (7).

POTENTIAL FACTORS INVOLVED IN THE PATHOGENESIS OF THROMBOTIC MICROANGIOPATHY

The kidneys of patients who are to be treated with BMT are repeatedly exposed to a large array of nephrotoxic agents. These include infiltrating tumor cells, chemotherapy, antibiotics, irradiation, infections, and GVHD. It is, therefore, impossible to determine the single agent responsible for BMT-associated TM. However, a critical review of the data has led to the conclusion that some of the suspected etiological agents are more likely than others to have a major role in the pathogenesis of the TM.

Malignancy

Leukemic cells as well as metastatic neuroblastoma can infiltrate the kidneys and compromise their function. However, the pathological characteristics of TM has not been described in the context of leukemic cell infiltration and, more importantly, none of the patients who presented with BMT-associated TM had evidence of their primary disease.

Infections

Hemolytic uremic syndrome has been associated with a number of infectious agents, especially *Escherichia coli* O157:H7. These compromised hosts are particularly susceptible to infections with many different organisms. The most consistent has been cytomegalovirus (CMV) viremia.

Patients suffering from CMV infection may have a marked fall in platelet and leukocyte counts in association with positive CMV cultures or a rise in anti-CMV antibody titers (20). If the infection is self-limiting, the platelet and leukocyte counts usually return to normal promptly. Furthermore, there are morphological similarities between the glomerular lesions of HUS and those described in renal allografts complicated by CMV viremia (21). However, because the etiology of renal transplantation-associated HUS is probably multifactorial, it is difficult to compare those histological findings with BMT-associated TM. In addition, definite causality has not been established between CMV infections and glomerular injury. Despite this caveat, it is important to note that there is high prevalence of CMV infection in reported cases of BMT-associated TM. In one small series (3) four of eight patients had a documented CMV infection, and two others had equivocal evidence of infection with asymptomatic seroconversions. In two cases (11), there was evidence of disseminated CMV infection, and one of three cases reported by Shulman et al. (6)

had CMV pneumonia. In another report (13), two of three cases had definite evidence of CMV infection, and the third had a rise in antibody titer. In the latter report, electron microscopy studies revealed electron-dense material in the walls of small arteries and arterioles that corresponded to the location of IgM and complement. This could be indicative of either nonspecific trapping of these molecules in areas of endothelial damage or, theoretically, might implicate a process involving immune complexes. It has been suggested that immunosuppression in BM recipients allows reactivation of herpes-viruses. This may then trigger a TM-type reaction either by a direct viral attack on endothelium, which is known to occur in CMV infection, or by immune complex damage.

A hypothesis that invokes the concept of "molecular mimicry," and that requires confirmation, is that the viral antigen inducing the immune response is cross-reactive with a renal endothelial antigen (22).

Because most of the reported cases did not show any evidence of CMV viremia, it seems unlikely that CMV has a pivotal role in the pathogenesis of TM. Nevertheless, it remains a possibility that CMV might render the endothelial cells more susceptible to injury by other agents.

Chemotherapeutic Drugs

Chemotherapy-associated HUS has been reviewed by Murgo (23) and is discussed in detail in Chapter 22. Mitomycin (formerly, mitomycin-C; MMC) is an anticancer agent that has been associated with microangiopathic hemolytic anemia, thrombocytopenia, and renal insufficiency (24). However, none of the patients who developed BMT-associated TM were treated with MMC.

Cyclosporine

Cyclosporine (formerly, cyclosporin A; CsA) is a fungal peptide with potent immunosuppressive properties (25). Unlike methotrexate, CsA is not myelotoxic and, therefore, permits faster engraftment. It also reduces the incidence of GVHD in BMT recipients (26). It has been suggested, on the basis of an animal model of the microangiopathic form of CsA nephrotoxicity, that the glomerular capillary thrombi probably result from an interaction between CsA and local and systemic inflammatory mediators that occur following transplantation (27) (see next section on GVHD). It seems that patients with HUS may have decreased levels of a plasma factor that sustains endothelial cell prostacyclin synthesis (28–29). This mechanism and an exaggerated renal thromboxane response have been implicated in the pathogenesis of CsA-associated cases of HUS (3). Therefore, it has been postulated that endothelial injury may be more likely to result in platelet aggregation if prostacyclin levels are reduced. Cyclosporine may also act synergistically as a noxious stimulus with other agents, such as infections or rejection, that can cause endothelial damage. It is particularly noteworthy that an HUS has not been described in patients with uveitis treated with CsA, despite that they may develop glomerular and tubulointerstitial diseases (31).

After having made a case for the potential role of CsA in the pathogenesis of the BMT-associated TM, it is important to observe that most of the patients were never treated with this agent, or that CsA was stopped before the onset of the renal symptoms. Hows et al. (12) described six patients who developed microangiopathic hemolytic anemia, thrombocytopenia, and increased serum creatinine concentrations in association with an increase in serum CsA levels. The abnormal findings were reversed when the CsA doses were decreased (12). Unfortunately, the other possible confounding factors were not defined well in that report.

Graft-Versus-Host Disease

Transplant glomerulopathy is a form of host versus graft disease that may occur in renal allografts. The glomerular endothelial damage seen in transplant glomerulopathy resembles that seen in HUS. It has been suggested, therefore, that BMT-associated TM may be a manifestation of GVHD (3). Graft-vs-host disease is T-cell-mediated. Although a mononuclear cell infiltrate is not usually observed in the kidneys of patients with TM, theoretically, it is possible that lymphokines secreted by T cells may act in concert with other agents to cause endothelial damage. Holler et al. (16) have found a high incidence of microangiopathic changes in patients who received HLA-identical HLA-identical bone marrow grafts and who were treated with CsA. The microangiopathic changes consisted of elevated serum LDH levels, fragmented red blood cells, low platelet counts, and elevated factor VIII receptor antigen (FVIIIR:Ag); serum creatinine concentrations were also increased. Endothelial damage was demonstrated as the central lesion by determination of FVIIIR:Ag. Elevation of FVIIIR:Ag has been attributed in renal transplant recipients to CsA nephrotoxicity (32). Cyclosporine nephrotoxicity is mediated by inhibition of endothelial cell prostacyclin synthesis (33). These authors claimed that their data demonstrated evidence of generalized endothelial damage that was distinct from the isolated nephrotoxicity, but they failed to provide corollary histological evidence to support the statement. However, they did find a correlation between the severity of GVHD and the severity of the microangiopathy. They speculated that, in the course of GVHD, activated lymphocytes secreted interferon gamma (IFN-γ), which then stimulated monocytes. The latter secreted interleukin-1 (IL-1) and tissue necrosis factor alpha (TNF-α) and caused endothelial damage that was associated with activation of coagulation and development of microangiopathic changes. They postulated that CsA failed to inhibit activation of GVH reactive cells in vivo and allowed subsequent release of cytokines and development of a microangiopathy. Although the suggested mechanism has intrinsic appeal, it needs to be challenged in an experimental model. Furthermore, since TM has been described in patients receiving autologous BMT and, therefore, who did not develop GVHD, it seems that other factors are essential for the development of this disease process.

Radiation

The patient's own marrow must often be ablated before a BMT, and this is usually achieved by total-body irradiation (TBI) in combination with chemotherapy. Total-body irradiation is potentially toxic to bone marrow, lungs, kidneys, gut, and so on. However, although BMT can rescue the patient from the hematopoietic toxicity of TBI, the total dose of TBI is limited by the tolerance of the nonhematopoietic tissues.

Radiation nephritis is an uncommon, but potentially devastating, complication of irradiation treatment (34). Renal tolerance is defined as the maximum dose that can be given to normal tissues in the irradiated volume without exceeding a 5% incidence of serious complications in the first 5 years after irradiation. The accepted renal tolerance is 2000 cGy (35). It is also believed that if one-third to one-half of the renal parenchyma is outside of the high-dose volume, unaccepted late renal consequences will not occur (34). This is only an approximation, and it has not been validated by clinical trials.

Luxton and Kunkler (36) identified four clinical syndromes associated with radiation nephritis: acute radiation nephritis, chronic radiation nephritis, malignant hypertension, and benign hypertension. Acute radiation nephritis can begin from 6 to 12 months after treatment. Unfortunately, there is a paucity of data on possible clinical, laboratory, and histological features that may be seen during this latent period. Studies of endothelial cell kinetics in vitro, and in normal and irradiated vasculature, have shown that capillary endothelial cells replicate every 2–3 months (37,38). This latent period reflects the slow turnover of the capillary endothelial cells. Endothelial cells do not proliferate after irradiation; this is in contrast with other types of radiation-induced injury. It has been suggested that irradiation damages the mitotic apparatus and that it may take longer than 2 months before a critical number of endothelial cells enter mitosis and die. This cell death may result in disruption of the normal endothelial cell barrier and allow platelet–basement membrane interaction and subsequent local activation of the coagulation system.

The clinical manifestations have included symptoms of volume overload and acute renal failure, such as the gradual development of edema, hypertension, dyspnea on exertion, and cardiomegaly. Laboratory findings may include microscopic hematuria, proteinuria, azotemia, and anemia (14).

The pathological findings in acute radiation nephritis are initially mainly in the glomeruli, but rapidly progress to include the interstitium and vessels (39). There are increases in mesangial cells and matrix, thickening and splitting of the glomerular capillary walls, and focal areas of tubular damage. In severely affected cases, glomerular capillary and arteriolar necrosis and thrombosis may be detected. The split appearance of the capillary wall is caused by interposition of the mesangial matrix between the endothelial cells and the glomerular basement membrane, as demonstrated by electron microscopic studies. The term *mesangiolysis* and *dissolution or attenuation of mesangial matrix and degeneration of mesangial cells,* as defined by Morita and Churg (18), describe these changes. In fact, in syndromes with thrombotic microangiopathy, the single changes that are almost always seen are detachment of the endothelium from the basement membranes, as well as edema, reticulation, and dissolution of the mesangial matrix (40). The morphological similarities among HUS, TTP, and acute radiation nephritis suggest a common pathogenetic mechanism: endothelial cell injury leading to localized intravascular coagulation within the kidney. The fact that anticoagulation reduces radiation injury in animals supports this concept (4). Furthermore, HUS has occurred after direct local irradiation of the kidney (42).

The sensitivity of the endothelial cell to radiation injury may be enhanced by chemotherapeutic agents. Cortisone (43), cyclophosphamide, doxorubicin (Adriamycin) and dactinomycin (formerly, actinomycin D) have been shown to potentiate radiation damage in animals (44,45) and may have similar effects in humans. It is noteworthy that not all of these agents have been evaluated as radiotoxic enhancers in the kidney, but have usually been studied in other organ systems, such as lungs, esophagus, or intestine. However, the possible clinical significance of the combination of chemotherapy and radiation in the induction of nephrotoxicity was demonstrated by Antignac et al. (7). They changed the conventional conditioning protocol from a single TBI dose plus cyclophosphamide, to a fractionated irradiation dosage, together with cytarabine (aracytidene; Ara-C) and melphalan. None of the ten children, followed for more than 6 months after BMT with the revised protocol, developed delayed renal disease. Although these were short-term results, it seemed that the elimination of cyclophosphamide from the conditioning regimen reduced the nephrotoxic potential. In addition, all ten patients treated at the Dana Farber Cancer Institute (8) by BMT after conditioning with cyclophosphamide and TBI, rather than with TBI, cyclophosphamide, teniposide (VM-26), and cisplatin or Ara-C, had normal serum creatinine concentrations, hematocrits, and haptoglobin levels 4 and 8 months posttransplant. This raises the possibility that adding other agents to the TBI and cyclophosphamide regimen causes sufficient tissue damage or sensitization to enable unexpected toxicity to occur with relatively low radiation doses.

Studies in young animals with growing kidneys, which have a more rapid rate of cell replication than adult kidneys, show greater injury following irradiation (46,47). Therefore, children may be more susceptible than adults to the toxic effects of radiation.

Only four patients have been reported who received a BMT after conditioning that did not include irradiation (12). Their clinical presentation with increasing serum creatinine concentrations, fragmented red blood cells, and thrombocytopenia, 5–36 weeks after transplantation, was associated with a significant rise in serum CsA levels. They all recovered normal kidney function once the dose of CsA was reduced. Renal tissue was unavailable for histological evaluation. With the exception of these patients, all the others received BMT after a conditioning regimen that included TBI and cyclophosphamide.

Because the preparative regimens and median ages do not differ between affected and unaffected patients, it is not yet possible to define a group of patients who may be at greatest risk for the development of this syndrome. In addition, it has not been possible to associated any particular dose, fraction size, or other parameters of TBI with the subsequent occurrence BMT-associated TM (9).

ACUTE RENAL FAILURE

For the sake of completion we are commenting on the occurrence of acute renal failure in the immediate after the BMT period. This has been studied retrospectively in a group of 272 patients who received transplants at the Fred Hutchinson Cancer Research Center during 1986 (48). Fifty-three percent of the patients had a twofold increase in the serum creatinine concentration, and 24% required dialysis. The degree of renal functional impairment had a dramatic impact on the patient mortality rates. Jaundice, weight gain, amphotericin B use, and elevated serum creatinine levels pretransplant were independently associated with the subsequent development of acute renal failure that required treatment with dialysis. Neither aminoglycoside, vancomycin, CsA use, nor GVHD correlated with the development of acute renal failure. Sixty-three percent of the patients who subsequently required dialysis had positive blood cultures and 39% developed hypotension, in the 48 hr period before their serum creatinine levels doubled. No clear explanation for the acute renal failure was apparent in kidney specimens studied at autopsy in most of these patients. It has been suggested that the renal functional impairment was usually the result of hemodynamic, rather than structural changes.

TREATMENT

There is no effective, specific treatment for BMT-associated TM. Treatment modalities that have been tried in patients with other forms of HUS or TTP have been applied to these patients. It is difficult to assess the benefits of individual types of treatment because of the few patients enrolled in each study, the fact that more than one modality was tried at a time, and treatments were initiated at different stages of the disease.

Several regimens that have been used to treat BMT-associated TM: plasma infusions (two patients), plasma exchange (four patients from different centers and in combination with other modalities), low-dose aspirin (two patients), ω-eicosapentaenoic acid (one patient), aspirin (acetylsalicylic acid) and dipyridamole (five patients each from two centers and in combination with other treatments). Most of the patients received only supportive therapy.

OUTCOME

Similar methodological problems render prognostications difficult in patients with BMT-associated TM. However, a few tentative conclusions may be derived from the available data.

Twenty-seven out of 44 patients died, usually during the acute event. However, 5 out of the 27 patients had relatively good kidney function before the relapse of their primary malignancy. On the other hand, only 2 patients recovered completely. The rest of the patients survived with variable degrees of kidney failure. Overall, it seems that patients who present with a rapidly progressive renal disease, which is more likely to be associated with a concurrent infection or severe GVHD, tend to do worse, and the likelihood of their survival is slim (6,10,11,13,14).

All the patients who survived, and who had had hemolytic anemia and thrombocytopenia, eventually had normal platelet counts and no evidence of hemolysis. When six affected patients with acute lymphocytic leukemia (ALL) were evaluated 12 months after the TM episode when they were in remission, they had a mean hematocrit value of only 26.5%. In contrast, seven ALL autologous BMT patients who did not have TM, and who were evaluated while in remission at 12 months after BMT, had mean hematocrits of 36.2% (8). This discrepancy cannot be solely attributed to difference in kidney function, as assessed by serum creatinine values. This raises two questions that have remained unanswered: (a) Does the serum creatinine concentration underestimate the severity of renal dysfunction? It is conceivable that the glomerular filtration rate (GFR) should be evaluated more precisely by methods such as ^{99}Tc-DTPA or ^{125}I-iothalamate. (b) Do we need to evaluate other aspects of renal function in addition to GFR? For example, erythropoietin secretion is probably independent of GFR, and changes in this may account for the difference between the mean hemoglobin concentrations of patients with and without TM. It has been suggested that chemotherapy may blunt the normal exponential relation between hematocrit and plasma erythropoietin titers (49).

One of the major caveats of the reported results is the extremely short-term follow-up (usually 1–2 years). This makes it impossible to predict the natural history of the renal involvement, although it seems likely that some of these patients will progress to end-stage renal disease.

In summary, we have reviewed TM in the context of BMT. This association is always characterized by various degrees of kidney dysfunction, and sometimes, by microangiopathic hemolytic anemia and thrombocytopenia. The pathological features are mesangiolysis and diffuse arteriolar necrosis. It seems that the pathogenesis is multifactorial, but early radiation nephritis, exacerbated by chemotherapy, seems to have an important role. No specific therapy has been defined, and the outcome is guarded. Physicians who take care of patients who have had a BMT must be aware of the symptoms of acute renal failure and should closely follow urinalyses, complete blood counts, and kidney function tests.

REFERENCES

1. Deeg, H. J., Storb, R., Thomas, E. D., Bone marrow transplantation: A review of delayed complications. *Br. J. Haematol., 57*: 185–208 (1984).
2. Symmers, W.St.C., Thrombotic microangiopathic haemolytic anemia (thrombotic microangiopathy). *Br. Med. J., 2*: 897–203 (1952).
3. Chappell, M. E., Keeling, D. M., Prentice, H. G., Sweny, P., Haemolytic uraemic syndrome after bone marrow transplantation: An adverse effect of total body irradiation? *Bone Marrow Transpl. 3*: 339–347 (1988).
4. Craig, J. I. O., Sheehan, T., Bell, K., The haemolytic uraemic syndrome and bone marrow transplantation. *Br. Med. J., 295*: 887 (1987).
5. Loomis, L. J., Aronson, A. J., Rudinsky, R., Spargo, B. H., Hemolytic uremic syndrome following bone marrow transplantation: A case report and review of the literature. *Am. J. Kidney Dis., 14*: 324–328 (1989).
6. Shulman, H., Striker, G., Deeg, H. J., Kennedy, M., Storb, R., Thomas, E. D., Nephrotoxicity of cyclosporin A after allogeneic marrow transplantation. *N. Engl. J. Med., 305*: 1392–1395 (1981).
7. Antignac, C., Gubler, M. C., Leverger, G., Broyer, M., Habib, R., Delayed renal failure with extensive mesangiolysis following bone marrow transplantation. *Kidney Int., 35*: 1336–1344 (1989).
8. Guinan, E. C., Tarbell, N. J., Niemeyer, C. M., Sallan, S. E., Weinstein, H. J., Intravascular hemolysis and renal insufficiency after bone marrow transplantation. *Blood, 72*: 451–455 (1988).
9. Tarbell, N. J., Guinan, E. C., Niemeyer, C., Mauch, P., Sallan, S. E., Weinstein, H. J., Late onset of renal dysfunction in survivors of bone marrow transplantation. *Int. J. Radiat. Oncol. Biol. Phys., 15*: 99–104 (1988).,
10. Spruce, W. E., Forman, S. J., Blume, K. G., et al., Hemolytic uremic syndrome after bone marrow transplantation. *Acta Haematol., 67*: 206–210 (1982).
11. Atkinson, K., Biggs, J. C., Hayes, J., et al., Cyclosporin A associated nephrotoxicity in the first 100 days after allogeneic bone marrow transplantation: Three distinct syndromes. *Br. J. Haematol., 54*: 59–67 (1983).
12. Hows, J. M., Chipping, P. M., Fairhead, S., Smith, J., Baughan, A., Gordon-Smith, E. C., Nephrotoxicity in bone marrow transplant recipients treated with cyclosporin A. *Br. J. Haematol., 54*: 69–78 (1983).
13. Marshall, R. J., Sweny, P., Haemolytic–uraemic syndrome in recipients of bone marrow transplants not treated with cyclosporin A. *Histopathology, 10*: 953–962 (1986).
14. Bergstein, J., Andreoli, S. P., Provisor, A. J., Yum, M., Radiation nephritis following total-body irradiation and cyclophosphamide in preparation for bone marrow transplantation. *Transplantation, 41*: 63–66 (1986).
15. Iskandar, S. S., Browning, M. C., Lorentz, W. B., Mesangiolytic glomerulopathy in a bone marrow allograft recipient. *Hum. Pathol. 20*: 290–292 (1989).
16. Holler, E., Kolb, H. J., Hiller, E., et al., Microangiopathy in patients on cyclosporine prophylaxis who developed acute graft-versus host disease after HLA-identical bone marrow transplantation. *Blood, 73*: 2018–2024 (1989).

17. Kaplan, B. S., Proesmans, W., The hemolytic uremic syndrome of childhood and its variants. *Semin. Hematol. 24*: 148–160 (1987).
18. Morita, T., Churg, J., Mesangiolysis. *Kidney Int. 24*: 1–9 (1983).
19. Witherspoon, R. P., Storb, R., Ochs, H. D., et al., Recovery of antibody production in human allogeneic marrow graft recipients: Influence of time post transplantation, the presence or absence of graft-versus-host disease, and anti-thymocyte globulin treatment. *Blood, 58*: 360–368 (1981).
20. Meyers, J. D., Flournoy, N., Thomas, E. D., Nonbacterial pneumonia after allogeneic marrow transplantation: A review of ten years' experience. *Rev. Infect. Dis., 4*: 1119–1132 (1982).
21. Richardson, W. P., Colvin, R. B., Cheeseman, S. H., et al., Glomerulopathy associated with cytomegalovirus viremia in renal allografts. *N. Engl. J. Med., 305*: 57–63 (1981).
22. Oldstone, M. B., Molecular mimicry as a mechanism for the cause and a probe uncovering etiologic agent(s) of autoimmune disorders. *Curr. Top. Microbiol. Immunol., 145*: 127–135 (1989).
23. Murgo, A. J., Thrombotic microangiopathy in the cancer patient including those induced by chemotherapeutic agents. *Semin. Hematol., 24*: 161–177 (1987).
24. Sheldon, R., Slaughter, D., A syndrome of microangiopathic hemolytic anemia, renal impairment and pulmonary edema in chemotherapy-treated patients with adenocarcinoma. *Cancer, 58*: 1428–1436 (1986).
25. Kahan, B. D., Cyclosporine. *N. Engl. J. Med., 321*: 1725–1738 (1989).
26. Deeg, H. G., Storb, R., Thomas, E. D., et al., Cyclosporine as prophylaxis for graft-versus-host disease: A randomized study in patients undergoing marrow transplantation for acute nonlymphoblastic leukemia. *Blood, 65*: 1325–1334 (1985).
27. Farco, P. R., Hewitson, T. D., Kincaid-Smith, P., An animal model for the study of the microangiopathic form of cyclosporine nephrotoxicity. *Transplantation, 51*: 1129–1131 (1991).
28. Remuzzi, G., Misiani, R., Marchesi, D., et al., Haemolytic–uraemic syndrome: Deficiency of plasma factor(s) regulating prostacyclin activity? *Lancet, 2*: 871–872 (1978).
29. Neild, G. H., Rocchi, G., Imberti, L., Effect of cyclosporine A on prostacycline synthesis by vascular tissue. *Thromb. Res., 32*: 373–379 (1983).
30. Ferico, N., Benigni, A., Zoja, C., Delaini, F., Remuzzi, G., Functional significance of exaggerated renal thromboxane A_2 synthesis induced by cyclosporine A. *Am. J. Physiol., 251*: F581–F587 (1986).
31. Palestine, A. G., Austin, H. A., Balow, J. E., et al., Renal histopathologic alterations in patients treated with cyclosporine for uveitis. *N. Engl. J. Med., 314*: 1293–1297 (1986).
32. Brown, Z., Neild, G. H., Willoughby, J. J., Somia, N. V., Cameron, S. J., Increased factor VIII as an index of vascular injury in cyclosporine nephrotoxicity. *Transplantation, 42*: 150–153 (1986).
33. Voss, B. L., Hamilton, K. K., Samara, E. N., McKee, P. A., Cyclosporine suppression of endothelial prostacyclin generation. A possible mechanism for nephrotoxicity. *Transplantation, 45*: 793–796 (1988).
34. Krochak, R. J., Baker, D. G., Radiation nephritis. Clinical manifestations and pathophysiologic mechanisms. *Urology, 27*: 383–393 (1986).
35. Rubin, P., Casarett, G. W., Concepts of clinical radiation pathology. In *Medical Radiation Biology*, G. Dalrymple, M. Gaulden, G. Kallomorgen, H. Vogel, eds., W. B. Saunders, Philadelphia, pp. 160–189 (1973).
36. Luxton, R. W., Kunkler, P. B., Radiation nephritis. *Acta Radiol., 2*: 169–178 (1964).
37. DeGowin, R. L., Lewis, L. J., Hoak, J. C., et al., Radiosensitivity of human endothelial cells in culture. *J. Lab. Clin. Med., 84*: 42–48 (1974).
38. Tannock, I. F., Hayashi, S., The proliferation of capillary endothelial cells. *Cancer Res. 32*: 77–82 (1972).

39. Keane, W. F., Crosson, J. T., Staley, N. A., et al., Radiation-induced renal disease—a clinicopathologic study. *Am. J. Med., 60*: 127–137 (1976).
40. Shigematsu, H., Dickman, S. H., Churg, J., et al., Mesangial involvement in hemolytic–uremic syndrome. A light and electron microscopic study. *Am. J. Pathol., 85*: 349–362 (1976)
41. Kinzie, J., Studer, R. K., Perez, B., et al., Noncytokinetic radiation injury: Anticoagulants as radioprotective agents in experimental radiation hepatitis. *Science, 175*: 1481–1483 (1972).
42. Cogan, M. G., Arieff, A. I., Radiation nephritis and intravascular coagulation. *Clin. Nephrol., 10*: 74–78 (1978).
43. Berdjis, C. C., Cortisone and radiation. III. Histopathology of the effect of cortisone on the irradiated kidney. *Arch. Pathol., 69*: 431–439 (1960).
44. Phillips, T. L., Wharam, M. D., Margolis, L. W., Modification of radiation injury to normal tissues by chemotherapeutic agents. *Cancer, 35*: 1678–1684 (1975).
45. D'Angio, G. J., Farber, S., Maddock, C. L., Potentiation of x-ray effects by actinomycin D. *Radiology, 73*: 175–177 (1959).
46. Guttman, P. H., Kohn, H. I., Age at exposure and acceleration of intercapillary glomerulosclerosis in mice. *Lab. Invest., 12*: 250–256 (1963).
47. Jaenke, R. S., Phemister, R. D., Norrdin, R. W., Progressive glomerulosclerosis and renal failure following perinatal gamma radiation in the beagle. *Lab. Invest, 42*: 643–655 (1980).
48. Zager, R. A., O'Quigley, J., Zager, B. K., et al., Acute renal failure following bone marrow transplantation: A retrospective study of 272 patients. *Am. J. Kidney Dis., 13*: 210–216 (1989).
49. Schapira, L., Antin, J. H., Rausil, B. J., et al., Serum erythropoietin levels in patients receiving intensive chemotherapy and radiotherapy. *Blood, 76*: 2354–2359 (1990).

IV
Causes of HUS

17
The Association of Verocytotoxins and the Classical Hemolytic Uremic Syndrome

Mohamed A. Karmali *The University of Toronto, Toronto, Ontario, Canada*

The hallmarks of "classical" hemolytic uremic syndrome (HUS), which is by far the most common variety of the syndrome, include an antecedent diarrheal illness which is usually bloody, a peak age incidence in early childhood, highest frequency during the summer and fall, the absence of significant fever, and a good prognosis (1–4).

The occurrence of outbreaks of classical HUS (1–4) lent support to a possible infectious etiology for the syndrome, and its occasional, but inconsistent, association with a wide range of different microbes fashioned the view that the cause was multifactorial (1, 2).

This multiple cause concept for classical HUS was challenged in 1983 (5) and subsequently (6) with reports of an association between infection by verocytotoxin (VT)-producing *Escherichia coli* (VTEC) and the syndrome, and the proposal that verocytotoxins are of direct significance in its genesis. The objective of this paper is to summarize current knowledge on the relationship between VTEC infection and human disease, with special reference to HUS, and to review evidence for a pathogenetic relationship between VTs and the syndrome.

VEROCYTOTOXIN-PRODUCING E. COLI (VTEC) AND HUMAN DISEASE

The term VTEC refers to strains of *E. coli* that produce one or both of at least two different VTs in their culture supernatants (5–8). These cytotoxins, first described by Konowalchuk and colleagues (7, 8) in Canada in the late 1970s, produce an irreversible cytopathic effect on a restricted number cell lines, which include Vero and HeLa (3, 9, 11). They are now known to be closely related, structurally and biologically, to Shiga toxin (9, 10), the exotoxin produced by *Shigella dysenteriae* type 1, a species known to be the cause of the worst forms of bacillary dysentery. For this reason, the toxins are also referred to a Shiga-like toxins (SLTs).

The clinical significance of VTEC remained uncertain until 1983 when a VTEC strain belonging to serotype O157:H7 became associated with two outbreaks of a hitherto poorly recognized bloody diarrheal syndrome, hemorrhagic colitis (12). At about the same time, VTEC belonging to several different serotypes, including O157:H7, became linked to sporadic cases of classical HUS (5).

It is now clear that VTEC are associated with a wide spectrum of illness that includes asymptomatic infection, mild uncomplicated diarrhea, hemorrhagic colitis, and HUS (3). Most of our knowledge about human VTEC infection comes from studies of a single serotype, O157:H7. This is largely because this serotype has a biochemical property (lack of sorbitol fermentation) that allows it to be readily distinguished from other fecal *E. coli* (13, 14), and thus makes recovery of this organism practical in most clinical laboratories (15). On the other hand, over 50 different OH serotypes have now been associated with human disease, and more information is beginning to emerge on the non-O157 serotypes (3, 11).

Hemorrhagic Colitis

Hemorrhagic colitis (ischemic colitis) (12, 16) is a distinct clinical syndrome that presents typically with abdominal cramps and watery diarrhea followed by a hemorrhagic discharge resembling lower gastrointestinal bleeding. It is distinguished from inflammatory colitis in that typically there is a lack of significant fever and an absence of an inflammatory exudate in the stools. In addition, in some patients, a barium enema examination may reveal a characteristic radiological picture of filling defects referred to as a thumbprinting or pseudotumor appearance (12, 16–18). These clinical and radiological features are also characteristic of the bloody diarrhea associated with HUS and emphasize the close relationship between the two syndromes (3).

In 1983 investigators from the Centers for Disease Control, Atlanta, published the results of a classic epidemiological and microbiological investigation of two outbreaks of hemorrhagic colitis in Michigan and Oregon (12). They identified 47 individuals with hemorrhagic colitis using a case definition of severe abdominal pain, grossly bloody diarrhea, and the lack of evidence of infection by recognized enteric pathogens. Case-control studies provided evidence that the illness was associated with ingestion of beef patties at outlets of a well-known fast-food restaurant chain. *E. coli* O157:H7 was recovered from the stools of about half the cases but from none of the healthy controls. Apparently the same strain of *E. coli* was isolated from a beef patty from a suspected lot of meat in Michigan. This seminal study attracted widespread attention and set the stage for several additional studies, mostly in North America, to understand better the magnitude of the problem. In Calgary, Pai and colleagues (19) isolated *E. coli* O157:H7 from 55 (40%) of 137 patients with bloody diarrhea presenting at the emergency departments of Calgary hospitals. Ratnam and March (20), in Newfoundland recovered the organism from seven (15%) of 47 patients with grossly bloody diarrhea. More studies followed, and it soon emerged that *E. coli* O157:H7 was by no means a "rare" serotype as initially thought but rather a fairly common isolate from patients with hemorrhagic colitis and unspecified bloody diarrhea (3, 21).

Hemolytic Uremic Syndrome

In 1980, my colleagues and I in Toronto became interested in the possible role of VTEC in HUS following the isolation of a VT^+ *E. coli* strain from the bowel of a fatal case. A search for VTEC was initiated in new cases of HUS by testing about 5–10 *E. coli* colonies from primary stool cultures for VT production. Initial results were negative, and this prompted us to examine fecal filtrates for the presence of VT activity. Interestingly, fecal VT (FVT) was detected in a number of cases that were negative for VTEC by culture, although a VT^+ *E. coli* strain was subsequently recovered from the stools of some of the cases when a much larger number of *E. coli* colonies were tested. A preliminary report of our findings (5) was followed up by the results of a prospective controlled study (6) involving 40 patients with classical HUS from Ontario and Quebec. In this study, fecal VTEC belonging to at least six different O serogroups (O26, O111, O113, O121, O145, and O157) or FVT or both were detected in 15 (60%) of the cases, but in none of age, sex, and season-matched controls. Ten of 15 cases with microbiological evidence of VTEC infection showed a four-fold or greater rise in VT-neutralizing antibody titer. However six additional patients who were negative for VTEC and FVT also showed significant serological responses giving a total of 30 (75%) who had evidence of VTEC infection. The results indicated not only that there was a close relationship between HUS and VTEC infection, but also suggested that VT was of direct pathogenetic significance because VT production was a common factor in an otherwise heterogeneous group of VTEC strains that belonged to at least 6 different serotypes including O157:H7; in vivo VT production (FVT activity) was demonstrated; and patients showed significant serological responses to VT.

Our findings have now been confirmed in sporadic cases of HUS by other investigators (11, 22, 23) as well as in outbreaks of VTEC-associated diarrhea and hemorrhagic colitis in which HUS occurred as a complication in one or more cases (24–28). In one outbreak of *E. coli* O157:H7–associated diarrhea in a day-care center (24), three (8.3%) of 36 symptomatic children developed HUS; in another affecting a group of kindergarten children after a farm trip (27), three (7%) of 42 symptomatic children developed the syndrome. In a family outbreak, all five (100%) affected children developed HUS (28). The most devastating outbreak of *E. coli* O157:H7 reported to date occurred in a Canadian nursing home (26) in which 12 (22%) of 55 affected residents developed HUS, which ended fatally in 11 cases. The latter outbreak emphasized that HUS, formerly thought to be a disease mostly of young children, should also be considered as a diagnosis in the elderly.

The association between VTEC infection and HUS has been recognized essentially with the classical form of the syndrome. The possible relationship of this infection to other forms of the syndrome is unclear, although Steele and colleagues (29) isolated a VTEC strain (serotype O6:H12) from the stools of a patient with postpartum HUS that was not preceded by a diarrheal illness; Stenger et al. (30) isolated a VTEC strain of serotype O111 from a young woman on oral contraceptives, which are a recognized risk factor for the development of HUS (31).

While HUS is now established as a complication in outbreaks of VTEC infection, controversy still exists as to the frequency of VTEC infection in sporadic cases of "classical" HUS. Recent findings from our laboratory (32) showed evidence of VTEC infection in 45 (88%) of 51 HUS cases; VTEC were isolated from only 23 (51%) of the 45 cases, the remainder being cases who were positive only for FVT. Interestingly, in five cases who were negative for VTEC but positive for FVT, VTEC were isolated from symptomatic family contacts. The OH serotype distribution of the 28 VTEC isolates (23 from index cases and 5 from symptomatic family contacts) was O2:H5 (1), O26:H11 (1), O91:H21 (1), O111:H- (4), O111:H8 (1), O113:H21 (1), O117:H4 (1),

O121:H19 (1), O145:H- (1), and O157:H7 (14); two isolates were untypable. Thus O157:H7 was clearly the most common serotype, accounting for 50% of VTEC isolates from our cases of HUS; the remaining 50% of the VTEC isolates were distributed among 9 different OH serotypes.

In a prospective 1-year study of HUS in the Northwest United States, Neill et al. (23) cultured *E. coli* O157:H7 from the stools of seven (58%) patients with classical HUS. These workers, however, did not examine their cases for FVT or for other VTEC serotypes.

In the United Kingdom (33), studies on patients with HUS were conducted using multiple diagnostic approaches including culture of VTEC, examination of FVT, and the use of colony hybridization with VT-specific DNA probes. Evidence of VTEC was found in 22 (33%) of 66 cases. VTEC strains which were isolated from the feces of 19 patients comprised 14 strains of serotype O157:H7, and one strain each of types O157:H-, O26:H11, O104:H2, O153:H25, and O163:H19.

A retrospective study in Argentina (34) on preserved stool samples from HUS patients presenting from November 1982 to May 1985 revealed that 15 (31%) of 49 patients had stools positive for FVT; this was probably an underestimate, because the test samples had already been diluted 1:10 for previous studies on virus isolation.

A further prospective case-control study (35) from Argentina, a country known to have one of the highest frequencies of HUS in the world, looked at the frequency of VTEC infection in three groups: 51 patients with HUS, 44 patients with diarrhea without HUS, and 25 patients without diarrhea or immunosuppression. The authors used tests for FVT, VT-neutralizing antibody, and detection of VTEC in primary fecal cultures using VT-specific DNA probes (although not all of these tests were performed in each case). They found that 15 (50%) of 31 HUS patients tested were positive for FVT, and most of the HUS patients had some evidence of VTEC infection when the results of all test categories were taken into consideration. Furthermore, about one third of the patients with diarrhea, but without HUS, also had evidence of this infection, whereas no evidence of this infection was found in the control patients without diarrhea. The authors concluded that the high frequency of HUS in Argentina is probably a reflection of the very high frequency of VTEC-associated diarrhea which they found in their population. This was contrasted with the low frequency of both HUS and VTEC-associated diarrhea in Thailand.

The differences in frequency of VTEC infection in HUS cases in various laboratories must be interpreted with caution, because the diagnosis of this infection is still at a developmental stage and optimal methods have yet to be defined and standardized. Note also has to be made of the fact that stools from HUS patients may not be received in laboratories until several days after the onset of the initial diarrheal illness. In our experience, the sensitivity of diagnostic tests declines as the interval between the onset of illness and examination of feces increases; furthermore, delays in transport, prolonged storage either at 4°C or at freezer temperatures (–20°C and –70°C), and repeat freezing and thawing also reduce the chances of a positive result.

VEROCYTOTOXINS

Human VTEC strains produce one or both of at least two distinct bacteriophage-mediated protein exotoxins, VT1 and VT2 (3, 7, 9, 11) that are closely related to Shiga toxin (9, 10). These toxins are cytopathic to a restricted number of cell lines (including Vero and HeLa), induce fluid accumulation in rabbit ileal loops, and are lethal in minute doses to various laboratory animals such as rabbits, rats, and mice (3, 9, 11). Structurally, they are all subunit toxins, being composed of an enzymatically active A subunit (MW ≈ 32,000) and several B subunits (MW ≈ 7,500) that allow binding of the toxin to a specific receptor which is probably the glycosphingolipid globotriosyl ceramide (Gb3) (36, 37). Binding is followed by the internalization, from coated pits (38), of the A subunit, which, after it is proteolytically nicked and reduced to the A1 fragment, inhibits protein synthesis through the catalytic inactivation of 60 S ribosomal subunits (9, 39). The precise mechanism involves inhibition of elongation factor 1-dependent aminoacyl-tRNA binding to the eukaryotic ribosome (40, 41). This is achieved through RNA *N* -glycosidase activity which cleaves the *N* -glycoside bond in the adenosine residue at position 4324 in 28 S rRNA of the 60S ribosomal subunit (42).

The structural genes for the three toxins (Shiga toxin, VT1 and VT2) have been cloned and characterized with respect to nucleotide sequence (3, 9, 11, 43, 44). The genes for VT1 and Shiga toxin are greater than 99% homologous. In contrast, the structural genes for VT1 and VT2 share about a 60% nucleotide sequence homology. Shiga toxin and VT1 are completely cross-neutralized by their respective antitoxins, but not by anti-VT2. Antisera to VT1 and Shiga toxin fail to neutralize VT2.

Head et al (45) have recently reported that toxins referred to as VT2 and SLT ll are not identical. They found that anti-VT2 (prepared against the toxin from VT2-producing strain E32511) completely neutralized the cytotoxic activity of SLT ll from the reference strain 933W as well as from other SLT ll-producing strains, whereas a monoclonal antibody to SLT ll only partically neutralized VT2. Oku et al. (46) have recently reported serological and physico-chemical differences between SLT ll (933W) and VT2 from strain B2F1 (originally isolated from one of our HUS patients), thus confirming that the toxins interchangeably reported as VT2 and SLT ll are heterogeneous.

Ostroff et al (47), using toxin-specific DNA probes, investigated the distribution of SLT l and SLT ll specifying genes in about 90 strains of *E. coli* O157:H7. They found that 76% of strains contained genes for both toxins, 20% contained genes for SLT ll alone, and 3% genes only for SLT l. In this study, SLT ll and VT2 were not necessarily distinguished.

We have studied the distribution of VT1 (H 30), VT 2 (E32511) and SLT ll (933W) among clinical VTEC isolates from patients with the hemolytic uremic syndrom (T. Morooka, M. Petric, G. S. Arbus, and M. A. Karmali; unpublished) using a neutralization assay. Of 21 VTEC strains belonging to serogroups O157:H7 or O157:H-, 18 (86%) elaborated both VT1 (SLT l) and SLT ll; 3 (14%) produced SLT ll alone, but none produced VT1 or VT2 alone. Of 13 non-serogroup O157 VTEC strains, 4 produced VT1 alone, 2, VT2 alone, 1, SLT ll alone, and 5 produced both VT1 and SLT ll. Strains from patients with the hemolytic uremic syndrome (HUS) included those which elaborated VT1, VT2, and SLT ll singly, and those which produced both VT1 and SLT ll, suggesting that all three toxin types are associated with HUS. The combinations of VT1 and VT2 was not observed.

A further VT (48) of considerable interest is that elaborated by porcine strains of *E. coli* that belong to a well-defined group of non-human serotypes that are associated with edema disease of pigs (49). The latter is a usually fatal condition of weanling pigs that is characterized by anorexia, edema of the eyelids, and neurological abnormalities. The VT (edema disease principle) produced by these strains has recently been shown to be closely related to SLT ll/VT2 and is referred to variously as VTE or SLT ll variant (SLT llv) (50). VTE differs from VT1, VT2 and SLT ll in that it is inactive on HeLa cells in contrast to VT1, VT2 and SLT ll which are active on this cell line. DeGrandis et al (51) have shown that VTE binds specifically to the glycolipid globotetraosylceramide (Gb4) and has reduced binding to Gb3. In contrast, Gb4 is not recognized by VT1, VT2, and SLT ll. This difference in glycolipid binding correlates with the differences in cell-line cytotoxicity between VTE and the other toxins. The differential binding of VTs to different glycolipid receptors has also been reported by Samuel et al (52).

VEROCYTOTOXINS AND THE HEMOLYTIC UREMIC SYNDROME

Evidence for the Role of VTs in the Genesis of HUS

Clinicopathological evidence that HUS is a toxemic disease includes the lack of significant fever and the occurrence of widespread sterile systemic lesions, which are characterized by microangiopathic changes in the kidney and other organs and tissues (1, 3, 53, 54).

Several observations made in patients with HUS support the role of VTs as the toxic agents in classical HUS: (a) they are produced in vivo (present in fecal filtrates); (b) patients develop rising levels of VT-neutralizing antibodies; and (c) VT production is a common factor in an otherwise serotypically heterogeneous group of VTEC strains (5, 6).

The availability of an experimental animal model of HUS in which the animal develops the classical syndrome following VTEC infection via the natural oral route would enable the specific role of VT to be elucidated in a direct manner. Unfortunately, such a model has not been described. On the other hand, a growing body of indirect evidence does support the role of VTs as the etiological agents of HUS. In an experimental rabbit model, Richardson and colleagues (55) observed that the injection of VT1 produces disease (mostly in the cecum and brain) whose underlying pathological features include microangiopathic lesions in the affected organs that are similar to the pathology seen in patients with VTEC-associated HUS (54). However, renal disease is not seen in rabbits. Nor do these animals develop thrombocytopenia or the characteristic hemolytic anemia.

When ^{125}I-VT1 is injected into rabbits (56), it is rapidly cleared (within minutes) from the circulation and accumulates at the sites of major histopathological change. This highly selective binding of the toxin to the sites of disease (mainly cecum and brain) supports the hypothesis that the underlying microangiopathy is related to the direct action of the toxin. Furthermore, the rapid clearance of the toxin provides an explanation of why the systemic toxin has not been demonstrated in patients with VTEC disease. The injection of ^{125}I-VT1 to rabbits immunized against VT1 prevents disease and binding of the toxin to the target tissues, thus further supporting the specific role of VT1.

Head et al. (57) found that rabbits challenged intravenously with VT2 develop overt hemorrhagic colitis that is much more severe than the disease elicited by VT1 administration. The possible relevance of this to human disease remains to be established. The possibility that the severity of human VT-associated disease correlates with specific toxin type remains to be established.

Additional animal experimental evidence for the vasotoxic action of VT comes from the work of Francis et al. (58), who challenged gnotobiotic piglets orally with VTEC O157:H7 strains that produced both SLT l and SLT ll, as well as strains that produced only one or other of the two toxins. They observed extensive vascular pathology in the brain and correlated this with the ability of strains to produce SLT ll. Interestingly, the vascular pathology, which included arteriolar necrosis and edema and platelet fibrin capillary thrombi, closely resembled the brain pathology seen in pig edema disease, an observation which Francis et al. (58) believe reflects the close similarity between SLT ll and SLT llv (edema disease principle) Gannon and colleagues (59), using extracts from recombinant SLT llv-positive and SLT llv-negative strains, have also reproduced the vascular brain pathology characteristic of edema disease by challenging pigs intravenously with toxin preparations. In comparative studies, Gannon et al. also observed vascular brain pathology in pigs challenged intravenously with SLT l and SLT ll preparations. These toxins also induced renal lesions characterized by cortical edema and hemorrhage and necrosis of renal tubules, but glomerular lesions characteristic of human HUS were not seen.

The mechanisms by which VTs gain systemic access to reach their ultimate target sites is not known. The present concept is that after the initiation of infection via the oral route, VTEC multiply and colonize the bowel. Evidence from several experimental animal models, including the rabbit (60), pig (61, 62), and calf (63), suggests that VTEC adhere to mucosal epithelial cells in a characteristic manner (64) that involves the destruction of the cell surface microvilli and an intimate effacing adherence of the bacteria to the epithelial cell membrane which forms cups or pedestals at the base of the attached bacterial cell. In animal models, this form of attachment is seen predominantly in the large bowel. The precise nature and site of VTEC colonization in humans remains to be established. It is possible that translocation of VT from the bowel to the circulation requires a specific interaction between VTEC and the epithelial cell. Alternatively there may be a specific mechanism that allows free VT in the bowel to traverse the mucosal barrier.

After gaining access to the circulation, VTs presumably bind to specific target cells which are thought to be vascular endothelial cells (1–3). Capillary endothelial cell damage is considered to be central to the pathogenesis of HUS (1–3). Ultrastructural studies of capillaries in tissues from patients with HUS reveal a characteristic swelling of endothelial cells accompanied by widening of the subendothelial space (1–3, 53). Similar appearances in rabbits challenged parenterally with VT1 (55) support the hypothesis that endothelial cells are primary target sites for the toxin. Additional supporting evidence for this view is that endothelial cells are susceptible to the cytotoxic action of VT1 in vitro (65–67), and, moreover, contain the specific receptor for the toxin, Gb3 (68), which has also been found in large quantities in the human kidney (69). Interestingly, the absence of renal microangiopathic lesions in rabbits challenged with VT1 has been corellated with the absence of Gb3 in rabbit kidneys (55, 69).

The pathophysiological abnormalities in HUS include not only endothelial cell damage but also a reduction in the platelet count, an increase in plasma platelet aggregating activity (70), and the occurrence of an abnormal factor VIII molecule in acute-phase plasma (71). The factor VIII molecule, or complex, consists of a low-molecular-weight portion which has the factor VIII anticoagulant activity, and a high-molecular-weight component referred to as factor VIII–related antigen (von Willebrand factor) (71). Factor VIII–related antigen is increased and has an abnormal multimer pattern in acute-phase HUS plasma, but usually returns to normal during convalescence. It has been suggested that abnormal factor VIII-related antigen leads to platelet aggregation and thrombocytopenia. The fact that factor VIII–related antigen is synthesized by endothelial cells suggests that the action of VT on these cells may be responsible for the factor VIII aberrations in patients with HUS. Research in the UK has demonstrated that VT promotes increased release of the antigen from cultured endothelial cells, which accords with this view (67).

The mechanism for the development of microangiopathic hemolytic anemia in HUS, and the possible role of VTs in its genesis, is not known.

HUS Associated with *Shigella dysenteriae* Type 1

The only other microbe which has been convincingly implicated in HUS is *Shigella dysenteriae* type 1 (Shiga's bacillus) (72). Shiga dysentery is the most severe form of bacillary dysentery; outbreaks have been associated with morbidity and mortality, particularly at the extremes of age. We (73) have suggested that VT/Shiga toxin may be the common denominator responsible for the genesis of HUS associated with both VTEC and *Shigella dysenteriae* type 1. The role of Shiga toxin in the genesis of bacillary dysentery in humans associated with Shiga's bacillus has been controversial. However, recently, on the basis of elegant experiments in macaque monkeys using a toxigenic strain of *Shigella dysenteriae* type 1 and a tox-mutant, Fontaine et al. (74) correlated the presence of the toxin with colonic vascular damage, and proposed that Shiga toxin influences the severity of dysentery by inducing such damage. This observation accords with the hypothesis that Shiga toxin has a primary vasotoxic effect. Vasotoxic activity of Shiga toxin and VT1 has been observed in vitro on cultured human umbilical vein endothelial cells (65–67).

The interplay between VTEC and *Shigella dysenteriae* type 1 in terms of eliciting antitoxic cross-immunity, and the part that this might play in the epidemiology and severity of both infections is an intriguing question that requires to be addressed.

Susceptibility to VTEC Infection and VT-Associated HUS

Little is known about factors that determine susceptibility to VTEC infection, and the risk factors for the development of systemic complications such as HUS.

If the peak age incidence (infants and young children) of "classical" HUS is a reflection of the age incidence of VTEC infection as a whole, it suggests that susceptibility to VTEC-associated HUS may, like to other specific infectious diseases of childhood, be due to the lack of specific immunity, possibly to VT. The increasing recognition of VTEC-associated HUS in the elderly would be consistent with waning immunity in that age group.

Patients with VTEC-associated HUS develop rising levels of VT-neutralizing antibodies (6). However, no definite information is available on the nature, class, and duration of these antibodies, or their relationship to long-term immunity.

Cohen et al. (75) reported that a number of different normal and transformed lymphoid and transformed cell lines tested, only B lymphoid cells were susceptible to VT cytotoxicity. They further showed that the majority of the sensitive B cells belonged to the IgG and IgA committed subset, whereas most IgM and IgM/D producing cells were resistant to VT toxicity. The relevance of this intriguing observation to the natural history of VTEC disease remains to be explored.

The development of systemic complications such as HUS could be a function of a variety of parasite traits such as more efficient colonizing ability or the expression of a specific type of VT. The inoculum size is likely to be a determinant of more severe disease, either directly or indirectly through factors such as the disruption of the gastric acid barrier. This is supported by the occurrence of a very high incidence of HUS among elderly residents in a large nursing home outbreak and the occurrence of more severe disease in those with previous gastrectomy (26).

On the other hand, the development of systemic complications such as HUS in susceptible individuals could be related to specific host factors such as the presence or absence of specific receptors (e.g., Gb3) in target tissues. Boyd and Lingwood (69) examined renal tissue from several patients in different age groups for the presence of Gb3. They found this substance to be a major component of the glycolipid fraction of all renal samples. The levels were higher in the cortex than in the medulla, thus correlating with the distribution of renal lesions in HUS. Tissue from two infants had significantly lower levels of Gb3 than did those from five adults, although the significance of this is unclear. Verotoxin binding was directly proportional to the renal Gb3 content. Of interest was the fact that in some of the tissues, VT also bound to a species consistent with pentaosyl ceramide, the P1 blood group antigen. This glycosphingolipid, like Gb3 (Pk antigen) also terminates in the disaccharide gal α1-4gal that is necessary for toxin binding. Since very few individuals are P1 antigen negative, Boyd and Lingwood concluded that there is probably heterogeneous expression of renal P1, and that this might play a role in susceptibility to renal injury during VTEC infection.

Taylor et al. (76) measured blood group P1 expression by direct agglutination in 32 patients who had previously had classical HUS and in 66 controls of similar ages who underwent venipuncture for other renal disorders. They observed that there was an excess of HUS patients with weak or absent expression of P1 and postulate that strong expression of P1 may promote binding of VT to red cells and thus reduce the dose to nucleated endothelial cells. Accordingly, they suggest that P1 positivity may be protective and P1 negativity a risk factor in HUS.

CONCLUDING REMARKS

There is now compelling evidence that VTEC are causally linked to classical HUS. What is unclear is whether VTEC are the sole cause or a major cause of this syndrome. A fundamental principle of the clinical science of infectious diseases is that a unique relationship exists between a microbe and a specific disease such that the microbial etiology can often be predicted on the basis of the presenting clinical or clinicopathological features. If this principle is applicable to VTEC infection and classical HUS, it would favor the concept that VTEC are the sole cause of classical HUS. This issue will be resolved when optimal methods of high sensitivity and specificity become widely established.

A growing body of evidence supports a direct role for VTs in the genesis of HUS. A variety of sophisticated experiments are under way in several laboratories to elucidate the precise mechanism of action of VTs in vivo and at the molecular level. Advances in our understanding of the pathogenesis of VT-associated HUS at the molecular level may open up possibilities for therapeutic intervention using pharmacological agents to prevent one or another stage in the action of the toxin. On the other hand, if future studies show that naturally acquired VTEC infection leads to long-term immunity, possibly antitoxic, then active immunization would be an option to altogether prevent the serious complication of HUS associated not only with VTEC, but also with Shiga dysentery. Candidate vaccines are already available for such an eventuality in the form of immunogenic synthetic Shiga toxin "B" subunit peptides (77). Rabbit antisera to these synthetic peptides are able to neutralize the biological activity of Shiga toxin in cell culture, and active immunization protects mice against the lethal effects of Shiga toxin.

REFERENCES

1. Fong, J.S.C., de Chadarevian, J-P., Kaplan, B. S. Hemolytic-uremic syndrome. Current concepts and management. *Pediatr. Clin. North. Am.*, *29*: 835–856 (1982).
2. Drummond, K. N. Hemolytic uremic syndrome—Then and now. *N Engl. J Med.*, *312*: 116–118 (1985).
3. Karmali, M. A. Infection by Verocytotoxin-producing *Escherichia coli*. *Clin. Microbiol. Rev.*, *2*: 15–38 (1989).
4. Levin, M., Walters, M.S.D., Barratt, T. M. Hemolytic uremic syndrome. *Adv. Pediatr. Infect. Dis.*, *4*: 51–82 (1989).
5. Karmali, M. A., Steele, B. T., Petric, M., Lim, C. Sporadic cases of haemolytic uraemic syndrome associated with faecal cytotoxin and cytotoxin-producing *Escherichia coli* in stools. *Lancet*, *1*: 619–620 (1983).
6. Karmali, M. A., Petric, M., Lim, C., Fleming, P. C., Arbus, G. S., Lior, H. The association between idiopathic hemolytic uremic syndrome and infection by verotoxin-producing *Escherichia coli*. *J. Infect. Dis.*, *151*: 775–782 (1985).
7. Konowalchuk, J., Speirs, J. I., Stavric, S. Vero response to a cytotoxin of *Escherichia coli*. *Infect. Immun.*, *18*: 775–779 (1977).
8. Konowalchuk, J., Dickie, N., Stavric, S., Speirs, J. I. Properties of an *Escherichia coli* cytotoxin. *Infect. Immun.*, *20*: 575–577 (1978).
9. O'Brien, A. D., Holmes, R. K. Shiga and Shiga-like toxins. *Microbiol. Rev.*, *51*: 206–220 (1987).
10. O'Brien, A. D., LaVeck, G. D., Thompson, M. R., Formal, S. B. Production of *Shigella dysenteriae* type 1-like cytotoxin by *Escherichica coli*. *J. Infect. Dis.*, *1446*: 763–769 (1982).
11. Smith, H. R., Scotland, S. M. Vero cytotoxin-producing strains of *Escherichia coli*. *J. Med. Microbiol.*, *26*: 77–85 (1988).
12. Riley, L. W., Remis, R. S., Helgerson, S. D., McGee, H. B., Wells, J. G., Davis, B. R., Hebert, R. J., Olcott, E. S., Johnson, L. M., Hargrett, N. T., Blake, P. A., Cohen, M. L. Hemorrhagic colitis associated with a rare *Escherichia coli* serotype. *N Engl. J. Med.*, *308*: 681–685 (1983).
13. Farmer, J. J., Davis, B. R. H7 antiserum-sorbitol fermentation medium: a single tube screening medium for detecting *Escherichia coli* O157:H7 associated with hemorrhagic colitis. *J. Clin. Microbiol.*, *22*: 620–625 (1985).
14. Krishnan, C., Fitzgerald, V. A., Dakin, S. J., Behme, R. J. Laboratory investigation of outbreak of hemorrhagic colitis caused by *Escherichia coli* O157:H7. *J. Clin. Microbiol.*, *25*: 1043–1047 (1987).
15. March, S. B., Ratnam, S. Sorbitol-MacConkey medium for detection of *Escherichia coli* O157:H7 associated with hemorrhagic colitis. *J. Clin. Microbiol.*, *23*: 869–872 (1986).
16. Riley, L. W. The epidemiologic, clinical, and microbiologic features of hemorrhagic colitis. *Ann. Rev. Microbiol.*, *41*: 383–407 (1987).
17. Clark, A. W., Lloyd-Mostyn, R.H.L., Sadler, M. R. deC. "Ischaemic colitis" in young adults. *Br. Med. J.*, *4*: 70–72 (1972).

18. Peterson, R. B., Meseroll, W. P., Sharago, G. G., Gooding, C. A. (1976). Radiographic features of colitis associated with the hemolytic uremic syndrome. *Radiology, 118*: 667–671 (1976).
19. Pai, C. H., Gordon, R., Sims, H. V., Bryan, L. E. Sporadic cases of hemorrhagic colitis associated with *Escherichia coli* O157:H7. *Ann. Intern. Med., 101*: 738–742 (1984).
20. Ratnam, S., March, S. B. Sporadic occurrence of hemorrhagic colitis associated with *Escherichia coli* O157:H7 in Newfoundland. *Can. Med. Assoc. J. 134*: 34–45 (1986).
21. Pai, C. H., Ahmed, N., Lior, H., Johnson, W. M., Sims, H. V., Woods, D. E. Epidemiology of sporadic diarrhea due to verocytotoxin-producing *Escherichia coli*: a two-year prospective study. *J. Infect. Dis., 157*: 1054–1057 (1988).
22. Gransden, W. R., Damm, M.A.S., Anderson, J. D., Carter, J. E., Lior, H. Further evidence associating hemolytic uremic syndrome with infection by Verotoxin-producing *Escherichia coli* O157:H7. *J. Infect. Dis., 154*: 522–524 (1986).
23. Neill, M. A., Tarr, P. I., Clausen, C., Christie, D. L., Hickman, R. O. *Escherichia coli* O157:H7 as the predominant pathogen associated with the hemolytic uremic syndrome: A prospective study in the Pacific Northwest. *Pediatrics, 80*: 37–40 (1987).
24. Spika, J. S., Parsons, J. E., Nordenberg, D., Wells, J. G., Gunn, R. A., Blake, P. A. Hemolytic uremic syndrome and diarrhea associated with *Escherichia coli* O157:H7 in a day-care center. *J. Pediatr., 109*: 287–291 (1986).
25. Ryan, C. A., Tauxe, R. V., Hosek, G. W., Well, J. G., Stoez, P. A. *Escherichia coli* O157:H7 diarrhea in a nursing home: clinical, epidemiological, and pathological findings. *J. Infect. Dis., 154*: 631–638 (1986).
26. Carter, A. O., Borczyk, A. A., Carlson, J.A.K., Harvey, B., Hockin, J. C., Karmali, M. A., Krishnan, C., Korn, D. A., Lior, H. A severe outbreak of *Escherichia coli* O157:H7-associated hemorrhagic colitis in a nursing home. *N. Engl. J. Med., 317*: 1496–1500 (1987).
27. Duncan, L., Mai, V., Carter, A., Carlson, J.A.K., Borczyk, A., Karmali, M. A. Outbreak of gastrointestinal disease—Ontario. *Can. Dis. Wkly. Rep., 13*: 5–8 (1987).
28. Karmali, M. A., Arbus, G. S., Ish-Shalom, N., Fleming, P. C., Malkin, D., Petric, M., Cheung, R., Louie, S., Humphreys, G. R., Strachan, M. A family outbreak of hemolytic-uremic syndrome associated with Verotoxin-producing *Escherichia coli* serotype O157:H7. *Pediatr. Nephrol., 2*: 409–414 (1988).
29. Steele, B. T., Goldie, J., Alexopoulou, I., Shimizu, A. Post-partum haemolytic uraemic syndrome and verotoxin-producing *Escherichia coli*. *Lancet 1*: 511 (1984).
30. Stenger, K-O., Windler, F., Karch, H., von Wulffen, H., Heesemann, J. Hemolytic-uremic syndrome associated with an infection by verotoxin-producing *Escherichia coli* O111 in a woman on oral contraceptives. *Clin. Nephrol., 29*: 153–158 (1988).
31. Brown, C. B., Robson, J. S., Thomson, D., Clarkson, A. R., Cameron, J. S., Ogg, C. S. Haemolytic uraemic syndrome in women taking oral contraceptives. *Lancet, 1*: 1479–1481 (1973).
32. Ish-Shalom, N., Arbu, G. S., Karmali, M. A., Petric, M. "Clinical and Prognostic Features of Verotoxin-Producing *E. coli*-Associated Hemolytic Uremic Syndrome." Abs HUS-11. Presented at an International Symposium and Workshop on Verocytotoxin-producing *Escherichia coli* infections, Toronto, July 12–15 (1987).
33. Scotland, S. M., Rowe, B., Smith, H. R., Willshaw, G. A., Gross, R. J. Verocytotoxin-producing strains of *Escherichia coli* from children with haemolytic uraemic syndrome and their detection by specific DNA probes. *J. Med. Microbiol., 25*: 237–243 (1988).
34. Novillo, A. A., Voyer, L. E., Cravioto, R., Freire, M. C., Castaño, G., Wainstein, R., Binztein, N. Haemolytic uraemic syndrome associated with faecal cytotoxin and verotoxin neutralizing antibodies. *Pediatr. Nephrol., 2*: 288–290 (1988).
35. Lopez, E. L., Diaz, M., Grinstein, S., Devoto, S., Mendilaharzu, F., Murray, B. E., Ashkenazi, S., Rubeglio, E., Woloj, M., Vasquez, M., Turco, M., Pickering, L. K.,

Cleary, T. G. Hemolytic uremic syndrome and diarrhea in Argentine children: the role of Shiga-like toxins. *J. Infect Dis., 160*: 469–475 (1989).

36. Lindberg, A. A., Brown, J. E., Strömberg, N., Westling-Ryd, M., Schultz, J. E., Karlsson, K-A. Identification of the carbohydrate receptor for Shiga toxin produced by Shigella dysenteriae type 1. *J. Biol. Chem., 262*: 1779–1785 (1987).
37. Lingwood, C. A., Law, H., Richardson, S. E., Petric, M., Brunton, J. L., de Grandis, S., Karmali, M. Glycolipid binding of natural and recombinant *Escherichia coli* produced Verotoxin in-vitro. *J. Biol. Chem., 262*: 8834–8839 (1987).
38. Sandvig, K., Olsnes, S., Brown, J. E., Peterson, O. W., van Deurs, B. Endocytosis from coated pits of Shiga toxin: a glycolipid-binding protein from Shigella dysenteriae type 1. *J. Cell Biol., 108*: 1331–1343 (1989).
39. Reisbig, R., Olsnes, S., Eiklid, K. The cytotoxic activity of Shigella toxin. Evidence for catalytic inactivation of the 60S ribosomal subunit. *J. Biol. Chem., 256*: 8739–8744 (1981).
40. Brown, J. E., Obrig, T. G., Ussery, M. A., Moran, T. P. Shiga toxin from Shigella dysenteriae 1 inhibits protein synthesis in reticulocyte lysates by inactivation of aminoacyl-tRNA binding. *Microb. Pathogenesis, 1*: 325–334 (1986).
41. Obrig, T. G., Moran, T. P., Brown, J. E. The mode of action of Shiga toxin on peptide elongation of eukaryotic protein synthesis. *Biochem. J., 244*: 287–294 (1987).
42. Endo, Y., Tsurugi, K., Yutsudo, T., Takeda, Y., Ogasawara, T., Igarashi, K. Site of action of verotoxin (VT2) from *Escherichia coli* O157:H7 and of Shiga toxin on eukaryotic ribosomes: RNA N-glycosidase activity of the toxins. *Eur. J. Biochem., 171*: 45–50 (1988).
43. Calderwood, S. B., Auclair, F., Donohue-Rolfe, A., Keusch, G. T., Mekalanos, J. J. Nucleotide sequence of the Shiga-like toxin genes of *Escherichia coli*. *Proc. Nat. Acad. Sci., 84*: 4364–4368 (1987).
44. Jackson, M. P., Neill, R. J., O'Brien, A. D., Holmes, R. K., Newland, J. W. Nucleotide sequence analysis and comparison of the structural gene for Shiga-like toxin I and Shiga-like toxin II encoded by bacteriophages from *Escherichia coli* 933J. *FEMS Microbiol. Letts., 44*: 109–114 (1987).
45. Head, S. C., Karmali, M. A., Roscoe, M. E., Petric, M., Strockbine, N. A., Wachsmuth, I. K. Serological differences between Verocytotoxin 2 and Shiga-like toxin II. *Lancet, 2*: 751 (1988).
46. Oku, Y., Yutsudo, T., Hirayama, T., O'Brien, A. D., Takeda, Y. Purification and some properties of a vero toxin from a human strain of *Escherichia coli* that is immunologically related to Shiga-like toxin II (VT2) *Microb. Pathogen., 6*: 113–122 (1989).
47. Ostroff, S. M., Tarr, P. I., Neill, M. A., Lewis, J. H., Hargrett-Bean, N., Kobayashi, J. M. Toxin genotypes and plasmid profiles as determinants of systemic sequelae in *Escherichia coli* O157:H7 infections. *J. Infect. Dis., 160*: 994–998.
48. Dobrescu, L. New biological effect of edema disease principle (*Escherichia coli* neurotoxin) and its use as an in-vitro assay for this toxin. *Am. J. Vet. Res., 44*: 31–34 (1983).
49. Timoney, J. F. Oedema disease of Swine. *Vet. Rec., 68*: 849–851 (1956).
50. Marques, L.R.M., Peiris, J.S.M., Cryz, S. J., O'Brien, A. D. *Escherichia coli* strains isolated from pigs with edema disease produce a variant of Shiga-like toxin II. *FEMS Microbiol. Letts., 44*: 33–38 (1987).
51. DeGrandis, S., Law, H., Brunton, J., Gyles, C., Lingwood, C. A. Globotetraosylceramide is recognized by the Pig Edema Disease Toxin. *J. Biol. Chem., 264*: 12520–12525.
52. Samuel, J. E., Perera, L. P., Ward, S., O'Brien, A. D., Ginsburg, V., Krivan, H. C. Comparison of the glycolipid receptor specificites of Shiga-like toxin type II and Shiga-like toxin II variants. *Infect. Immun., 58*: 611–618 (1990).
53. Vitsky, B. H., Suzuki, Y., Strauss, L., Churg, J. The hemolytic uremic syndrome: a study of renal pathologic alternations. *Am. J. Pathol. 57*: 627 (1969).
54. Richardson, S. E., Karmali, M. A., Becker, L. E., Smith, C. R. The histopathology of the hemolytic uremic syndrome associated with verocytotoxin-producing *Escherichia coli* infections. *Hum. Pathol., 19*: 1102–1108 (1988).

55. Richardson, S. E., Jagadha, V., Smith, C. R., Becker, L. E., Petric, M., Karmali, M. A. Comparative pathology of the hemolytic uremic syndrome associated with Verotoxin-producing *Escherichia coli* infection and experimental disease in rabbits produced by parenteral VT challenge. Abstract AMV-5. Presented at an International Symposium and Workshop on Verocytotoxin-producing *Escherichia coli* infections, Toronto, July 12–15 (1987).
56. Richardson, S. E., Petric, M., Karmali, M. A. Site-specific localization of ^{125}I-Verocytotoxin 1 in rabbits. Abs B-35. Presented at the 88th Annual Meeting of the American Society of Microbiology, Miami Beach, 8–13 May (1988).
57. Head, S. C., Petric, M., Richardson, S. E., Roscoe, M. E., Karmali, M. A. Purification and characterization of Verocytotoxin 2. *FEMS Microbiol. Letts., 51*: 211–216 (1988).
58. Francis, D. H., Moxley, R. A., Andraos, C. Y. Edema disease-like brain lesions in gnotobiotic piglets infected with *Escherichia coli* serotype O157:H7. *Infect. Immun., 57*: 1339–1341 (1989).
59. Gannon, V.P.J., Gayles, C. L., Wilcock, B. P. Effects of *Escherichia coli* Shiga-like toxins (Verotoxins) in Pigs. *Can. J. Vet. Res., 53*: 306–312 (1989).
60. Sherman, P., Soni, R., Karmali, M. A. Attaching and effacing adherence of verocytotoxin-producing *Escherichia coli* to rabbit intestine in-vivo. *Infect. Immun., 56*: 756–761 (1988).
61. Francis, D. H., Collins, J. E., Duimstra, J. R. Infection of gnotobiotic pigs with an *Escherichia coli* O157:H7 strain associated with an outbreak of hemorrhagic colitis. *Infect. Immun., 51*: 953–956 (1986).
62. Tzipori, S., Karch, H., Wachsmuth, I. K., Robins-Browne, R. M., O'Brien, A. D., Lior, H., Cohen, M. L., Smithers, J., Levine, M. M. The role of a 60-Md plasmid and shiga-like toxins in the pathogenesis of infection caused by enterohemorrhagic *Escherichia coli* O157:H7 in gnotobiotic piglets. *Infect. Immun., 55*: 3117–3125 (1987).
63. Moxley, R. A., Francis, D. H. Natural and experimental infection with an attaching and effacing strain of *Escherichia coli* in calves. *Infect. Immun., 53*: 339–346 (1986).
64. Moon, H. W., Whipp, S. C., Arzenio, R. A., Levine, M. M., Gianella, R. A. Attaching and effacing activities of rabbit and human enteropathogenic *Escherichia coli* in pig and rabbit intestines. *Infect. Immun., 41*: 1340–1351 (1983).
65. Obrig, T. G., Del Vecchio, P. J., Karmali, M. A., Petric, M., Moran, T. P., Judge, T. K. Pathogenesis of hemolytic uremic syndrome. *Lancet 2*: 687.
66. Obrig, T. G., del Vecchio, P. J., Brown, J. E., Moran, T. P., Rowland, B. M., Judge, T. K., Rothman, S. W. Direct cytotoxic action of Shiga toxin on human vascular endothelial cells. *Infect. Immun., 56*: 2373–2378.
67. Kavi, J., Chant, I., Maris, M., and Rose, P. E. Cytopathic effect of Verotoxin on endothelial cells. *Lancet, 2*: 1035 (1987).
68. Moran, T., Lingwood, C. A., Branca, A., del Vecchio, P., Brown, J. E., Obrig, T. Analysis of Shiga toxin receptors on human vascular endothelial cells. Abs B-93. Presented at the 89th Annual Meeting of the American Society of Microbiology, New Orleans, 14–18 May (1989).
69. Boyd, B., Lingwood, C. A. Verotoxin receptor glycolipid in human renal tissue. *Nephron., 51*: 207–210 (1989).
70. Monnens, L., van de Meer, W., Langenhuysen, C., van Munster, P., and van Oostrom, C. Platelet aggregating factor in the epidemic form of hemolytic uremic syndrome in childhood. *Clin. Nephrol., 24*: 135–137 (1985).
71. Rose, P. E., Enayat, S. M., Sunderland, R., Short, P. E., Williams, C. E., Hill, F.G.H. Abnormalities of Factor VIII related protein multimers in the hemolytic uremic syndrome. *Arch. Dis. Child., 59*: 1135–1140 (1984).
72. Koster, F., Levin, J., Walker, L., Tung, K.S.K., Gilman, R. H., Rahaman, M. M., Majid, M. A., Islam, S., Williams, R. C. Hemolytic uremic syndrome after shigellosis.

Relation to endotoxemia and circulating immune complexes. *N. Engl. J. Med.*, *298*: 927–933 (1977).

73. Karmali, M. A., Petric, M., Lim, C., Fleming, P. C., Steele, B. T. *Escherichia coli* cytotoxin, hemolytic uremic syndrome, and hemorrhagic colitis. *Lancet* 2: 1299–1300 (1985).
74. Fontaine, A., Arondel, J., Sansonetti, P. J. Role of Shiga toxin in the pathogenesis of bacillary dysentery, studied by using a tox- mutant of Shigella dysenteriae type 1. *Infect. Immun.*, *56*: 3099–3109 (1988).
75. Cohen, A., Madrid-Marina, V., Estrov, Z., Freedman, M. H., Lingwood, C. A., Dosch, H-M. Expression of glycolipid receptors to Shiga-like toxin on human B lymphocytes: a mechanism for the failure of long-lived antibody response to dysenteric disease. *International Immunol.*, *2*: 1–8 (1990).
76. Taylor, C. M., Milford, D. V., Rose, P. E., Roy, T.C.F., and Rowe, B. The expression of blood group P1 in post-enteropathic hemolytic uremic syndrome. *Pediatr. Nephrol.*, *4*: 59–61 (1990).
77. Harari, I., Donohue-Rolfe, A., Keusch, G., Arnon, R. Synthetic peptides of Shiga toxin B subunit induce antibodies which neutralize its biological activity. *Infect. Immun.*, *56*: 1618–1624.

18
Hemolytic Uremic Syndrome in Families

Bernard S. Kaplan and Paige Kaplan *Children's Hospital of Philadelphia and University of Pennsylvania, Philadelphia, Pennsylvania*

The familial occurrence of HUS in siblings was first reported by Fison in 1956 (1). Fison's patients undoubtedly had HUS, despite the title "Acute Glomerulonephritis in Infancy." The first child became symptomatic at 5 months and 3 weeks in February 1951 and died a month later. Her brother became ill at 5 months in May 1952 and died 2 weeks later. Thirteen years later their male cousin died at age 5 months as a result of HUS (personal communication, Dr. T. H. Hughes-Davies and Dr. M. Brain). Clement et al. (1957) described the occurrence of "purpura thrombotique thrombocytopenique (maladie de Moschcowitz)" in three siblings aged 10, 13, and 10 months, who all died (2). A number of remarkable traits were noted in the index patient by the authors: thrombi were seen only in the kidneys, and there were no neurologic signs (2). HUS in twins was first reported in 1965: They were monozygotic, aged 5 months at onset, the prodrome was an upper respiratory tract infection with vomiting, and both died (3). Chan et al. (4) described the occurrence, almost at the same time, of HUS in two nonrelated adopted siblings; neither died.

Gervais et al. (5) and Kaplan et al. (6) described a family in which three siblings had HUS in 1969, 1970, and 1974 at 9, 8, and 6 months. Each died within 1 month of onset of illness. The parents had adopted two unrelated children between the death of their second biological child and the birth of their third child; neither of the two adopted children has ever had features of HUS. As a result of their experience with this family, Kaplan et al. (6) obtained information on 41 families with 83 affected siblings by carefully reviewing published reports of HUS and by requesting information from pediatricians and nephrologists from many countries. An analysis of this data revealed that there were two groups of families: Group 1 consisted of siblings in whom the onset of HUS occurred within days to weeks of each other. Their prognosis was relatively good, with a mortality rate of 19%, and none had recurrences. Most of these families lived in regions in which HUS was considered, at that time, to be endemic. Group 2 consisted of siblings in whom onset of HUS was separated by more than 1 year. Some patients had recurrent episodes, and prognosis was poor, with a mortality rate of 68%. Most of these patients had lived in areas in which HUS occurred infrequently. The authors speculated that patients in Group 1 had acquired HUS as a result of an environmental insult, whereas those in Group 2 seemed to have had a genetic predisposition to develop the syndrome. An autosomal recessive mode of inheritance was postulated for patients in Group 2. It is now recognized that there are hereditary forms of HUS (7); however, this concept has not gained universal acceptance, perhaps because the notion of heterogeneity is not always appreciated.

Subsequent studies, and personal observations, indicate that familial occurrence of HUS (especially Group 1) is not unusual (8–14). Evidence supporting the theory that HUS in Group 1 is induced by exogenous factors has been provided by several reports that include Shiga toxin–associated HUS in five siblings (14) and *Campylobacter*-associated HUS in a mother and her 27-month-old daughter (15).

It has also become clear that some patients inherit HUS in an autosomal dominant mode (16–22). In addition to recessive and dominant inheritance, the complexity of this problem is further complicated by the fact that, although most probands contain affected members with only HUS (recessive or dominant), some have HUS and TTP (recessive or dominant), and others have only TTP (recessive). The patterns that have occurred in families with inherited forms of HUS, TTP, or HUS, and TTP are shown in Table 1. In families with both HUS and TTP, the features more often resemble those seen in TTP than HUS. Therefore, the terms HUS/TTP, or perhaps hereditary thrombotic microangiopathy, could be used for patients from families with inherited HUS and TTP. The features of the different forms of familial (acquired versus inherited) HUS are summarized in Table 2.

THE REGISTRY FOR INHERITED CASES OF HUS

The prevalence, phenotype, expression, and outcome are not well delineated because most reports are of single kindreds, and many affected families have not been

Table 1 Hemolytic Uremic Syndrome in Families

Group	Postdiarrheal	Recessive	Dominant
Interval	Very short	More than 1 year	Many years
Patients' ages	Asynchronous	Synchronous	Usually adults
	Occasionally	Occasionally	Usually
Seasonal onset	Yes	No	No
Prodrome	Diarrhea	No/respiratory	No/pregnancy
Onset	Sudden	Gradual	Gradual
"TTP-like"	No	At times	Often
Renal pathology	Glomerular	Arteriolar	Arteriolar
Relapse	Very rare	Common	Occasional
End-stage renal failure	Uncommon	Common	Very common
Death	Uncommon	Common	Very common
	$< 10\%$	65%	$> 90\%$

Table 2 Patterns of Inherited HUS and TTP

Autosomal recessive	HUS-HUS-
Autosomal recessive	HUS-TTP-
Autosomal recessive	TTP-TTP-
Autosomal dominant	HUS
	HUS
Autosomal dominant	HUS
	TTP
Twins with HUS	Monozygous
	Dizygous

reported. We therefore established a registry for inherited cases of HUS and TTP under the auspices of the International Registry for HUS to collect demographic data on these families. We have also contacted authors of reported cases for additional information. Kindreds are classified as shown in Table 1. By December 1989, 68 kindreds were listed in the Registry.

AUTOSOMAL RECESSIVE HUS

Forty-three families are known to have had between two and six affected siblings (1, 2, 6, 23–36; personal communications: W. Balfe, T. Baliah, J. Belabradkova, J. Bergstein, M. DeBeukelaer, B. Gauthier, F. Harley, J. Herrin, M. Honda, K. Itaka, M. Levy, C. Loirat, E. Lieberman, J-G. Mongeau, C. Piel, G. Remuzzi, H. Repetto, S. Querin, P. Swee, A. Wasserstein). The interval between onset of HUS in successively affected siblings ranged from 11 months (27) to 10 years (24). The total number of affected patients was 98, of whom 45 were males and 51 were females. An autosomal recessive mode of inheritance is suggested by the occurrence in siblings, with both sexes affected equally and as frequently, with unaffected parents and other unaffected siblings, and onset of the disease at different times but at similar ages in each patient within a sibship.

There are, however, several kindreds with apparent autosomal recessive inheritance of HUS in whom cousins were affected (29, Dr. M. Brain, personal communication). In one kindred, two sisters and two of their nephrews had HUS (31).

In 1986 HUS occurred in a girl aged 2 years after a prodrome of bloody diarrhea. She developed chronic renal failure after several recurrences of HUS that were not associated with bloody diarrhea. Her maternal aunt died from HUS at age 6 months in 1969. Examination of the kidneys by light microscopy revealed unequivocal evidence of a thrombotic microangiopathy (Kaplan and O'Regan, personal observations).

The age of onset within a family is often similar, although there have been notable exceptions. The age of onset has, however, varied markedly among families (Table 3). Most of the patients were children, but onset has occurred as early as 2 weeks (23) and in patients as old as 35 years (32). Some of the patients had no

Table 3 Ages of Onset of HUS in Selected Families

References						
1.	Sex	F		M	Cousin	M
Brain[a]	Age at onset	5 mo, 3 wk		5 mo		5 mo
	Outcome	Died		Died		
23.	Sex	M		M		
	Age at onset	1 mo		.5 mo		
	Outcome	Died		Died		
25.	Sex	F		F		
	Age at onset	2 yr		2 yr		
	Outcome	Died		Died		
6.	Sex	M		F	M	
	Age at onset	8 mo		7 mo	6 mo	
	Outcome	Died		Died	Died	
Lieberman[a]	Sex	M		F		
	Age at onset	36 mo		36 mo		
	Outcome	Died		Died		
24.	Sex	F		F		
	Age at onset	6 yr		6 yr		
	Outcome	Alive 13 yr		12 yr		
	Recurrences	+		−		
24.	Sex	F		M		
	Age at onset	16 mo		16 mo		
	Outcome	Died		Died		
31.	Nephews					
	Sex	M		M		
	Age at onset	5 mo		5 mo		
	Outcome	Died		Died		
	Aunts					
	Sex	F		F		
	Age at onset	23 yr		26 yr		
	Outcome	Died		Died		
Gauthier[a]	Sex	M		F	M	M
	Age at onset	6 mo	<TWINS>	6 mo	12 mo	12 mo
	Outcome	Died		Died	Died	Alive
	Recurrence				+	
34.	Sex	F		F	F	
	Age at onset	11.5 mo		12 mo	16 mo	
	Outcome	Died		Died	Died	Died

[a]Personal communication.

apparent prodromal illness, whereas others had minor prodromal illnesses which usually consisted of an upper respiratory infection with or without vomiting. Two patients were taking oral contraceptives prior to the onset of HUS (27; S. Querin, personal communication). One patient had HUS associated with pregnancy (26). Pirson et al. (32) described the occurrence of HUS in three male siblings aged 27 to 35 years. Each progressed to end-stage renal failure and received successful cadaver allografts. There have been no recurrences of HUS. Two sisters have not had HUS; both have used oral contraception.

The total number of patients alive at the last determination was 34/98 (35%). Only nine of the survivors were well (9/98, 9%). Twelve were either in chronic renal failure or had been transplanted (17%). Recurrent episodes occurred in 14 patients (14%). Some patients had as many as 12 recurrences of HUS. The mortality rate was 65% (63/98). The mortality rate has not changed since 1975, despite the introduction of new types of treatment such as infusions of fresh frozen plasma and plasmapheresis.

FAMILIES WITH HUS AND TTP

There have been several reports of HUS in one sibling and TTP in another (26, 37–39). Hellmann et al. (38) described the occurrence of HUS in a male aged 19 years, and TTP in his HLA-identical twin brother 6 years later. Although these twins had virtually identical illnesses, a diagnosis of HUS was made in the first twin and one of TTP in the second. Elias et al. (39) reported a family with nonconsanguineous parents in whom there were three affected siblings and seven healthy sisters. The findings in these siblings are shown in Table 4. Case 1 initially had no evidence of renal involvement but subsequently developed proteinuria and red blood cell casts. The diagnosis of TTP is tenable because the central nervous system injury was the major problem and the features of clinical renal disease were minor. Case 2, a brother, also had a recurrent episode of TTP with onset at age 2 months. The third sibling presented at 18 months with a similar clinical picture to his siblings. These three patients appear to have had variable expression of the same genetic defect. In this context the appellations HUS and TTP serve to confuse the issue. These patients as well as others that have been reported or that are known to us may not have had "HUS" or "TTP" but a different mutation that produced illnesses that resemble the phenotypes of HUS and TTP.

Table 4 HUS/TTP

	Case 1	Case 2	Case 3
Age at onset	12 mo	2 mo	18 mo
Sex	F	M	M
Prodrome	Vomiting, diarrhea	Fever, lethargy	Fever, lethargy
Anemia	Yes	Yes	Yes
Thrombopenia	Yes	Yes	Yes
Azotemia	No	No	No
Proteinuria	Yes	Yes	Yes
Hematuria/casts	Yes	No	Yes
CNS	Hemiplegia, convulsions	Confusion	Confusion
Recurrences	2	3	3
Outcome	Died, 22 mo	Alive, 15 mo	5 yr
Diagnosis	TTP	TTP	HUS

Source: Ref. 39.

AUTOSOMAL RECESSIVE TTP

Simultaneous and non-simultaneous onset of TTP have occurred within families. Onset of TTP has been simultaneous in two sisters (40) and within months of each other in a husband and wife (41).

We are aware of six families in which two to four siblings have had TTP (42–45; B. Wiedermann, personal communication). The ages at onset ranged from 8 months to 25 years; 11 were under 17 years and four were over age 19 years at onset. Six were male and nine were female. Ten patients died; six (including two survivors) had recurrent episodes. TTP was associated with systemic lupus in two sisters (42) and with pregnancy in two other sisters in another kindred (44).

AUTOSOMAL DOMINANT HUS

We are aware of 13 families with dominant transmission of HUS (16–22, 46–48; A. J. Williams, J. Berns, personal communications). These patients present many problems of assessment and interpretation because there are marked differences in expression within and among families. Ascertainment is also a problem because only a presumptive diagnosis of HUS can be made in cases who died many years ago and in whom complete records are unavailable or postmortems were not done. Because of these difficulties, we have chosen to summarize the findings in several kindreds so that attention can be directed at particular points. The cases reported by Farr et al. (17) are summarized briefly:

Case 1, patient X, died in 1946 at the age of 57 years with hypertension and uremic pericarditis. Postmortem tissue was not available for study.

Case 2, patient E, (son of X and brother of A), died in 1953 at the age of 45 years with hypertension and uremia. Thrombi were seen in glomeruli, afferent arterioles, intralobular arteries, segmental arteries of the kidneys, and in some small arterioles of the myocardium at postmortem.

Case 6, patient A (father of A2 and A4), presented in 1973 at age 45 years with hypertension, hemolysis, fragmented erythrocytes, thrombocytopenia, and uremia. Renal biopsy showed thickening of glomerular capillary loops, concentric proliferative endarteritis, severe narrowing of arterial lumens, fibrin deposition, and fibrinoid necrosis in smaller arteries and arterioles.

Case 4, A4 (son of A) had HUS in 1963 at 5 years and died soon after admission to hospital. The HUS was preceded by measles. Postmortem examination of kidneys showed enlarged and congested glomeruli with splitting of basement membranes; subendothelial fibrin deposits; increased mesangial matrix; thrombi in many afferent arterioles; endothelial cell proliferation; and, in larger vessels, thrombi and subintimal fibroblastic proliferation.

Case 5, patient A2 (sister of A4, daughter of A) had HUS in 1972 at age 19 years and died the same year. She had been taking Norinyl® 1 for 6 weeks. The prodromal illness was vague ill health, anorexia, and a 24-hour period of diarrhea. Renal biopsy and postmortem studies showed necrosed glomeruli, fibrin thrombi in capillary loops, widened subendothelial spaces, and fibroblastic proliferation of larger vessels.

Case 3, patient D2 (nephew of A) became ill with an influenza-like illness in 1954 at age 7 years. He rapidly developed purpura, hypertension, hemolytic anemia, thrombocytopenia and, uremia, and died 9 days after admission. Postmortem examination showed similar changes to those seen in Case 6.

With the exception of the grandmother (X), each of the patients had good evidence of HUS, although Case 2 had features of TTP, as evidenced by the presence of thrombi in multiple stages of organization in two organs. Only one patients survive the illness (Case 6). Both males and females were affected, apparently with equal severity. The ages of onset varied markedly from 5–45 years (and possibly 57 years). None had a typical prodromal illness of bloody diarrhea; one had been on an oral contraceptive agent for 6 weeks.

The family reported by Hogewind et al. (19) is remarkable because HUS occurred in five females in two generations; four developed HUS within 6 weeks postpartum; four died; the only survivor received a renal allograft; four were between 18 and 40 years of age and one was aged 5 years; one patient had been given stilbestrol before the onset of HUS.

Perret et al. (46) described HUS in a boy aged 4 years; four adults in his family (two males and two females, in three generations) also had HUS; two patients died, and the remaining three developed chronic renal failure.

In the family reported by Karlsberg et al., there were four affected males aged 27–47 years. Three died and one developed chronic renal failure (18).

Details of the cases of the mother and daughter reported by Kirchner et al. (21) are summarized in Table 5 to highlight the fact that, although the diagnosis was said

Table 5 "TTP" in a Mother, "HUS" in Her Daughter

	Mother	Daughter
Age at onset	27 y	24 y
		Headache
		Fever
		Pregnant
	Abdominal pain	
	Hematuria	
	220/130	160/210
	Papilledema	
	Hepatosplenomegaly	Hepatosplenomegaly
	Ecchyumoses	
Hemoglobin	6.6	14%
Platelets	75,000	15,000
WBC count	11,111	
Fragment cells	+	+
Urine		
Protein	5.4 g	4+
Blood	++	+
BUN	32	58
Creatinine	2.1	
Seizures	+	
BP control	Poor	Good
CRF	Yes	Yes
Outcome	Death	Hemodialysis
Histologic diagnosis		
BUT	TTP	HUS
	Thrombi in kidneys	Thrombi in kidneys and spleen

Source: Ref. 21.

to be TTP in the mother and HUS in her daughter, they had virtually identical illnesses which began at almost the same ages.

The kindred reported by Carreras et al. (20) has been referred to in detail in the Chapter 13, "Recurrent Hemolytic Uremic Syndrome" but is summarized again because of a number of instructive points. A woman aged 32 years had a spontaneous abortion in July 1975. She then used oral contraceptives for 4 months; 1 month after she stopped taking the oral contraceptives, she had anorexia, lassitude, headaches, vomiting, myalgias, and pallor. In December 1977 she had another episode of HUS that started 10 days after onset of an *Escherichia coli* urinary tract infection which was treated with gentamicin. Serum C3 was persistently low and C3A was slightly decreased. Many family members had low C3 concentrations and evidence of alternate pathway activation. The patient developed end-stage renal failure. Her daughter, aged 7 months, had several episodes of HUS; C3 concentrations were depressed. She died, and thrombotic microangiopathy was diagnosed postmortem. A nephew aged 2 years had onset of HUS after an upper respiratory tract infection. He recovered and was also found to have hypocomplementemia. Another important common factor in this family was the demonstration of the HLA haplotype A3, B7 in affected patients and in the family members who had evidence of complement activation.

HUS in two families was reported by Camba et al. (47). The posita aged 17 years in one family developed chronic renal failure. She had been treated with plasmapheresis. Her father and maternal uncle had also had HUS. In a second family, the father aged 50 years had chronic renal failure after treatment failure with plasmapheresis; two daughters also had HUS.

The report of Merrill et al. (22) is of interest because of the rare occurrence of HUS in blacks. In addition, this report draws attention again to the facts that the diagnosis of thrombotic microangiopathy was missed in the past, and that inherited causes of renal disease constitute up to 20% of all patients in chronic renal failure.

Case I-1 was a 61-year-old black woman who died from chronic renal failure, hypertension, and vascular disease. Case II-2 was a 41-year-old male who died with severe hypertension. Case II-6 was a 31-year-old female who had hypertension and renal failure prior to her death. None had evidence of HUS, but neither did they not have HUS. It seems likely that II-6 had HUS because her twin sister had histological evidence of thrombotic microangiopathy at autopsy. Case II-7 was the twin of II-6. She was a 32-year-old female who had a history of hypertension during pregnancy, renal failure. Postmortem examination revealed evidence of thrombotic microangiopathy.

Case II-10 was a 39-year-old female who presented in 1983 with severe hypertension and renal failure. She had hemolysis with schistocytes as well as thrombocytopenia. A renal biopsy revealed a diagnosis of thrombotic microangiopathy. She developed end-stage renal failure.

Grottum et al. (16) described a family in whom the diagnosis of HUS also is not unequivocal. A brief summary of this very complicated family follows:

Case 1. Female aged 20 years presented with edema and proteinuria. At age 24, while pregnant, developed severe edema, hypertension, oliguria, microangiopathic hemolytic anemia, and thrombocytopenia. After delivering a stillbirth, her condition improved. Three weeks later she became severely ill, had a bilateral nephrectomy and splenectomy, recovered rapidly, and was transplanted. Case 2 was her 28-year-old brother, who presented in 1971 with edema, proteinuria, hypertension, severe microangiopathic hemolytic anemia, and thrombocytopenia. His condition improved after a bilateral nephrectomy and splenectomy. Case 3 was another brother aged 31 years who in 1966 had proteinuria and hypertension. In 1972 he developed edema, malignant hypertension, nonoliguric renal failure, microangiopathic hemolytic anemia, and thrombocytopenia. Bilateral nephrectomy and splenectomy were followed by a renal transplant. Case 4 was a cousin aged 24 years who developed proteinuria and hypertension in 1963, "chronic glomerulonephritis" in 1966, and died in oliguric renal failure in 1968.

Ten family members out of 174 in five generations died from uremia; two women died at 26 and 34 years from renal disease during pregnancy. The authors speculated that this was an autosomal dominant trait with incomplete penetrance in females and that the renal histologic findings in case 3 were suggestive of TTP.

Williams (personal communication) has provided information on a family in which the father died in the 1960s of renal failure complicated by acute hemolytic anemia and thrombocytopenia. His daughter died in the 1970s of renal failure complicated by acute hemolytic anemia. A son aged 26 years has had three failed renal transplants for treatment of end-stage renal failure caused by HUS.

HUS IN TWINS

HUS has been reported in monozygotic and in dizygotic twins (3, 35; H. Altman, C. Piel, personal communication). HUS occurred in one and TTP in the other of HLA-identical twins (38). Katz (personal communication) has provided data on twin boys whose onset of HUS was in infancy; both have had two additional episodes of HUS.

PATHOGENESIS OF INHERITED HUS

The pathogenesis of inherited HUS is unknown. Mattoo et al. (36) provided unequivocal evidence of autosomal recessive inheritance (if any doubters still exist) by describing an unfortunate experiment of nature in a polygamous marriage. The father had two wives, one of whom was a first cousin. All the members of this family lived together. None of the children of the nonconsanguineous wife had HUS. However, four of the children of the cousin-wife definitely had HUS and two others died of renal failure. Remuzzi et al. (49) have speculated that these patients may have a defect in the metabolism or function of prostacyclin (50, 51). They found a persistent defect in the capacity of the plasma of a 54-year-old woman with HUS to stimulate prostacyclin activity; a similar abnormality could be demonstrated in her two sons but not in her two daughters. Deficiency of a plasma factor stimulating vascular prostacyclin production was also found in a 2-year-old girl with HUS and in her unaffected mother; the ability of the father's plasma to stimulate protacyclin production was normal (50).

Platelet-aggregating activity or abnormal vWF:FVIII multimers could not be detected in patients with dominant inheritance of HUS (22).

There are a few kindreds with complement abnormalities. Hypocomplementemia was associated with a HLA A3, B7 haplotype in one family (20). In another, in vivo complement activation could be shown before and after nephrectomy and a serum C3 degrading factor could be detected (by Grottum et al. (16)).

In view of the abnormal complement profiles that have been demonstrated in some families with inherited HUS or TTP, and in many patients with relapsing HUS, we recommend that a serum C3 concentration and CH50 activity be done in all patients in these contexts.

TREATMENT OF HEREDITARY HUS, TTP, AND HUS/TTP

At least five extremely difficult questions arise in the management of patients with inherited forms of HUS or TTP and their families:

1. *Diagnosis in the first affected member*. The diagnosis of an inherited form of HUS or TTP is easy if another family member has already had either condition. The diagnosis in a proband with a negative family history cannot be made with certainty at this time. Clues that indicate the possibility of an inherited form are listed in Table 6.

2. *Acute treatment*. There is no effective treatment for patients with the inherited forms of HUS or TTP. Because of the small numbers of patients it has not been possible to design any prospective trials of therapy. Infusions of fresh frozen plasma have been advocated (49) but there is no evidence that they have been efficacious. Plasmapheresis has also been suggested but, again, evidence favoring its use is also lacking. Despite these caveats, it has been our practice to recommend treatment with fresh frozen plasma and plasmapheresis, although we are cognizant of the lack of any proof that they are helpful.

3. *Genetic counseling*. If an inherited form of HUS or TTP is suspected, it is incumbent upon the physician to offer genetic counseling in the event that further pregnancies are planned. Unfortunately no markers have yet been identified that might enable the heterozygous state to be determined. Nor can antenatal diagnosis be done by amniocentesis or chorionic villus biopsy.

4. *Prognosis*. The prognosis is grim. Many patients die or have a progressive course, or have relapses, or require dialysis. Some have recurrences after renal transplantation. There are as yet no guidelines as to whether or not living related kidney transplants should be done in this context.

5. *Use of oral contraceptives, risks of pregnancy*. There are anecdotal reports of HUS or TTP following the use of an oral contraceptive agent. We recommend that they not be used by women who have had a positive family history of HUS or TTP or by those who have had an atypical nondiarrhea associated form of the syndrome. There is, however, no scientific basis for this opinion.

The problem of pregnancy is more vexing. Clearly, in families in which HUS or TTP has occurred in association with pregnancy, it might be prudent to recommend that pregnancy be avoided, preferably by methods other than the use of an oral contraceptive agent.

Table 6 Clues to the Diagnosis of an Inherited form of HUS, TTP, or HUS/TTP

1. A previously affected family member at a remote time
2. An atypical, nondiarrheal prodrome *or* no definable prodromal illness
3. A slowly progressive course
4. Recurrent episodes
5. Predominantly arteriolar changes in the kidney
6. Recurrence after renal transplantation

REFERENCES

1. Fison, T. N. Acute glomerulonephritis in infancy. *Arch. Dis. Child, 3*: 101–109 (1956).
2. Clement, R., Bernard, J., Papainnou, A., Mathe, G., Habib, R., Designolle, M. Purpura thrombotique thrombocytopenique (maladie de Moschcowitz) chez un enfant de dix mois. *Press. Med., 65*: 2144–2146 (1957).
3. Campbell, S., Carre, I. J. Fatal haemolytic uraemic syndrome and idiopathic hyperlipidemia in monozygotic twins. *Arch. Dis. Child, 40*: 654–658 (1965).
4. Chan, J.C.M., Eleff, M. G., Campbell, R. A. The hemolytic-syndrome in nonrelated adopted siblings. *J. Pediatr., 75*: 1050–1053 (1969).
5. Gervais, M., Richardson, J. B., Chiu, J. M., and Drummond, K. N. Immunofluorescent and histologic findings in the hemolytic uremic syndrome. *Pediatrics, 47*: 352–359 (1971).
6. Kaplan, B. S., Chesney, R. W., Drummond, K. N. Hemolytic uremic syndrome in families. *N. Engl. J. Med., 292*: 1090–1093 (1975).
7. Kaplan, B. S., Kaplan, P. Hemolytic-uremic syndrome. In: *Birth Defects Encyclopedia*. (M. L. Buyse, ed.) Center for Birth Defects Information Services, Inc. Dover, Mass. (in press)
8. Ray, C. G., Tucker, V. L., Harris, D. J., Cuppage, F. E., Chin, T.D.Y. Enteroviruses associated with the hemolytic-uremic syndrome. *Pediatrics, 46*: 378–388 (1970).
9. Vildosola, S.M.J., Bravo, R. I., Emparanza, Del, S. E. Sindrome hemolitico-uremico en la infancia. *Pediatria, 5*: 292–307 (1962).
10. Tune, B. M., Groshong, T., Plumer, L. B., and Mendoza, S. A. The hemolytic-uremic syndrome in siblings: A prospective survey. *J. Pediatr., 85*: 682–683 (1974).
11. Arenson, E. B. Jr., August, C. S. Preliminary report: Treatment of the hemolytic-uremic syndrome with aspirin and dipyridamole. *J. Pediatr., 86*: 957–961 (1975).
12. Larke, R.P.B., Preiksaitis, J. K., Devine, R.D.O. Hemolytic uremic syndrome: Clustering of ten cases and association with multiple viral infections. *Soc. Serv. Commun. Health, 4*: 2–5 (1980).
13. Vecilla, M. C., Morena, M. R., Bernacer, M., Rocandio, S.C.L. Sindrome hemolitico uremico familiar associado a infeccion por Coxsachie B. *An. Esp. Pediatr., 20*: 369–374 (1984).
14. Karmali, M. A., Arbus, G. S., Ish-Shalom, N., Fleming, P. C., Malkin, D., Petric, M., Cheung, R., Louie, S., Humphreys, G. R., Srachan, M. A familial outbreak of hemolytic-uremic syndrome associated with verotoxin-producing *Escherichia coli* serotype O157:H7. *Pediatr. Nephrol., 2*: 409–414 (1987).
15. Chamovitz, B. N., Hartstein, A. I., Alexander, S. R., Terry, A. B., Short, P., Katon, R. Campylobacter jejuni-associated hemolytic-uremic syndrome in a mother and daughter. *Pediatrics, 71*: 253–256 (1983).
16. Grottum, K. A., Flatmark, A., Myhre, E., Jansen, H., Teisberg, P., Oystese, B., Husby, G., and Hovig, T. Immunologic hereditary nephropathy. *Acta. Med. Scand.,* 571 (Suppl): 1–27 (1974).
17. Farr, M. J., Roberts, S., Morley, A. R., Dewar, P. J., Roberts, D. F., and Uldall, P. R. The haemolytic-uraemic syndrome—a family study. *Q. J. Med., 44*: 161–188 (1975).
18. Karlsberg, R. P., Lacher, J. W., Bartecchi, C. E. Adult hemolytic-uremic syndrome. Familial variant. *Arch. Int. Med., 137*: 1155–1157 (1977).
19. Hogewind, B. L., de la Riviere, G. B., van Es, L. A., Veltkamp, J. J. Familial occurrence of the haemolytic uraemic syndrome. *Acta Med. Scand., 207*: 73–77 (1980).
20. Carreras, L., Romero, R., Requesens, C., Oliver, A. J., Carrera, M., Clavo, M., Alsina, J. Familial hypocomplementemic hemolytic uremic syndrome with HLA-A3, B7 haplotype. *J.A.M.A., 245*: 602–604 (1981).
21. Kirchner, K. A., Smith, R. M., Gockerman, J. P., Luke, R. G. Hereditary thrombotic thrombocytopenic purpura: Microangiopathic hemolytic anemia, thrombocytopenia, and renal insufficiency occuring in consecutive generations. *Nephron, 30*: 28–30 (1982).

22. Merrill, C. H., Knupp, C. L., Jennette, J. C. Familial thrombotic microangiopathy. *Q. J. Med.*, *57*: 749–759 (1985).
23. Anthony, P. P., Kaplan, A. B. Fatal haemolytic-uraemic syndrome in two sibs. *Arch. Dis. Child*, *43*: 316–318 (1968).
24. Belobradkova, J., Nozicka, Z. Hemolyticko-uremicky syndrom. *Cas. Lek. Ces.*, *111*: 85–90 (1972).
25. Bohle, A., Gartner, H-V., Laberke, H-G., Krucke. *In Der Niere*. F. K. Schattauer, Stuttgart, Germany, p. 384. (1984).
26. Ekberg, M., Nilsson, I. M., Dennenberg, T. Coagulation studies in hemolytic uremic syndrome and thrombotic thrombocytopenic purpura. *Acta. Med. Scand.*, *196*: 373–382 (1974).
27. Bergstein, J., Michael, A. Jr., Kjellstrand, C., Simmons, R., Najarian, J. Hemolytic-uremic syndrome in adult sisters. *Transplantation*, *17*: 487–489 (1974).
28. Blattler, W., Wegmann, W., Herold, H., Straub, P. W. Familiares hamolytisch-uramisches syndrom. Untersuchungen zur pathogenese bei den uberlebenden. *Schweiz. med. Wschr.*, *105*: 1773–1774 (1975).
29. Courtecuisse, V., Dommergues, J-P., Rivron, J., Chaon, P. Syndrome hemolytique et uremique familial avec biopsie renale normale. *Arch. Fr. Pediatr.* *32*: 749–755 (1975).
30. Quazi, Q. H., Schutta, E. J. Familial hemolytic-uremic syndrome in siblings. *Pediatr. Res.* (Abstract), *9*: 377 (1975).
31. Edelsten, A. D., Tuck, S. Familial haemolytic uraemic syndrome. *Arch. Dis. Child*, *53*: 255–256 (1978).
32. Pirson, Y., Lefebvre, C., Arnout, C., de Strihou, C. Y. Hemolytic uremic syndrome in three adult siblings: a familial study and evolution. *Clin. Nephrol.*, *28*: 250–255 (1987).
33. Monn, E. Hemolytic-uremic syndrome in two sisters due to a deficiency in prostacyclin metabolism. *Eur. J. Pediatr.* (Abstract), *140*: 199 (1983).
34. Feldhoff, C., Pistor, K., Bachmann, H., Horacek, U., Obling, H. Hemolytic uremic syndrome in 3 siblings. *Clin. Nephrol.*, *22*: 44–46 (1984).
35. Loirat, C., Sonsino, E., Moreno, A. V., Pillion, G., Mercier, J. C., Beaufils, F., Mathieu, H. Hemolytic-uremic syndrome: An analysis of the natural history and prognostic features. *Acta. Paediatr. Scand.*, *73*: 505–514 (1984).
36. Mattoo, T. J., Mahmood, M. A., Al-Harbi, M. S., Mikail, I. Familial, recurrent hemolytic-uremic syndrome. *J. Pediatr.*, *114*: 814–816 (1989).
37. Hagge, W. F., Holley, K. E., Burke, E. G., Stickler, G. B. Hemolytic-uremic syndrome in two siblings. *N. Engl. J. Med.*, *277*: 138–139 (1967).
38. Hellman, R. M., Jackson, D. V., Buss, D. H. Thrombotic thrombocytopenic purpura and hemolytic-uremic syndrome in HLA-identical siblings. *Ann. Intern. Med.*, *93*: 283–284 (1980).
39. Elias, M., Horowitz, J., Tal, I., Kohn, D., Flatau, E. Thrombotic thrombocytopenic purpura and haemolytic uraemic syndrome in three siblings. *Arch. Dis. Child*, *63*: 644–646 (1988).
40. Paz, R. A., Elijovich, F., Barcat, J. A., Sanchez-Avalos, J. C. Fatal simultaneous thrombocytopenic purpura in siblings *Br. Med. J.*, *2*: 727–728 (1969).
41. Watson, C. G., Cooper, W. M. Thrombotic thrombocytopenic purpura. Concomitant occurrence in husband and wife. *J.A.M.A.*, *215*: 1821–1823 (1971).
42. Norkin, S. A., Freedman, H. H., Evans, G. W. Thrombotic thrombocytopenic purpura in siblings. *Am. J. Med.*,—: 294–303 (1967).
43. Wallace, D.C., Lovric, A., Clubb, J. S., Carseldine D. B. Thrombotic thrombocytopenic purpura in four siblings. *Am. J. Med.*, *58*: 724–734 (1975).
44. Fuchs, W. E., George, J. N., Dotin, L. N., Sears, D. A. Thrombotic thrombocytopenic purpura. Occurrence two years apart during late pregnancy in two sisters. *J.A.M.A.*, *235*: 2126–2127 (1976).

45. Waage, A., Siegel, J., Thornstensen, K., Lamvik, J. Thrombotic thrombocytopenic purpura in 2 siblings: Defective platelet function and plasma factor deficiency occurring simultaneously. *Scand. J. Haematol., 36*: 55–57 (1986).
46. Perret, B., Gaze, H., Zimmermann, A., Oetliker, O. Syndrome hemolytique uremique familial nonendemique: Nephrectomie et transplantation. *Helv. Paediatr. Acta., 34*: 167–176 (1979).
47. Camba, L., Al-Hilali, M. M., Shulji, M.M.H., Joyner, M. V., Feest, T. G. Haemolytic-uraemic syndrome with renal failure: the effect of plasmapheresis. *Haematologica, 70*: 341–344 (1985).
48. Halgreen, M., Andersen, R. H., Jorgensen, J-I. D. Familiaert haemolytisk uraemisk syndrom. *Ugeskr. Laeger, 149*: 662–663 (1987).
49. Remuzzi, G., Marchesi, D., Misiani, R., Misiani, R., Mecca, G., de Gaetano, G., Donati, M. B. Familial deficiency of a plasma factor stimulating vascular prostacyclin activity. *Thromb. Res., 16*: 517–525 (1979).
50. Jorgensen, K. A., Pedersen, R. S. Familial deficiency of prostacyclin production stimulating factor in the hemolytic uremic syndrome of childhood. *Thromb. Res., 21*: 311–315 (1981).
51. Wiles, P. G., Solomon, L. R., Lawler, W., Mallick, N. P. Inherited plasma factor deficiency in haemolytic-uraemic syndrome. *Lancet, 2*: 1105–1106 (1981).

19
An Analysis of the Association of the Hemolytic Uremic Syndrome and the Birth Control Pill

Bernard S. Kaplan *Children's Hospital of Philadelphia and University of Pennsylvania, Philadelphia, Pennsylvania*

The occurrence of the hemolytic uremic syndrome (HUS) in women using estrogen-containing birth control pills (BCP) led to the belief that there is a causal relationship between the BCP and the occurrence of HUS (1–3). This association has not been examined in critical detail and remains a hypothesis. Arguments advanced to support the connection include the line of reasoning that because HUS is uncommon in adults, the association between adult HUS and contraceptive agents seemed to be valid (4, 5). This contention has been supported by quoting the papers of Brown et al. (1), who described five cases with no control population, and the case report of Giromini and Lamperrouza (6). This unproven assertion is typical of those that creep unchallenged into the medical literature; as a result, the concept of an association as defined by the apposition of two things that are put side by side may become accepted as a union, and then as cause and effect. An association in this context may mean the mental connection between an object and ideas, but because its usage may also extend to examples of similarity, contrariety, contiguity, and causation (7), it may be advisable to introduce modifiers or to impose a moratorium on its unqualified use in medical papers. A clear definition of association is rendered more ambiguous by the inclusion of contrariety as an example provided by a dictionary (7).

We are not exempt from the criticism that this word has been used too loosely in describing the possible causes of the HUS (9). Under Causes of Hemolytic Uremic Syndrome we have stated previously that hemolytic uremic syndrome can occur in women using oral contraceptives or other agents containing estrogen (8). We also quoted the reports of others (1, 10) to support this statement. Brown et al. (1) described the occurrence of HUS in nine women, five of whom had been on oral contraceptives for periods that ranged from 3 weeks to 10 years. Bohle et al. (10) described the occurrence of secondary malignant nephrosclerose (sic) in 45 patients, 26% of whom were taking oral contraceptives. Insufficient information was available for further analysis. Only a small percentage of these patients developed HUS.

This association has been reexamined by studying published reports; it seems from this analysis that firm evidence favoring the idea that the BCP is a cause of the HUS is lacking.

METHODS

A large number of reports of HUS and thrombotic thrombocytopenic purpura (TTP) were studied to find cases of HUS or TTP in whom use of oral contraceptives was noted in at least one patient. Some cases may have been omitted inadvertently. The reports have been classified under five sub-headings:

1. Evidence of preexisting diseases + BCP + HUS;
2. Prodromal illnesses + BCP + HUS;
3. Familial HUS + BCP;
4. Recurrent episodes of HUS + BCP;
5. No other predisposing factors noted.

The combinations and permutations of HUS and TTP and the BCP are listed in Table 1.

CASE REPORTS

Evidence of Preexisting Diseases

Giromini and Lamperrouza (6) noted that proteinuria was detected during evaluation of irregular menses in spring 1968 in a woman aged 23 years. She was then treated with an ovulatory suppressant because of the menstrual irregularity. In October 1968 she had sudden onset of fever, myalgia, vomiting, diarrhea, and headache. HUS was diagnosed. Both kidneys were removed and histologic studies revealed thrombi in preglomerular arteries and in a small number of glomeruli. There were no sub-endothelial deposits. The patient had preexisting renal disease (proteinuria) and a flu-like prodrome prior to onset of HUS.

Causative factors possibly responsible for the hemolytic uremic syndrome (11)

Table 1 HUS/TTP BCP Combinations and Permutations

HUS	+ BCP
HUS	+ BCP + pregnancy
HUS	+ BCP + pregnancy + recessive inheritance
HUS	+ BCP + pregnancy + dominant inheritance
HUS	+ BCP + recurrences
HUS	+ BCP + recurrences without BCP
HUS	+ BCP + malignancy
HUS	+ BCP + flu-like prodrome
HUS	+ BCP + VTEC
TTP	+ BCP
TTP	+ BCP + husband + TTP

BCP = birth control pills
VTEC = verocytotoxin-producing *E. coli*

were present in 21 of 31 patients: previous hypertension, 9; multiple systemic sclerosis, 4; pregnancy, 3; acute promyelocytic leukemia, 1; pulmonary hypertension, 1; and oral contraceptives, 2. Two patients (cases 5 and 9) took BCPs for 1 month and 30 months. In case 5, HUS began after pregnancy, while she was taking BCPs. Case 9 was in remission for acute myelocytic leukemia and had HUS while taking BCPs. Case 5 died, and case 9 had residual mild chronic renal failure. Each of these patients had other variables, including pregnancy and leukemia.

Bonsib et al. (12) described recurrent thrombotic microangiopathy in a renal allograft. The patient was a 20-year-old woman who presented with HUS after a week of nausea, vomiting, diarrhea, mental confusion, and obtundation. She had been taking oral contraceptives since a therapeutic abortion at age 18 years. Nineteen days after transplantation, thrombotic microangiopathy developed in the allograft. The authors concluded that several factors may have been responsible for the recurrence but favored a role played by donor-specific antimonocyte antibody.

Prodromal Illnesses

Brown et al. (1) treated 11 patients with HUS between 1970 and 1972. Two were male and nine were female. Five females developed HUS while using estrogen-containing oral contraceptives. The age of each patient and the duration of ingestion of the BCPs were: case 1, 47 years old, BCP use for 2 years; case 2, 65 years old, BCP use for 3 weeks; case 3, 32 years old, BCP use for 5 years; case 4, 39 years old, BCP use for 10 years; and case 5, 19 years old, BCP use for 11 months. Each patient was ill for a month before admission with nausea, vomiting, edema, and dyspnea. No viral or bacterial pathogens were identified. The authors concluded that, if substantiated, the observation that estrogen-containing drugs predispose women to this serious and often fatal condition may provide a clue to its pathogenesis.

A 22-year-old women who had been on anovulatory pills for 8 months presented with malaise, fatigue, nausea, and vomiting (13). Her blood pressure was known to have been normal the previous month, but on admission to hospital it was $^{170}/_{90}$ mm Hg. The renal biopsy findings were occasional segmental glomerular necrosis, mucinous intimal thickening, and bland necrosis of arteries; thrombi were present in some arteries, arterioles, and glomerular capillaries. She was diagnosed as having chronic renal failure and was treated with hemodialysis. There seemed to be an antecedent viral prodrome of malaise, nausea, vomiting, and fatigue. She presented with severe hypertension and features consistent with a histopathologic diagnosis of malignant nephrosclerosis.

Ponticelli et al. (14) described the case of a 28-year-old woman who had a normal pregnancy in 1969. The same year she commenced ethinyl estradiol and Norgestrel and within 1 month presented with fever, vomiting, edema, dyspnea, and increasing oliguria. In a renal biopsy specimen some arterioles showed fibrinoid necrosis of the walls; there were no thrombi or acute tubular necrosis. The patient also had an antecedent flu-like illness and recovered uneventfully.

Five months prior to admission, a 52-year-old woman developed an atrophic vaginitis which was treated with Premarin® (conjugated estrogens) vaginal cream (15). Four months before admission she became hypertensive and was treated with hydrochlorothiazide and triamterine. A month later she was found to have a benign uterine leiomyoma and was then given Premarin® (conjugated estrogens) tablets. Six weeks before admission she developed nausea, vomiting, malaise, headache, edema, weakness, and oliguria. A renal biopsy revealed fibrinoid necrosis of afferent arterioles and thrombosis of most small arteries and arterioles. The patient died. Variables in this patient included Premarin®, uterine leiomyoma, and prodrome of nausea and vomiting. A second patient (15), aged 72 years, had used Premarin® for years. Eighteen months before admission, she had a normal physical examination, urinalysis, and blood chemical analysis. She then had increasing nausea and vomiting for several months. A renal biopsy showed thrombi and fibrinoid necrosis. She died. These authors concluded that a flu-like illness along with onset of hypertension in women taking oral contraceptives or conjugated estrogens should alert the physician to the possibility that these women may be susceptible to the development of HUS.

A woman aged 22 years had been taking oral contraceptives for four years when she developed HUS. VTEC (verocytotoxin-producing *Escherichia coli*) 0111 was isolated from her stool (16).

Familial HUS + BCP

Two sisters had HUS (17). The first, aged 17 years, had an upper respiratory infection, nausea, and vomiting. HUS was diagnosed 8 days later. A renal biopsy revealed glomerular capillary dilatation and thrombosis, endothelial proliferation, and focal thickening of the glomerular basement membranes. An A-matched kidney allograft from a sister had to be removed because of apparent rejection. A second allograft from a second sister was also rejected. The second sister, aged 21 years, was well until 2 weeks after donating the her kidney; then developed nausea, lethargy, vomiting, and diarrhea. HUS was diagnosed. The authors noted that it was of interest, in view of the recent association between estrogen-containing drugs and HUS, that both patients were taking estrogen-containing oral contraceptives at the onset of their illnesses. It is also of interest that both sisters had an antecedent flu-like illness before onset of HUS.

A 19-year-old girl died of HUS after presenting with a grand mal convulsion, depression, diarrhea, headaches, and anorexia while on Norinyl 1 for 6 weeks (18). Her father and brother died from HUS, and it is likely that her grandmother and several relatives also did so.

The findings in the two sisters reported by Edelsten and Tuck (19) are shown in Table 2. These sisters had two nephews who died at age 5 months from HUS in 1974 and 1976. It is difficult to ascribe the occurrence of the HUS in the first sister to the BCP.

Table 2 HUS in Two Sisters with and without BCP Use

Two sisters	Case 3	Case 4
Age at onset	26 years	23 years
Year	1966	1963
Pregnancy	5 weeks before admission	No
BCP	Stilbestrol × 10 days	No
History	For 1 week	Nausea, vomiting
Died	Yes	Yes
Histology	Thrombi	Thrombi

BCP = birth control pills

Carreras et al. (20) reported familial occurrence of HUS. Case 1, a woman aged 32 years, had a spontaneous abortion in July 1975. She then used BCPs for 4 months and had anorexia, lassitude, headaches, vomiting, myalgias, and pallor a month after stopping the BCP. In December 1977 she had a recurrence of HUS that started 10 days after an *E. coli* urinary tract infection which was treated with gentamicin. She had a persistently low serum C3 concentration and a slightly low C3A value. Many members of her family had low C3 concentrations and evidence of alternate pathway activation. This patient required hemodialysis. Case 2 was a daughter, aged 7 months, who had several episodes of HUS; C3 concentrations were depressed. She died and the pathologic report was that of thrombotic microangiopathy. Case 3 was the 2-year-old nephew of case 1, who had HUS after an upper respiratory tract infection. He recovered and was also found to have hypocomplementia. Were it not for the occurrence of HUS in the daughter and the nephew, and the recurrence of HUS in the mother when she was not on the BCP, it might have been suggested that the HUS in this woman was caused by the BCP.

Recurrent Episodes of HUS

At the age of 3 years, a girl reported by Rifle et al. (21) had an upper respiratory tract infection (URTI) followed by HUS. A second episode of HUS was associated with measles, a third with varicella, and a fourth with a URTI. There were no sequelae, and no specific treatment was given. At age 17 years she had another episode of HUS, 15 days after a bacterial infection (angine bactrerienne). This occurred after she had been using oral contraceptives for 4 months. She also had a low serum C3 concentration, a reduced factor B level, and a positive C3NeF. Despite the occurrence of HUS with a variety of infections, the title of the paper is "Irreversible Cortical Necrosis While on oestro-progestifs."

A 17-year-old girl had headaches and oliguria (22). She had been taking Microgynon for 14 months. Two years later her initial symptoms recurred 3 weeks after restarting Microgynon and again presented with severe headaches and dyspnea. On the basis of the available evidence, this is the clearest indication of an association between BCP and HUS reported to date.

Five months after delivery of her normal second child, a 23-year-old woman was admitted to hospital with acute renal failure and features of HUS (3). She had been given ergotamine and estrogen after delivery and was then prescribed an oral contraceptive (Sequens). Four months prior to admission she had complained of weakness and vomiting. A renal biopsy revealed a few thrombi in the tufts, interlobular, and afferent arteriolar thromboses; subintimal bleeding; and mucinous thickening of the intima. In December 1972 she had a cadaveric transplant and was kept on progestogen. In April 1977 she was given estro-progestogen. In February 1978 she experienced feverishness and weakness and had a recurrence of HUS. Viral antibody titers revealed a 4-fold rise for influenza A, herpes simplex, and cytomegalovirus. A repeat biopsy showed changes similar to the first biopsy. She had a second transplant and was well 2 years later. This patient had a recurrence of HUS associated with the BCP and well-documented viral infections.

No Apparent Predisposing Factors

Boyd et al. (2) studied three groups of patients in whom there seemed to be a relationship between the occurrence of hypertension, renal disease, or HUS, and the use of oral contraceptives. Group 1 consisted of five patients aged 33–46 years who had been normotensive before taking BCPs (estrogen + progesterone) for 10 months to 10 years (mean 4.8 years) before documentation of hypertension. One woman had minimal renal failure; one had thrombocytopenia; none had hemolysis.

Group 2 comprised two women aged 23 and 48 years who were previously normotensive but became hypertensive after pregnancies complicated by hypertension, edema, and proteinuria. Each was started on BCPs immediately after pregnancy and had been taking them for 9 and 12 months when they developed thrombocytopenia, uremia, and intrarenal microthrombi. After the BCPs were stopped, there was a fall in blood pressure, an increase in platelet count, and an improvement in renal function.

Group 3 contained two women, aged 22 and 31 years, who had acute oliguric renal failure after being on BCPs for 6 months and 2 years, respectively. They also had anemia and thrombocytopenia. Discontinuation of the BCP was associated with normalization of intravascular coagulation and incomplete improvement in renal function. Histologic examination of their kidneys revealed extensive microthrombi in glomerular capillaries, afferent arterioles, and larger cortical arteries. Angiograms revealed abnormalities of peripheral renal vessels in all cases. This is an important paper (2). Unfortunately there are no age-matched controls. Furthermore there is scanty information on the presence, absence, or nature of prodromal illnesses. The abnormalities seen on the renal angiograms may have been the result of severe hypertension and may not be specific for HUS, nor can it be deduced that these changes were caused by the BCP.

Ponticelli et al. (23) studied 11 patients aged 23–42 years; nine were females, two were males. One of the women was aged 28 years and had been using oral contraceptives for 2 years. Renal histological studies revealed evidence of tubular necrosis, but no fibrinoid thrombi, no focal sclerosis, and no focal necrosis.

A 44-year-old woman who had been using oral contraceptives for 18 years, except during four pregnancies (24) developed HUS. This patient had an antecedent episode of "grippe intestinale" but seemed to have been ill with dyspnea and tiredness prior to onset of vomiting and had lost 7 kg during the previous 3 weeks.

THROMBOTIC THROMBOCYTOPENIC PURPURA AND BIRTH CONTROL PILLS

Forty-eight unselected cases of TTP were analyzed by Kennedy et al. (25); 26 were females, 22 were males; one female was taking BCPs. Rosove et al. (26) described 19 patients aged 18–71 years, of whom 14 were female. One postmenopausal and three premenopausal women were taking an estrogen-containing medication at the time of diagnosis of TTP. Twelve patients were reported by Glas-Greenwalt et al. (27), of whom nine were female. Case 2 was a 30-year-old female who died and had a history of taking BCPs. Cuttner (28) reported 20 cases of TTP, four of whom had been on BCPs; unfortunately the details that have been provided are scanty.

CASE REPORTS

Paz et al. (29) described the occurrence of fatal TTP in a 29-year-old woman and her 31-year-old sister. The first patient was taking an oral contraceptive (Sequens) at the onset of her illness, often used analgesics, complained of urticaria after eating certain foods, and said she was intolerant to certain unspecified drugs. She had severe renal failure and the kidneys were small, with intimal thickening, fibrinoid necrosis, and acute tubular necrosis. She died. Another sister had died of hypertension and uremia. Case 2, the 31-year-old sister of case 1, had two normal pregnancies and had been using Sequens since her last pregnancy the previous year. They lived in the same house. She had no known allergies but had an episode of angioneurotic edema in hospital. She also died and had platelet aggregates in many vessels and similar changes in her kidneys to case 1. The authors concluded that the sisters shared many items of diet, cosmetics, and household remedies, as well as taking the same type of oral contraceptives—any of which could have been the causative factor.

TTP occurred in a man aged 36 years who was hospitalized in September 1968 with a 1-week history of illness and died soon after (30). There were widespread small-vessel occlusions with hyaline thrombi. His wife, aged 35 years, was hospitalized in March 1969 with a 6-month history of metromenorrhagia. Twelve years previously, she had been treated for colitis and 4 years before had pleuritis and arthritis. She also had sporadic recurrences of nonbloody diarrhea. Shortly before onset of TTP, an oral contraceptive (Ortho-Novum®) was prescribed to control menorrhagia. She was also given meprobamate. A splenectomy was performed and the histology was in keeping with a diagnosis of TTP. She also died.

A 43-year-woman was hospitalized in February 1976 and died one week later (31). She had been well until August 1975 and stopped taking BCPs in October 1975. In February 1976, she had fever and chills. The illness began after an acute febrile, "flu-like" episode which, in turn, was superimposed on a several-month history of easy tiring. A possible role for the BCP was not mentioned.

Jackson et al. (32) described the sudden onset of severe hypertension with headaches, nausea, vomiting, anorexia, and malaise associated with ingestion of Serial C (ethinyl estradiol 100 mcg) in a woman on the day that she started taking this dose of oral contraceptive.

A 22-year-old woman with hirsutism was treated for a year with ethinyl estradiol (50 mg) and ethynodiol acetate (33). She was given Ortho-Novum® 1/80 and developed TTP 5 weeks later. Treatment with a variety of agents was successful. She recovered from the TTP but relapsed when plasma exchanges were discontinued after four weeks.

A woman aged 28 years had taken Ortho-Novum® for 7 years before presenting with fever, headaches, and petechiae following a flu-like illness. She had a splenectomy and 15 months later was found to have a cholangiocarcinoma (34).

Vesconi (35) described the case of a woman aged 22 years who developed TTP a few days after an episode of hyperpyrexia. She had been taking oral contraceptives (ethinyl estradiol 0.05 mg, norgestrel 0.5 mg) for 13 cycles. These authors concluded that "it is conceivable that drugs containing estrogens may predispose . . . to . . . microangiopath[y], especially if combined with other vascular risk factors such as viral or bacterial infections (as suggested in our patient by the fever episode. . . .) (35).

A 27-year-old woman developed TTP in the 12th week of her first pregnancy (36) and had relapses with reductions in platelet count and haptoglobin levels. These were noted with and without the use of a contraceptive pill and sometimes coincided with menstrual cycles. The association between relapses of TTP and menstrual cycles, as well as with pregnancy, and the BCP makes this a unique case, but it is unclear how firm the evidence is for periodicity. Subsequently, these authors described the occurrence of TTP in a woman aged 28 years and a 16-year-girl who had been on BCPs prior to the onset of TTP (37). The girl attained a complete remission, but the woman died.

An 18-year-old woman had high fever, tachycardia, left-sided paresis, diffuse abdominal pains, nausea, vomiting, dizziness, and anxiety. She had been on oral contraceptive (Microgynon-30) for two weeks before admission to hospital (38).

DISCUSSION

An attempt has been made in this review to answer a number of questions. However, although many questions can be asked, regrettably few have answers.

1. How commonly is a prodromal illness, variously described as an upper respiratory tract infection or a "flu-like" illness, reported prior to the onset of HUS in women who are on the BCP?
2. How frequently have other possible causal agents been demonstrated in these cases?
3. If the BCP is a cause of HUS, why do so few women on the BCP develop HUS?
4. Is there a genetic predisposition to develop HUS while on BCP?
5. Can a predisposition to the development of HUS (if such a predisposition exists in nonfamilial cases) be anticipated?
6. What is the extent of ascertainment bias with respect to reporting cases of HUS in women?
7. Is there a trend in the reporting of cases of HUS that is biased in favor of reports of women on oral contraceptives?
8. Do the histopathological appearances differ between HUS associated with the BCP, and HUS not associated with the BCP?
9. For HUS to occur, is it sufficient for there to be intake of BCPs, or is it also necessary for the patient to have had a viral infection—i.e., is there an analogy with Reye's syndrome and aspirin?
10. Why does the latent period vary so much, and why may it take as long as 10 years for something so catastrophic and rapidly progressive to have its onset?
11. Do BCPs alter coagulation, and is there any evidence that altered coagulation factors are found in patients who develop HUS while using oral contraceptives?
12. Do BCPs perturb prostacyclin, and has this been demonstrated in patients with HUS associated with BCPs?
13. Are there any reasons to extrapolate from pregnancy-associated HUS to BCP-associated HUS?

The most convincing evidence for an association in an individual case would be the tendency for HUS to recur when the woman is challenged by a BCP.

There are 26 case reports in which an antecedent "flu-like illness" was mentioned (sudden onset of fever, myalgia, vomiting, diarrhea, and headache). Eighteen patients (69%) had symptoms that occur in viral illnesses. These included nausea and vomiting, fever, diarrhea, lassitude, and myalgias. In one case relapses were associated with well-defined illnesses such as measles and varicella (21), in a second with an

E. coli urinary tract infection (20), in a third with several organisms including cytomegalovirus (3), and in a fourth with a VTEC gastroenteritis prodrome (16).

A genetic predisposition toward HUS may have been operative in five of the patients (17–21). These cases are particularly challenging because they introduce so much confusion into the subject. One of the sisters described by Edelsten and Tuck (19) had HUS in association with pregnancy, diarrhea, vomiting, and BCP use; neither her affected sister nor their affected male cousins were exposed to BCPs or pregnancy. Similarly, in the case described by Farr et al. (18), several male members of a woman's family were afflicted by HUS. The patients reported by Carreras et al. (20) and Rifle et al. (21) yield additional interesting information because they had a complement abnormality. There have been other reports of the association of HUS with hypocomplementemia, serum C3Nef, and recurrent episodes of HUS (39).

Five of the 26 cases had recently been pregnant. In each case, however, there were additional possible predisposing factors such as "flu" or familial HUS.

Published data on the prevalence of HUS in women who are taking the BCP are lacking. Fifty-three adult patients from three series have been analyzed (1, 11, 23). In each study there was a definite mention of at least one patient having been on the BCP prior to onset of the HUS. It is unclear how rigorously this information was sought in each case so that the true prevalence may have been higher, but each of the authors was aware of a possible association. Eight of 53 adults (15%) had been on the BCP prior to onset of HUS. The sex of the patients was mentioned in only two reports (22 patients), so that 30% of the women in the studies developed the HUS while on the BCP. These studies were from Britain and Italy. A population-based study of HUS directed mainly at children and adolescents was undertaken in Oregon (40). No figures are available for the prevalence of HUS in any adult population, but those for the 15–18-year age range in the Oregon study was 0.11 based on a single case out of 178,761 people in the same age range in the population. Most of the reported cases of HUS associated with ingestion of BCPs were aged between 17 and 34 years. Figures are available for the prevalance of BCP use in females aged 15–34 years from 1971–1980 in the United States (41). The percentage of women using the BCP was as high as 37.4 in the 20–24-year age group from 1971–1974. From this data it does not seem as though the percent of women who use the BCP and develop HUS is far out of line when compared with those who use the BCP in the population.

More pertinent, however, is the difficulty that one is faced with when one attempts to make sense of this apparent association. HUS is a rare condition in adults. Many adult females take the BCP. Some women who are on the BCP develop the HUS. Sixty-nine percent of these have had a prodromal illness. Others have an apparent genetic predisposition toward HUS. Men develop HUS. So do children. Furthermore, a 12-year-old boy with HUS was treated with ethylestrenol in a dose of 2 mg/day for 84 days; it was concluded that, although one should not draw conclusions from a single case, this patient improved despite treatment with ethylestrenol (42).

In the past it was thought that the pathogenesis of HUS was due in part to the occurrence of intravascular coagulation. This view is no longer held by most authors. The BCP appears to produce a hypercoagulable state; therefore it has been assumed that this is why the HUS may occur in women taking the BCP. Although the BCP is mentioned as a cause of a hypercoagulable state in one review (43), the HUS is not mentioned at all. Thrombotic thrombocytopenic purpura, however, is listed as a secondary hypercoagulable state. Although there is some controversy as to whether or not HUS and TTP are the same or different entities, there is information to support the notion that typical cases of HUS differ from typical cases of TTP (44). In TTP thrombi of different ages are found in many organs—in contrast to HUS, in which the kidney is usually the only organ that is affected. Thrombi are always found in patients with TTP; thrombi are sometimes found in patients with HUS.

IF the BCP is associated with adult HUS, then one may argue that there should be an even more frequent or tighter association with TTP because these patients have a more generalized form of vascular injury. Furthermore, the theories of the pathogenesis of TTP more closely approximate those advanced for that of HUS associated with the BCP. These include vessel wall injury and platelet consumption at the site of injury. In view of this possibility, the prevalence of TTP associated with BCP has also been analyzed in some detail. Use of oral contraceptives is mentioned in four series consisting of a total of 99 cases, of whom 69 were female (25–28). Ten out of 99 patients of both sexes (10%) and 15.9% of women were on the BCP prior to the onset of TTP. These figures are even lower than those estimated for an association between HUS and oral contraception.

Ten studies (from 1979–1986) contained more than four cases of TTP per paper. Seventy of 91 patients were females. The BCP was not mentioned in any of these papers. If it can be assumed that the BCP was not mentioned because it was not being taken, then 139 women are included in series of more than four cases. Ten women with TTP (7.5%) were using the BCP, but as noted above, 15–30% of women in the general population may be taking the BCP. Therefore, although TTP is uncommon, only 19 patients with TTP have been reported in whom there was a history of oral contraceptive use.

It has been suggested that there are similarities between HUS associated with the BCP and HUS associated with pregnancy, and that this may be further evidence of a causal relationship between HUS and the BCP (4). Although disturbances of blood coagulation have been described in normal pregnancy and in women on oral contraceptives, convincing evidence of a causal relationship between oral contraceptives and thromboembolic complications has not been found (45). It remains possible that a combination of coagulation disturbances and infection precipitates HUS in some women (46). This argument may be logically correct but scientifically fallacious because no proof of an association between the BCP and HUS has been forthcoming. Grunfeld et al. (47) have stated that it is not always clear whether HUS should, in certain cases, be ascribed to pregnancy or to the oral contraceptive agents; that there is no good evidence that post-BCP and postpartum renal failure share similar pathogenetic mechanism(s); that a similar dissociation has been noted between pregnancy-associated hypertension and post-BCP hypertension (48); and that a genetic predisposition may be involved. In addition, not all cases of HUS in which a relationship has been attributed to pregnancy are necessarily related to the state of pregnancy itself.

From these analyses it would seem that a differential diagnosis that includes BCP does not ipso facto mean that oral contraception is a cause of HUS. An association is mentioned so that, if enough cases accumulate, proof of cause and effect may be forthcoming. However, more solid epidemiological or laboratory research is required to prove cause and effect. Anecdotal reports, although useful and potentially important, remain anecdotes.

REFERENCES

1. Brown, C. B., Robson, J. S., Thomson, D., Clarkson, A. R., Cameron, J. S., Ogg, C. S. Haemolytic Uraemic syndrome in women taking oral contraceptives. *Lancet, 1*: 1479–1481 (1973).
2. Boyd, W. N., Burden, R. P., Aber, G. M. Intrarenal vascular changes in patients receiving oestrogen-containing compounds—A clinical, histological and angiographic study. *Q. J. Med., 44*: 415–432 (1975).
3. Hauglustaine, D., van Damme, B., Vanrenterghem, Y., Michielsen, P. Recurrent hemolytic uremic syndrome during oral contraception. *Clin. Nephrol., 15*: 148–153 (1981).
4. Hayslett, J. P. Postpartum renal failure. *N. Engl. J. Med., 312*: 1556–1559 (1985).
5. Humphreys, M. H., Alfrey, A. C. Vascular diseases of the kidney. In: *The Kidney*, ed. 3, vol. II. (B. M. Brenner, F. C. Rector, eds.) W. B. Saunders Co. Philadelphia, pp. 1185–1186 (1986).
6. Giromini, M., Laperrouza, C. Prolonged survival after bilateral nephrectomy in an adult with haemolytic-uraemic syndrome. *Lancet, 2*: 169–170 (1969).
7. Onions, C. T. *The Oxford Universal Dictionary on Historical Principles*, ed. 3. Oxford at the Clarendon Press, London, p. 11. (1953).
8. Kaplan, B. S., Drummond, K. N. The hemolytic-uremic syndrome is a syndrome. *N. Engl. J. Med., 298*: 964–966 (1978).
9. Fong, J.S.C., de Chadarevian, J-P., Kaplan, B. S. Hemolytic-uremic syndrome. Current concepts and management. *Pediatr. Clin. N. Am., 29*: 835–856 (1982).
10. Bohle, A., Helmchen, U., Grund, K. E., Gartner, H. V., Meyer, D., Bock, K. D., Bulla, M., Bunger, P., Diekmann, L., Frotscher, U., Hayduk, K., Kasters, W., Srauch, M., Scheler, F., Christ, H. Malignant nephrosclerosis in patients with hemolytic uremic syndrome (primary malignant nephrosclerosis). *Curr. Topics Pathol., 65*: 81–113 (1977).
11. Morel-Maroger, L. Adult hemolytic-uremic syndrome. *Kidney Int., 18*: 125–134 (1980).
12. Bonsib, S. M., Ercolani, L., Ngheim, D., Hamilton, H. E. Recurrent thrombotic microangiopathy in a renal allograft. case report and review of the literature. *Am. J. Med., 79*: 520–527 (1985).
13. Schoolwerth, A. C., Sandler, R. S., Klahr, S., Kissane, J. M. Nephrosclerosis postpartum and in women taking oral contraceptives. *Arch. Intern. Med., 136*: 178–185 (1976).
14. Ponticelli. C., Maestri, O., Imbasciati, E., Brancaccio, D., Rossi, E. Late recovery of renal function in a woman with the hemolytic uremic syndrome. *Clin. Nephrol., 8*: 367–370 (1977).
15. Ashouri, O. S., Marbury, T. C., Fuller, T. J., Gaffney, E., Grubb, W. G., Cade, J. R. Hemolytic uremic syndrome in two postmenapausal women taking a conjugated estrogen preparation. *Clin. Nephrol., 17*: 212–215 (1982).
16. Stenger, K-O., Windler, F., Karch, H., von Wulfen, H., and Heesemann, J. Hemolytic-uremic syndrome associated with an infection by verotoxin producing *Escherichia coli* 0111 in a woman on oral contraceptives. *Clin. Nephrol., 29*: 153–158 (1988).
17. Bergstein, J., Michael, A. Jr., Kjellstrand, C., Simmons, R., and Najarian, J. Hemolytic-uremic syndrome in adult sisters. *Transplantation, 17*: 487–489 (1974).
18. Farr, M. J., Roberts, S., Morley, A. R., Dewar, P. J., Roberts, D. F., and Uldall, P. R. The haemolytic-uraemic syndrome—a family study. *Q. J. Med., 44*: 161–188 (1975).
19. Edelsten, A. D., Tuck, S. Familial haemolytic uraemic syndrome. *Arch. Dis. Child, 53*: 255–256 (1978).

20. Carreras, L., Romero, R., Requesens, C., Oliver, A. J., Carrera, M., Clavo, M., Alsina, J. Familial hypocomplementemic hemolytic uremic syndrome with HLA-A3,B7 haplotype. *J.A.M.A.*, *245*: 602–604 (1981).
21. Rifle, G., Chalopin, J. M., Genin, R., Justrabo, E., Severac, J., Balte, F. Syndrome hemolytique et uremique recidivant. Necrose cortical irreversible sous oestro-progestatifs. *J. Urol. Nephrol. (Paris)*, *85*: 331 (1979).
22. Hoorntje, S. J., Prins, E.J.l., Smit, A. J., Donker, AB.J.M. Reversal of long-standing renal insufficiency by captopril in a patient with relapsing hemolytic uremic syndrome due to an oral contraceptive. *Ann. Intern. Med.*, *94*: 355–357 (1981).
23. Ponticelli, C., Rivolta, E., Imbasciati, E., Rossi, E., Mannucci, P. M. Hemolytic uremic syndrome in adults. *Arch. Intern. Med.*, *140*: 353 (1980).
24. Schillinger, F., Montagnac, R., Birembaut, P., Hopfner, C. Syndrome hemolytique et uremique au decours d'une contraception orale. *Rev. Fr. Gynecol. Obstet.*, *81*: 721–725 (1986).
25. Kennedy, S. S., Zacharski, L. R., Beck, J. R. Thrombotic thrombocytopenic purpura: analysis of 48 unselected cases. *Semin. Thromb. Hemost.*, *6*: 341–349 (1980).
26. Rosove, M. H., Ho, W. G. Goldfinger, D. Ineffectiveness of aspirin and dipyridamole in the treatment of TTP. *Ann. Intern. Med.*, *96*: 27–33 (1982).
27. Glas-Greenwalt, P., Hall, J. M., Panke, T. W., Kant, K. S., Allen, C. M., Pollak, V. E. Fibrinolysis in health and disease: Abnormal levels of plasminogen activator, plasminogen activator inhibitor, and protein C in thrombotic thrombocytopenic purpura. *J. Lab. Clin. Med.*, *108*: 415–422 (1986).
28. Cuttner, J. Thrombotic thrombocytopenic purpura: a ten year experience. *Blood*, *56*: 302–306 (1980).
29. Paz, R. A., Elijovich, F., Barcat, J. A., Sanchez-Avalos, J. C. Fatal simultaneous thrombocytopenic purpura in siblings. *Br. Med. J.*, *2*: 727–728 (1969).
30. Watson, C. G., Cooper, W. M. Thrombotic thrombocytopenic purpura. Concomitant occurence in husband and wife. *J.A.M.A.*, *215*: 1821–1823 (1971).
31. Cryer, P., Kissane, J. M. Anemia, Thrombocytopenia, proteinuria, and central nervous system dysfunction. *Am. J. Med.*, *63*: 789–798 (1977).
32. Jackson, B., Clarkson, A. R., Seymour, A. E. The haemolytic uraemic syndrome and oral contraceptives. *Aust. N.Z. J. Med.*, *6*: 580–582 (1976).
33. McShane, P. M., Bern, M. M., Schiff I. Thrombotic thrombocytopenic purpura associated with oral contraceptives: a case report. *Am. J. Obstet. Gynecol.*, *145*: 762–763 (1983).
34. Caggiano, V., Chosney, B., Way, L. W. Thrombotic thrombocytopenic purpura, cholangiocarcinoma, and oral contraceptives. *Lancet*, *2*: 365 (1980).
35. Vesconi, S., Langer, M., Rossi, E., Mondonico, P., Cambiaghi, G. Thrombotic thromboctopenic purpura during oral contraceptive treatment. *Thromb. Hemost.*, *40*: 563–564 (1978).
36. Holdrinet, R.S.G., de Pauw, B. E., Haanen, C. Hormonal dependent thrombotic thrombocytopenic purpura (TTP). *Scand. J. Haematol.*, *30*: 250–256 (1983).
37. Holdrinet, R.S.G., Namdar, Z., Haanen, C. Thrombotic thrombocytopenic purpura: clinical course and response to therapy in twelve patients. *Neth. J. Med.*, *33*: 113–132 (1988).
38. Snir, M., Cohen, S. Ben-Sira, I., Buckman, G. Retinal manifestations of thrombotic thrombocytopenic purpura (TTP) following use of contraceptive treatment. *Ann. Ophthal.*, *17*: 109–112 (1985).
39. Kaplan BS: Hemolytic uremic syndrome with recurrent episodes: an important subset. *Clin. Nephrol.*, *8*: 495–498 (1977).
40. Rogers, M. F., Rutherford, G. W., Alexander, S. R., DiLiberti, J. H., Foster, L., Schonberger, L. B., Hurwitz, E. S. A population-based study of hemolytic-uremic syndrome in Oregon, 1979–1982. *Am. J. Epidemiol.*, *123*: 137–142 (1986).

41. Russell-Briefel, R., Ezzatti, T., Perlman, J. Prevalence and trends in oral contraceptives use in premenopausal females ages 12–54 years, United States, 1971–1980. *Am. J. Public Health, 75*: 1173–1176 (1985).
42. Mandal, B. K., McNulty, M. Treatment of haemolytic-uraemic syndrome with phenformin and ethyloestrenol. *Lancet, 2*: 1036 (1971).
43. Schaffer, A. I. The hypercoagulable states. *Ann. Intern. Med., 102*: 814–828 (1985).
44. Vedaranayanan, V. V., Preus, M., Kaplan, B. S. An Application of cluster analysis as an objective method of syndrome differentiation hemolytic uremic syndrome and thrombotic thrombocytopenic purpura. In *Recent Advances in Pediatric Nephrology*. (K. Murakami, T. Kitagawa, K. Yabuta, T. Sakai, eds.) Excerpta Medica, Amsterdam. 1987. pp 573–576.
45. Beller, F. K., Ebert, C. Effects of oral contraceptives on blood coagulation. A review. *Obstet. Gynecol. Survey, 40*: 425–436 (1985).
46. Haemolytic uraemic syndrome of young women (editorial). *Lancet, 2*: 943–944 (1976).
47. Grunfeld, J-P., Ganeval, D., Bournerias, F. Acute renal failure in pregnancy. *Kidney Int., 18*: 179–191 (1980).
48. Pritchard, J. A. and Pritchard, S. A. Blood pressure response to estrogen-progestin oral contraceptive after pregnancy-induced hypertension. *Am. J. Obstet. Gynecol., 129*: 733–739 (1978).

20
Hemolytic Uremic Syndrome in Association with Pregnancy

Claudine Saltiel, Christophe Legendre, and Jean-Pierre Grünfeld *Hôpital Necker, Paris, France* **Jean-Michel Descamps** *Centre Hospitalier Georges Renon, Niort, France* **Michel Hecht** *Centre Hospitalier Henri Duffaut, Avignon, France*

The triad of microangiopathic hemolytic anemia, acute renal failure, and often thrombocytopenia may develop during pregnancy or in the postpartum period. These manifestations may be divided into three main clinical entities which can be schematically differentiated on the following criteria:

1. The hemolytic uremic syndrome (HUS) occurs mostly in the immediate postpartum period. Severe acute renal failure is the prominent finding.
2. Thrombotic thrombocytopenic purpura (TTP) develops in the second or third trimester of pregnancy. Renal involvement is usually mild, whereas extrarenal features predominate (fever, hematological disturbances, and fluctuating neurological involvement). Both HUS and TTP are characterized by a similar basic histopathological lesion, thrombotic microangiopathy.
3. Hemolytic anemia with red blood cell fragmentation, thrombocytopenia, and reversible acute renal failure are not uncommon findings in severe preeclampsia/eclampsia (1). Recently, the so-called HELLP syndrome (*H*emolysis, *E*levated *L*iver enzymes, and *L*ow *P*latelet count) has been described. This is not a separate disorder and probably represents the extreme of the spectrum of severe preeclampsia (2).

Diagnosis of these three separate entities may be difficult because of clinical overlap in some cases. However, as will be discussed below, patient management depends in part on a classification that is as precise as possible.

Since the 1970s, there has been a dramatic decrease in the incidence of acute renal failure in pregnancy in Western countries. The current estimate of the incidence of acute renal failure necessitating dialysis during pregnancy is less than 0.01% (3, 4). Among the causes of pre- and postpartum renal failure, the exact incidence of HUS is unknown and is obviously very low. Sixty-two cases had been identified in 1989 by Weiner (5) in the English language literature. Many cases, however, have probably not been reported. In our 1957–1979 series, idiopathic postpartum acute renal failure (which includes HUS) represented approximately 9% of the cases (6).

POSTPARTUM HEMOLYTIC UREMIC SYNDROME

Postpartum HUS is characterized by acute renal failure associated with microangiopathic hemolytic anemia and thrombocytopenia, typically following normal pregnancy and delivery after a symptom-free interval, and unrelated to a specific obstetric problem. This entity was described by Robson et al. in 1968 as "irreversible postpartum renal failure," but the term "postpartum HUS" should be restricted to cases with unequivocal microangiopathic hemolytic anemia.

Clinical Presentation

The mean maternal age was 27 years (5). The diagnosis was made postpartum in 94% of cases after a mean symptom-free interval of 27 days (5). Typically, this syndrome affects previously healthy women between 48 hours and 1 month after normal pregnancy (without hypertension) and delivery. The patients usually present with an influenza-like syndrome, rapidly followed by acute oliguric or often anuric renal failure. Blood pressure is either normal or mildly elevated at the onset, but severe or even malignant hypertension frequently develops as the disease progresses. Congestive heart failure and generalized seizures are common findings.

About 75% of cases involve features of microangiopathic Coombs'-negative hemolytic anemia (anisocytes, schizocytes, high reticulocyte count, low serum haptoglobin, and elevated lacticodehydrogenase enzyme levels) and thrombopenia (3, 7). Importantly, routine clotting tests such as prothrombin time and partial thromboplastin time, thrombin time and fibrinogen concentration are normal. Antithrombin III activity is normal (5). In contrast, fibrin split products are often increased as a result of fibrinogen rather than fibrin degradation. Serum complement levels are usually normal.

Atypical cases have also been described. In a few women, the syndrome has begun during a pregnancy, which has often been ectopic (8, 9). Symptoms preceded delivery in 14% of the cases reviewed by Weiner (5). The syndrome has also been reported as occurring as late as 7 months postpartum (6), but in such cases the role of pregnancy may be seriously questioned.

Histological Findings

Renal histopathological changes affect glomeruli, afferent arterioles, and intralobular arteries. Glomerular lesions are characterized by thickening of the capillary walls due to endothelial swelling and subendothelial deposition of a pale, granular, fibrin-like material leading to capillary obstruction (Fig. 1a). Other findings include capillary thrombi and, occasionally, proliferative changes. Intimal swelling, subintimal deposits and fibrinoid necrosis with thrombosis in the lumen are found in the arterioles. In other patients, however, renal changes most closely resemble those found in malignant nephrosclerosis or scleroderma. The glomerular lesions are of the ischemic type with retracted tufts and wrinkled membranes, and vascular changes involve intralobular arteries (Fig. 1b). Immunofluorescent studies usually show fibrin and

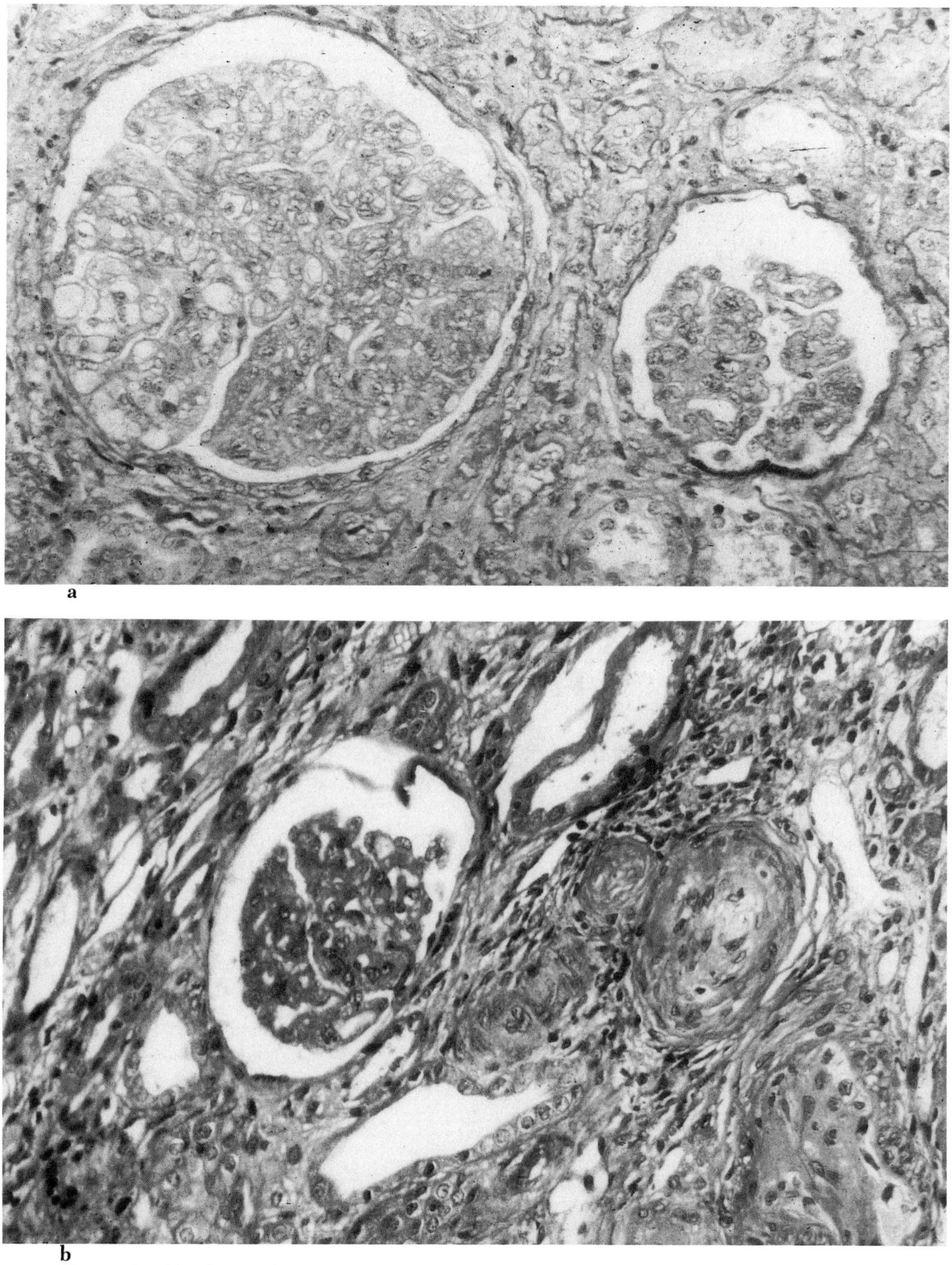

Figure 1 (a) Glomerular involvement in thrombotic microangiopathy. Hypertrophy of the intracapillary cells, involving mainly the endothelial cells. Capillary walls are thickened by "double contour," and some wrinkled membranes are present. (b) Ischemic glomerular changes with few visible capillary lumina and large urinary space. Mucinous intimal thickening is present in several sections of preglomerular arterioles. The lesion is sparsely cellular and consists mainly of lucent, faintly basophilic-staining, amorphous material (Trichrome × 400).

occasionally C3 in the mesangium, capillary walls, and arterioles (5). These two types of glomerular lesions may represent successive stages of the disease and may well coexist in the same biopsy specimen. The ischemic type of lesion, however, predominates in postpartum HUS. Scattered areas of cortical necrosis may be demonstrated on the renal biopsy specimen. Morel-Maroger et al. (10) have shown that severe arterial involvement carries a poor prognosis, whereas glomerular changes have no prognostic value.

A relatively high prevalence of severe postbiopsy bleeding has previously been emphasized. This occurred in hypertensive patients, especially when heparin therapy was instituted a few days after renal biopsy (7). However, this complication has become much more uncommon because antihypertensive therapy allows better blood pressure control and heparin is no longer indicated.

Evolution

The prognosis of postpartum HUS is poor; the overall maternal mortality rate was 55%, and nearly half of the survivors were on dialysis or were in severe renal failure. Five women subsequently required kidney transplantations (5). However, this pessimistic view should probably be modified because there has been improvement in symptomatic management and the introduction of plasma therapy seems to have reduced the acute mortality. The possibility of bilateral renal cortical necrosis should be contemplated in patients with prolonged anuria. Surprisingly, this risk is rarely emphasized in most studies on postpartum HUS, despite the fact that both HUS and pregnancy are predisposing factors to cortical necrosis (7). In our series, three of five patients with postpartum HUS had patchy cortical necrosis (6). The extent of cortical necrosis can be evaluated from renal arteriography or preferentially from computed tomography (6, 11, 7). According to Weiner, there was only one report of a woman with postpartum HUS who recovered and had a subsequent normal pregnancy (5). Conversely, recurrent postpartum HUS was reported in a woman at 18 and at 23 years of age who was symptom-free in the interval between pregnancies (12). Renal transplantation may be successful, although recurrence of the lesion of HUS in kidney allografts has occasionally been observed (11, 7).

Etiology

As in HUS in nonpregnant patients, various causes or triggering factors may be found in postpartum HUS. Some women had an influenza-like illness a few days before the onset of the disease. A role for verotoxin producing *Escherichia coli* has been suggested in cases of postpartum HUS (13–15), as have other pathogenic agents such as *Shigella* (16) and *Streptococcus* (17).

Drugs used during delivery, such as ergotamine compounds or oxytoxic agents, have been incriminated, but conclusive evidence is lacking (18). In contrast, the occurrence of HUS in women taking oral contraceptives is well documented (19). Severe hypertension is often present, but there are exceptions to the rule (16). Some of the patients with late postpartum HUS were taking contraceptives, and the respective role of pregnancy and of oral contraceptive agents is an open question (19). Postpartum HUS has been reported after the use of beta-estradiol benzoate, a hormonal compound aimed at blocking lactation (18). Renal histopathological changes in post-pill HUS resemble those found in postpartum HUS and range from malignant nephrosclerosis to thrombotic microangiopathy. Surprisingly, despite prominent and severe hypertension, glomerular changes mimicking those of childhood HUS, were found in four of 15 cases in which renal biopsies were available in our series (6); arteriolar lesions were more diffuse. There is no evidence that post-pill and postpartum HUS share similar pathogenic mechanisms. Cases have been reported when hypertension and severe renal failure followed oral contraceptive administration, whereas pregnancies had been uneventful in these women, and a dissociation between pregnancy-induced hypertension and post-pill hypertension has also been noted (6).

A genetic predisposition has contributed to the expression of the disease in some cases. HUS (20), as well as TPP (21), have been reported in siblings taking oral contraceptives; in two sisters, TTP developed during oral contraception; in two other sisters, TTP developed during late pregnancy, 2 years apart (22). One of two HLA identical sisters developed postpartum HUS while the other developed post-pill HUS (23). It is possible that a genetic susceptibility may have a relation to familial HUS (24).

THROMBOTIC THROMBOCYTOPENIC PURPURA

Clinical Presentation

It is well established that the first manifestations of TTP often appear during pregnancy. The onset of pregnancy-related TTP occurred in about 90% of the cases during pregnancy. In the review of 65 cases by Weiner (5), the mean maternal age was 23 years and the mean gestational age at onset was 23.5 weeks, predominating at or before 24 weeks. In only 10% of the cases did the first symptoms appear in the immediate postpartum period.

Thrombocytopenic purpura is a common finding. The decrease in platelet count is usually more pronounced than in HUS. Thrombocytopenia may antedate the development of Coombs'-negative, microangiopathic hemolytic anemia. A prolonged bleeding time may be seen before the platelet count begins to decrease. Of interest, all clotting tests, including fibrin-split products and antithrombin III activity, are completely normal. The renal disease is usually mild (with proteinuria and hematuria), although occasionally it may be more severe, leading to acute renal failure. Proteinuria and hypertension may coexist in a pregnant TTP patient, simulating preeclampsia; preeclampsia-related glomerular changes may also be superimposed on a TTP kidney. Neurological manifestations and fever are frequently observed, and may raise problems of differential diagnosis (see below).

Evolution

Because TTP occurs early in pregnancy, it clearly jeopardizes its course. Only 25% of maternal-infant pairs survived, and 80% of the infants died (5). However, when TTP develops late in pregnancy, a better prognosis can be achieved for the fetus and the neonate. Weiner (5), in a review of TTP in pregnancy found that the overall maternal mortality rate was 45%; however, he also noted that the mortality rate was 0% when patients were treated with plasma and 60% when this treatment was not used.

One of us (J.M.D.) has observed a case of "recurrent TTP" in a 19-year-old woman. The main features are summarized in Table 1. During the first pregnancy,

Table 1 Case 1: Summary of Main Features Observed in One Case of Recurrent TTP During Pregnancy

Age (yr)	Pregnancy	Time of onset (wk)	Clinical manifestations	Laboratory tests	Treatment
19	1st	26	Fever, hematuria, vomiting, jaundice, purpura	Serum creatinine level: 170 μmol/L Serum uric acid: 690 μmol/L Proteinuria	Induction of labor Death in utero
				Anemia Ht 15% Hb 5.6 g/dL platelets: 10,000/mm^3	Antiplatelet agents: aspirin, dipyramidole
				Schizocytes + serum aminotransferase activity mildly elevated	Plasma infusion Blood transfusion
21	2nd	29	Hypertension, hematuria abdominal symptoms	Serum creatinine level: 110 μmol/L Serum uric acid: 431 μmol/L Anemia Ht: 25% Hb 9.2 g/dL	Antihypertensive drugs dihydralazine Cesarean section at 31 weeks of pregnancy;
				Platelets 10,000/mm^3	baby alive
				Schizocytes + serum aminotransferase activity highly elevated	Aspirin Plasma infusion Blood transfusion

she developed microangiopathic hemolytic anemia, severe thrombocytopenia, and slight renal involvement without hypertension. All abnormalities and symptoms disappeared after delivery. Two years later, she again developed microangiopathic hemolytic anemia and thrombocytopenia but had no renal involvement; the serum liver enzyme concentrations were elevated. Hypertension was present. This case is an example of the difficulties of exact classification. Among possible diagnoses are severe recurrent preeclampsia (but the blood pressure was normal during first pregnancy), recurrent HUS (but the syndrome occurred during pregnancy and renal failure was mild), and recurrent TTP.

A similar case was brought to our attention (M.H.). The main findings are indicated in Table 2. At the end of the patient's second pregnancy, rupture of a subcapsular hematoma of the liver occurred. This complication is well documented in severe preeclampsia (2). All symptoms cleared after the first two deliveries. In contrast, after her third pregnancy and delivery in April 1990, acute pyelonephritis and acute transient renal failure developed and thrombocytopenia recurred, necessitating plasma infusion. The platelet count was restored to 200,000/mm^3. However, 1 month after the patient ended plasma therapy, severe thrombocytopenia developed again. This showed clearly that this disease was not restricted to pregnancy, and it indicated the TTP might be a more reasonable diagnosis.

Table 2 Case 2: Summary of Main Features Observed in Second Case of Recurrent TTP During Three Successive Pregnancies and Persistence of Thrombocytopenia After the Third Pregnancy

Age (years)	Pregnancy	Time of onset (weeks)	Clinical manifestations	Laboratory tests	Treatment
25	1st	27	Hypertension 170/100 mmHg Abdominal pain Seizures	Serum creatinine level 128 μmol/l Proteinuria Anemia Hb 6 g/dl Platelets 10,000/mm^3 Haptoglobin level ↓ Clotting tests normal	Cesarean section: fetal death
26	2nd	33	No hypertension	Anemia Hb 8.5 g/dl Platelets 10,000 mm^3	Cesarean section: baby alive
30	3rd	28	Severe hypertension	Proteinuria Anemia Hb 7 g/dl Platelets 15,000/mm^3 Schizocytes 8% Serum aminotransferase activity elevated	Aspirin, dipyridamole Cesarean section: fetal death

Table 3 Differential Diagnosis of TTP and HUS Associated with Pregnancy: Clinical Manifestations

	HUS	TTP	HELLP	Severe pure preeclampsia
Time of Onset	Postpartum	Any time	3rd trimester	3rd trimester
Symptoms				
Abdominal pain	0	0	++ to +++	+ to +++
Signs				
Hypertension	+ to +++	+	0 to +++	+ to +++
Fever	0	+	0	0
Neurological features (confusion, coma, seizures)	0	+ to +++	0 to +	0 to +++

Differential Diagnosis

The main features concerning the differential diagnosis are summarized in Tables 3, 4, and 5.

Severe Preeclampsia

Severe preeclampsia should be differentiated from the TTP/HUS complex. Preeclampsia is a clinical entity that is usually diagnosed in the third trimester of

Table 4 Differential Diagnosis: Renal, Hematological, and Hepatic Tests

	HUS	TTP	HELLP	Severe pure preeclampsia
Renal function				
Proteinuria	+ to 4 +	0 + to 4 +	1 + to 4 +	1 + to 4 +
Serum creatinine level	↑ ↑ ↑	Nl to ↑ ↑	Nl to ↑ ↑	Nl to ↑ ↑
Serum uric acid level	↑	Nl	↑	↑
Renal histology	Thrombotic microangiopathy	Thrombotic microangiopathy	Glomerular endotheliosis	Glomerular endotheliosis
Hematology				
White blood cells	Nl to ↑	Nl to ↑	Nl to ↑	Nl to ↑
Schizocytes	+++	+++	+ to +++	+ to +++
Platelets	↓ to ↓ ↓	↓ to ↓ ↓	↓ to ↓ ↓	Nl to ↓
Partial thromboplastin time	Nl	Nl	Nl to ↓ ↓ ↓	Nl to ↓
Antithrombin III	Nl	Nl	↓	↓
Liver function				
Bilirubin	↑ ↑ indirect	↑ ↑ indirect	Nl to ↑	Nl to ↑
Serum aminotransferase	Nl to ↑	Nl to ↑	↑ to ↑ ↑	Nl to ↑

Table 5 Differential Diagnosis: Prognosis and Treatment

	HUS	TTP	HELLP	Severe pure preeclampsia
Maternal prognosis				
Mortality	0–55%[a]	0–45%[a]	2%	2%
Renal failure	100%	20%	10–50%	20%
Need of temporary dialysis	100%	10%	< 10%	< 1%
End-stage renal failure	15%	0%	0%	0%
Fetal prognosis	Good in postpartum cases	Poor	Poor	Poor
Perinatal mortality		75%	10 to 60%	33%
Treatment	Plasma infusion or exchange	Plasma infusion or exchange	Delivery	Delivery

[a]Mortality is probably much lower presently than in the 1970s (35).
The figures indicated are approximate, taking into account recent and less recent data in the literature (31, 35).

pregnancy, primarily in primigravidas, and is characterized by hypertension and proteinuria. The disease is occasionally seen in multiparas, especially with multifetal pregnancy or with coexisting renal disease, hypertension, or diabetes. Severe preeclampsia includes a diastolic blood pressure of greater than 110 mm Hg, massive proteinuria, elevated serum creatinine, thrombocytopenia, increased serum aminotransferase activity, and fetal growth retardation. The association with convulsions defines eclampsia (which can also develop within the first 48 hours after delivery). Acute renal failure complicates the course of severe preeclampsia in approximately 20% of cases, preferentially in older multiparas (3). In pure preeclampsia, acute renal failure often develops in the immediate postpartum period (25). Thrombocytopenia ($<$100,000 platelets/mm^3) occurs in about 10% of preeclamptic women. Red blood cell fragmentation has not been studied prospectively in women with severe preeclampsia, but some authors have indicated that it is found frequently (26); typical microangiopathic hemolytic anemia has been described in this context (1).

On occasion it is impossible to distinguish severe preeclampsia from either TTP or HUS on clinical grounds. A renal biopsy is usually not performed in preeclamptic women, and it is contraindicated in thrombocytopenic patients. An accurate diagnosis is of importance because patients with TTP need not deliver immediately. Many pregnant women reported to have had TTP or HUS that resolved quickly after delivery (now recognized in this setting) were likely in retrospect to have had preeclampsia. Conversely, some women with TTP were originally considered to have preeclampsia, leading to a delay in therapy and unnecessary delivery of a premature infant; the correct diagnosis was made only when the patient failed to improve.

Measurement of plasma antithrombin activity is of interest. Multiple studies have shown a significant reduction in antithrombin III in women with preeclampsia. The decline was proportional to the severity of the disease, and perinatal mortality was inversely proportional to the extent of the reduction. Decreased antithrombin activity has been related to the destruction of the vascular endothelium. The sensitivity and specificity for preeclampsia were 76% and 91%, respectively (27). The value of this test, however, has recently been challenged in preeclamptic women with heavy proteinuria (28, 29).

The HELLP Syndrome

The HELLP syndrome (*H*emolysis, *E*levated *L*iver enzymes, *L*ow *P*latelet count) was first described by Pritchard et al. in 1954 (30). It represents approximately 10% of the cases of preeclampsia and affects multiparous women. Occurrence is usually between 34 and 36 weeks of pregnancy. Most affected women have vomiting (84%), epigastric pain (86%), and right upper quadrant tenderness (86%). Decreased renal function is found in approximately 50% and frank acute renal failure in 10% of the patients (31, 32). The HELLP syndrome is associated with a poor prognosis; maternal mortality is about 2% and perinatal mortality ranges from 10–60%. In most cases, there is spontaneous progressive regression of the syndrome after delivery, with platelet counts reaching more than 100,000/mm^3 within 72 hours (2, 33). The clearcut increase in serum aminotransferase activity helps to differentiate HELLP syndrome from TTP/HUS (Table 4).

Acute Fatty Liver of Pregnancy (AFLP)

AFLP is a rare and severe complication of pregnancy characterized by microvesicular fatty infiltration of centrilobular hepatocytes, unaccompanied by inflammatory cell infiltration or hepatocellular necrosis. The first manifestations appear after the 35th week of pregnancy, often in primigravidas, particularly those carrying twins. Initial symptoms are fatigue, abdominal pain and vomiting, followed by jaundice, bleeding, encephalopathy, and coma. Mild preeclampsia is found in 50% and acute renal failure, usually mild, in 60% of the cases.

Thrombocytopenia and microangiopathic hemolytic anemia may be found. The plasma antithrombin III level may be depressed. In early AFLP, serum aminotransferase levels may be only moderately elevated and the differential diagnosis includes HELLP syndrome or TTP. It is of interest that the white blood cell count is elevated in AFLP. Ultrasonography or computed tomography may demonstrate increased liver fat content. A liver biopsy with specific staining for fat should be performed to confirm the diagnosis. In addition to supportive therapy, immediate delivery is advocated as soon as the diagnosis of AFLP is ascertained.

Bilateral Renal Cortical Necrosis

Bilateral renal cortical necrosis used to be a frequent and severe complication of obstetric acute renal failure, mainly associated with abruptio placentae, prolonged intrauterine fetal death, and postpartum hemorrhage. Early detection and adequate therapy of these complications have considerably reduced the prevalence of cortical necrosis in industrialized countries (6), but it has not been eradicated in less developed regions. Confusion with TTP/HUS is possible when signs of disseminated intravascular coagulation, including thrombocytopenia, are prominent.

PATHOPHYSIOLOGY

Increasing evidence indicates that endothelial cell damage has a central role in TTP/HUS regardless of the triggering factor (see Chapter 27). It has been stated that the primary renal microvascular lesion was similar in preeclampsia, TTP, and idiopathic postpartum acute renal failure, the only difference being the extent and severity of the pathological changes (5, 6, 27). Preeclampsia is characterized by features of chronic disseminated intravascular coagulation, whereas TTP/HUS are not (5). It is of note that aspirin in high-risk subjects has a preventive effect on preeclampsia, whatever the mechanisms involved.

Pregnancy and the postpartum period potentiate the deleterious effects of the endothelial damage. Normal pregnancy is accompanied by an enhanced capacity to produce fibrin, whereas removal activity is depressed. The decreased fibrinolytic activity returns to normal between half an hour and 1 hour after delivery of the placenta. The placenta itself is a very potent source of thromboplastin, which is a key factor in triggering coagulation. Features suggesting intravascular coagulation have been found in abruptio placentae and prolonged intrauterine fetal death. These coagulation disturbances most probably predispose to bilateral renal cortical necrosis. It has long been known that only one injection of endotoxin was required to elicit the generalized Shwartzman's reaction (with renal cortical necrosis) in pregnant animals (34).

In addition to coagulation disorders, other predisposing factors may contribute during pregnancy. Conger et al. (35) have shown that 10-day postpartum rats exhibited the same predisposition toward acute renal failure after a single injection of endotoxin. In the early phase, the decrease in single nephron glomerular filtration rate resulted from a decrease in both glomerular plasma flow and capillary pressure, whereas fibrin deposition within the kidneys was minimal. These functional hemodynamic changes preceded fibrin occlusion of vessels and are probably mediated by neurohormonal substances that result from endotoxin challenge or consumption coagulopathy. In these experiments, the infusion of an angiotensin II antagonist prior to endotoxin administration protected the glomerular filtration rate, despite the fact that the occurrence of glomerular fibrin deposition and consumptive coagulopathy was similar to the control rats (35).

The results of Raij et al. (34) also point to the conclusion that endothelial damage is primary and that thrombi subsequently form in situ. These authors have shown that in the unilateral renal Shwartzman reaction, the initial event in the genesis of renal cortical necrosis was a specific local effect of endotoxin on the vascular endothelium (34, 36).

Kincaid-Smith et al. (34) observed the association of renal disease and recurrent abortion in 12 women with a circulating coagulation inhibitor (lupus "anticoagulant"). Only a few of these 12 had serological evidence of systemic lupus. The renal biopsies showed lesions which were essentially the same as those of thrombotic microangiopathy that had been described previously in postpartum renal failure. These cases raise the question of the frequency of the involvement of the lupus anticoagulant in "idiopathic" postpartum renal failure. It would be worth testing for the presence of lupus anticoagulant and antiphospholipid (anticardiolipin) antibody in cases of postpartum renal failure (37).

TREATMENT

Supportive Therapy

Supportive therapy is necessary regardless of the diagnosis. Symptomatic management of acute renal failure and hypertension are indicated. Both peritoneal dialysis and hemodialysis have been used in gravidas. During hemodialysis, anticoagulation and fluid balance should be carefully monitored. The peritoneal dialysis catheter should be inserted high in the abdomen under direct vision through a small incision (6). Severe preeclampsia requires anticonvulsant and antihypertensive therapy. In the United States, magnesium sulfate administered parenterally is currently used as an anticonvulsant, whereas in Europe diazepam, chlormethiazole, and phenytoin are favored. Few comparative trials are available (38). Hydralazine or dihydralazine is the drug of choice for controlling hypertension.

Monitoring of fetal well-being and placental function is crucial. The choice between vaginal delivery and cesarean section is beyond the scope of this chapter.

Supportive management is also indicated in postpartum acute renal failure. Angioteusin converting enzyme inhibitors, alone or in association with dihydropyridine derivatives are of great value for controlling the hypertension.

Specific Therapy

Specific therapy is based on precise identification of the disease. In severe preeclampsia and HELLP syndrome, rapid delivery is indicated, since a cure requires the expulsion or removal of the trophoblast. However, in approximately 5% of patients with HELLP syndrome, severe microangiopathic hemolytic anemia and thrombocytopenia fail to show improvement within 72 hours of delivery; this is usually accompanied by maternal deterioration involving the central nervous system, the kidneys, cardiopulmonary function, and/or the coagulation system, suggestive of ongoing thrombotic microangiopathy. In these cases, a trial of plasma exchanges with fresh frozen plasma has been advocated (39, 40).

In TTP, plasma therapy, whether by infusion or by plasmapheresis with donor plasma, is the first line therapy (4, 41). One plasma volume is recommended over the first 24 hours. Glucocorticoids have been recommended by some authors, but no specific conclusion has been reached in pregnant patients. Antiplatelet agents have been used in association with other therapy. Splenectomy should probably be considered only as a last measure if other forms of treatment are ineffective. In HUS, plasma therapy, associated with the management of renal failure and hypertension, is also indicated, but the results are much less rewarding than in TTP. Definitive data are, however, lacking in postpartum HUS. In anuric patients, only plasmapheresis should be considered so that cardiocirculatory overload can be prevented. The question of heparin therapy in postpartum HUS has long been debated (3, 6), but there is no strong evidence for its use. The risk of bleeding from the genital tract and from the renal biopsy site also must be considered seriously. With potent antihypertensive therapy, bilateral nephrectomy is no longer required. Successful renal transplantation without recurrence of the disease may be envisaged in patients with chronic renal failure due to postpartum HUS (3, 6). It should be emphasized that the lines of demarcation between the various disorders overlap considerably. These entities are probably closely related, and the rational choice of therapy remains difficult in some cases.

REFERENCES

1. Brain, M. C., Kuau, K. B., Dixon, H. G. Heparin treatment of hemolysis and thrombocytopenia in preeclampsia. *J. Obstet. Gynecol. Br. Cwlth.*, *74*: 702–711 (1967).
2. Sibai, B., Taslimi, M., El-Nazer, A., Amon, E., Mabie, B., Ryan, G. Maternal perinatal outcome associated with the syndrome of hemolysis, elevated liver enzymes and low platelets in severe preeclampsia eclampsia. *Am. J. Obstet. Gynecol.*, *155*: 501–509 (1986).
3. Grünfeld, J. P., Pertuiset, N. Acute renal failure in pregnancy. *Am. J. Kidney Dis.*, *9*: 359–362 (1987).
4. Krane, N. K. Acute renal failure in pregnancy. *Arch. Intern. Med.*, *148*: 2347–2357 (1988).
5. Weiner, C. Thrombotic microangiopathy in pregnancy and the postpartum period. *Semin. Hematol.*, *24*: 119–129 (1987).
6. Grünfeld, J. P., Ganeval, D., Bournerias, F. Acute renal failure in pregnancy. *Kidney. Int.*, *18*: 179–191 (1980).
7. Pertuiset, N., Grünfeld, J. P. Acute renal failure in pregnancy. *Bailliéres. Clin. Obstet. Gynaecol.*, *1*: 873–890 (1987).
8. Creasy, G., Morgan, J. Hemolytic uremic syndrome after ectopic pregnancy: Postectopic nephrosclerosis. *Obstet. Gynecol.*, *69*: 448–449 (1987).
9. Judlin, P., Bollaert, P. E., Bauer, P., Laprévote-Heully, M. C., Lambert, H., Larcan, A. Syndrome urémo-hémolytique survenant au décours d'une grossesse extra-utérine. A propos d'un cas. *Rev. Fr. Gynécol. Obstét.*, *83:* 557–559 (1988).
10. Morel-Maroger, L., Kanfer, A., Solez, K., Sraer, J. D., Richet, G. Prognostic importance of vascular lesions in acute renal failure with microangiopathic hemolytic anemia (hemolytic-uremic syndrome): Clinicopathologic study in 20 adults. *Kidney Int.*, *15*: 548–558 (1979).
11. Pertuiset, N., Ganeval, D., Grünfeld, J. P. Acute renal failure in pregnancy: An update. *Semin. Nephrol.*, *4*: 232–239 (1984).
12. Gomperts, E. D., Sessel, L., du Plessis, V., Hersch, C. Recurrent post-partum haemolytic uraemic syndrome. *Lancet*, *1*: 48 (1978).
13. Coratelli, P., Buongiorno, E., Passavanti, G. Endotoxemia in hemolytic uremic syndrome. *Nephron*, *50*: 365–367 (1988).
14. Karmali, M., Petric, M., Lim, C., Fleming, P., Arbus, G., Lior, H. The association between idiopathic hemolytic uremic syndrome and infection by verotoxin producing *Escherichia coli*. *J. Infect. Dis.* *151*: 775–782 (1985).
15. Steele, B. T., Goldie, J., Alexopoulou, I., Shimizu, A. Postpartum hemolytic uremic syndrome and verotoxin producing *Escherichia coli*. *Lancet*, *1*: 511 (1984).
16. Zacherle, B. J., Richardson, J. A. Irreversible renal failure secondary to hypertension induced by oral contraceptives. *Ann. Intern. Med.*, *77*: 83–85 (1972).
17. Bollaert, P. E., Bauer, P., Judlin, P., Laprevote-Heully, M. C., Lambert, H., Larcan, A. Hemorrhagic colitis with *Streptococcus pyogenes* preceding hemolytic uremic syndrome during early pregnancy. *Nephron*, *52*: 103–104 (1989).
18. Stratta, P., Canavese, C., Colla, L., Goia, F., Cavalli, G., Vercellone, A. Postpartum hemolytic uremic syndrome (HUS) following β-orthoestradiol benzoate and dimethylergonovine therapies. *Biol. Res. Pregnancy*, *7*: 171–175 (1986).
19. Hauglustaine, D., van Damme, B., Vanrenterghem, Y., Michielsen, P. Recurrent hemolytic uremic syndrome during oral contraception. *Clin. Nephrol.*, *15*: 148–153 (1981).

20. Bergstein, J., Michael, A., Kjellstrand, C., Simmons, R., Najarian, J. Hemolytic-uremic syndrome in adult sisters. *Transplantation, 17*: 487–490 (1974).
21. Paz, R. A., Elijovich, F., Barcat, J. A., Sanchez-Avalos, J. C. Fatal simultaneous thrombocytopenic purpura in siblings. *Br. Med. J., 4*: 727–728 (1969).
22. Fuchs, W., George, J., Dotin, L., Sears, D. Thrombotic thrombocytopenic purpura: Occurrence two years apart during late pregnancy in two sisters. *J.A.M.A., 235*: 2126–2127 (1976).
23. Modesto, A., Durand, D., Orfila, C., Suc, J. M. Syndrome hémolytique urémique chez deux germains HLA identiques. *Néphrologie, 5*: 47–48 (1984).
24. Pirson, Y., Lefebvre, C., Arnout, C., van Ypersele de Strihou, C. Hemolytic uremic syndrome in three adult siblings: a familial study and evolution. *Clin. Nephrol., 28*: 250–255 (1987).
25. Sibai, B., Villar, M., Mabie B. Acute renal failure in hypertensive disorders of pregnancy. Pregnancy outcome and remote prognosis in thirty-one consecutive cases. *Am. J. Obstet. Gynecol. 162*: 777–783 (1990).
26. Spencer, C., Crane, F., Kumar, J., Alving, B. Treatment of postpartum hemolytic uremic syndrome with plasma exchange. *J.A.M.A., 247*: 2808–2809 (1982).
27. Weiner, C. The clinical spectrum of preeclampsia. *Am. J. Kidney Dis., 9*: 312–316 (1987).
28. Aghai, E., Brunstein, J., Quitt, M., Abramovici, H., Froom, P. Antithrombin III levels in preeclampsia. *Isr. J. Med. Sci., 26*: 140–143 (1990).
29. Brenner, B. Antithrombin III and preeclampsia. *Isr. J. Med. Sci., 26*: 121–122 (1990).
30. Pritchard, J., Weisman, R., Ratnof, O., Vosburgh, G Intravascular hemolysis, thrombocytopenia and other hematologic abnormalities associated with severe toxemia of prenancy. *N. Engl. J. Med., 250*: 89–98 (1954).
31. Dantzer, M., Rigaud, P., Agnani, G., Maillet, R., Colette, C. Le "HELLP syndrome" peut précéder l'apparition de l'hypertension artérielle au cours de la toxémie gravidique. *Rev. Fr. Gynécol. Obstét., 82*: 243–245 (1987).
32. Weinstein, L. Preeclampsia/eclampsia with hemolysis, elevated liver enzymes, and thrombocytopenia. *Obstet. Gynecol., 66*: 657–660 (1985).
33. Monnier, J. C., Vaksmann, S., Vinatier, D., Patey-Savatier, P., Maunoury-Lefebvre, C. Faut-il individualiser le HELLP syndrome? *J. Gynécol. Obstet. Biol. Reprod., 16*: 765–771 (1987).
34. Raij, L., Keane, W., Michael, A. Unilateral Shwartzman reaction: Cortical necrosis in one kidney following *in vivo* perfusion with endotoxin. *Kidney Int., 12*: 91–95 (1977).
35. Conger, J., Falk, S., Guggenheim, S. Glomerular dynamics and morphologic changes in the generalized Shwartzman reaction in the postpartum rats. *J. Clin. Invest., 67*: 1334–1346 (1981).
36. Remuzzi, G., Garella, S. HUS and TTP: Variable expression of a single entity. *Kidney Int., 32*: 292–308 (1987).
37. Kincaid-Smith, P., Kenneth, F., Kloss, M. Lupus anticoagulant associated with renal thrombotic microangiopathy and pregnancy-related renal failure. *Q. J. Med., 69*: 795–815 (1988).
38. Crowther, C. Magnesium sulphate versus diazepam in the management of eclampsia: A randomized controlled trial. *Br. J. Obstet. Gyneaecol., 97*: 110–117 (1990).
39. Martin, J., Files, J., Blake, P., Norman, P., Martin, R., Hess, W., Morrison, J., Wiser, W. Plasma exchange for preeclampsia. *Am. J. Obstet. Gynecol., 162*: 126–137 (1990).
40. Schwartz, M. Possible role for exchange plasmapheresis with fresh frozen plasma for maternal indications in selected cases of preeclampsia and eclampsia. *Obstet. Gynecol., 68*: 136–139 (1986).
41. Conte, F., Meroni, M., Battini, G., Ferrario, G., Tommasi, A., Volpi, A., Sessa, A. Plasma exchange in acute renal failure due to postpartum hemolytic uremic syndrome. *Nephron, 50*: 167–168 (1988).

21
Inborn Errors of Cobalamin Metabolism and the Hemolytic Uremic Syndrome

Pierre A. Russo *Hôpital Ste-Justine, Montreal, Quebec, Canada* **Josée Doyon** *Université de Montréal, Montreal, Quebec, Canada* **Elise Sonsino and Hélène Ogier** *Hôpital Robert Debré, Paris, France* **Jean-Marie Saudubray** *Hôpital Necker–Enfants Malades, Paris, France*

The hemolytic uremic syndrome rarely occurs in the neonate or within the first few months of life (1, 2). A dearth of anatomical data, incomplete clinical manifestations, and the frequent absence of a typical prodomal illness have only added to our lack of insight into the etiology of microangiopathy in this age group.

Conversely, renal abnormalities have rarely been documented in association with disorders of vitamin B_{12} metabolism and/or methylmalonic acidemia. Imerslund (3) and Grasbeck (4) described persistent proteinuria in association with a defect in intestinal absorption of vitamin B_{12}. Interstitial nephritis in association with renal failure has been noted with methylmalonic acidemia, (5, 6) perhaps related to hyperuricemia (7). Proximal renal tubular acidosis has also been described with methylmalonic acidemia (8–10) without, however, the complete biochemical characteristics of the Fanconi syndrome.

There are a few reports of a renal microangiopathy in a subset of patients with a congenital intracellular defect of vitamin B_{12} metabolism (11–13). These infants have usually manifested severe illness within the first several weeks of life; most have died before age 5 months.

OVERVIEW OF VITAMIN B_{12} METABOLISM

An understanding of vitamin B_{12} metabolism (14, 15) is required to allow speculation on the pathophysiology of these cases. Vitaimin B_{12} (cobalamin) is a series of organometallic substances consisting of a central cobalt atom bonded to four pyrrole rings via their nitrogen groups, constituting the corrin ring (Fig. 1). A fifth substituent of the cobalt atom is a dimethyl benzimidazole derivative, whereas the sixth substituent can be either -CH_3, OH- or 5'-deoxyadenosyl. Only two chemical reactions in the mammalian system have been unequivocally demonstrated to require the

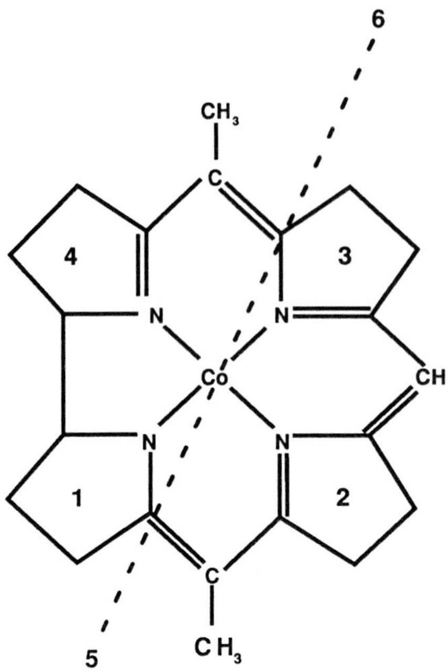

Figure 1 The corrin ring, with a central cobalt atom bonded to four pyrrole rings, represents the core chemical structure of cobalamin. A fifth chemical group bonded to cobalt is a dimethyl benzimidazole derivative, whereas group 6 can be $-CHM_3$, $-OH$, or 5'deoxyadenosyl.

participation of cobalamin as a coenzyme (Fig. 2): The first is the conversion of homocysteine to methionine via the enzyme methyl transferase, using methyltetrahydrofolate as a methyl donor; the second is the conversion of methylmalonyl CoA to succinyl CoA by the mutase enzyme.

Cobalamin is obtained exclusively from the diet. Cobalamin binds to intrinsic factor (IF), a glycoprotein secreted by gastric parietal cells, and penetrates the ileal enterocyte as a complex via an endocytotic mechanism. This complex is dissolved

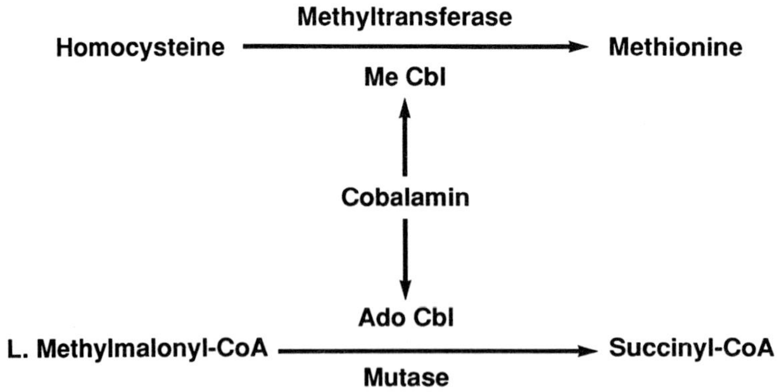

Figure 2 The two major chemical reactions in the mammalian system catalyzed by cobalamin: the conversion of homocysteine to methionine and that of methylmalonyl-CoA to succinyl-CoA.

within the enterocyte and enters the portal venous system bound to transcobalamin II (TC II). It is then rapidly taken up by a wide variety of cells, TC II being recognized by a specific, high-affinity surface receptor, thus facilitating entry of cobalamin within the cell. Smaller amounts of cobalamin circulate in the plasma bound to transcobalamin I and III (TC I and TC III), constituting a slow turnover pool.

The Imerslund-Grasbeck syndrome is believed to be caused by a defect in ileal uptake of B_{12} bound to IF. In this syndrome, renal disease is manifested by persistent proteinuria and accompanied by megaloblastic anemia that can be corrected by parenteral vitamin B_{12}. The clinical course is indolent (16). Proteinuria could be caused by a defect in the synthesis of the matrix of the glomerular basement membrane (17, 18).

Once within the cell, cobalamin is either converted within the cytoplasm to methylcobalamin, which will catalyze the methylation of homocysteine to methionine or will penetrate the mitochondrion, to be converted to adenosylcobalamin and effect the conversion of methylmalonyl CoA to succinyl-CoA (Fig. 3). Although the various steps in these conversions are incompletely understood, defects in the sequence have been characterized so far as a series of complementation groups (A–G). These various defects are defined by complementation studies, the cultured

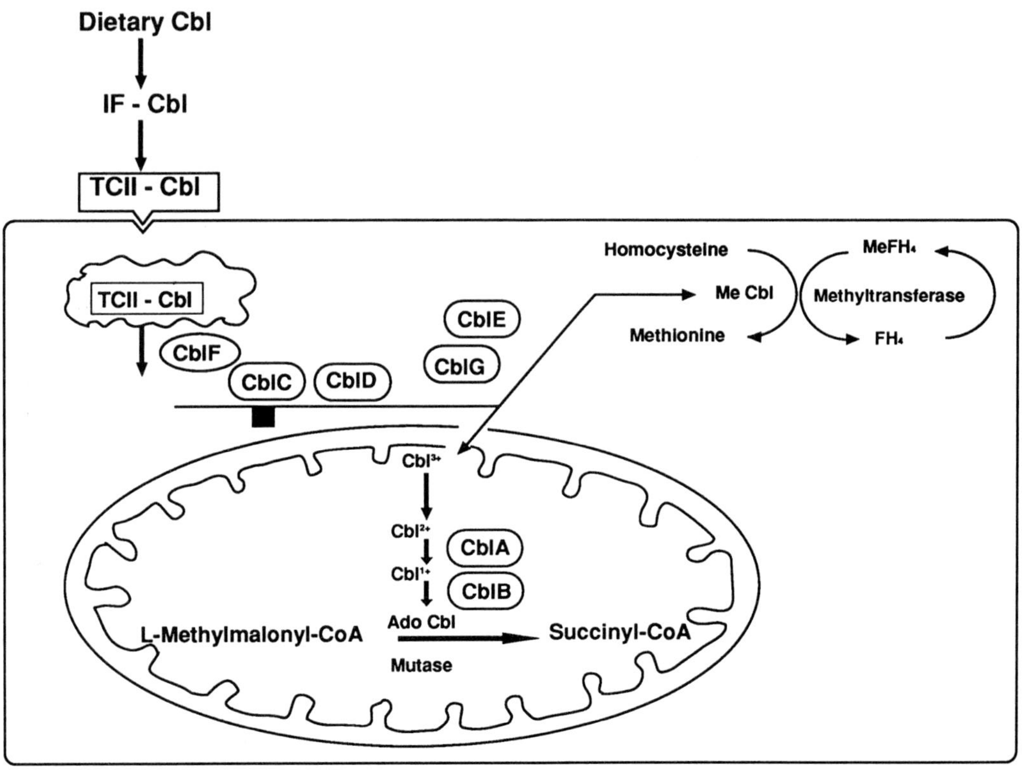

Figure 3 The intracellular conversion of cobalamin to either methylcobalamin or adenosylcobalamin occurs via a graded series of steps; mutations identified along the pathways have been classified alphabetically as mutation groups CblA–CblG, respectively.

fibroblasts from an affected patient being assigned to one group based on their ability to correct the metabolic defect in a mixed culture with a series of reference cell lines (19). Thus, deficiencies in the conversion of cobalamin to adenosylcobalamin have been defined as CblA and CblB, resulting in methylmalonic acidemia without homocystinuria, approximately half of which are corrected by pharmacologic doses of vitamin B_{12}.

Defective synthesis of both adenosylcobalamin and methylcobalamin results in both methylmalonic acidemia and homocystinuria. These have been divided into three different groups. Complementation group C (CblC) comprises the largest number of patients, whereas only a few isolated cases have been described in the CblD and CblF groups.

CASES OF CONGENITAL VITAMIN B_{12} DEFICIENCY AND HUS

All the cases reported with clinical and laboratory evidence of HUS have belonged to CblC. The first case was reported by Baumgartner and colleagues (11). Since then, five additional cases have been described (12, 13, 20). All presented with strikingly similar clinical profiles (Table 1), characterized by neonatal onset with failure to thrive, poor feeding, and vomiting. Lethargy and hypotonia, without localizing neurological findings, usually were prominent physical findings. Pancytopenia, hypoproteinemia, and decreased coagulation factors were major laboratory findings that manifested early in the course of hospitalization. The hypoproteinemia in three of the cases was resistant to albumin infusions. Rapid deterioration with the onset of refractory metabolic acidosis, gastrointestinal bleeding, hemolytic episodes, and renal failure have further characterized the last weeks of life of these patients. Three of the cases were also observed to have developed severe respiratory failure with radiological evidence of interstitial lung disease. All reported cases have died within the first 4 months of life. The clinical course was not improved by pharmacological doses of parenteral vitamin B_{12}.

The multisystemic nature of the disease and its early onset led to the suspicion of a metabolic disorder. Screening urine for amino and organic acids revealed the presence of both methylmalonic acid and homocysteine. In four cases the deficit was further characterized by complementation studies of the patients' fibroblasts. Two of the cases (4 and 5, Table 1) were diagnosed retrospectively based on their clinical and histological similarities with the others; partial metabolic investigation of urine revealed homocystinuria and methylmalonic aciduria in keeping with a diagnosis of CblC deficiency. These two cases were siblings born to parents who were consanguineous to the fourth degree.

Approximately 20 cases of CblC disease have been documented in the literature, and although initially it was believed that the condition manifested soon after birth, some have had their onset in adolescence. All reported cases have had abnormal neurological or psychiatric signs. A comparison of these cases with those demonstrating microangiopathy is presented in Table 2. Of 10 cases of CblC disease with a neonatal onset but without evidence of HUS, three have died in early infancy. One had pancytopenia, convulsions, and gastrointestinal hemorrhage (21, 22), whereas the clinical picture in the second was dominated by cor pulmonale (23). In the other

Table 1 CblC Disease—Major Clinical and Laboratory Features of Cases with HUS

	Pretreatment biochemistry							Age at onset				
Case No	Ref.	Onset	Death	MHA	Homo-cysteine	Anemia	Hepatic failure	Meta-bolic acidosis	GI bleeding	Respi-ratory failure	Hemo-lysis	Renal failure
1	11	2 wks	4 mo	*u* 8.9–61.9 mM/g creat	*u* 2.38–12.65 mM/g creat	7 wks		3 mo			3 mo	3.5 mo
2	12, 13	Nn	35 d	*u* 0.91 mM/g creat	*u* 0.26 mM/g creat *pl* 88 mM/L	28 d	28 d	28 d	30 d		30 d	30 d
3	12, 13	Nn	40 d	*u* 1.39 mM/g creat	*u* 0.043 mM/g creat *pl* 64 mM/L	30 d	39 d	30 d	30 d		30 d	30 d
4	12, 13	Nn	44 d	*u* 1.62 mM/g creat		36 d	35 d	10 d	30 d	36 d		36 d
5	12, 13 (sibling of above)	Nn	52 d	*u* ++	*u* ++	11 d	11 d	38 d	14 d	38 d	38 d	NR
6	20	1 mo	3 mo				30 d			60 d		60d

Nn = neonatal period
MA = methylmalonic acid
u = urine
pl = plasma
NR = not reported

Table 2 A Comparison of Major Clinical and Laboratory Features of CblC Cases with and Without HUS

	Cases with HUS	Cases Without HUS
Clinical features		
Sex (M/F)	3/3	7/7
Neonatal onset	6/6	10/14
Failure to thrive	6/6	5/14
Hypotonia/lethargy	6/6	5/14
Seizures	6/6	4/14
Respiratory difficulties	3/6	1/14
Retinal pigmentation	NR	3/14
GI bleeding	5/6	2/14
Death ≤4 mo of age	6/6	2/14
Laboratory findings		
Anemia	6/6	7/14
Thrombocytopenia	6/6	1/14
Hemolytic episode(s)	6/6	1/14
Acidosis	6/6	
Hematuria	5/6	2/14

NR = not reported

cases (8, 9, 24–31) with neonatal onset, a partial, or, rarely, a complete remission of the megaloblastic anemia and biochemical abnormalities was obtained with injections of vitamin B_{12}. However, all cases had neurologic or developmental sequelae. One patient died at 7 years of age on treatment (24, 25). Other cases have presented in later infancy (27, 32, 33) and up to 14 years of age (34).

Pathological changes in the six cases with HUS revealed many similarities (Table 3A). Glomerular and arterial thrombi were seen in four of the six cases (Fig. 4). Although no fresh thrombi were noted in case 6, ultrastructural examination revealed widespread subendothelial thickening with accumulation of granular, slightly electron-dense material and endothelial degeneration, characteristic of endothelial injury (Fig. 5). Thromboemboli were also detected in the lungs of cases 3, 4, and 6 (Fig. 6), accompanied by thickening of arterial and arteriolar walls and interstitial pneumonitis. This accounted for the severe respiratory difficulties which were a dominant clinical feature of cases 4–6. Hepatic changes were characterized by steatosis and hemosiderosis in all cases.

In five cases, the gastric mucosa revealed inflammation, varying degrees of atrophy, and striking cystic changes with marked atypia of epithelial nuclei (Figs. 7, 8). Occasional intranuclear inclusions diagnostic of cytomegalovirus (CMV) infection were detected in the gastric epithelium of one patient (Fig. 8). The gastric mucosa in all these cases was further characterized by a complete absence of parietal and chief cells. No abnormalities were detected throughout the rest of the gastrointestinal tract, although atrophic duodenal villi were reported by Baumgartner (11).

Table 3A Major Autopsy Findings: CblC Disease (Cases with HUS)

Case No.	Age at Death	Kidneys	Lungs	Liver	Extraparenchymal vessels	Bone marrow	GI tract	CNS
1	4 mo	Glomerular and arterial thrombi	Edema	Steatosis Hemosiderin Sinusoidal thrombi	Initimal proliferation destruction of inner elastica		Short and atrophic duodenal villi	No changes
2	35 d	Glomerular and arterial thrombi		Steatosis		Megaloblastosis		
3	40 d	Glomerular and arterial thrombi subendothelial widening	Occult thromboemboli	Steatosis Hemosiderosis			Cystic atrophic gastritis	Normal
4	44 d	Glomerular and arterial thrombi	Interstitial pneumonitis Arterial + arteriolar thickening	Steatosis Hemosiderosis			Cystic atrophic gastritis	Normal
5	52 d			Steatosis				
6	3 mo	Glomerular capillary subendothelial widening	Interstitial pneumonitis Arteriolar thickening	Steatosis Hemosiderosis	Normal	Megaloblastosis	Cystic atrophic gastritis	Normal

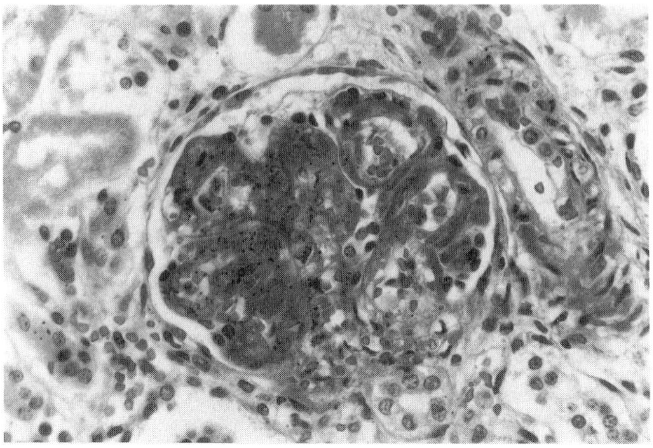

Figure 4 Thrombi occlude glomerular capillaries (hematoxylin-phloxine-safran; × 500).

Anatomical data are available for comparison in two patients who died in early infancy without evidence of HUS (Table 3B). The first reported case of CblC disease (21) revealed steatosis and "gastric mucosal atrophy with cystic change." The case reported by Brandstetter et al. (23) died as a result of respiratory failure, a cardinal clinical feature in three of the six cases with HUS. Pulmonary thromboemboli were

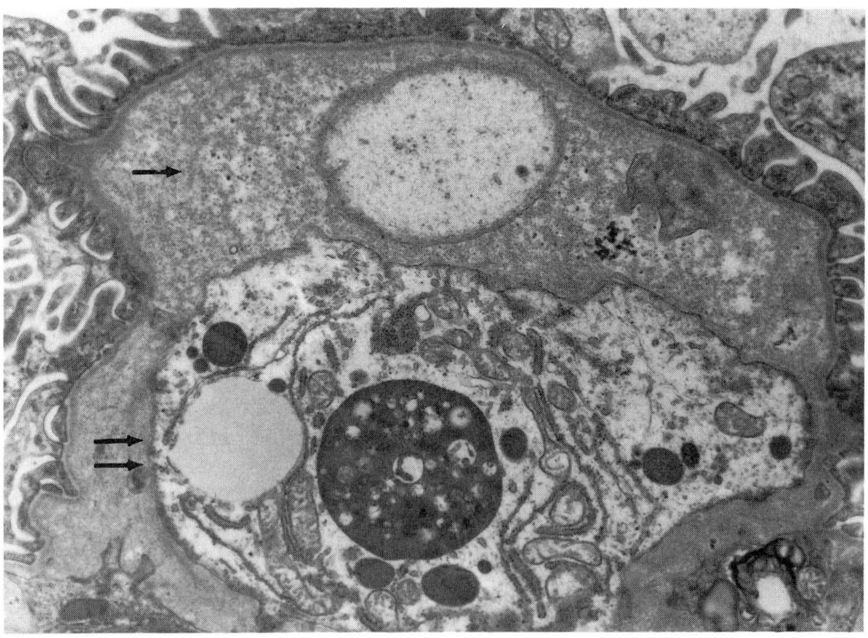

Figure 5 Ultrastructural examination of kidney reveals the presence of floculent granular material in the subendothelial space (arrow) and degenerative changes in the endothelial cell (below). Uranylacetate-lead citrate (× 7000).

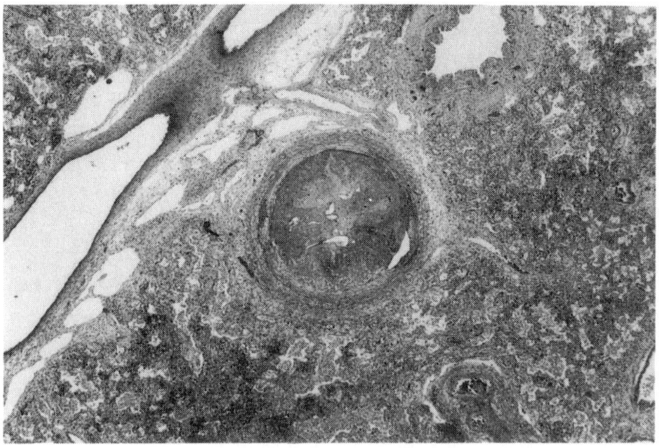

Figure 6 Thrombus present in pulmonary artery (HPS; × 30).

found at autopsy; there were hepatic steatosis and extensive glomerulosclerosis, although no renal arteriolar or glomerular thrombi were detected.

It is of interest that few CNS changes were noted except in two cases; that of Levy et al. (21), in which vascular damage accompanied the white matter changes, and a second, that of a child dying at 7 years of age (24, 25), in whom demyelinating changes were detected, similar to those reported in acquired vitamin B_{12} deficiency.

A remarkable degree of clinical and morphological homogeneity is apparent in

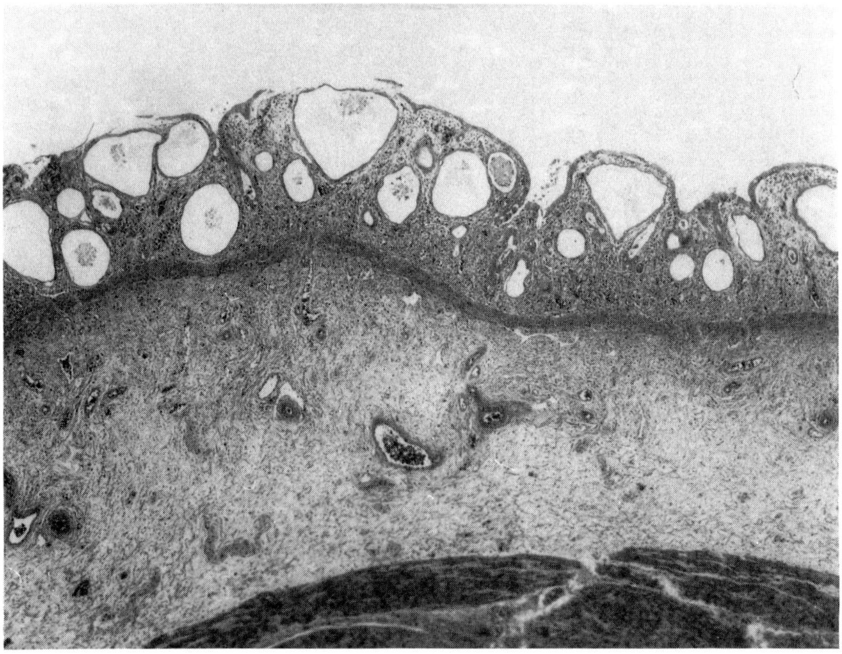

Figure 7 Severe atrophy of the stomach mucosa with the presence of cysts. (HPS; × 30).

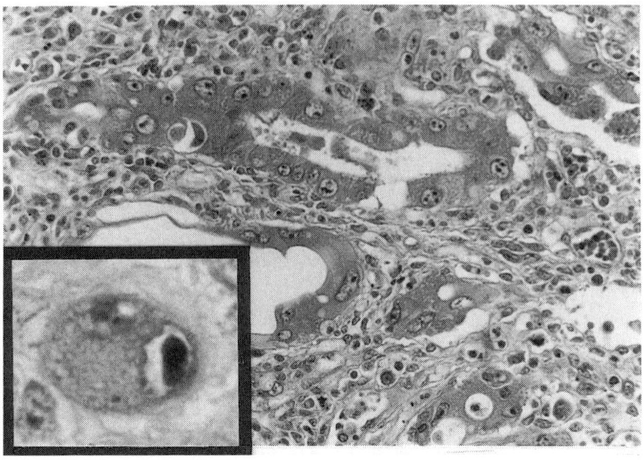

Figure 8 Marked atypia of nuclei of gastric epithelial lining and the presence of inflammation characterized the gastric mucosa. No parietal or chief cells could be visualized (HPS; × 300). Inset reveals intranuclear inclusions diagnostic of CMV infection, noted in one of the cases (HPS; × 800).

the cases with HUS when compared with other reported cases of CblC disease. Their early onset and severe multisystem involvement are distinguishing features. Although most reported cases of CblC disease had their onset in the neonatal period or early infancy, cases without HUS have been characterized mainly by neurologic and, in some, ophthalmologic findings, and most have pursued an indolent clinical course.

PATHOPHYSIOLOGICAL CONSIDERATIONS

Do these cases constitute a distinct syndrome within the subgroup of CblC disease? If so, what pathophysiologic mechanisms underlie the widespread morphological damage?

The elevated levels of plasma homocysteine in these patients provide the first clue. Thromboembolism occurring at any age is the major cause of morbidity and death in patients with cystathionine synthase deficiency (classical homocysteinuria), which results in elevated plasma and urinary levels of homocysteine and methionine (35). Extraparenchymal peripheral veins and arteries are most commonly affected, and postmortem examinations have revealed atherosclerotic lesions in most large and medium-sized arteries (36). Elevated levels of homocysteine due to methylenetetrahydrofolate reductase deficiency, a rarer cause of elevated plasma homocysteine, also result in vascular pathology (37).

In the present series of cases with HUS, vascular damage was also evident in the lungs (two cases) and extraparenchymal vessels (one case) as well as the kidneys. Even in cases without renal angiopathy, pulmonary thromboemboli were prominent in one case, whereas vasculitis was detected in arterioles of the brain in another (Table 3B).

Experimentally, homocysteine induces endothelial cell detachment and injury in vitro (38, 39), an effect which may be mediated by the generation of hydrogen peroxide (40). Furthermore, endothelial cells derived from an obligate heterozygote

Table 3B Major Autopsy Findings: CblC Disease (Cases Without HUS)

Ref.		Age at Death	Kidneys	Lungs	Extra-parenchymal vessels	Hepatic	Bone marrow	GI tract	CNS
21, 22	7.5 wk	NR	Broncho-pneumonia	Steatosis	NR	Myeloid hyperplasia		Atypical mucosal atrophy of stomach	Craniosynostosis "White matter changes"
24, 25	7 yrs	Normal	Diffuse pulmonary fibrosis	Moderate steatosis	NR		Megaloblastosis	Normal	Multiple foci of demyelination Arteriolar damage
23	17 wk	Glomerulosclerosis	Hyaline membranes Widened septa Occasional thromboemboli	Steatosis				Gastric mucosal congestion	Microcephaly Micromyelia

NR = not reported

for homocystinuria appear to be more susceptible to homocysteine-mediated injury than normal cells (41). The damage induced by homocysteine in endothelial cells is similar to that caused by endotoxin in vitro (42, 43). Parenthetically, endothelial damage appears to be, in the endotoxemia model of HUS, the most proximal event in the generation of renal microangiopathy (44).

In vivo, homocysteine produces endothelial injury in baboons and rats (45, 46) and pulmonary thrombi in mice (47). Homocysteine also appears to stimulate prostaglandin metabolism in platelets (48), abnormalities of which may subtend some cases of HUS (49).

Mild to moderate homocystinuria also occurs in patients with chronic renal disease, a population with an increased risk of premature vascular disease; these patients also have many other biochemical abnormalities (50). Renal transplant patients are also known to have some elevation of plasma homocysteine, and it is tempting to speculate as to the role of this metabolite, especially over long periods of time, in the development of "de novo" hemolytic uremic syndrome or in transplant glomerulopathy, in which there is ultrastructural evidence of endothelial injury, in these patients when factors such as cyclosporine, rejection, or severe hypertension are not operative (51).

A further concomitant of homocysteine-induced damage is the finding of hepatic steatosis, common to all the cases in the present series, even those without HUS, and in virtually all patients with cystathionine synthase deficiency (36). However, renal microangiopathy was not observed in a recent international survey of patients with homocysteinuria due to cystathionine synthase deficiency, despite the documentation of numerous vascular episodes (36). Furthermore, the plasma levels of homocysteine are usually much higher in that disease than is reported in cases of CblC disease. To date, vascular abnormalities have not been reported in patients with CblE and CblG disease, which only involve deficient methylcobalamin synthesis (15). Finally, microangiopathy and vascular disease have not been documented in patients with severe nutritional deficiency of vitamin B_{12}, despite the presence of hematological and neurological disease (52), indicating that factor(s) other than elevated homocysteine or in combination with the latter are necessary to induce vascular damage.

The occurrence of proteinuria in cases of Imerslund-Grasbeck syndrome has also led to speculation concerning the role of vitamin B_{12} deficiency in the causation of renal injury. However, the nonspecific nature of the renal histologic changes, the persistence of proteinuria despite parenteral therapy effective enough to correct the hematological anomalies, and the absence of documented renal damage in pernicious anemia (16–18) cast doubt on a direct cause and effect relationship between vitamin B_{12} deficiency and renal damage.

Another puzzling feature of the cases of CblC disease presenting with renal microangiopathy has been the presence of a severe cystic gastritis, which was well documented in four cases (Table 3A). Furthermore, no parietal or chief cells were detected histologically despite thorough sampling of gastric mucosa at autopsy. Case 1, reported by Baumgartner et al. (11) has atrophic duodenal villi, though no mention is made of gastric changes. Gastric mucosal atrophy with cystic change was also present in the case reported by Levy et al. (21) and separately by McCully (22). These changes are similar to those reported in adult patients with severe long-standing atrophic gastritis and pernicious anemia, in adult Menetrier's disease (53), arising in gastrojejunostomy stomas (54), or as an isolated finding with or without defects in other organ systems (55). Although cystic changes in the gastric mucosa are a concomitant of pediatric hypertrophic gastropathy—a disease with an indolent clinical course—the gastric mucosa in that condition is usually thickened, and parietal and chief cells have always been preserved (53). To our knowledge, such changes have never been reported in the pediatric literature in association with other diseases.

The striking nature of these changes, their almost uniform occurence, and the relative sparing of the rest of the gastrointestinal tract are highly suggestive of a selective assault on the gastric mucosa, although the etiology of these changes is unknown.

CONCLUSIONS

Cases of CblC disease can be divided into two major groups: The first is characterized by neonatal onset, a fulminant lethal clinical course unresponsive to parenteral vitamin B_{12} therapy, death in the first months of life, and widespread organ damage including renal microangiopathy and cystic gastritis. The second has onset from neonatal period to adolescence and an indolent course with neurological damage. The occurrence in two siblings of consanguineous parents suggests an autosomal recessive inheritance.

A congenital deficiency of vitamin B_{12} metabolism, particularly of the CblC group, must be considered in the differential diagnosis of renal microangiopathy in the neonate. The clinical course is fulminant and is unresponsive to administration of pharmacological doses of vitamin B_{12}.

ACKNOWLEDGMENTS

The authors wish to thank Danielle Roy for devoted secretarial assistance, and Claude Guilbeault for expert photographic help.

This work was supported in part by the Téléthon des étoiles and by the Fondation de l'hôpital Ste-Justine, and was presented in part at the Society for Pediatric Pathology Meeting, Boston, March 4th, 1990.

REFERENCES

1. Kaplan, B. S., Proesmans, W. The hemolytic uremic syndrome of childhood and its variants. *Semin. Hematol.*, *24*: 148–160 (1987).
2. Gianantonio, C. A., Vitacco, M., Mendilaharzu, F., Gallo, G. E., Sojo, E. T. The hemolytic-uremic syndrome. *Nephron*, *11*: 174–192 (1973).
3. Imerslund, O. Idiopatic chronic megaloblastic anemia in children. *Acta Pediatr.*, (suppl) *119*: 1 (1960).
4. Grasbeck, R., Godin, R., Kantero, I., Kuhlback, B. Selective vitamin B_{12} malabsorption and proteinuria in young people: a syndrome. *Acta Med. Scand.*, *167*: 289 (1960).
5. Shelan, D. T., Ryan, E., Spate, M., Morris, M., Hurley, R. M., Hill, R. Methylmalonic acidemia: 6 years' clinical experience with two variants unresponsive to vitamin B_{12} therapy. *Can. Med. Assoc. J.*, *19*: 1230–1235 (1978).
6. Walter, J. H., Michalski, A., Wilson, W. M., Leonard, J. V., Barratt, T. M., Dillon, M.

J. Chronic renal failure in methylmalonic acidaemia. *Eur. J. Pediatr.*, *148*: 344–348 (1989).

7. Broyer, M., Guesry, P., Burgess, E.-A., Charpentier, C., Lemonnier, A. Acidémie methyl malonique avec néphropathie hyperuricémique. *Arch. Fr. Pediatr.*, *31*: 543–552 (1978).
8. Wolff, J. A., Strom, C., Griswold, W., Sweetman, F., Kulovich, S., Prodanos, C., Nyhan, W. L. Proximal renal tubular acidosis in methylmalonic acidemia. *J. Neurogenetics*, *2*: 31–39 (1985).
9. Ribes, A., Vilaseca, M. A., Briones, P., Maya, A., Sabater, J., Pascual, P., Alvarez, L., Ros, J., Pascual, E. G. Methylmalonic aciduria with homocystinuria. *J. Inher. Metab. Dis.*, *2*: 129–130 (1984).
10. Ribes, A., Briones, P., Vilaseca, M. A., Lluch, M., Rodes, M., Maya, A., Campistol, J., Pascual, P. Methylmalonic aciduria with homocystinuria: biochemical studies, treatment, and clinical course of a Cbl-C patient. *Eur. J. Pediatr.*, *149*: 412–415 (1990).
11. Baumgartner, E. R., Wick, H., Maurer, R., Egli, N.., Steinmann, B. Congenital defect in intracellular cobalamin metabolism resulting in homocystinuria and methylmalonic aciduria. I. Case report and histopathology. *Helv. Paediatr. Acta.*, *34*: 465–482 (1979).
12. Sonsino, E., Ogier, H., Mercier, J. C., Devictor, D., Bloch, D., Grangeponte, M. C., Nivet, H. Hemolytic-uremic syndrome (HUS) secondary to vitamin b12 metabolism anomaly. *International Journal of Pediatric Nephrology 6*: Abstracts from the Annual Meeting of the French Club of Pediatric Nephrology (A). (1985).
13. Sonsino, E., Ogier, H., Mercier, J. C., Devictor, D., Ferkdadji, L., Bocquet, L. Anomalie congénitale du métabolisme de la vitamine B_{12}. *Arch. Anat. Cytol. Pathol.*, *33*: 98–99 (1985).
14. Cooper, B. A., Rosenblatt, D. S. Inherited defects of vitamin B_{12} metabolism. *Ann. Rev. Nutr.*, *7*: 291–320 (1987).
15. Fenton, W. A., Rosenberg, L. E. Inherited disorders of cobalamin transport and metabolism. In *The Metabolic Basis of Inherited Disease*, ed. 6. (C. R. Scriver, A. L. Beaudet, W. S. Sly, D. Vallee, eds.) McGraw-Hill, New York, pp 2065–2082 (1989).
16. Broch, H., Imerslund, O., Monn, E., Hovig, T., Seip, M. Imerslund-Grasbeck Anemia. A long-term Follow-up Study. *Acta Paediatr. Scand.*, *73*: 248–253 (1984).
17. Collin, Y., Lahdevirta, J., Jokinen, E. J. Selective Vitamin B_{12} Malabsorption with Proteinuria. Renal Biopsy Study. *Nephron*, *23*: 297–303 (1979).
18. Rumpelt, H. J., Michl, W. Selective vitamin B12 malabsorption with proteinuria (Imerslund-Najman-Grasbeck-syndrome): Ultrastructural examination on renal glomeruli. *Clin. Nephrol.*, *11*: 213–217 (1979).
19. Gravel, R. A., Mahoney, M. J., Ruddle, F. H., Rosenberg, L. E. Genetic complementation in heterokaryons of human fibroblasts defective in cobalamin metabolism. *Proc. Nat. Acad. Sci. USA*, *72*: 3181–3185 (1975).
20. Doyon, J., Russo, P., Sonsino, E., Ogier, H. Congenital anomaly of vitamin B12 metabolism—an analysis of three cases (abstract). *Lab. Invest.*, *62*: 3P (1990).
21. Levy, H. L., Mudd, S. H., Schulman, J. D., Dreyfus, P. M., Abeles, R. H. A derangement in B_{12} metabolism associated with homocystinemia, cystathioninemia, hypomethioninemia and methylmalonic aciduria. *Am. J. Med.*, *48*: 390–397 (1970).
22. McCully, K. S. Vascular pathology of homocysteinemia: implications for the pathogenesis of arteriosclerosis. *Am. J. Pathol.*, *56*: 111–123 (1969).
23. Brandstetter, Y., Weinhouse, E., Splaingard, M. L., Tang, T. T. Cor pulmonale as a complication of methylmalonic acidemia and homocystinuria (Cbl-C Type). *Am. J. Med. Genet.*, *36*: 167–171 (1990).
24. Dillon, M. J., England, J. M., Gompertz, D., Goodey, P. A., Grant, D. B., Hussein, H.A-A., Linnell, J. C., Matthews, D. M., Mudd, S. H., Newns, G. H., Seakins, J.W.T., Uhlendorf, B. W., Wise, I. J. Mental retardation, megaloblastic anaemia, methylmalonic

aciduria and abnormal homocysteine metabolism due to an error in vitamin B12 metabolism. *Clin. Sci. Mol. Med.*, *47*: 43–61 (1974).

25. Dayan, A. D., Ramsey, R. B. An inborn error of vitamin B_{12} metabolism associated with cellular deficiency of coenzyme forms of the vitamin. Pathological and neurochemical findings in one case. *J. Neuro. Sci.*, *23*: 117–128 (1974).
26. Carmel, R., Bedros, A. A., Mace, J. W., Goodman, S. I. Congenital methylmalonic aciduria-homocystinuria with megaloblastic anemia: Observations on response to hydroxocobalamin and on the effect of homocysteine and methionine on the deoxyuridine suppression test. *Blood*, *55*: 570–579 (1980).
27. Mitchell, G. A., Watkins, D., Melançon, S. B., Rosenblatt, D. S., Geoffroy, G., Orquin, J., Barsoum Homsy, M., Dallaire, L. Clinical heterogeneity in cobalamin C variant of combined homocystinuria and methylmalonic aciduria. *J. Pediatr.*, *108*: 410–415 (1986).
28. Linnell, J. C., Miranda, B., Bhatt, H. R., Dowton, S. B., Levy, H. L. Abnormal cobalamin metabolism in a megaloblastic child with homocystinuria, cystathioninuria and methylmalonic aciduria. *J. Inher. Metabol. Dis.*, *6* (suppl) 2: 137–139 (1983).
29. Mamlok, R. J., Isenberg, J. N., Rassin, D. K., Norcross, K., Tallan, H. H. A cobalamin metabolic defect with homocystinuria, methylmalonic aciduria and macrocytic anemia. *Neuropediatrics*, *17*: 94–99 (1986).
30. Robb, R. M., Dowton, S. B., Fulton, A. B., Levy, A. L. Retinal degeneration in vitamin B_{12} disorder associated with methylmalonic aciduria and sulfur amino acid abnormalities. *Am. J. Ophthal.*, *97*: 691–696 (1984).
31. Ravindranath, Y., Krieger, I. Vitamin B-12 (Cb) and folate interrelationship in a case of homocystinuria-methylmalonic acid (HC-MMA)—uria due to genetic co-factor deficiency (abstract). *Pediatr. Res.*, *18*: 247A (1984).
32. Cogan, D. G., Schulman, J., Porter, R. J., Mudd, S. H. Epileptiform ocular movements with methylmalonic aciduria and homocystinuria. *Am. J. Ophthal.*, *90*: 251–253 (1980).
33. Anthony, M., McLeay, A. C. A unique case of derangement of vitamin B_{12} metabolism. *Proc. Austrl. Assoc. Neurol.*, *13*: 61–65 (1976).
34. Shinnar, S., Singer, H. S. Cobalamin C mutation (methylmalonic aciduria and homocytinuria) in adolescence. A treatable cause of dementia and myelopathy. *N. Engl. J. Med.*, *311*: 451–454 (1984).
35. Mudd, S. H., Skovby, Fl., Levy, H. L., Pettigrew, K. D., Wilcken, B., Pyeritz, R. E., Andria, G., Boers, G.H.J., Bromberg, I. L., Cerone, R., Fowler, B., Grobe, H., Schmidt, H., Schweitzer, L. The natural history of homocytinura due to cytathionine B-synthase deficiency. *Am. J. Hum. Genet.*, *37*: 1–31 (1985).
36. Ueland, P. M., Refsum, H. Plasma homocysteine, a risk factor for vascular disease: Plasma levels in health, disease, and drug therapy. *J. Lab. Clin. Med.*, *114*: 473–501 (1989).
37. Baumgartner, R., Wick, H., Ohnacker, H., Probst, A., Maurer, R. Vascular lesion in two patients with congenital homocystinuria due to different defects of remethylation. *J. Inher. Metab. Dis.*, *3*: 101–103 (1980).
38. Wall, R. T., Harlan, J. M., Harker, L. A., Striker, G. E. Homocysteine-induced endothelial cell injury in vitro: a model for the study of vascular injury. *Thrombos. Res.*, *18*: 113–121 (1980).
39. Dudman, N.P.B., Hicks, C., Piddington, S. K., Wilcken, D.E.L. The attachment and detachment of human endothelial cells (abstract). *J. Mol. Cell. Cardiol.*, *18*: (suppl 1): 63 (1986).
40. Starkebaum G., Harian, J. M. Endothelial cell injury due to Copper-catalyzed hydrogen peroxyde generation from homocysteine. *J. Clin. Invest.*, *77*: 1370–1376 (1986).
41. De Groot, P. G., Willems, Ch., Boers, G.H.J., Gonsalves, M. D., Van Aken, W. G., van Mourik, J. A. Endothelial cell dysfunction in homocystinuria. *Eur. J. Clin. Invest.*, *13*: 405–410 (1983).

42. Bertani, T., Abbate, M., Zoja, C., Corna, D., Remuzzi G. Sequence of glomerular changes in experimental endotoxemia: A possible model of hemolytic uremic syndrome. *Nephron, 53*: 330–337 (1989).
43. McGrath, J. M., Stewart, G. J. The effects of endotoxin on vascular endothelium. *J. Exp. Med., 129*: 833–848 (1969).
44. Harlan, J. M., Harker, L. A., Reidy, M. A., Gajdusek, C. M., Schwartz, S. M., Striker, G. E. Lipopolysaccharide-mediated bovine endothelial cell injury in vitro. *Lab. Invest., 48*: 269–274 (1983).
45. Harker, L. A., Slichter, S. J., Scott, C. R., Ross, R. Homocysteinemia: Vascular injury and arterial thrombosis. *N. Engl. J. Med., 291*: 537–543 (1974).
46. Hladovec, J. Experimental homocysteinemia, endothelial lesions and thrombosis. *Blood Vessels, 16*: 202–205 (1979).
47. McCully, K. S., Vezeridis, M. P. Histopathological effects of homocysteine thiolactone on epithelial and stromal tissues. *Exp. Mol. Pathol., 51*: 159–170 (1989).
48. Graeber, J. E., Slott, J. H., Ulane, R. E., Schulman, J. D., Stuart, M. J. Effect of homocysteine and homocystine on platelet and vascular arachidonic acid metabolism. *Pediatr. Res., 16*: 490–493 (1982).
49. Walters, M.D.S., Levin M., Smith, C., Nokes, T.J.C., Hardisty, R. M., Dillon, M. J., Barratt, T. M. Intravascular platelet activation in the hemolytic uremic syndrome. *Kidney Int., 33*: 107–115 (1988).
50. Wilcken, D.E.L., Dudman, N.P.B. Mechanisms of thrombogenesis and accelerated atherogenesis in homocystinaemia. *Haemostasis, 19* (suppl 1): 14–23 (1989).
51. Chavers, B. M., Wells, T. G., Burke, B. A., Mauer, S. M. De novo hemolytic uremic syndrome following renal transplantation. *Pediatr. Nephrol., 4*: 62–64 (1990).
52. Higginbottom, M. C., Sweetman, L., Nyhan, W. L. A syndrome of methylmalonic aciduria, homocytinuria, megaloblastic anemia and neurologic abnormalities in a vitamin B_{12}-deficient breast-fed infant of a strict vegetarian. *N. Engl. J. Med., 299*: 317–323 (1978).
53. Chouraqui, J. P., Roy, C. C., Brochu, P., Gregoire, H., Morin, C. L., Weber, A. M. Ménétrier's disease in children: report of a patient and review of sixteen other cases. *Gastroenterology, 80*: 1042–1047 (1981).
54. Qizilbash, A. H. Gastritis cystica and carcinoma arising in old gastrojejunostomy stoma. *Can. Med. Assoc. J., 112*: 1432–1433 (1975).
55. Lipper, S., Kahn, L. B. Superficial cystic gastritis with alopecia. *Arch. Pathol. Lab. Med., 101*: 432–436 (1977).

22
Cancer- and Chemotherapy-Associated Thrombotic Microangiopathy

Anthony J. Murgo *Center for Drug Evaluation and Research, Food and Drug Administration, Rockville, Maryland*

Microangiopathic hemolytic anemia (MAHA), typical of that seen in a variety of disorders affecting small blood vessels, such as thrombotic thrombocytopenic purpura (TTP), hemolytic uremic syndrome (HUS), malignant hypertension, and vasculitis, is an occasional complication of neoplastic disease (1). There are several different clinical settings in which this may occur. Certain vascular tumors, such as giant hemangioma and hemangioendothelioma, may cause MAHA (2–5). MAHA may occasionally occur in disseminated intravascular coagulation (DIC), a common complication of sepsis and certain types of malignancies, such as prostate cancer, pancreatic carcinoma, and acute promyelocytic leukemia (6). However, there are two conditions in the cancer patient in which thrombotic microangiopathy (TMA) and MAHA are characteristic features. The first was initially described by Brain et al. in 1962 (1), in patients with widely metastatic carcinoma. MAHA associated with carcinoma may be considered a variant of DIC in which TMA and MAHA are the most prominent findings, often overshadowing the coagulopathy (7–9). The other syndrome is a more recently recognized complication of chemotherapy that resembles HUS and occurs most frequently in patients who have been treated with mitomycin (formerly mitomycin C; MMC) (8, 10, 11). The purpose of this chapter is to review the clinical and pathological features of these two distinctly different syndromes, TMA being common to both. Since MAHA is the most prominent feature of TMA associated with carcinoma, and renal involvement is the most characteristic feature in patients with TMA induced by chemotherapy, these syndromes are designated in this chapter as carcinoma-associated TMA/MAHA and chemotherapy-associated TMA/HUS, respectively.

This chapter was authored by Dr. Murgo in his private capacity. No official support or endorsement by the Food and Drug Administration is intended or should be inferred.

CARCINOMA-ASSOCIATED THROMBOTIC MICROANGIOPATHY/MICRANGIOPATHIC HEMOLYTIC ANEMIA

Incidence

Carcinoma is a common cause of erythrocyte fragmentation (12). The presence of increased numbers of peripheral blood schistocytes in patients with metastatic carcinoma is strongly indicative of MAHA (13). In a large prospective study, evidence of MAHA was found in 5.7% of patients with metastatic carcinoma (13). Furthermore, the detection of MAHA in a cancer patient is a strong indication of disseminated disease (13).

Since the first description of TMA/MAHA associated with carcinoma (1), there have been several extensive reviews of this syndrome (7, 8, 14). The first was published in 1979, by Antman et al. (7). These authors reviewed 55 published cases of MAHA and neoplasia, including 4 patients from their own institution; cases of giant hemangiomas and related vascular tumors producing the Kasabach–Merritt syndrome were excluded. Since then, at least 26 additional cases of carcinoma-associated TMA/MAHA have been reported (8, 14–22).

Most of the patients with carcinoma-associated TMA/MAHA are between the ages of 40 and 70 years (range 16–83). The incidence in males and females is approximately equal. Gastric carcinoma is by far the most common malignancy associated with TMA/MAHA, accounting for almost half the reported cases (Table 1). Breast and lung cancer make up 17 and 10%, respectively. With rare exception (21), patients with this syndrome have evidence of widely metastatic disease.

Pathologically, the most common types of tumors associated with TMA/MAHA are the mucin-producing adenocarcinomas (7, 13, 23); however, carcinoma-associated TMA/MAHA has been described in patients with squamous cell carcinoma of the anus (24), poorly differentiated epidermoid lung cancer (25), and undifferentiated metastatic carcinoma of unknown primary (26). Davis et al. (18) reviewed the peripheral blood smears of 167 consecutive patients with newly diagnosed small-cell undifferentiated carcinoma of the lung and identified three patients (1.8%) with MAHA. All three of these patients had extensive stage disease.

Table 1 Tumors in Carcinoma-Associated TMA/MAHA[a]

Tumor origin	Percent of cases
Gastric	47
Breast	17
Lung	10
Unknown primary	7
Prostate	4
Pancreas	4
Colon	4
Ovarian	2
Other (hepatoma, biliary, anal, seminal vesicle)	5

[a]From 81 published cases (see text).

Rauch et al. (27) reported a case of MAHA in a patient with a large mediastinal thymoma. However, such cases of TMA/MAHA associated with a nonvascular malignancy other than carcinoma are rare.

Clinical Features

The clinical onset of carcinoma-associated TMA/MAHA may be overshadowed by the symptoms of progressive malignancy (25–29). However, most patients with this syndrome present with a hemolytic anemia of abrupt onset. There are well-documented cases in which severe anemia emerged within a 2-week period (30, 31). In almost all patients, metastatic carcinoma is apparent clinically or established at necropsy. However, rare cases of localized tumors causing MAHA that improve following surgical resection have been reported (21, 27). In about a third of cases, the diagnosis of metastatic cancer is made after the patient presents with MAHA (7, 8, 14, 32).

The most common presenting symptoms of carcinoma-associated TMA/MAHA are secondary to anemia; these include fatigue, malaise, dizziness, dyspnea, and pallor. Bleeding and bruising are also common at presentation. Purpura, hematuria, and gastrointestinal bleeding occur frequently. Gastrointestinal hemorrhage may be severe, resulting in shock and death (33). Intracranial hemorrhage is a frequent complication, but usually as a preterminal or terminal event (13, 22, 29, 31, 34–36). The presenting symptoms are sometimes not clearly related to hemolysis or bleeding. The complaints of back or abdominal pain are not uncommon (7, 13, 23, 25, 29, 31, 33, 36). Occasionally, the clinical features are characteristic of chronic DIC, and venous thromboses may be prominent (6, 7, 23, 24).

The physical findings usually represent the manifestations of both the TMA/MAHA and the underlying malignancy. Fever is uncommon and usually low grade (17, 37, 38). At least a third of the patients become icteric; this is usually the result of hemolysis or liver infiltration with tumor or of an extrahepatic biliary obstruction. Severe cardiopulmonary abnormalities are unusual at presentation and are not characteristic features of this syndrome. Dyspnea commonly occurs because of anemia or intrathoracic metastasis. Tachycardia secondary to anemia is a frequent finding. However, hypertension occurs in only a small fraction of the patients (17, 23 35). Hypotension and shock may occur as a terminal event in some cases (16, 17, 38). Examination of the heart and lungs is usually unremarkable at the time of presentation; however, systolic murmurs (16, 26, 35) and x-ray evidence of cardiomegaly (16, 17) may be noted in a few patients. Hypoxemia is uncommon and usually not an early complication of the syndrome (7, 16). Hepatomegaly is a common finding, but this is often due to infiltration with metastatic disease (7, 26, 33–35, 38). Splenomegaly is less common and usually mild.

Neurological abnormalities occur quite frequently during the course of the syndrome. Headache may be a prominent complaint in some patients, occasionally at presentation (21, 33, 34, 36). Other neurological findings may include mild confusion (7, 32), obtundation (26, 34), hemiparesthesias (32, 37) hemiplegia or hemiparesis (13, 24, 39) and, terminally, coma (31, 34). Intracranial bleeding, such as subdural, subarachnoid, and intracerebral hemorrhage, is a not uncommon cause of death (13, 22, 26, 35, 36). In addition, it has been suggested that the neurological abnormalities in some patients simulate those of TTP (29).

In distinction to chemotherapy-associated TMA/HUS, renal failure is not a characteristic feature of carcinoma-associated TMA/MAHA. Rarely, the clinical picture resembles HUS (21, 40), but the pathogenesis of TMA in these patients may be distinct from typical cases of carcinoma-associated TMA/MAHA.

Laboratory Findings

The most prominent laboratory findings are those of MAHA, with or without overt evidence of intravascular coagulation. Anemia is almost always severe or moderately severe. At presentation, the hemoglobin level in more than half the patients is less than 8 g/dl and, in some, it is lower than 5 g/dl (14, 17, 23, 24, 38); rarely is the hemoglobin value in the normal range (14, 26). The peripheral smear always shows red cell fragmentation, characteristic of a microangiopathic process (e.g., schistocytes, burr cells, and helmet cells). The proportion of fragmented erythrocytes is variable, but may account for more than 20% of the total circulating red cells (13). Reticulocytosis, poikilocytosis, and polychromasia are common. Nucleated red cells are frequently seen, sometimes is great numbers (7, 16, 39). The platelet count is characteristically decreased: fewer than 50,000/μl in about half the patients at presentation. Rarely, the platelet count is in the normal range (13, 14, 23, 31); but platelet survival is probably shortened in all patients (13, 41). Most patients have a mild to moderate leukocytosis. A leukoerythroblastic blood picture, consisting of nucleated red cells, myelocytes, and metamyelocytes is a common finding (13, 16, 17, 21, 22, 36–38). Rarely, malignant cells are found in the peripheral blood smear (14).

Additional evidence of hemolysis may include an increase in indirect bilirubin values and marked elevation of serum lactic dehydrogenase levels. The serum haptoglobin concentration is usually decreased or absent, and the plasma hemoglobin level may be increased. Results of the Coombs' test (both direct and indirect) are characteristically negative. The urine may be positive for hemoglobin, and some patients have gross or microscopic hematuria or have proteinuria (7, 16, 21).

Although mild azotemia is not an uncommon finding, renal failure is not characteristic of carcinoma-associated TMA/MAHA. In some patients, the azotemia could be attributed to gastrointestinal bleeding or to genitourinary complications of malignancy, such as ureteral obstruction (31). Rarely, renal failure is a prominent feature, and the picture resembles HUS (21, 40). Serum complement levels may be normal, but data on other immunological factors are unavailable for most reported cases (27, 39).

The results of coagulation studies may be difficult to interpret. Prolongation of the prothrombin time or partial thromboplastin time, or of both, may be related to underlying liver disease or to a consumptive coagulopathy. The findings in about half the reported cases are consistent with DIC (7, 13, 14, 17, 22, 29, 33). Fibrin and fibrinogen degradation products (FDP) are usually elevated, but it is not uncommon to find no FDP or only a slight increase (i.e., <40 μg/ml) (7, 14, 23). Test results for fibrin monomers may be positive in cases in which intravascular coagulopathy is evident (22, 29). Plasma fibrinogen levels are commonly low or are in the normal range (7, 13, 23). Occasionally, fibrinogen levels are elevated, but this is not unexpected in such seriously ill patients (7, 13, 14). However, fibrinogen metabolism is probably increased in all patients, even those with normal or high levels of plasma fibrinogen (23).

Bone marrow examination usually shows erythroid hyperplasia and normal to increased numbers of megakarycotes. Malignant cells are seen in the bone marrow biopsy in about two-thirds of the cases (8, 14, 36, 38). In those patients with bone marrow invasion, normal hematopoietic precursors may be decreased (36, 38).

AUTOPSY FINDINGS

Many reported cases of carcinoma-associated TMA/MAHA include autopsy findings. Necropsy usually confirms the presence of widespread metastases, often evident on gross examination. Liver, lymph nodes, lung, bone, and bone marrow are common sites of metastases. The adrenal glands, brain, meninges, and spleen are also frequently involved. Histologically, almost all of the tumors are mucin-producing adenocarcinomas; however, exceptions have been well documented (18, 24, 26). Extramedullary hematopoiesis and hemosiderosis in the spleen and liver are frequent findings (13).

Extensive involvement of blood and lymphatic vessels is the most characteristic pathological feature. Although these lesions may be widespread (14, 16, 26, 34), the pulmonary vessels are the most frequently involved (7, 13, 14, 23). Microvascular abnormalities can be found in about 90% of patients. In about 60% of the cases, tumor emboli are seen within small pulmonary vessels, including the arterioles and the alveolar capillaries. Fibrin microthrombi are found in about half the cases, and they may be more widespread than tumor emboli. However, the most common site for fibrin microthrombi involvement is also the lung. Other common sites are the myocardium (13, 24, 29, 39) and kidneys (7, 13, 23, 33, 35, 37). Rarely are the kidneys the only site of microthrombi involvement (13), and renal involvement is usually not as extensive as in HUS (23, 42). The adrenal glands and brain are also frequently involved (13, 23, 35, 37, 39). Fibrin thrombi are often seen in close association with tumor emboli (16, 30, 33–35); however, sometimes, they can be found in organs in which tumor emboli are not observed (13, 23, 29, 37). Light and scanning electron microscopy of the microthrombi may reveal fine fibrin strands (0.2–25 μm in diameter), commonly twisted and matted together (30). These microclots frequently contain tumor cells, red cells, and white cells; however, platelets may not be apparent (30). Fibrin microthrombi that become arrested at such sites as the arteriolar–capillary junctions may not completely occlude blood flow, but they impart mechanical damage to circulating red cells (30, 43).

Another characteristic vascular feature of carcinoma-associated TMA/MAHA is hypertrophy associated with intimal hyperplasia of the small pulmonary arteries and arterioles (7). Rarely, intimal hyperplasia can be seen in tissues other than the lung (44). The prevalence of these lesions in patients with carcinoma-associated TMA/MAHA is not precisely known; however, they are described much less commonly than tumor emboli or microthrombi. Since only a small proportion of vessels may be affected, the prevalence of these lesions may be underestimated (7). Intimal hyperplasia may be seen in association with tumor emboli (7, 17, 24, 44) or fibrin thrombi (32, 37). Tumor cells may be found within the proliferating intima (7); however, pulmonary vascular hyperplasia may be absent, even in patients in whom tumor emboli and fibrin microthrombi are pronounced (7, 16).

Pathogenesis

The red cell changes in carcinoma-associated TMA/MAHA are indistinguishable from those seen in TTP, HUS, DIC, and other macrovascular disorders, such as malignant hypertension, renal cortical necrosis, and microscopic polyarteritis nodosa (1). Erythrocyte fragmentation results from direct contact of circulating red cells with fibrin microthrombi, tumor cells, and affected small arteries, arterioles, or capillaries. Thrombocytopenia can occur because of the accumulation of platelets at the site of small-vessel involvement (1, 45). Some damaged red cells and platelets are removed by the reticuloendothelial system (13, 41).

The pathogenesis of carcinoma-associated TMA-MAHA is distinguishable from other variants of DIC. Although DIC is a common complication of cancer, extensive thrombotic microangiopathy and severe hemolytic anemia is not a common feature of DIC (6, 9, 46, 47). Also, there is a discrepancy between the types of tumors that frequently cause DIC and those that are associated with MAHA. In a review by Sack et al. (6) of 182 cases of neoplasms associated with chronic DIC, the relative incidence of primary malignancies was as follows: pancreatic cancer (24%); carcinoma of the lung (20%), prostate (13%), and stomach (12%); acute leukemia (9%); carcinoma of the colon (5%), ovary (4%), and breast (0.5%). Laboratory evidence of MAHA was not a prominent finding in this series. In contrast, gastric carcinoma is by far the most common neoplasm associated with MAHA, reported in 47% of cases, whereas pancreatic and prostate cancer account for only 4% each. Finally, laboratory findings indicative of DIC are not evident in all patients with carcinoma-associated TMA/MAHA and, often, the clinical courses of DIC and MAHA are not parallel (7). In some patients, the hemolytic process progresses, despite improvement in the DIC picture with heparin therapy (25, 29).

The exact pathogenesis of TMA in carcinoma-associated TMA-MAHA is unknown. In a report by Lohrmann et al. (13), microvascular changes were identified in all of the seven patients with carcinoma-associated MAHA studied, and fibrin thrombi were found in six. These microscopic lesions resemble those seen in TTP, but are usually not as widespread (1). In six patients, mutliple tumor emboli were found within small pulmonary vessels. Similar microvascular changes have been found in most other patients reported with this syndrome (1, 7, 14, 16, 17, 23, 26, 32, 33, 35–37).

Both tumor emboli and fibrin thrombi probably play essential roles in the pathogenesis of the syndrome. Fragmentation of erythrocytes is likely to occur as they pass through arterioles containing fine fibrin strands (30, 43). However, fibrin thrombi have not been identified in every case, suggesting that other mechanisms of red cell fragmentation may be involved (7). It is conceivable that red cells are damaged by direct contact with tumor cell aggregates, but this alone is not likely responsible for the severe hemolysis that occurs. A more probable explanation for the absence of fibrin microthrombi in some specimens is that microthrombi formed in carcinoma-associated TMA/MAHA are very sensitive to fibrinolysis that occurs during the period between death and autopsy (23, 30).

Besides microthrombi and tumor emboli, other microvascular changes have been described that may contribute to red cell fragmentation. Antman et al. (7) found pronounced intimal proliferation with luminal occlusion and angiomatoid vascular formation in small pulmonary vessels containing tumor emboli. Intimal proliferation may result from endothelial cell injury that is locally induced by tumor emboli and microthrombi (48, 49). The changes are most prominently seen in the pulmonary vasculature probably because the lung is the most frequent location for tumor embolization. Also, the types of cancers most commonly associated with MAHA are those that frequently result in pulmonary tumor emboli, such as carcinoma of the stomach, breast, and lung (50, 51). Although this provides further evidence that tumor emboli play an important role in the pathogenesis of the vascular lesions and of hemolysis, other factors must be involved, since the incidence of tumor emboli at necropsy is much higher than that of MAHA (50, 51).

The development of intravascular tumor cell aggregates may be the earliest event leading to the formation of fibrin thrombi. The adhesion of tumor cells to vessel walls is essential for invasion (i.e., conversion of an embolus to a hematogenously derived metastasis). The interaction of tumor cells with the coagulation system, platelets, and inflammatory cells can promote the formation of a fibrin thrombus, which is probably necessary for adhesion (52–54). von Willebrand factor protein can bind directly to some types of tumor cells and provide a bridge between tumor cells, platelets, and the subendothelial tissue (56). The inhibition of tumor metastasis with the use of anticoagulants or by preinducing thrombocytopenia provides additional evidence for the interactive involvement of these different components (52, 57, 58).

There are several mechanisms by which tumor emboli can promote the local formation of microthrombi (Table 2). Cancer cells and their products can have profound effects on platelets and the coagulation system (52, 55, 58–61). Tumor cells produce a variety of procoagulant and platelet-activating factors that can initiate the formation of local fibrin thrombi (59, 60, 62). Some tumor cells produce substances with both procoagulant and platelet-aggregating properties (59, 63). Most tumors associated with MAHA are of the mucin-producing type, and the procoagulant properties of mucus may play an important role in fibrin thrombi formation (64). The enhanced procoagulant activity of monocytes near tumor cell aggregates may also be involved (65). Finally, the release of platelet-activating factors, possibly adenosine diphosphate (ADP), by trapped red cells may contribute to the propagation of thrombi within the microvasculature (66).

The simulation of carcinoma-associated TMA/MAHA by using experimental models in laboratory animals has helped understand the functional abnormalities of

Table 2 Pathogenesis of Carcinoma-Associated TMA/MAHA

Possible contributing factors
Microvascular tumor emboli
Tumor cell-derived procoagulants and platelet activators
Monocyte-derived procoagulants
Release of platelet activators from trapped red cells
Microvascular endothelial cell injury
Impaired local fibrinolysis

this syndrome. The intravenous inoculation of Walker carcinosarcoma 256 tumor cells into rats results in acute intravascular hemolysis (45). The discovery of tumor emboli associated with both fibrin and platelets within pulmonary arterioles and capillaries simulates the necropsy findings seen in patients with carcinoma-associated TMA/MAHA (43). Hemolysis in these animals is accompanied by a decrease in platelets and the appearance of fibrin monomers, and it is alleviated by heparin administration (45). Although only a slight decrease in plasma fibrinogen occurs, tracer studies with ^{125}I-fibronogen have shown that fibrinogen accumulates in the lungs and decreases in the plasma (45). Similarly, the catabolic rate of fibrinogen in cancer patients with MAHA is about two to three times that seen in metastatic carcinoma patients without hemolysis (23). Taken together, these results suggest that the fibrin thrombi, produced by intravascular coagulation locally at the site of tumor cell lodgment, are responsible for the MAHA associated with metastatic carcinoma.

The severe degree of TMA and hemolysis in carcinoma-associated TMA/MAHA suggests that the ability of the fibrinolytic system to counteract intravascular coagulation and to limit the formation of fibrin thrombi within the microcirculation is impaired. It has been proposed that defective local fibrinolysis may be an important mechanism by which microthrombi persist in TTP (67). Depressed activity of tissue plasminogen activator, decreased levels of protein C antigen, and increased plasminogen activator inhibitor have been found in the plasma of TTP patients (68). Tumor emboli that form in carcinoma-associated TMA/MAHA can cause local microvascular injury, resulting in a decrease in endothelial cell production of tissue plasminogen activator. Furthermore, tumor cells produce factors that can directly inhibit fibrinolysis (69). In addition, platelet antithrombin activity is decreased in about 50% of patients with advanced cancer (70). Another potential, yet unproved, mechanism for local intravascular coagulation in carcinoma-associated TMA-MAHA is vascular injury caused by tumor-related immune complexes.

In conclusion, the pathogenesis of carcinoma-associated TMA/MAHA is not clearly known. The formation of tumor cell emboli may be the earliest event leading to a complex interaction between tumor cells, coagulation factors, platelets, inflammatory cells, and vascular endothelium. The fibrin microthrombi that are formed because of this interaction are responsible for red cell fragmentation and hemolysis. Defective local fibrinolysis may be responsible for the persistence of fibrin thrombi.

Prognosis and Treatment

Patients with carcinoma-associated TMA/MAHA have an extremely poor prognosis, and most of them die within a few weeks, despite aggressive blood product support (7, 8, 14). Many patients require daily transfusions with packed cells, in the attempt to maintain adequate hemoglobin levels (13). In contrast to the high incidence of complications from blood transfusions reported in patients with chemotherapy-associated TMA/HUS (71), there is no evidence that this occurs in patients with carcinoma-associated TMA/MAHA, and withholding transfusions on this basis is unwarranted (34).

There is convincing evidence that plasma transfusions and heparinization may transiently improve coagulation parameters, platelet counts, and bleeding diatheses and, possibly, stabilize hemaglobin levels (22, 25, 29, 39). Although heparin treatment usually does not appear to affect the hemolytic process (13), this should be strongly considered in those patients with overt laboratory evidence of intravascular coagulation. ϵ-Aminocaproic acid (EACA) should not be administered, since this agent has not been clinically effective (25, 35), and it has exacerbated the hemolytic process in animal studies (45). The effects of fibrinolytic agents, such as tissue plasminogen activator and urokinase, have not been well studied in carcinoma-associated TMA/MAHA. Treatment with steroids is usually not beneficial (13, 16, 24, 25, 32, 33), but should be considered in patients with steroid-sensitive tumors. Aspirin does not seem effective; however, experience with this agent is very limited (16). In the rare cases that resemble HUS, treatment with antiplatelet agents and plasma may be effective (40). Patients with renal failure may benefit from hemodialysis.

Every possible effort should be made to reduce the tumor burden, since this is currently the only effective means of aborting the hemolytic process. Rarely, this can be accomplished surgically (21, 27). However, almost all patients have widely metastatic carcinoma that is not amenable to local therapy. If systemic treatment is indicated for the underlying malignancy, it should be initiated as soon as possible. Patients with hormone-sensitive tumors may respond to hormonal agents or manipulation. In responding patients, improvements in red cell and platelet survival may accompany tumor reduction (23, 41). Hormonal therapy may be preferable to potentially myelosuppressive cytotoxic agents in patients with metastatic breast cancer who have hormone receptor-positive tumors. However, hematological improvement has been observed in patients with a variety of cancers sensitive to chemotherapy (7, 18–20, 24).

Since the response to antitumor agents may not be immediate, clinical trials of potentially beneficial supportive measures are needed. Therapies that warrant further investigation include plasma exchange or immunoperfusion (72), administration of vincristine (73) or immunoglobulin (74), and other modalities that have shown some activity in the treatment of other types of thrombotic microangiopathy, such as TTP and HUS (68, 75). Such therapy, if successful, may temper the thrombotic and hemolytic process pending the response to specific antitumor therapy.

CHEMOTHERAPY-ASSOCIATED THROMBOTIC MICROANGIOPATHY/HEMOLYTIC UREMIC SYNDROME

Etiology and Incidence

Thrombotic microangiopathy clinically resembling HUS, and less commonly TTP, has been described in cancer patients treated with antineoplastic drugs. Chemotherapy-associated TMA/HUS is most commonly associated with the alkylating agent mitomycin. This agent accounts for at least 152 published cases of chemotherapy-associated TMA/HUS (Table 3). Although often administered in combination with fluorouracil and doxorubicin, mitomycin has been implicated as the responsible component, since use of these other agents alone has not been associated with chemotherapy-associated TMA/HUS. Also, TMA/HUS has occurred in patients who have received MMC in combination with different cytotoxic drugs (71, 76, 106, 108, 114, 120) or hormonal agents (110, 111) and MMC alone (107). Furthermore, in large randomized controlled trials, HUS occurred in patients who received an MMC-containing regimen, but not in those treated with a regimen without MMC or with placebo alone (78, 101).

Table 3 Published Cases of Mitomycin-Associated TMA/HUS

Tumor type	Number of cases	Refs.
Gastric	61	71,76–95
Colorectal	37	71,79,84,89,93,94,96–105
Breast	20	71,76,84,94,96,101,106–112
Unknown primary	7	71,84,113,114
Pancreas	6	84,104,115,116
Lung	6	84,88,102,114,117
Prostate	3	84,99
Biliary	3	90,99,104
Hepatoma	3	94,104,118
Other (hypernephroma, cervix, anal, ileal carcinoid, urinary bladder, lymphoma)	6	76,90,94,119,120
Total	152	

Source: Adapted from Ref. 8.

Chemotherapy-associated TMA/HUS can occur in patients with various types of malignancy. The most common types of malignancy associated with mitomycin-induced TMA/HUS are carcinoma of the stomach, colorectum, and breast (see Table 3); this is probably a reflection of the relative frequency in which these tumors are treated with this agent. The mediun age of patients with mitomycin-induced TMA/HUS is 52 years and there is a slight female preponderance (1.9:1).

The reported incidence of TMA/HUS following treatment with mitomycin varies from fewer than 2% to as high as 10% (78, 96, 104, 113, 116, 117, 121, 122). The incidence appears to be dose-related, rarely occurring in patients who have received less than 30 mg/m^2 or fewer than two cycles of therapy (109, 115, 122). Another, less likely, possibility is that the effect is time-dependent, rather than dose-dependent, but more of the drug is administered incidentally during a hypothetical lag period (123). The incidence of chemotherapy-associated TMA/HUS may also depend upon the specific schedule of administration (11). In fact, a protocol involving the administration of the standard total dose of MMC, but in equal fractions daily for 4 consecutive days, was discontinued because the first three patients treated developed HUS (81).

Thrombotic microangiopathy resembling HUS or TTP can occur following the administration of chemotherapeutic agents other than mitomycin. The types of malignancies in these cases vary from those associated with chemotherapy-associated TMA/HUS caused by mitomycin, a reflection of the spectrum of antitumor activity of these other agents. Platinum- and bleomycin-containing combinations are particularly common (Table 4). In patients in whom these two drugs are given in combination, it is not clear which of the two agents is responsible. Thrombotic microangiopathy has occurred following regimens containing bleomycin, but not cisplatin (130, 131) and has been reported in a patient following single-agent treatment with the cisplatin analogue, carboplatin (133). There are also rare reports of TMA occurring in association with combination chemotherapy consisting of daunorubicin, and cytarabine (cytosine arabinoside) (134); cyclophosphamide, doxorubicin, and vincristine (135,

Table 4 TMA/HUS Induced by Bleomycin- and Platinum-Containing Regimens

Regimen[a]	Number of cases	Refs.
Bleo, Vlb, Plat	5	124–126
Bleo, Vcr, Plat	4	125,127,128
Bleo, Plat	1	129
Bleo, Vlb, Vcr, Dox, Dact, Dacarb	1	130
Bleo, Vcr, Vind, Dacarb, CCNU	1	131
Bleo, Vcr, Plat, Mtx, LV, FU	1	132
Carboplatin	1	133

[a]Bleo, bleomycin; Vlb, vinblastine; Vcr, vincristine; Plat, cisplatin; Dox, doxorubicin; Dact, dactinomycin; Dacarb, dacarbazine; Vind, vindesine; Mtx, methotrexate; LV, leucovorin; FU, fluorouracil.
Source: Adapted from Ref. 8.

136); and following the administration of the investigational agents chlorozotocin (85), zinostatin (neocarcinostatin) (71), and semustine (methyl-CCNU) (137). The causal relationship of the drug or drugs to these events needs to be established.

TMA/HUS is a recently recognized complication of bone marrow transplantation (138, 139). However, it is unclear whether TMA in these cases is induced by the ablative chemotherapy regimen or by various other factors, such as cyclosporine, infectious agents, or immune phenomena. Thrombotic microangiopathy associated with bone marrow transplantation is discussed in detail in Chapter 16. The reported incidence of TMA induced by chemotherapeutic agents may increase as more clinicians become aware of this potential complication of cancer treatment.

Clinical Characteristics

The onset of mitomycin-induced TMA/HUS is usually within 4–8 weeks from the last dose of chemotherapy, but in as many as 25% of cases, there is a latent period of 4–9 months between the last dose of treatment and the onset of symptoms (11, 76, 80, 81, 91, 99, 125). The median time from the beginning of therapy to the onset of TMA/HUS is about 11.5 months (123). Most patients who develop this syndrome are in a state of clinical remission (11, 71, 94). In many patients, the chemotherapy is instituted as adjuvant treatment following surgical resection of a primary tumor (78). Patients with advanced cancer often have recently experienced tumor regression in response to chemotherapy (71, 101). It is much less common for the syndrome to occur in patients who have clinical evidence of progressive cancer (8, 11).

The clinical syndrome is characterized by the triad of MAHA, thrombocytopenia, and renal insufficiency. In addition, most patients have systemic hypertension and, frequently, develop pulmonary edema at sometime during their clinical course. The exacerbation of the hemolytic process and other features of the syndrome by blood transfusions is also a characteristic feature. Neurological abnormalities occur inconsistently, and fever is not common. The clinical syndrome that occurs with agents other than mitomycin is usually quite similar, but frequently, the picture resembles TTP more than HUS (125, 133, 134). Some patients with TMA caused by bleomycin-based regimens also experience Raynaud's phenomena (124, 125).

The initial symptoms of chemotherapy-associated TMA/HUS are variable, but usually result from severe anemia and frequently include mild dyspnea, weakness, and fatigue. Evidence of hemolytic anemia, thrombocytopenia, and azotemia are the most frequent objective findings at presentation. Rarely, mitomycin causes severe renal changes indicative of TMA, without associated MAHA (140, 141). Although thrombocytopenia may be severe, significant bleeding other than purpura is an unusual presenting feature. Oliguria is a common finding, and rarely, this can progress to anuria (107). The severity of renal insufficiency at onset is variable, but renal failure is usually progressive, and as many as a third of the patients will require supportive hemodialysis (71). Renal ultrasonography is usually unremarkable and commonly shows normal-sized kidneys (88, 99, 103, 124, 141).

Cardiopulmonary abnormalities are quite frequent and may result in significant morbidity and mortality. Systemic hypertension is often found at presentation (83, 103, 104). Severe elevations in blood pressure are common, particularly following blood transfusions or in association with worsening renal failure (71, 76, 82, 114). However, some patients with chemotherapy-associated TMA-HUS do not develop hypertension (76, 96).

Congestive heart failure has been reported frequently, particularly later in the course of the illness and often in association with worsening renal function (77, 85, 89, 105, 111, 119). Atrial arrhythmias, systolic murmurs, gallop rhythms, cardiomegaly, small pericardial effusions, pericardial friction rubs, and dependent edema have also been reported (71, 80, 98, 105, 107). Pulmonary abnormalities are quite common, especially pulmonary edema. Severe dyspnea and hypoxemia may occur, particularly following blood transfusions (71, 81, 97, 111); this has been reported to result from the administration of as little as 150 ml of packed red cells (98). Associated pulmonary findings usually include the presence of rales on physical examination and bilateral interstitial infiltrates on x-ray examination (71, 91, 97, 98, 110). The nature of the pulmonary insufficiency is not clear and is often unrelated to congestive heart failure (89, 97, 107, 110). In fact, noncardiogenic pulmonary edema is considered a characteristic feature of chemotherapy-associated TMA/HUS (71, 81, 98). Subtle pulmonary abnormalities may antecede the onset of HUS by 3–9 months (102).

The degree of central nervous system involvement with TMA is not often clinically apparent. Headache, mental confusion, and nausea are frequent symptoms (71, 77, 82, 89, 103, 107, 112); however, these symptoms may be due to severe anemia, hypertension, or renal failure. Other objective neurological findings are less consistently seen. As with other features of the syndrome, neurological abnormalities appear to be exacerbated by blood transfusions (71). Cerebral edema has been suspected in several cases (77, 82). Seizures and transient cortical blindness have been reported and may occur in association with accelerated hypertension (71, 88, 109). However, focal neurological deficits are not common, and results of computed tomographic head scans are usually negative (71, 88).

Laboratory and Pathological Findings

The hematological findings in chemotherapy-associated TMA/HUS are typical of MAHA. Anemia is usually moderately severe to severe; about 50% of patients have a hemoglobin level of 7 g/dl or less (8, 11). The peripheral smear almost always shows evidence of red cell fragmentation, with prominent schistocytosis; rarely, schistocytes are not evident (124). Additional evidence of intravascular hemolysis includes reticulocytosis, decreased plasma haptoglobin values, and elevated serum lactic dehydrogenase levels; the latter abnormality correlates very well with the hemolytic process. The serum bilirubin concentration may be normal or slightly increased, and results of the Coombs' test are characteristically negative. The white blood cell count is usually within normal limits; circulating nucleated red cells are unusual (107, 134). Almost all patients present with thrombocytopenia, and platelet counts commonly fall further during the course of the illness. Platelet counts may vary, but almost all patients have counts below 100,000/μl; in about 50% of cases the platelet count falls below 70,000/μl (8, 11). Rarely, the platelet count can be in the normal range (81, 124, 125). Bone marrow aspiration and biopsy usually show erythroid hyperplasia and normal to increased numbers of megakaryocytes, without tumor involvement. Occasionally, the marrow cellularity may be decreased, possibly because of previous chemotherapy (103, 111).

Unlike patients with carcinoma-associated TMA/MAHA, most patients with chemotherapy-associated TMA/HUS do not have evidence of disseminated intravascular coagulation (11). Prothrombin times, partial thromboplastic times, and fibrinogen levels are characteristically normal. Fibrin/fibrinogen degradation product values may be normal or only slightly increased, usually less than 40 μg/ml. Thrombin time is usually normal or mildly prolonged (71). Antithrombin III levels have been normal in the few patients studied (81, 119). Test results for fibrin monomers, such as protamine sulfate or ethanol gelation, are usually negative (81, 107, 119). Factor VIII-related antigen (von Willebrand factor) may be markedly elevated (133).

Typically, the serum creatinine is elevated at presentation, and further deterioration in renal function tests occurs during the course of the syndrome. Serum renin levels may be extremely high, consistent with reduced renal blood flow (92). Urinalysis characteristically shows microscopic hematuria and proteinuria. Granular or hyaline casts and microscopic pyuria may occasionally be seen. The amount of proteinuria may vary, but excretion of greater than 1 g in 24 h may occasionally occur (88, 106, 131). In some cases, the abnormalities in urinalysis clearly precede the onset of HUS (82, 88, 98, 137).

Usually, results of serological studies for antinuclear antibodies and rheumatoid factor are negative, and serum complement levels, including total, C3, and C4, are in the normal range (84, 86, 103, 105, 111, 131, 137). Results for antiplatelet antibodies and platelet-associated IgG may be positive (92, 101, 102, 111). Circulating immune complexes are elevated in almost all cases (11, 71, 84, 85, 101, 102). The Raji assay may be the most sensitive test for immune complexes in these patients (84), and differences in techniques may explain the negative results that are sometimes reported (79, 92, 97, 135).

Gingival biopsies are not helpful for diagnosis, since this procedure has yielded normal results in all five patients previously reported (82, 86, 111, 119). The diagnostic value of skin biopsies is unclear; in the one patient for whom the result of this test was reported, immunofluorescence was positive for fibrin (82).

Renal biopsies have been performed on many patients with TMA/HUS associated with mitomycin (80, 88, 90, 94, 103, 105). The histological changes observed in autopsy specimens are similar to those seen in the material obtained from percutaneous biopsies (71, 77, 81, 85, 100, 114). The characteristic features of TMA are present in every case and are similar to those seen in HUS from other causes. These changes are also seen in cases of chemotherapy-associated TMA/HUS associated with agents other than mitomycin (118, 125, 130, 133, 134). Light microscopy reveals microthrombi occluding a variable proportion of the glomerular capillaries and afferent arterioles. These thrombi are cytochemically reactive with special stains for fibrin (141). There is narrowing of the lumina of glomerular capillaries, arterioles, and small arteries. The glomerular tufts may appear hypocellular and shrunken and may contain focal or segmental infarcts. Wrinkling and reduplication or double contouring of the glomerular basement membrane is usually evident, and mesangial expansion and interposition are common. Endothelial and mesangial cell atypia is sometimes seen. Intimal hyperplasia and fibrinoid necrosis of arterioles are very common findings. The degree of glomerular and microvascular involvement is variable. Interstitial fibrosis, arteriosclerosis, and glomerulosclerosis may be prominent features in some patients (103, 119, 125). Tubules may contain proteinaceous casts and appear dilated and atrophic. The tubulointerstitial changes are often seen in association with marked vascular involvement. Immunofluorescence studies often demonstrate fibrin/fibrinogen deposition within damaged vessel walls and lumina, and within Bowman's space. Staining for complement components and immunoglobulin is usually nonspecific and, surprising, negative for immune complexes (80, 81, 85, 88, 103, 105, 111, 118, 119, 124). The most prominent change seen on electron microscopy is marked expansion of the glomerular basement membrane lamina rara interna (subendothelial space) with electron-lucent material (85, 103, 125, 141). Electron-dense deposits of fibrin are also often seen, particularly on the subendothelial side next to the lamina densa (Fig. 1). Aggregates of platelets, neutrophils, red blood cell frag-

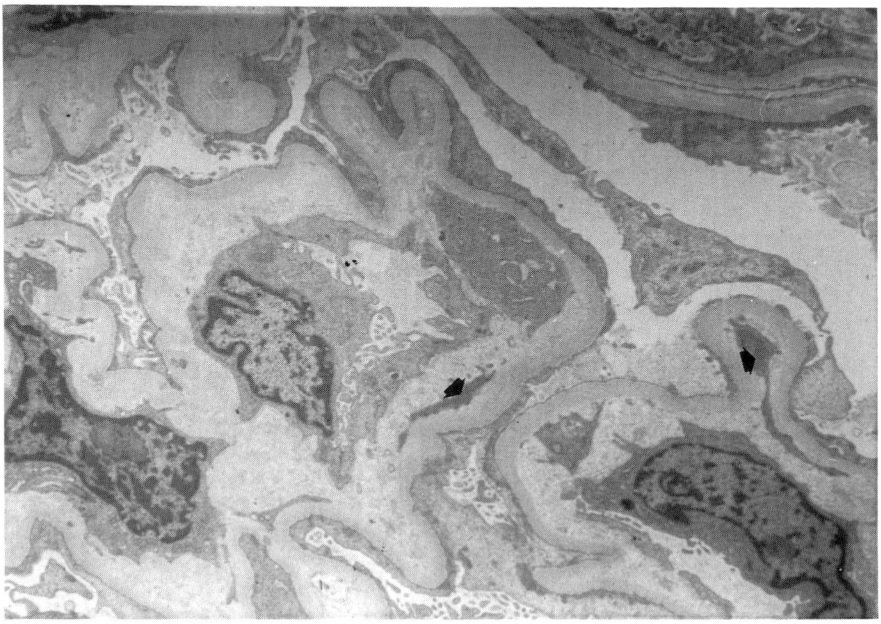

Figure 1 Electron micrograph of a glomerulus from a patient with mitomycin-induced TMA/HUS, showing pronounced widening of the lamina rara interna (subendothelial space) and narrowing of the capillary lumen. Focal osmophilic aggregates of fibrin (arrows) are noted within the lamina rara adjacent to the lamina densa (×6300). (From Ref. 108.)

ments, and other cellular debris may be seen within the subendothelial space and lumina of arterioles and capillaries (71, 80, 85, 125).

Autopsies usually reveal little or no evidence of residual cancer in most patients (71, 77, 81, 82, 85, 125); sometimes only necrotic tumor is found (118, 125). One of the most consistent findings at autopsy is pulmonary congestion; pleural effusion, hepatic congestion, and cerebral edema are not uncommon. The gross appearance of the kidneys is usually normal. Occasionally, the kidneys are symmetrically either small or swollen, and the cortical surfaces sometimes appear mottled (77, 89, 105).

The microvascular abnormalities in chemotherapy-associated TMA/HUS preponderantly involve the kidneys; occasionally, the kidneys are the only organs involved. Infrequently, the degree of extrarenal involvement is minimal, with the lung and brain being the most common sites. In a few cases, extrarenal involvement with microthrombi is widespread and severe, with associated microinfarcts and hemorrhages in the involved tissues (81, 125, 134). Pulmonary arteriolar intimal hyperplasia and septal capillary angiomatoid changes may be prominent in some cases, but interstitial pneumonitis and fibrosis are unusual (71, 77, 89, 97, 110).

Pathogenesis

The pathogenesis of chemotherapy-associated TMA/HUS is unclear. However, it can be distinguished from that of carcinoma-associated TMA/MAHA, since tumor microemboli are probably not involved, and many patients with chemotherapy-associated TMA/HUS have minimal or no evidence of residual cancer at the onset of the syndrome. Also, the chemotherapy-related syndrome is characterized by distinctly different clinical manifestations, such as renal failure, pulmonary edema, and adverse reactions to blood transfusions. The mechanism by which blood transfusions exacerbate the syndrome is as yet unclear; but there is suggestive evidence that transfusions trigger intravascular coagulation, which enhances the development of microvascular lesions (115). However, DIC is not likely to be the precipitating event, because coagulation studies are characteristically normal in patients with this syndrome. There is considerable evidence to suggest that the pathogenesis of TMA in chemotherapy-associated TMA/HUS involves a combination of factors that cause microvascular injury. These include the formation of cancer-related host factors, such as immune complexes, and drug toxicity.

Mitomycin, which is the most common agent associated with this syndrome, is an alkylating agent with activity against a variety of gastrointestinal tumors, non-small–cell lung cancer, breast cancer, transitional cell carcinoma of the bladder, and several types of squamous cell malignancies (142). The major toxic effects of mitomycin include bone marrow suppression, interstitial pneumonitis, and renal failure. However, interstitial pneumonitis or fibrosis does not usually occur in chemotherapy-associated TMA/HUS. The nature of noncardiogenic pulmonary edema, which is common in patients with chemotherpay-associated TMA/HUS, remains unclear; however, it is conceivable that chemotherapy toxicity and local fibrin formation contribute to pulmonary vascular endothelial cell injury, resulting in edema (85). The incidence of nephrotoxicity from mitomycin is 8–10% and appears to be dose-related; about 50% of patients with renal toxicity develop the other manifestations of HUS (100, 104, 143).

The etiological role of MMC in chemotherapy-associated TMA/HUS is supported by an animal model in which the perfusion of the drug into the isolated rat kidney results in lesions that resemble the TMA of HUS (144). Furthermore, mitomycin may have direct effects on endothelial cell function. Treatment of human umbilical cord endothelial cells in vitro with nonlethal concentrations of MMC decreases thrombin-induced synthesis of prostacyclin (145). Decreased prostacyclin production may play a role in the pathogenesis of thrombotic microangiopathy by promoting platelet aggregation and local intravascular coagulation (146). The role of other abnormalities affecting prostacyclin activity, such as the degree of binding to plasma components and the presence of plasma factors inhibiting production, requires further investigation (147).

Theoretically, endothelial cell damage by chemotherapeutic agents such as mitomycin can cause a decrease in tissue plasminogen activator or an increase in plasminogen activator inhibitor; this can result in defective fibrinolysis and the promotion of local fibrin deposition. The finding of elevated levels of von Willebrand factor antigen in the plasma of patients who have received antineoplastic agents that potentially induce TMA is further evidence that these drugs can cause endothelial cell perturbation (129, 133). Additional studies are required to determine whether abnormalities in von Willebrand factor patterns play a role in the pathogenesis of chemotherapy-associated TMA/HUS, as proposed for some cases of HUS from other causes or chronic relapsing TTP (75). Likewise, it is not known if other clotting factors are involved. The treatment of breast cancer patients with combination chemotherapy consisting of cyclophosphamide, methotrexate, and flourouracil results in decreased plasma levels of protein C and protein S, which may explain the increased incidence of thrombosis observed in this population (148). Whether a depression in the levels of these natural anticoagulants plays a role in the pathogenesis of chemotherapy-associated TMA/HUS has not been established.

Mitomycin and other agents associated with TMA/HUS, such as bleomycin- and cisplatin-containing regimens, have been reported to cause renal vascular changes, without evidence of TMA or MAHA (10, 100, 124, 149). It is proposed that factors besides direct drug-induced microvascular injury are involved in the pathogenesis of chemotherapy-assocated TMA/HUS. These other factors may be immunological. Plasma levels of immune complexes may be higher in patients with mitomycin-associated TMA/HUS than in patients with carcinoma who do not have the syndrome (71). The formation of these immune complexes probably precedes the syndrome and, presumably, levels increase when tumor burden (antigen) diminishes in response to chemotherapy or after surgery (150). These complexes are made up of IgG, complement, and a glycoprotein antigen. Antibodies eluted from these complexes do not bind to MMC; however, they react specifically with adenocarcinoma cells, but not with normal tissue (71, 150). Immune complexes obtained from patients with chemotherapy-associated TMA/HUS, but not those from patients with adenocarcinoma without the syndrome, cause the aggregation of normal platelets in vitro (71, 84). These circulating immune complexes may result in the in vitro aggregation of platelets and participate in endothelial cell injury and microvascular thrombosis. Furthermore, endothelial cell damage by circulating immune complexes can decrease tissue plasminogen activator and stimulate plasminogen activator inhibitor, resulting in a net impairment of fibrinolysis, thereby promoting local microthrombi formation (151). However, the exact role that circulating immune complexes play in the pathogenesis of chemotherapy-associated TMA/HUS requires further study.

Prognosis and Treatment

The case fatality rate of TMA/HUS induced by mytomycin is 60–70%, and the median time to death is about 4 weeks (8, 11, 89). Early deaths, such as those occurring within the first few months, are usually related to direct complications of the syndrome, especially severe renal or pulmonary failure (8, 11, 71, 81, 88, 97, 110). The development of pulmonary edema portends a very poor prognosis (89). Sepsis may be responsible for the death of some patients (71, 88, 89, 105). Many of the patients who succumb early are found to be without residual tumor! Some of the patients who survive longer may undergo a partial or complete amelioration of the hemolytic process and thrombocytopenia, but often renal insufficiency continues, and maintenance hemodialysis is required (76, 87, 99, 103, 119). A few patients may experience a complete recovery without recurrence of HUS (92, 96, 99, 135, 150). Some of the long-term survivors of the syndrome may later develop recurrent cancer and die of metastatic disease (76, 92, 96, 99).

Because the prognosis may be better for those patients with chemotherapy-associated TMA/HUS in whom the diagnosis is made early (76), the responsible agent should be stopped at the earliest indication of the syndrome. In patients receiving mitomycin, renal function should be monitored closely; this especially applies to patients who have received relatively large cumulative doses of the drug. Urinalysis may be useful, since the development of proteinuria or hematuria may be the earliest indication of nephrotoxicity and precede other signs of TMA/HUS (82, 88, 98, 137). The peripheral smear should be observed for the presence of schistocytes, which may signal the onset of MAHA.

In patients with chemotherapy-associated TMA/HUS, red blood cell transfusions should be avoided, since these usually do not result in a sustained improvement in hematocrit and are likely to exacerbate the syndrome; this also applies to the transfusion of washed cells (96). If transfusions with red cells are deemed necessary, they should be administered slowly, and the patient should be monitored very carefully. The value of low-dose heparin in the prevention of transfusion complications has been suggested, but warrants further investigation (115); otherwise, the administration of heparin appears to be ineffective in the treatment of the syndrome (81, 100). Given our current understanding of the pathogenesis of this disorder, platelet transfusions generally should be avoided.

Many cases demand intensive medical management, especially those patients with severe pulmonary and renal failure. Dialysis is often required. Antihypertensive drugs are indicated for the treatment of accelerated high blood pressure (71); diuretics and inotropic agents should be tried in patients with pulmonary edema (98). Angiotensin-converting enzyme inhibitors may be effective in improving the blood pressure and urine output in patients with severe renal failure, particularly when the serum renin levels are very high (92).

Therapy of chemotherapy-associated TMA/HUS has been minimally effective. Treatment modalities that have been studied in other forms of HUS and TTP have also been used empirically in patients with chemotherapy-associated TMA/HUS, with questionable success. The benefits of individual types of treatments are difficult to assess for several reasons. First, the number of patients treated with any particular regimen has been too small, and controlled studies have not been done. Second, since most patients have been treated with a combination of modalities, it is often not possible to evaluate the effects of the individual agents. Lastly, the various treatments have been administered at different stages in the course of the syndrome, making historical data difficult to interpret.

Treatment with steroids is usually not beneficial (82, 88, 92, 98, 102, 108, 109, 141, 150). However, it has been suggested that the administration of steroids concomitantly with mitomycin may lower the risk of developing HUS (152); whether or not steroids are protective needs to be confirmed with prospective randomized, controlled trials. The role of immunomodulatory agents in the treatment of chemotherapy-associated TMA/HUS is not clear; it has been suggested that azathioprine and low-dose cyclophosphamide may be beneficial in some patients (108, 150). The vinca alkaloid, vincristine, may hold some promise in the treatment of this syndrome (99), but the mechanism of action and effectiveness and safety of this agent for this condition requires further investigation. Single-agent treatment with antiplatelet agents, such as aspirin, sulfinpyrazone, and dipyridamole, is probably not very beneficial (71, 76, 79, 86, 102, 130), but the effectiveness of these drugs should be further investigated in combination with other modalities.

Since elevated levels of circulating immune complexes may play an important role in the pathogenesis of this syndrome, it is conceivable that the removal of these complexes would be beneficial. Although plasmapheresis can successfully reduce the level of circulating immune complexes (71), a complete reversal of all of the manifestations of the syndrome is not usual (71, 76, 86–88, 98, 103, 111, 119, 125, 150). Plasma exchange has been reported to reverse the hematological abnormalities, including a rapid rise in platelet count and stabilization of hemoglobin levels; these changes may, or may not, be accompanied by a reduction in schistocytes (103). However, renal failure is not reversed in most patients, despite hematological recovery (71, 86, 103, 119). Possibly, plasma exchange would have a better chance of improving renal function if it is instituted before irreversible renal vascular lesions develop (153). Nevertheless, the survival of those patients with severe renal failure may be improved with maintenance dialysis.

Another form of plasma therapy that may be very effective in removing circulation immune complexes is immunoperfusion (11, 72, 84). This procedure involves the perfusion of autologous plasma over filters containing staphylococcal protein A (SPA), covalently bound to polyacrylamide beads; the treated plasma is then reinfused into the patient. Korec et al. (84) initially reported the results of a study of this treatment in 11 patients with chemotherapy-associated TMA/HUS. There was complete clearance of circulating immune complexes in 8 patients. A significant rise in the platelet and erythrocyte counts was achieved in 9 of the 11 patients, and stabilization of progressive renal impairment occurred in 6; above all, long-term responses were observed in 7 patients. Similar beneficial effects of SPA immunoperfusion have been reported in 21 patients (11). The median survival of patients with chemotherapy-associated TMA/HUS treated with SPA immunoperfusion is about 6 months (11). Patients with no clinical evidence of residual cancer may respond better than those with large tumors. Unfortunately, SPA immunoperfusion, as with the other therapies reported, does not appear to reverse significant renal impairment (11, 72, 84), which remains as a major cause of morbidity. In any event, the results with SPA immunoperfusion may be better than those of conventional plasma exchange. Whether this indicates a true superiority of immunoperfusion or simply a reflection of selecting

Table 5 Summary of Clinicopathological Features of Cancer- and Chemotherapy-Associated TMA

Distinguishing features	Carcinoma-associated TMA/ MAHA	Chemotherapy-associated TMA/HUS
Most common tumors	Gastric, breast, lung	Gastric, colon, breast
Tumor status	Usually widely metastatic	Clinical remission common
Principal site of microvascular lesions	Lung	Kidney
Renal failure	Unusual	Characteristic
Severe hypertension	Uncommon	Common
Pulmonary edema	Unusual	Common
Adverse reactions to red cell transfusions	Not described	Common
Leukoerythroblastic picture	Common	Unusual
Laboratory evidence of DIC	Common	Usually absent
Proposed initiating factor(s)	Tumor microemboli-derived factors	Endothelial cell damage from chemotherapeutic agent and circulating immune complexes

Source: Adapted from Ref. 8.

less severely affected patients earlier in the course of the syndrome requires further study in larger groups of patients, preferably in randomized controlled trials.

CONCLUSION

Carcinoma-associated TMA/MAHA and chemotherapy-associated TMA/HUS represent two distinct syndromes in the cancer patient in whom the major pathological lesion is TMA. The distinguishing clinical and pathological features of these disorders are outlined in Table 5. The incidence of carcinoma-associated TMA/MAHA may decrease with the availability of more effective antitumor agents. For chemotherapy-associated TMA/HUS, further research is necessary to identify those individuals who are at particular risk and to discover more effective means of prevention and therapy of this often fatal complication of cancer treatment.

REFERENCES

1. Brain, M. C., Dacie, J. V., Hourhiane, D. O'B., Microangiopathic hemolytic anemia: The possible role of vascular lesions in pathogenesis. *Br. J. Haematol.*, *8*: 358–374 (1962).
2. Alpert, L.. L., Benisch, B., Hemangioendothelioma of the liver associated with microangiopathic hemolytic anemia: Report of four cases. *Am. J. Med. 48*: 624–628 (1970).
3. Case Records of the Massachusetts General Hospital (case 4-1980). *N. Engl. J. Med.*, *302*: 283–289 (1980).
4. Donald, D., Dawson, A. A., Microangiopathic haemolytic anaemia associated with malignant haemangioendothelioma. *J. Clin. Pathol.*, *24*: 456–459 (1971).

5. Inceman, S., Tangun, Y., Chronic defibrination syndrome due to a giant hemangioma associated with microangiopathic hemolytic anemia. *Am. J. Med., 46:* 997–1002 (1969).
6. Sack, G. H., Levin, J., Bell, W. R., Trousseau's syndrome and other manifestations of chronic disseminated coagulopathy in patients with neoplasms: Clinical, pathophysiologic, and therapeutic features. *Medicine, 56:* 1–37 (1977).
7. Antman, K. H., Skarin, A. T., Mayor, R. J., Hargreaves, H. K., Canellos, G. P., Microangiopathic hemolytic anemia and cancer: A review. *Medicine, 58:* 377–384 (1979).
8. Murgo, A. J., Thrombotic microangiopathy in the cancer patient including those induced by chemotherapeutic agents. *Semin. Hematol., 24:* 161–177 (1987).
9. Colman, R. W., Rubin, R. N., Disseminated intravascular coagulation due to malignancy. *Semin. Oncol. 17:* 172–186 (1990).
10. Doll, D. C., Ringenberg, O. S., Yarbro, J. W., Vascular toxicity associated with antineoplastic agents. *J. Clin. Oncol., 4:* 1405–1417 (1986).
11. Lesesne, J. V., Rothschild, N., Erickson, B., Korec, S., Sisk, R., Keller, J., Arbus, M., Woolley, P. B., Chiazze, L., Schein, P. S., Neefe, J. R., Cancer-associated hemolytic–uremic syndrome: Analysis of 85 cases from a national registry. *J. Clin. Oncol. 7:*781–789 (1989).
12. Forshaw, J., Harwood, L., Poikilocytosis associated with carcinoma. *Arch. Intern. Med., 117:* 203–205 (1966).
13. Lohrmann, H.-P., Adam, W., Heymer, B., Kubanek, B., Microangiopathic hemolytic anemia in metastatic carcinoma: Report of eight cases. *Ann. Intern. Med., 79:* 368–375 (1973).
14. Hügli, A., Beris, P., Eleven cases of neoplastic microangiopathy. *Nouv. Rev. Fr. Hematol. 31:* 223–230 (1989).
15. Brinch, L., Emblem, R., Hoel, P. S., Mikrangiopatisk hemolytisk anemi ved metastasert adenocarcinoma cardiae. *Tidsskr. Nor. Laegeforen., 104:* 739–741 (1984).
16. Case Records of the Massachusetts General Hospital (case 26-1984). *N. Engl. J. Med., 310:* 1728–1736 (1984).
17. Clinicopathologic Conference, Microangiopathic anemia and disseminated intravascular coagulation in an elderly woman. *Am. J. Med., 74:* 1052–1060 (1983).
18. Davis, S., Rambotti, P., Gringnani, F., and Steinhouse, K., Microangiopathic hemolytic anemia and pulmonary small cell carcinoma. *Ann. Intern. Med., 103:* 638 (1985).
19. Essers, U., Angelkort, B., Mikroangiopathische haemolytisch–thrombozytopenische purpura bei metastasierendem mammakarzinom erfolgreiche behandlung durch chemotherapie. *Blut, 40:* 157–159 (1980).
20. Horne, M. K., Cooper, B., Microangiopathic hemolytic anemia with metastatic adenocarcinoma: Response to chemotherapy. *South. Med. J., 75:* 503–504 (1982).
21. Marcos, O. O., Escuin, E., Miguel, J. L., Fernàndez, P. G., Fontàn, M. P., Selgas, R., Sicilia, L. S., Hemolytic syndrome in a patient with gastric adenocarcinoma: Partial recovery of renal function after gastrectomy. *Clin. Nephrol., 24:* 265–268 (1985).
22. Takeuchi, R., Kuto, M., Katayama, N., Kamio, N., Tsuda, M., Nagano, T., Wada, H., Murashima, S., Deguchi, K., Shirakawa, S., A case of carcinomatosis associated with microangiopathic hemolytic anemia (MHA) and disseminated intravascular coagulation (DIC) occurring after 12 years of operation for gastric cancer. *Rinscho Ketsueki, 24:* 1423–1429 (1983).
23. Brain, M. C., Azzopardi, J. G., Baker, L. R. I., Pineo, G. F., Roberts, P. D., Dacie, J. V., Microangiopathic haemolytic anemia and mucin-forming adenocarcinoma. *Br. J. Haematol., 18:* 183–193 (1970).
24. Tapp, E., Ralson, A., Thrombotic microangiopathy associated with squamous carcinoma. *Br. Med. J., 4:* 209–210 (1969).
25. Miller, S. P., Davison, T., Defibrination syndrome in cancer: Treatment with heparin. *N.Y. State J. Med., 67*: 452–459 (1967).
26. Clinicopathologic Conference, Congenital hemolytic jaundice corrected by splenectomy

followed twenty-six years later by bleeding tendency, hepatomegaly and sudden death. *Am. J. Med., 38:* 257–267 (1965).
27. Rauch, A. E., Tartaglia, A. P., Kaufman, B., Kausel, H., RBC fragmentation and thymoma. *Arch. Intern. Med., 144:* 1280–1282 (1984).
28. Case Records of the Massachusets General Hospital (Case 30-1987). *N. Engl. J. Med., 317:* 225–235 (1987).
29. Goodnight, S. H., Bleeding and intravascular clotting in malignancy: A review. *Ann. N.Y. Acad. Sci., 230:* 271–288 (1974).
30. Bull, B. S., Kuhn, I. N., The production of schistocytes by fibrin strands (a scanning electron microscope study). *Blood, 35:* 104–111 (1970).
31. Landaw, S. A., Hemolytic anemia as a complication of carcinoma: Case report and review of the literature. *J. Mt. Sinai Hosp., 31:* 167–178 (1964).
32. Stratford, E. C., Ranaka, K. R., Microangiopathic hemolytic anemia in metastatic carcinoma. *Arch. Intern. Med., 116:* 346–350 (1965).
33. Joseph, R. R., Day, H. J., Sherwin, R. M., and Schwartz, H. D., Microangiopathic haemolytic anaemia associated with consumption coagulopathy in a patient with disseminated carcinoma. *Scand. J. Haematol., 4:* 271–282 (1967).
34. Cohan, M., Pittman, G., Hoffman, G. C., Hemolytic anemia, tumor cell emboli, and intravascular coagulation. *Arch. Pathol., 93:* 305–307 (1972).
35. Seligsohn, U., Weber, H., Yoran, C., Horowitz, A., Ramot, B., Microangiopathic hemolytic anemia and defibrination syndrome in metastatic carcinoma of the stomach. *Isr. J. Med., 4:* 69–75 (1968).
36. Lynch, E. C., Bakken, C. L., Casey, T. H., Alfrey, C. P., Microangiopathic hemolytic anemia in carcinoma of the stomach. *Gastroenterology, 52:* 88–93 (1967).
37. Brook, M., Konwaler, B. E., Thrombotic thrombocytopenic purpura: Association with gastric carcinoma and a possible auto-immune disorder. *Calif. Med., 102:* 222–227 (1965).
38. Ballas, S. K., Rubin, R. N., Case report: Microangiopathic hemolytic anemia and thrombocytopenia with disseminated cancer. *Postgrad. Med., 60:* 180–181 (1976).
39. Rodriguez, J. M., Stevenson, T. D., Chronic intravascular coagulation and microangiopathic hemolytic anemia in a patient with carcinoma of the lung. *Ohio State Med. J., 65:* 1010–1016 (1969).
40. Milutinovic, J., Irby, S., Fisher, M., Hemolytic uremic syndrome and metastatic malignancy. *South. Med. J., 75:* 1409–1411 (1982).
41. Propp, R., Microangiopathic anemia and thrombocytopenia in disseminated breast cancer. *Clin. Res., 14:* 324 (1966).
42. Vitsky, B. H., Suzuki, Y., Strauss, L., Churg, J., The hemolytic–uremic syndrome: A study of renal pathologic alternations. *Am. J. Pathol. 57:* 627–647 (1969).
43. Bull, B. S., Rubenberg, M. L., Dacie, J. V., Brain, M. C., Microangiopathic haemolytic anemia: Mechanisms of red-cell fragmentation: In vitro studies. *Br. J. Haematol., 14:* 643–652 (1968).
44. Sakamoto, S., Shibata, A., Onodera, S., Miuri, A. B., Suzuki, A., Suzuki, C., Mouri, T., A case of microangiopathic hemolytic anemia due to disseminated metastasis of gastric cancer. *Acta Haematol. (Jpn)., 31:* 307–317 (1968).
45. Hilgard, P., Gordon-Smith, E. C., Microangiopathic haemolytic anaemia and experimental tumour-cell emboli. *Br. J. Haematol., 26:* 651–659 (1974).
46. Jacobson, R. J., Jackson, D. P., Erythrocyte fragmentation in defibrination syndromes. *Ann. Intern. Med., 81:* 207–209 (1974).
47. Sun, N. C. J., Bowie, E. J. W., Kazmire, F. J., Elveback, L. R., Owen, C. A., Blood coagulation studies in patients with cancer. *Mayo Clin. Proc., 49:* 636–641 (1974).
48. Case Records of the Massachusetts General Hospital (case 43-1980). *N. Engl. J. Med., 303:* 1049–1056 (1980).
49. Malik, A. B., Thrombin-induced endothelial injury. *Semin. Thromb. Hemost., 12:* 184–196 (1986).

50. Gonzalez-Vitale, J. C., Garcia-Bunuel, R., Pulmonary tumor emboli and cor pulmonali in primary carcinoma of the lung. *Cancer, 38:* 2105–2110 (1976).
51. Winterbauer, R. H., Elfenbein, I. B., Ball, W. C., Incidence and clinical significance of tumor embolization to the lungs. *Am. J. Med., 45:* 271–290 (1968).
52. Gasic, G. J., Gasic, T. B., Galanti, N., Johnson, T., Murphy, S., Platelet-tumor cell interactions in mice. The role of platelets in the spread of malignant disease. *Int. J. Cancer., 11:* 704–718 (1973).
53. Ketcham, A. S., Sugerbaker, E. V., Ryan, J. J., Orme, S. K., Clotting factors and metastasis. *Am. J. Roentgenol. Radium Ther. Nucl. Med., 3:* 42–47 (1971).
54. Warren, B. A., Vales, O., The adhesion of thromboplastic tumour emboli to vessel walls in vivo. *Br. J. Exp. Pathol. 53:* 301–313 (1972).
55. Zacharski, L. R., Memoli, V. A., Rousseau, S. M., Coagulation–cancer interaction in situ in renal cell carcinoma. *Blood, 68:* 394–399 (1986).
56. Floyd, C. M., Irani, K., Kessler, C. M., von Willebrand factor protein (vWF) interacts specifically with human tumor cells (TCs). *Blood, 68*(Suppl. 1): *346*a (1986).
57. Maat, B., Hilgard, P., Anticoagulants and experimental metastases: Evaluation of antineoplastic effects in different model systems. *J. Cancer Res. Clin. Oncol., 101:* 275–283 (1981).
58. Rickles, F. R., Hancock, W. W., Edwards, R. L., Zacharski, L. R., Antimetastatic agents. I. Role of cellular procoagulants in the pathogenesis of fibrin deposition in cancer and the use of anticoagulants and/or antiplatelet drugs in cancer treatment. *Semin. Thromb. Hemost. 14:* 88–94 (1988).
59. Grignani, G., Falanga, A., Pacchiarini, L., Alessio, M. G., Zucchella, M., Fratino, P., Donati, M. B., Human breast and colon carcinomas express cysteine proteinase activities with pro-aggregating and pro-coagulant properties. *Int. J. Cancer, 42:* 554–557 (1988).
60. Mohanty, D., Hilgard, P., A new platelet aggregating material (PAM) in an experimentally induced rat fibrosarcoma. *Thromb. Haemost. 51:* 192–195 (1984).
61. Grignani, G., Jamieson, G. A., Platelets in tumor metastasis: Generation of adenosine diphosphate by tumor cells is specific but unrelated to metastatic potential. *Blood, 71:* 844–849 (1988).
62. Rickles, F. R., Edwards, R. L., Activation of blood coagulation in cancer: Trousseau's syndrome revisited. *Blood, 62:* 14–31 (1983).
63. Cavanaugh, P. G., Sloane, B. F., Honn, K. V., Role of the coagulation system in tumor-cell–induced platelet aggregation and metastasis. *Hemostasis, 18:* 37–46 (1988).
64. Pineo, G. F., Brain, M. C., Gallus, A. S., Hirsh, J., Hatton, M. W. C., Regoeczi, E., Tumors, mucus production, and hypercoagulability. *Ann. N.Y. Acad. Sci., 230:* 262–270 (1974).
65. Morgan, D., Edwards, R. L., Rickes, F. R., Monocyte procoagulant activity as a peripheral marker of clotting activation in cancer patients. *Hemostasis, 18:* 55–65 (1988).
66. Valles, J., Santos, M. T., Aznar, J., Marcus, A. J., Martinez-Sales, V., Portoles, M., Broekman, M. J., Safier, L. B., Erythrocytes metabolically enhance collagen-induced platelet responsiveness via increased thromboxane production, adenosine diphosphate release and recruitment. *Blood, 78:* 154–162 (1991).
67. Kwaan, H. C., The pathogenesis of thrombotic thrombocytopenic purpura. *Semin. Thromb. Hemost., 3:* 184–198 (1979).
68. Glas-Greenwalt, P., Hall, J. M., Panke, T. W., Kant, K. S., Allen, C. M., Pollak, V. E., Fibrinolysis in health and disease: Abnormal levels of plasminogen activator, plasminogen activator inhibitor, and protein C in thrombotic thrombocytopenic purpura. *J. Lab. Clin. Med., 108:* 415–422 (1986).
69. Yuen, P., Kwaan, H. C., Fibrinolytic activity in human tumor tissues. *Cancer Invest., 1:* 369–378 (1983).

70. Sloand, E. M., Kenney, D. M., Choa, F. C., Lawler, J., Tulis, J. L., Platelet antithrombin defect in malignancy: Platelet protein alterations. *Blood, 69:* 479–485 (1987).
71. Cantrell, J. E., Phillips, T. M., Schein, P. S., Carcinoma-associated hemolytic–uremic syndrome: A complication of mitomycin-C chemotherapy. *J. Clin. Oncol., 3:* 723–734 (1985).
72. Mittelman, A., Bertram, J., Henry, D. H., Snyder, H. W., Messerschmidt, G. L., Ciavarella, D., Ainsworth, S., Kiprov, D., Arlin, Z., Treatment of patients with HIV thrombocytopenia and hemolytic uremic syndrome with protein A (Prosorba column) immunoadsorption. *Semin. Hematol., 26*(Suppl. 1): 15–18 (1989).
73. Gutterman, L. A., Stevenson, T. D., Treatment of thrombotic thrombocytopenic purpura with vincristine. *JAMA, 247:* 1433–1436 (1982).
74. Wong, P., Itoh, K., Yoshida, S., Treatment of thrombotic thrombocytopenia purpura with intravenous gamma globulin. *N. Engl. J. Med., 314:* 385–386 (1986).
75. Byrnes, J. J., Moake, J. L., Thrombotic thrombocytopenic purpura and haemolytic–uremic syndrome: Evolving concepts of pathogenesis and therapy. *Clin. Haematol., 15:* 413–442 (1986).
76. Chow, S., Roscoe, J., Cattran, D. C., Plasmapheresis and antiplatelet agents in the treatment of hemolytic uremic syndrome secondary to mitomycin. *Am. J. Kidney Dis., 7:* 407–412 (1986).
77. Crocker, J., Jones, E. L., Haemolytic–uraemic syndrome complicating long-term mitomycin C and 5-fluorouracil therapy for gastric carcinoma. *J. Clin. Pathol., 36:* 24–29 (1983).
78. Fielding, J. W. L., Fagg, S. L., Jones, B. G., Ellis, D., Hockey, M. S., Minawa, A., Brookes, V. S., Craven, J. L., Mason, M. C., Timothy, A., Waterhouse, J. A. H., Wrigley, P. F. M., An interim report of a prospective, randomized, controlled study of adjuvant chemotherapy in operable gastric cancer: British Stomach Cancer Group. *World J. Surg., 7:* 390–399 (1983).
79. Ito, S., Hirono, S., Two cases with microangiopathic hemolytic anemia caused by anti-cancer drugs who improved rapidly after administration of aspirin and dipyridamole. *Rinsho Ketsueki, 23:* 730–735 (1982).
80. Jao, W., Manaligod, J. R., Renal disease associated with mitomycin therapy. *Ultrastruct. Pathol., 5:* 83–88 (1983).
81. Jolivet, J., Giroux, L., Laurin, S., Gruber, J., Bettez, P., Band, P. R., Microangiopathic hemolytic anemia, renal failure, and non-cardiogenic pulmonary edema: A chemotherapy induced syndrome. *Cancer Treat. Rep., 67:* 429–434 (1983).
82. Jones, B. G., Fielding, J. W., Newman, C. E., Howell, A., Brookes, V. S., Intravascular haemolysis and renal impairment after blood transfusion in two patients on long-term 5-fluorouracil and mitomycin-C. *Lancet, 1:* 1225–1226 (1980).
83. Karlin, D. A., Stroehlein, J. E., Rash, nephritis, hypertension, and haemolysis in patient on 5-fluorouracil, doxorubicin, and mitomycin-C. *Lancet, 2:* 534–535 (1980).
84. Korec, S., Schein, P. S., Smith, F. P., Neefe, J. R., Woolley, P. V., Godberg, R. M., Phillips, T. M., Treatment of cancer-associated hemolytic syndrome with staphylococcal protein A immunoperfusion. *J. Clin. Oncol., 4:* 210–215 (1986).
85. Kressel, B. R., Ryan, K. P., Duong, A. T., Berenberg, J., Schein, P. S., Microangiopathic hemolytic anemia, thrombocytopenia, and renal failure in patients treated for adenocarcinoma. *Cancer, 48:* 1738–1745 (1981).
86. Lempert, K. D., Haemolysis and renal impairment syndrome in patients on 5-fluorouracil and mitomycin-C. *Lancet, 2:* 369–370 (1980).
87. Lyman, N. W., Michaelson, R., Viscuso, R. L., Winn, R., Mulgoankar, S., Jacobs, M. G., Mitomycin-induced hemolytic-uremic syndrome: Successful treatment with corticosteroids and intense plasma exchange. *Arch. Intern. Med., 143:* 1617–1618 (1983).

88. Peterson, K. B., Smith, W. E., Mitomycin induced hemolytic-uremic syndrome. *Samaratan Med., 2:* 17–20 (1984).
89. Sheldon, R., Slaughter, D., A syndrome of microangiopathic hemolytic anemia, renal impairment, and pulmonary edema in chemotherapy-treated patients with adenocarcinoma. *Cancer, 58:* 1428–1436 (1986).
90. Simon, P., Hervé, J.-P., Ramee, M.-P., Leroy, J. P., Ang, K. S., Leguy, P., Vignoud, J., Cledes, J., La nephrotoxicité de la mitomycine C: Trois nouvelles observations et revue de la litterature. *Nephrologie, 3:* 152–157 (1982).
91. Van Spreeuwel, J. P., Hemrika, M. H., De Maat, C. E. M., Nadorp, J. H. S. M., Letters to the editor. *Neth. J. Med., 26:* 287–288 (1983).
92. Verwey, J., Boven, E., van der Meulen, J., Pinedo, H. M., Recovery from mitomycin C-induced hemolytic uremic syndrome: A case report. *Cancer, 54:* 2878–2881 (1984).
93. Nicolàs, J. M., Villalta, J., Gonzàlez-Clemente, J. M., Antùnez, E., Almirall, J., Bosch, J., Torras, A., Urbano-Màrquez, Y. A., Mitomycin C induced hemolytic uremic syndrome. Presentation of a series of 5 cases and literature review. *Rev. Clin. Esp., 186:* 166–170 (1990).
94. Cordonnier, D., Vert-Pré, F. C., Bayle, F., Alix, J. L., Couderc, P., La Néphrotoxicité de la mitomycine C (à propos de 25 observations). *Néphrologie, 6:* 19–26 (1985).
95. Giroux, L., Bettez, P., Giroux, L., Mitomycin-C nephrotoxicity: A clinico-pathologic study of 17 cases. *Am. J. Kidney Dis., 6:* 28–39 (1985).
96. Bruntsch, U., Groos, G., Tigges, F.-J., Gallmeier, W. M., Microangiopathic hemolytic anemia, a frequent complication of mitomycin therapy in cancer patients. *Eur. J. Cancer Clin. Oncol., 20:* 905–909 (1984).
97. Chang-Poon, V. Y.-H., Hwang, W. S., Wong, A., Berry, J., Klassen, J., Poon, M.-C., Pulmonary angiomatoid vascular changes in mitomycin C-associated hemolytic–uremic syndrome. *Arch Pathol. Lab. Med., 109:* 877–878 (1985).
98. Claycomb, C. L., Berkovic, M., Microangiopathic hemolytic anemia, noncardiac pulmonary edema, and renal failure after treatment of metastatic adenocarcinoma of the colon with 5-fluorourcil and mitomycin-C: Report of a case. *J. Am. Osteopath. Assoc., 86:* 499–503 (1986).
99. Grem, J. L., Merrit, J. A., Carbone, P. P., Treatment of mitomycin-associated microangiopathic hemolytic anemia with vincristine. *Arch. Intern. Med., 146:* 566–568 (1986).
100. Hanna, W. T., Krauss, S., Regester, R. F., Murphy, W. M., Renal disease after mitomycin C therapy. *Cancer, 48:* 2588–2588 (1981).
101. Proia, A. D., Harden, E. A., Silberman, H. R., Mitomycin-induced hemolytic uremic syndrome. *Arch. Pathol. Lab. Med., 108:* 959–962 (1984).
102. Laufman, L., Courter, S., Pritchard, J., Fatal mitomycin C (MMC) syndrome heralded by pulmonary symptoms. *Proc. Am. Soc. Clin. Oncol., 2:* 197 (1983).
103. Price, T. M., Murgo, A. J., Keveney, J. J., Miller-Hardy, D., Kasprisin, D. O., Renal failure and hemolytic anemia associated with mitomycin C. *Cancer, 55:* 51–56 (1985).
104. Valavaara, R., Nordman, E., Renal complications of mitomycin C therapy with special reference to the total dose. *Cancer, 55:* 47–50 (1985).
105. Willie, G. R., Levy, S. M., Michaels, R. S., Zirkin, R. M., Hemolytic–uremic syndrome in a patient receiving mitomycin C and 5-fluorouracil. *Henry Ford Hosp. Med. J., 31:* 104–109 (1983).
106. Bayle, F., Vialtel, P., Bastrenta, F., Swiercz, P., Dechelette E., Pin, I., Carpentier, P., Mousseau, M., Schaerer, R., Couderc, P., Cordonnier, D. Microangiopathie thrombotique et insuffisance renale chronique par la mitomycine c chez 4 femmes traitees pour cancer du sein. *Nouv. Presse Med., 11:* 2300–2301 (1982).
107. Boven, E., Pinedo, H. M., Mitomycin-C: Interstitial pneumonitis and haemolytic–uremic syndrome: A report of two cases and review of the literature. *Neth. J. Med., 26:* 153–155 (1983).

108. Hug, V., Burgess, A., Blumenshein, G., Hortobagyi, G., Cohen, A. G., Effects of cyclophosphamide on the mitomycin-induced syndrome of thrombotic thrombocytopenic purpura. *Cancer Treat. Rep., 69:* 565–566 (1985).
109. Khojasteh, A., Reynolds, R. D., Garcia, A. R., Walter, J., Hemolytic uremic-like syndrome following a single dose of mitomycin-C. *Proc. Am. Soc. Clin. Oncol., 3:* 4 (1984).
110. Loprinzi, C. L., Mitomycin C-induced pulmonary and renal toxicities. *Wis. Med. J., 83:* 16–17 (1984).
111. Rabaldi, S. J., Khandekar, J. D., Miller, H. J., Mitomycin-induced hemolytic uremic syndrome: Case presentation and review of the literature. *Cancer Treat. Rep., 66:* 1244–1247 (1982).
112. Rumpf, K. W., Rieger, J., Lankisch, P. G., von Heyden, H. W., Nagel, G. A., Scheler, F., Mitomycin-induced haemolysis and renal failure. *Lancet, 2:* 1037–1038 (1980).
113. Goldberg, R. M., Smith, F. P., Ueno, W., Ahlgren, J. D., Schein, P. S., 5-Fluorouracil, Adriamycin, and mitomycin in the treatment of adenocarcinoma of unknown primary. *J. Clin. Oncol., 4:* 395–399 (1986).
114. Pavy, M. D., Wiley, E. L., Abeloff, M. D., Hemolytic–uremic syndrome associated with mitomycin therapy. *Cancer Treat. Rep., 66:* 457–461 (1982).
115. Agnelli, G., Greseli, P., Nenci, G. G., Clotting activation after blood transfusion in patients receiving 5-fluorouracil and mitomycin-C treatment. *Cancer Chemother. Pharmacol., 5:* 205–206 (1981).
116. Krauss, S., Sonoda, T., Solomon, A., Treatment of advanced gastrointestinal cancer with 5-fluorouracil and mitomycin C. *Cancer, 43:* 1598–1603 (1979).
117. Chahinian, A. P., Perlow, L., Goldberg, J., Johnson, J., Holland, J. F., Alternating combinations (MEPH-MACC) in advanced lung cancer, cell types other than small cell. *Proc. Am. Soc. Clin. Oncol., 2:* 198 (1983).
118. Harada, L., Makisaka, Y., Nishimura, H., Okuda, K., Complete necrotization of hepatocellular carcinoma by chemotherapy and subsequent intravascular coagulation: A case report. *Cancer, 42:* 67–73 (1978).
119. Gulati, S. C., Sordillo, P., Kempin, S., Reich, L., Magill, G. B., Scheiner, E., Clarkson, B., Microangiopathic hemolytic anemia observed after treatment of epidermoid carcinoma with mitomycin C and 5-fluorouracil. *Cancer, 45:* 2252–2257 (1980).
120. Tannock, I. F., Methotrexate and mitomycin for patients with metastatic transitional cell carcinoma of the urinary tract. *Cancer Treat. Rep., 67:* 503–504 (1983).
121. Richards, F., Case, L.D., White, D. R., Muss, H. B., Spurr, C. L., Jackson, D. V., Cooper, M. R., Zekan, P., Cruz, J., Stuart, J. J., Capizzi, R. L., McCulloch, J. H., McFarland, J. A., Kincaid, W. R., Harding, R. W., Pope, E., McMahan, R., Wells, H. B., Combination chemotherapy (5-fluorouracil, methyl-CCNU, mitomycin C) versus 5-fluorouracil alone for advanced previously untreated colorectal carcinoma. A phase III study of the Piedmont Oncology Association. *J. Clin. Oncol., 4:* 565–570 (1986).
122. Verwey, J., Vreis, E. G. E., Pinedo, H. M., Mitomycin C-related renal toxicity, a dose-dependent side effect. *Eur. J. Cancer Clin. Oncol., 23:* 195–199 (1987).
123. Lesesne, J. B., Chiazze, L., Erickson, B., Korec, S., Sisk, R., Keller, J., Arbus, M., Schein, P. S., Neefe, J. R., First analysis of 102 cases from a registry of cancer associated hemolytic uremic syndrome (C-HUS). *Proc. Am. Soc. Clin. Oncol., 5:* 82 (1986).
124. Harrell, R. M., Sibley, R., Vogelzang, N. J., Renal Vascular lesions after chemotherapy with vinblastine, bleomycin, and cisplatin. *Am. J. Med., 73:* 429–433 (1982).
125. Jackson, A. M., Rose, B. D., Graff, L. G., Jacobs, J. B., Schwartz, J. H., Strauss, G. M., Yang, J. P. S., Rudnick, M. R., Elfenbein, I. B., Narins, R. G., Thrombotic microangiopathy and renal failure associated with antineoplastic chemotherapy. *Ann. Intern. Med. 101:* 41–44 (1984).

126. Van der Meer, J., de Vreis, E. G. E., Vriesendorp, R., Willemse, P. H. B., Donker, A. J. M., Aalders, J. G., Hemolytic uremic syndrome in a patient on cis-platinum, vinblastine and bleomycin. *J. Cancer Res. Clin. Oncol., 110:* 119–122 (1985).
127. Gardner, G., Mesler, D., Gitelman, H. J., Hemolytic uremic symdrome following cisplatin, bleomycin, and vincristine chemotherapy: A report of a case and a review of the literature. *Renal Failure, 11:* 133–137 (1989).
128. Angiola, G., Bloss, J. D., DiSaia, P. J., Warner, A. S., Manetta, A., Berman, M. L., Hemolytic–uremic syndrome associated with neoadjuvant chemotherapy in the treatment of advanced cervical cancer. *Gynecol. Oncol., 39:* 214–217 (1990).
129. Licciardello, J. T. W., Moake, J. L., Rudy, C. K., Karp, D. D., Hong, W. K., Elevated plasma von Willebrand factor levels and arterial occlusive complications associated with cisplatin-based chemotherapy. *Oncology, 42:* 296–300 (1985).
130. Boccia, R. V., Gelman, E. P., Baker, C. C., Marti, G., Longo, D. L., A hemolytic–uremic-syndrome with the acquired immunodeficiency syndrome. *Ann. Intern. Med. 101:* 716–717 (1984).
131. Desablens, B., Fievet, P., Pruna, A., Claisse, J. F., Westeel, P. F., Tolani, M., Fournier, A., Hemolytic–uremic syndrome after cancer chemotherapy without mitomycin C. *Nephron, 42:* 343–344 (1986).
132. Fields, S. M., Lindley, C. M., Thrombotic microangiopathy associated with chemotherapy: Case report and review of the literature. *Drug. Intell. Clin. Pharm., 23:* 582–588 (1989).
133. Walker, R. W., Rosenblum, M. K., Kempin, S. J., Christian, M. C., Carboplatin-associated thrombotic microangiopathic hemolytic anemia. *Cancer, 64:* 1017–1020 (1989).
134. Byrnes, J. J., Barquerinzo, H., Gonzalez, M., Hensely, H., Thrombotic thrombocytopenic purpura subsequent to acute myelogenous leukemia chemotherapy. *Am. J. Hematol., 21:* 299–304 (1986).
135. Avvento, L., Gordon, S., Silberberg, J. M., Zarrabi, M. H., Zucker, S., Hemolytic uremic syndrome in a patient with small cell lung cancer. *Am. J. Hematol., 27:* 221–223 (1988).
136. Case Records of the Massachusetts General Hospital (case 16-1988). *N. Engl. J. Med., 318:* 1047–1057 (1988).
137. Laffay, D. L., Tubbs, R. R., Valenzuela, R., Hall, P. M., McCormack, L. J., Chronic glomerular microangiopathy and metastatic carcinoma. *Hum. Pathol., 10:* 433–438 (1979).
138. Spruce, W. E., Forman, S. J., Blume, K. G., Bearman, R. M., Bixby, H., Ching, A., Drinkard, J., San Marco, A., Hemolytic uremic syndrome after bone marrow transplantation. *Acta Haematol., 67:* 206–210 (1982).
139. Loomis, L. J., Aronson, A. J., Rudinsky, R., and Spargo, B. H., Hemolytic uremic syndrome following bone marrow transplantation: A case report and review of the literature. *Am. J. Kidney Dis., 14:* 324–328 (1989).
140. Poch, E., Gonzàlez-Clemente, J. M., Torras, A., Darnell, A., Botey, A., Revert, L., Silent renal microangiopathy after mitomycin-C therapy. *Am. J. Nephrol., 10:*514–517 (1990).
141. Hamner, R. W., Varani, R., Weinman, E. J., Mitomycin-associated renal failure: Case report and review. *Arch. Intern. Med., 143:* 803–807 (1983).
142. Doll, D. C., Weiss, R. B., Issell, B. F., Mitomycin: Ten years after approval for marketing. *J. Clin. Oncol., 3:* 276–286 (1985).
143. Liu, K., Mittelman, A., Sproul, E. E., Elias, E. G., Renal toxicity in man treated with mitomycin C. *Cancer, 28:* 1314–1320 (1971).
144. Cattell, V., Mitomycin-induced hemolytic uremic kidney: An experimental model in the rat. *Am. J. Pathol., 121:* 88–95 (1985).

145. Duperray, A., Tranqui, L., Alix, J. L., Manoeuvrier, M., Cordonnier, D., The effect of mitomycin C on the biosynthesis of prostacyclin by primary cultures of human umbilical cord vein endothelial cells. *Proc. Int. Congr. Nephrol., 9:* 448A (1984).
146. Remuzzi, G., Zoja, C., Rossi, E. C., Prostacyclin in thrombotic microangiopathy. *Semin. Hematol., 24:* 110–118 (1987).
147. Siegler, R. L., Smith, J. B., Linch, M. B., Mohammad, S. F., In vitro prostacyclin production in the hemolytic–uremic syndrome. *West. J. Med., 144:* 165–168 (1986).
148. Rogers, J. S., Murgo, A. J., Fontana, J. A., Raich, P. C., Chemotherapy for breast cancer decreases plasma protein C and protein S. *J. Clin. Oncol., 6:* 276–281 (1988).
149. Mazzucco, G., Fornari, G., Monga, G., Severe glomerular mesangiolysis in a patient with rectal adenocarcinoma treated with cytotoxic drugs. *Virchows Arch. [A],* (Pathol Anat) *398:* 197–203 (1982).
150. Zimmerman, S. E., Smith, F. P., Phillips, T. M., Coffey, R. J., Schein, P. S., Gastric carcinoma and thrombotic thrombocytopenic purpura: Association with plasma immune complex concentrations. *Br. Med. J., 284:* 1432–1434 (1982).
151. Tannenbaum, S. H., Barnathan, E., Vanderkeyl, H., Kuo, A., Murray, S., Cines, D. B., Aggregated IgG stimulates the fibrinolytic inhibitory activity of human endothelial cells. *Blood, 68*(Suppl. 1): 119a (1986).
152. Blanco, R., Griffin, J., Radice, P., Mitomycin-C pulmonary toxicity protective measures. *Proc. Am. Soc. Clin. Oncol., 5:* 48 (1986).
153. Taft, E. G., Thrombotic thrombocytopenic purpura and dose of plasma exchange. *Blood, 54:* 842–849 (1979).

23
Hemolytic Uremic Syndrome and Thrombotic Thrombocytopenic Purpura Associated with Human Immunodeficiency Virus Infection and Acquired Immunodeficiency Syndrome

Jeffrey S. Berns *University of Pennsylvania School of Medicine and The Graduate Hospital, Philadelphia, Pennsylvania* **John E. Tomaszewski** *University of Pennsylvania Medical Center, Philadelphia, Pennsylvania*

Hemolytic uremic syndrome in a homosexual man with acquired immunodeficiency syndrome (AIDS) was first reported by Boccia and colleagues in 1984 (1). Since then, microangiopathic hemolytic anemia with thrombocytopenia and varying degrees of renal involvement, diagnosed as either hemolytic uremic syndrome (HUS) or thrombotic thrombocytopenic purpura (TTP), has become a well-described occurrence in patients with human immunodeficiency virus (HIV) infection (2–18).

The nomenclature of the thrombotic microangiopathic hemolytic anemias is a matter of some confusion and debate (19). Thrombotic microangiopathic hemolytic anemia with fever and prominent neurologic manifestations is likely to be diagnosed as TTP. HUS is more likely to be diagnosed in children, and in persons with a diarrheal prodrome or significant renal failure. However, the clinical distinction between HUS and TTP can be imprecise or the terms may be used loosely. For example, a patient reported by Boccia and colleagues with "HUS" had fever, headaches, and dizziness, but only mild renal failure until the terminal phase of the illness (1). In a patient to be described below, fever and tonic-clonic seizures suggested a diagnosis of TTP, while a gastrointestinal prodrome and progressive renal failure were compatible with a diagnosis of HUS. For the purposes of this discussion, patients reported with a diagnosis of HUS, TTP, or simply (and perhaps preferably) thrombotic microangiopathic hemolytic anemia will be considered together.

AN ILLUSTRATIVE CASE

A 30-year-old woman tested positive for HIV in 1989. She had a history of *Pneumocystis carinii* pneumonia which was being treated with zidovudine (3'-azido-2'-3'-dideoxythymidine, AZT). She was admitted to the hospital in October 1990 with fever, nausea, vomiting, diarrhea, and abdominal pain. Other than hepatomegaly, her physical examination was unremarkable. The stool was positive for occult blood. The hematocrit was 31%, platelets were 321,000/mm^3, and the serum creatinine was 1.1 mg/dL. Urinalysis showed 2+ protein and 2–5 wbc/hpf. Routine stool cultures were negative for enteric pathogens. Her symptoms resolved over a few days. Although her hematocrit had fallen to 22% she was discharged from hospital, but was readmitted 1 week later with recurrent symptoms and marked hypertension (BP 172/119 mm Hg.). The hematocrit subsequently decreased to 15%, the platelet count dropped to 30,000/mm^3, and the serum creatinine rose to 6.9 mg/dL. The AST and ALT were slightly elevated, the bilirubin was 3.0 mg/dL, and the LDH was over 2,000 IU/L. There were many schistocytes on the peripheral blood smear. The prothrombin time, partial thromboplastin time, and fibrinogen level were normal. The reticulocyte count was 0.9%. A 24-hour urine collection had 2 grams of protein. The CD4 count was 3/mm^3, with a total lymphocyte count of 300/mm^3. Colonoscopy showed hemorrhagic colitis with diffuse mucosal petechiae. She had a generalized tonic-clonic seizure; a CT of the brain was, however, normal.

A diagnosis of TTP was made. A gingival biopsy was normal. A renal biopsy showed numerous fibrin thrombi in arterioles, interlobular arteries, and glomerular capillaries, along with myxoid intimal proliferation and focal fibrinoid necrosis of the vessels (Fig. 1). Fragmented red blood cells were seen in glomeruli and the walls of arterioles (Fig. 2). Occasional platelet thrombi were also seen. There were tubular ectasia, interstitial fibrosis, and mild diffuse mesangial sclerosis. Immunofluorescent staining was positive in glomeruli and arteriolar walls for IgA, IgM, C3, kappa and

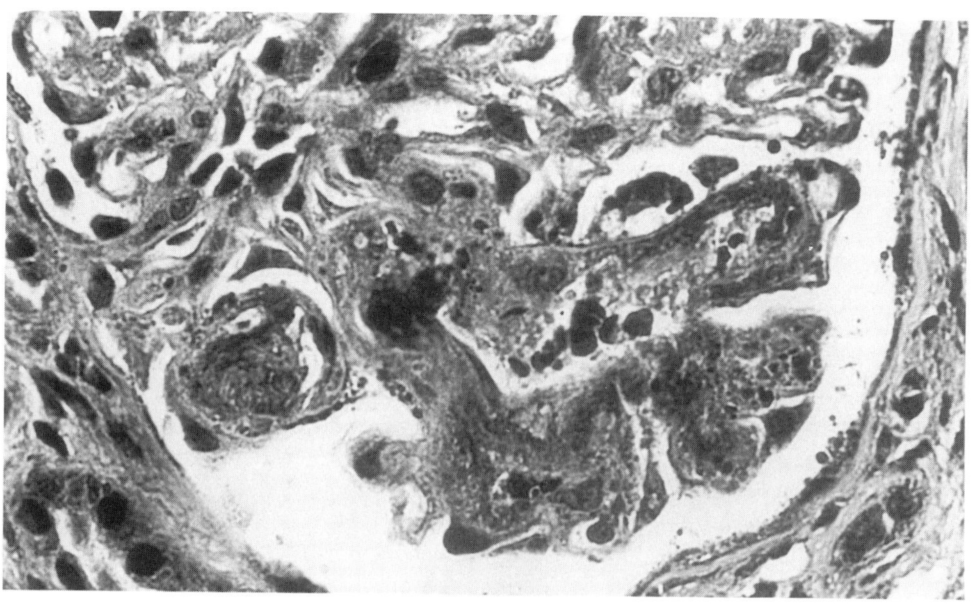

Figure 1 Glomerulus with capillary fibrin thrombi.

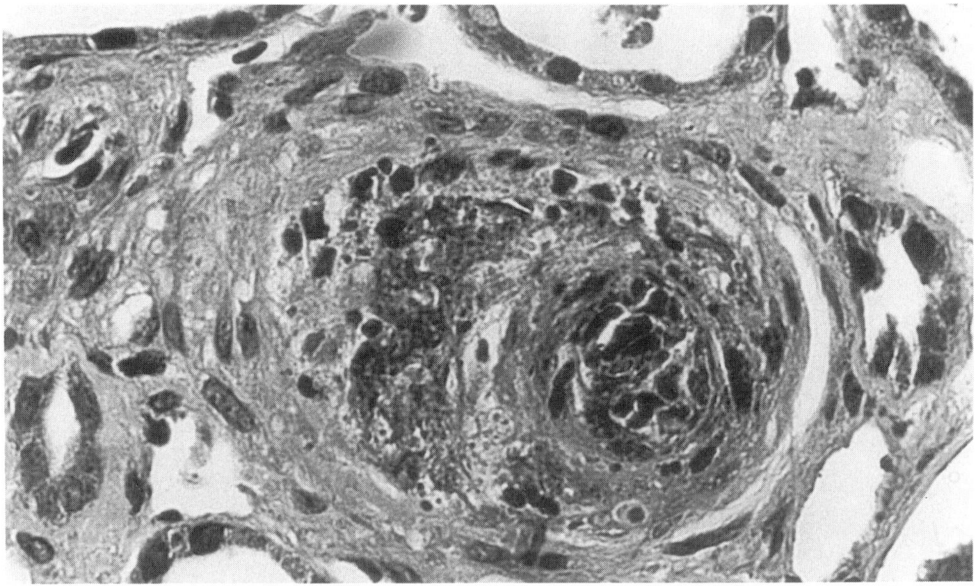

Figure 2 Renal arteriole with fibrin thrombus and fragmented red blood cells in arteriolar wall.

lambda light chains, and fibrinogen. On electron microscopy, there was partial collapse of the glomerular tuft and ischemic wrinkling of the glomerular basement membrane, with endothelial cells focally lifted off the basement membrane. Tubuloreticular bodies were seen in endothelial cell cytoplasm (Fig. 3). No immune complex deposits were seen.

Plasmapheresis with fresh frozen plasma replacement was performed daily for 2 weeks, with improvement in the platelet count to 104,000/mm^3, hematocrit 29%, and creatinine of 4.2 mg/dL. Within a few days of stopping plasmapheresis, however, the platelet count fell to 18,000/mm^3 with worsening of the hemolytic anemia and development of oliguric renal failure. Her course was complicated by staphylococcal and *Klebsiella pneumoniae* sepsis. Hemodialysis was initiated, but progressive neurologic deterioration resulted in coma, and the patient died.

In addition to renal arteriolar and glomerular hyaline thrombi with acute tubular necrosis, an autopsy revealed disseminated invasive aspergillosis with infarction of the heart, lungs, and gastrointestinal tract.

EPIDEMIOLOGY

HUS has been reported in two patients with HIV infection or AIDS (1, 12), while TTP or thrombotic microangiopathy (TMA) has been reported in over 30 patients (2–11, 13–18). Karpatkin (5) indicated that five cases of HIV-associated TTP reported from his institution in 1988 represented one third of all cases of TTP seen there over a 3-year period, at a time when about 2% of their hospitalized patient population had AIDS (20). The precise incidence of HUS and TTP among various patient populations

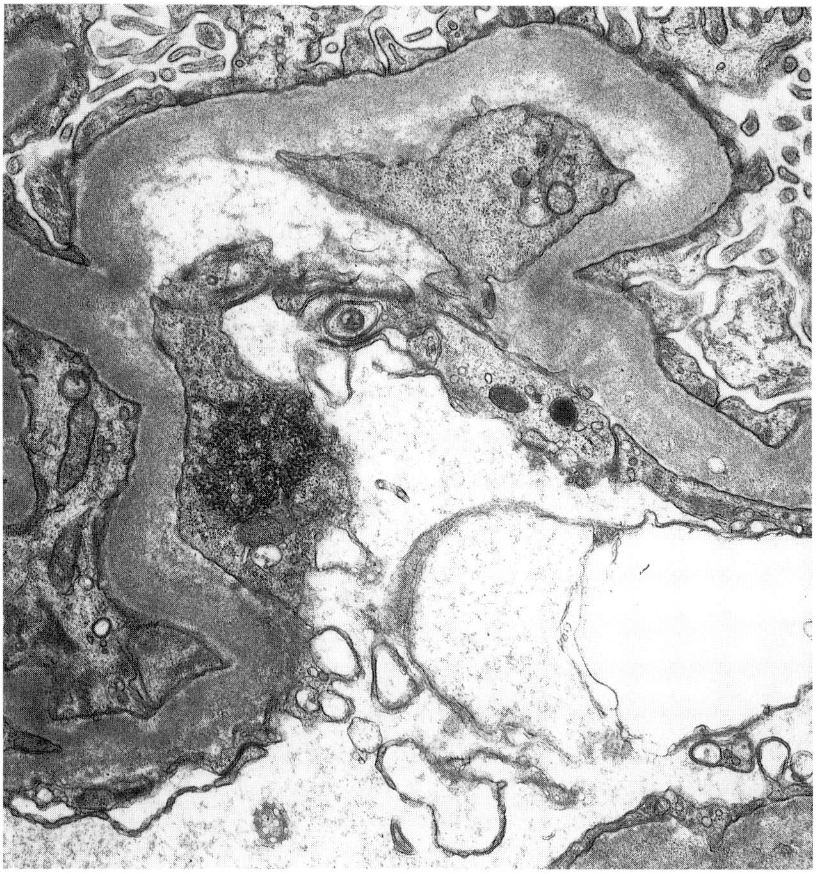

Figure 3 Electron micrograph demonstrating tubuloreticular inclusions in glomerular capillary endothelial cell cytoplasm.

with HIV infection is not known. However, even allowing for many unreported cases, HIV-associated HUS/TTP appears to be an uncommon occurrence among the more than 179,000 cases of AIDS diagnosed in the United States between 1981 and 1990 (21) or the millions of individuals around the world who are infected with HIV. In fact, it remains to be proven that the incidence of the HUS/TTP disorders is any higher in HIV-infected patients than in the general population.

The male-to-female ratio of reported cases is about 9:1, reflecting the demographics of HIV infection and AIDS. In contrast, others have noted a female predominance in adults with TTP which is not related to HIV infection (22, 23). In fact, the striking male predominance of HIV-associated HUS/TTP is perhaps one of the only pieces of epidemiologic evidence available which suggests a specific relationship between HIV infection and these disorders. Also reflecting the underlying demographics of HIV infection is a mean age of about 35 years, with a range of 23–51 years. We are aware of one case of HIV-associated HUS/TTP in a child (M. E. Turner, personal communication). Most of the patients have been homosexual men or intravenous drug users, although men and women with apparent heterosexually acquired HIV infection have also developed HUS/TTP syndromes. HUS/TTP has developed in patients with AIDS (opportunistic infections and serologic evidence of HIV infection), as well as in patients with known but previously asymptomatic HIV infection. In several patients, the HUS/TTP disorder was the presenting illness which led to the initial diagnosis of HIV infection. A few patients with a clinical diagnosis of AIDS without serological confirmation of HIV infection may in fact have had "idiopathic" TTP (5, 8).

CLINICAL MANIFESTATIONS

The clinical features of HIV-related HUS/TTP are similar to those of the idiopathic disorders (22, 23). The most common presenting symptoms include fever, headache, abdominal pain, nausea, vomiting, diarrhea, weight loss, malaise, and lethargy. A number of patients have had bleeding manifestations, such as petechiae of the skin and oral mucosa, easy bruising, epistaxis, rectal bleeding, gross hematuria, subconjunctival hemorrhage, and gingival bleeding. Neurologic symptoms are often present, including dizziness, paresthesias, aphasia, blurred vision, confusion, tonic-clonic seizures, behavioral disturbances, and hemiparesis.

Physical examination may reveal findings of HIV infection, such as oral thrush or Kaposi sarcoma. Severe hypertension has been infrequent. The most notable physical findings include fever, pallor, ecchymoses, petechiae, and jaundice. A number of patients have had lymphadenopathy, hepatomegaly, and splenomegaly, as have also been noted in idiopathic TTP (23).

LABORATORY FEATURES

The platelet counts are often as low as 8,000–10,000/mm^3. The hemoglobin ranges from 5–6 g/dL, but it may be as low as 3 g/dL or as high as 10 g/dL. Fragmented red blood cells, spherocytes, and other abnormal red blood cell forms are seen on peripheral blood smears. Despite the severe hemolytic anemia, which is Coombs'-test negative, the reticulocyte count is usually not elevated. This may be due to impaired hematopoiesis because of HIV infection, treatment with zidovudine, malnutrition, bone marrow infiltrative disorders, and chronic infection (24). The prothrombin time and partial thromboplastin time are usually normal, although occasional patients have had mild abnormalities of these tests, and fibrin degradation products may be elevated. The serum LDH and bilirubin are usually elevated, and the haptoglobin is low in keeping with hemolysis. Liver function tests may be mildly abnormal. Elevated levels of platelet-associated IgG, C3, C4, and IgM have been reported, which are probably a feature of an immune-mediated thrombocytopenia seen in many HIV-infected individuals (24–28). Lymphocyte marker studies in the few patients in whom they have been reported have revealed reduced helper T-lympocyte (OKT4, CD4) counts. Hypergammaglobulinemia is also common with HIV infection (24) and has been described in some patients with HIV-related HUS/TTP.

Urinalysis has usually revealed 1–3+ proteinuria, microscopic hematuria, low-grade pyuria, and granular casts, but may also be normal. Gross hematuria has occurred rarely. Nephrotic range proteinuria has been reported (17), and one patient had a prior history of nephrotic syndrome with focal glomerulosclerosis (6), which may have been caused by HIV-associated nephropathy (29). Renal function has been normal or only moderately reduced at presentation in the majority of patients, with serum creatinine levels usually between 1.0 and 2.5 mg/dL and BUN concentrations of 15–50 mg/dL. A few patients have had more severe renal failure (3, 5, 8), and one presented with oliguric renal failure which needed to be treated with dialysis (12). It should be kept in mind that BUN and creatinine levels in patients with poor nutrition and reduced muscle mass due to AIDS-related cachexia may cause one to underestimate significantly the actual extent of renal functional impairment (30). Worsening of renal function during an acute illness may be directly related to the HUS/TTP process, or due to superimposed volume depletion, sepsis, nephrotoxic drug administration, glomerulonephritis, or interstitial nephritis (29, 31, 32).

PATHOLOGY

Bone Marrow

Findings on bone marrow biopsies can reflect the response to the acute thrombotic thrombocytopenic hemolytic anemia, as well as effects of HIV infection, its treatment, and opportunistic infections which can involve the marrow (24). As in other patients with HUS/TTP disorders, the marrow typically shows erythroid and megakaryocyte hyperplasia. However, normal or even reduced megakaryocyte numbers may also be seen, and the marrow may be normocellular or show megaloblastic changes. Hyaline, fibrin, and platelet thrombi, suggestive of a thrombotic microangiopathy, may be seen in the vessels of bone marrow biopsy specimens (2, 15).

Kidneys

Aside from the case described above, detailed reports of renal histopathology in HIV-related HUS/TTP are available from only two other patients with TTP. In a postmortem renal biopsy specimen, Charasse et al. (17) found ischemic glomerular changes and basement membrane thickening. There was "onion-skin" arteriolar proliferation, with fibrin deposition, intimal edema, and endothelial cell swelling. There was also interstitial fibrosis, tubular atrophy, and epithelial cell necrosis. Immunofluorescent studies showed fibrin, Clq, C3, and IgM deposits. Segal et al. (16) described enlarged, swollen kidneys in one case at autopsy. Many eosinophilic thrombi were seen occluding glomerular vascular poles, and there were findings of acute tubular necrosis. On electron microscopy, there was separation of glomerular capillary endothelial cells from the basement membrane by granular material.

The findings in these three cases are similar to those noted in other patients with renal involvement in TMA (33). Additional features seen in the biopsy of our patient were fragmented red blood cells in arterioles and glomerular capillaries (33), and tubuloreticular bodies in endothelial cell cytoplasm. These tubuloreticular structures are common in glomerular endothelial cells (34–36) and other cell types (37, 38) from patients with HIV infection. It has been suggested that these structures, which are similar to those seen in other disorders such as systemic lupus erythematosus, may be induced by systemic or local production of alpha-interferon (37, 38).

Other Tissues

Gingival biopsies have shown capillary microthrombi in about one third of reported patients. Fibrin or hyaline thrombi have also been seen in lymph nodes, brain, heart, pancreas, thyroid, liver, spleen, and the adrenal glands, as well as in the vessels of the lesions of Kaposi sarcoma (13).

ETIOLOGY AND PATHOGENESIS

Little is known about the specific etiologic factors and pathophysiologic mechanisms of HUS/TTP in patients with HIV infection, nor whether they differ from others with these disorders. Diarrheal prodromes, which are common with childhood HUS (39), have been described in four patients. In the patient described above, routine stool cultres were negative, and in one patient they were positive for *Salmonella* Group D12 (15), which is probably not specifically related to the development of HUS/TTP (40). However, verocytotoxin-producing *Escherichia coli,* associated with occurrences of both HUS and TTP (40–44), was isolated from stool cultures of one patient (12). A Shiga toxin produced by *Shigella dysenteriae* and some strains of *Shigella flexneri,* which was isolated from another patient who had recently travelled to Nepal (11) has also been described in cases of HUS (40, 45). Thus, toxin-producing enteric pathogens may be involved in the development of HUS/TTP in some patients with HIV infection. These enterotoxins are thought to induce endothelial injury with subsequent disturbances of prostacyclin and factor VIII/von Willebrand factor homeostasis, increased production of interleukin-1 and tumor necrosis factor, release of proteases, and platelet activation (40, 46).

Several other patients have also had previously recognized "risk factors" for HUS/TTP, other than HIV infection or AIDS. Of the few women reported with HIV-associated HUS/TTP, one was 8 weeks pregnant when she was diagnosed with TTP. She developed ophthalmic herpes zoster about 1 month later and was found to be HIV positive (7). Others have also reported TTP developing in early pregnancy unrelated to HIV infection (47, 48). The patient described by Boccia and colleagues (1) was undergoing chemotherapy with vinblastine, doxorubicin, dactinomycin, bleomycin, vincristine, and dacarbazine for Kaposi sarcoma when he developed thrombocytopenia, hemolytic anemia, and renal insufficiency. One of the patients reported by Leaf and colleagues (5) had Stage IIIB nodular sclerosing Hodgkin's disease, which had been treated with combination chemotherapy about one year prior to his developing TTP. Although neither of these patients had received mitomycin-C, which is the antineoplastic agent most frequently associated with cancer-related HUS/TTP (49–51), other drugs have also been implicated (52).

Because many patients with HIV-associated HUS/TTP have histories of illicit drug use, the case report by Tumlin and colleagues (53) is noteworthy. A 28-year old woman who was HIV negative developed microangiopathic hemolytic anemia, thrombocytopenia, and severe renal failure following inhalation of "crack" cocaine. Histopathologic changes compatible with a TMA were seen on a renal biopsy specimen. Cocaine-induced endothelial damage and a hypercoagulable state were postulated as possible mechanisms for this occurrence. Another report is that of a 55-year-old Japanese Hawaiian who, after being diagnosed with TTP, was found to be infected with a different retrovirus, human T-lymphotrophic virus type 1 (HTLV-1)

(54). These cases point out the difficulty in definitively establishing a specific causal relationship between HIV infection and HUS/TTP. Further epidemiologic studies are needed to determine whether there is in fact an actual etiologic role of HIV infection in the development of the HUS/TTP disorders, or if these cases simply represent the chance association of two unrelated disease processes.

Only limited information is available regarding the pathogenesis of the HUS/TTP disorders in patients with HIV infections. As mentioned above, immune thrombocytopenia with elevated levels of platelet-associated IgG, C3, and C4 complement occurs commonly in patients with AIDS, as well as in those with asymptomatic HIV infection and acute HIV seroconversion (20, 24, 28). Elevated levels of platelet-associated antibodies have also occasionally been detected in patients with HIV-related TTP (5, 6). In one patient, these were shown to decrease during successful treatment which included plasmapheresis (6). However, the level of antiplatelet antibodies rebounded after plasmapheresis was stopped, yet the patient remained in remission with a normal platelet count. Another patient developed immune thrombocytopenia while in remission from TTP (6). Others have not detected specific platelet-associated antibodies (2). Platelet-aggregating activity in patient serum, which has been associated with idiopathic TTP (55, 56) and epidemic childhood HUS (57), has not been detected in the few HIV patients tested (4, 20). It is likely that HUS and TTP in patients with HIV infection are not directly related to these factors associated with HIV-immune thrombocytopenia, although increased platelet-associated IgG has been reported in non-HIV TTP (58), and TTP has rarely developed in the setting of autoimmune thrombocytopenia (59).

Abnormalities of factor VIII/von Willebrand factor have been implicated in the pathophysiology of non-HIV HUS and TTP (56, 60–63) and have also been investigated in patients with HIV infection. Segal and colleagues (16) performed immunostaining using a polyclonal antibody directed at factor VIII-related antigen (vWF) of postmortem tissues from a patient with AIDS who died with TTP. Vascular thrombi in various organs were reported to show "moderately intense vWF activity." Immunofluorescent staining was also noted in glomerular thrombi using a monoclonal antibody to the platelet specific glycoprotein IIb/IIIa, which may interact with large vWF multimers to induce platelet aggregation (60, 64). The HIV-seropositive patient reported by Beris and colleagues (11), who developed TTP during an episode of *Shigella flexneri* rectosigmoiditis, was found during his acute illness to have decreased levels of factor VIII coagulant and ristocetin cofactor activity, with absence of high-molecular-weight vWF multimers. During remission, high-molecular-weight vWF multimers were detected, and factor VIII coagulant activity, ristocetine cofactor activity, and vWF antigen levels were all above normal (11). In contrast, Karpatkin (20) did not find abnormalities of von Willebrand factor multimers in either acute or convalescent plasma samples.

TREATMENT

Because there have been no controlled trials of treatment for HIV-related TTP/HUS, it is impossible to determine the specific effect of any therapy on patient outcome. Management has included the same treatments generally recommended, but used empirically, for other forms of HUS and TTP (60, 65–70). These include plasmapheresis with fresh frozen plasma replacement, or plasma infusions alone. Most patients also received aspirin, dipyridamole, and prednisone or other corticosteroids. Given the substantial morbidity and mortality associated with HUS/TTP in patients with HIV infection or AIDS, plasmapheresis is likely to remain the mainstay of therapy. However, the potential infectious complications of plasmapheresis in these already immunosuppressed patients should be kept in mind. Although one recent report (71) did not find an increased risk of infection due to plasmapheresis in patients with lupus nephritis, Wing and colleagues (72) reported severe infection in five of eight patients treated with plasmapheresis for rapidly progressive glomerulonephritis. In their series, two patients developed *P. carinii* pneumonia, already an important and common pathogen in HIV-positive patients (73). In fact, one patient reported to have AIDS-related TTP had no known risk factors for HIV infection and a diagnosis of AIDS was made, without serologic confirmation, only when he developed opportunistic infections after several weeks of treatment with steroids and exchange transfusions for TTP (8). Wing and colleagues (72) also noted cytomegalovirus infection, *Listeria monocytogenes* sepsis, *Candida albicans* and *Aspergillus fumigatus* infections, and other infectious complications for which HIV-positive patients are already at risk.

Additional therapies, which have also been used in other patients with HUS and TTP (19, 60, 65, 66, 69), have included vincristine (3, 6, 11, 18), intravenous gamma globulin (10, 18), and prostacyclin (11). In several of these reports, these additional therapies were felt to be useful in obtaining a remission; however, it is virtually impossible to draw any firm conclusions, since all of the patients received other forms of therapy concurrently. Treatment with *Staphylococcus aureus* protein A immunoadsorption, which has been reported to be successful in patients with HIV-related immune-thrombocytopenia and HUS associated with neoplastic disease and mitomycin-C (74, 75) has not yet been reported in HIV-associated HUS/TTP.

A patient with AIDS and relapsing TTP was treated initially with aspirin, Persantine® (dipyridamole), plasma infusions, plasmapheresis, folate, and intravenous gamma globulin (18). However, it was concluded that a sustained remission was maintained only after the addition of an adequate dose of the antiretroviral agent zidovudine. Another patient developed TTP shortly after zidovudine had been discontinued because of bone marrow suppression (16). In contrast to these reports, which suggest that zidovudine may have a therapeutic role in the management of HIV-related HUS/TTP, TTP developed in our patient and another patient (17) while they were being treated with zidovudine. Therefore, the role for this drug in the management of HIV-related TMA remains to be determined.

CLINICAL COURSE

The serious nature of the HUS/TTP process is underscored by the occurrence of several deaths prior to institution of therapy or shortly after therapy was initiated (5, 13, 16). Hematologic remissions were obtained in about two thirds of patients, although in some patients they were very slowly obtained or only partially successful. While some remissions were sustained for many months, relapses were reported in about 20% of patients. In many cases the duration of follow-up has been brief. Relapses may respond to further therapy (5, 8, 18), or they may be fatal (1).

Hemodialysis has been required in a few patients (8, 9, 12, 17), but was able to be discontinued following treatment in one patient with HUS (12). One patient with

Table 1 Differential Diagnosis of HUS and TTP in patients with HIV Infection or AIDS

Subacute bacterial endocarditis
Severe, acute reaction to rifampin (81,82) or dapsone (83)
Preeclampsia, eclampsia
Disseminated intravascular coagulation (DIC)
Sepsis
Septic abortion
Malignant hypertension
Cocaine abuse
Rhabdomyolysis with DIC (84)
Systemic vasculitis
Idiopathic
Collagen vascular disease
Intravenous drug abuse (85)
Multiple disorders which together cause features of HUS/TTP with: diarrhea (86), fever, neurologic manifestations (80), thrombocytopenia (24,28), anemia (24), and acute renal failure (29,31)

preexisting renal insufficiency due to focal glomerulosclerosis required permanent chronic hemodialysis while in a hematologic remission (6). Over one third of the patients died due to "cardiopulmonary arrest," complications of HUS/TTP, or septicemia. Overall, the clinical course and prognosis of HIV-related HUS/TTP does not appear to be too dissimilar from that of other series of TTP (22, 68, 69, 76). This may be better than that reported for adults with HUS of other etiologies (50, 77, 78).

CONCLUSION

As the HIV epidemic has expanded, the clinical spectrum of diseases associated with this infection has also grown. Many of the clinical and laboratory features of the thrombotic hemolytic microangiopathies overlap with the many hematologic (24), renal (29, 31, 32, 79), and neurologic (80) manifestations of HIV infection, its treatment, or associated opportunistic infections. For this reason, even when a patient is thought to have "classical" features of HUS or TTP, a careful evaluation is essential to exclude other disorders (or all too frequently in patients with HIV infection, combinations of disorders) which can mimic HUS/TTP (Table 1).

REFERENCES

1. Boccia, R. V., Gelmann, E. P., Baker, C. C., Marti, G., Longo, D. L. A hemolytic-uremic syndrome with the acquired immunodeficiency syndrome. *Ann. Intern. Med.*, *101:* 716–717 (1984).
2. Jokela, J., Flynn, T., Henry, K. Thrombotic thrombocytopenic purpura in a human immunodeficiency virus (HIV) seropositive homosexual man. *Am. J. Hematol.*, *25:* 341–3437 (1987).
3. Botti, A. C., Hyde, P., DiPillo, F. Thrombotic thrombocytopenic purpura in a patient who subsequently developed the acquired immunodeficiency syndrome (AIDS). *Ann. Intern. Med.*, *109:* 242–243 (1988).

4. Nair, J. M. G., Bellevue, R., Bertoni, M., Dosik, H. Thrombotic thrombocytopenic purpura in patients with the acquired immunodeficiency syndrome (AIDS)-related complex. A report of two cases. *Ann. Intern. Med., 109:* 209–212 (1988).
5. Leaf, A. N., Laubenstein, L. J., Raphael, B., Hochster, H., Baez, L., Karpatkin, S. Thrombotic thrombocytopenic purpura associated with human immunodeficiency virus type 1 (HIV-1) infection. *Ann. Intern. Med., 109:* 194–197 (1988).
6. Meisenberg, B. R., Robinson, W. L., Mosley, C. A., Duke, M. S., Rabetoy, G. M., Kosty, M. P. Thrombotic thrombocytopenic purpura in human immunodeficiency (HIV)-seropositive males. *Am. J. Hematol., 27:* 212–215 (1988).
7. Besalduch, J., Altes, J., Morey, M., Villalonga, C. Thrombotic thrombocytopenic purpura with human immunodeficiency virus infection. *Medicina Clinica, 92:* 795–796 (1989).
8. Platanias, L. C., Paiusco, D., Bernstein, S., Murali, M. R. Thrombotic thrombocytopenic purpura as the first manifestation of human immunodeficiency virus infection. *Am. J. Med., 87:* 699–700 (1989).
9. Kuong, M. A., DeTruchis, P., Oksenhendler, E., Matteron, S., Dosquet, P., Clauvel, J. P. Thrombotic microangiopathy and HIV infection (abstract). *International Conference on AIDS,* p. 263 (1989).
10. DeNobriga, J., Chu-Fong, A., Elizalde, A. Thrombotic thrombocytopenic purpura (TTP) in a human immune deficiency virus (HIV)-positive patient: successful treatment with high dose gamma globulin (HDGG) (abstract). *Proc. Ann. Mtg. Am. Soc. Clin. Oncol., 8:* A21 (1989).
11. Beris, P., Dunand, V., Isoz, C., Reynard, C. Association of thrombotic thrombocytopenic purpura and human immunodeficiency virus infection. *Nouv. Rev. Fr. Hematol., 32:* 277–280 (1990).
12. Farina, C., Gavazzeni, G., Caprioli, A., Remuzzi, G. Hemolytic uremic syndrome associated with verocytotoxin-producing *Escherichia coli* infection in acquired immunodeficiency syndrome. *Blood, 75:* 2465 (1990).
13. Bell, M. D., Barnhart, J. S., Martin, J. M. Thrombotic thrombocytopenic purpura causing sudden, unexpected death—a series of eight patients. *J. Forens. Sci., 35:* 601–613 (1990).
14. Kiprov, D. D., Kwiatkowska, B. J., Miller, R. G. Therapeutic apheresis in human immunodeficiency virus-related syndromes. *Curr. Stud. Blood Transf., 57:* 184–197 (1990).
15. Pachon, J., Viciana, P., Espigado, I., Fernandez-Alonso, J. Thrombotic thrombocytopenic purpura in a patient with acquired immunodeficiency syndrome. *Revista Clinica Española, 187:* 41–42 (1990).
16. Segal G. H., Tubbs, R. R., Ratliff, N. B., Miller, M. L., Longworth, D. L. Thrombotic thrombocytopenic purpura in a patient with AIDS. *Cleve. Clin. J. Med., 57:* 360–366 (1990).
17. Charasse, C., Michelet. C., LeTulzo, Y., Liegaux, J.-M., Camus, C., Thomas, R., Cartier, F., Ramee, M.-P. Thrombotic thrombocytopenic purpura with the acquired immunodeficiency syndrome: a pathologically documented case report. *Am. J. Kidney Dis., 17:* 80–82 (1991).
18. Salem, G., Terebelo, H., Raman, S. Human immunodeficiency virus associated with thrombotic thrombocytopenic purpura: Successful treatment with zidovudine. *South. Med. J., 84:* 493–495 (1991).
19. Remuzzi, G. HUS and TTP: variable expression of a single entity. *Kidney Int., 32:* 292–308 (1987).
20. Karpatkin, S. HIV-1-related thrombocytopenia. *Clin. Haematol., 3:* 115–138 (1990).
21. Centers for Disease Control. Update: Acquired immunodeficiency syndrome—United States, 1981–1990. *M.M.W.R., 40:* 358–369 (1991).

22. Ridolfi, R. L., Bell, W. R. Thrombotic thrombocytopenic purpura. Report of 25 cases and review of the literature. *Medicine, 60:* 413–428 (1981).
23. Amorosi, E. L., Ultmann, J. E. Thrombotic thrombocytopenic purpura: report of 16 cases and review of the literature. *Medicine, 45:* 139–159 (1966).
24. Hoxie, J. A. Hematologic manifestations of AIDS. In: *Hematology, Basic Principles and Practice*. (R. Hoffman, E. J. Benz, S. J. Shattil, B. Furie, and H. J. Cohen, eds.) Churchill Livingstone, New York (1991).
25. Morris, L., Distenfeld, A., Amorosi, E., Karpatkin, S. Autoimmune thrombocytopenic purpura in homosexual men. *Ann. Intern. Med., 96*(Pt. 1): 714–717 (1982).
26. Ratnoff, O. D., Menitove, J. E., Aster, R. H., Lederman, M. M. Coincident classic hemophilia and "idiopathic" thrombocytopenic purpura in patients under treatment with concentrates of antihemophilic factor (factor VIII). *N. Engl. J. Med., 308:* 439–442 (1983).
27. Walsh, C. M., Nardi, M. A., Karpatkin, S. On the mechanism of thrombocytopenic purpura in sexually active homosexual men. *N. Engl. J. Med., 311:* 635–639 (1984).
28. Ratner, L. Human immunodeficiency virus-associated autoimmune thrombocytopenic purpura: A review. *Am. J. Med. 86:* 194–198 (1989).
29. Bourgoignie, J. J. Renal complications of human immunodeficiency virus type 1. *Kidney Int., 37:* 1571–1584 (1990).
30. Levey, A. S., Perrone, R. D., Madias, N. E. Serum creatinine and renal function. *Ann. Rev. Med., 39:* 465–490 (1988).
31. Valeri, A., Neusy, A.-J. Acute and chronic renal disease in hospitalized AIDS patients. *Clin. Nephrol., 35:* 110–118 (1991).
32. Berns, J. S., Cohen, R. M., Stumacher, R. J., Rudnick, M. R. Renal aspects of therapy for human immunodeficiency virus and associated opportunistic infections. *J. Am. Soc. Nephrol., 1:* 1061–1080 (1991).
33. Churg, J., Goldstein, M. H., Bernstein, J. Thrombotic microangiopathy including hemolytic-uremic syndrome, thrombotic thrombocytopenic purpura, and postpartum renal failure. In *Renal Pathology with Clinical and Functional Correlations*. (C. G. Tisher, B. M. Brenner, eds.) J. B. Lippincott Company, Philadelphia (1989).
34. Chander, P., Soni, A., Suri, A., Bhagwat, R., Yoo, J., Treser, G. Renal ultrastructural markers in AIDS-associated nephropathy. *Am. J. Pathol., 126:* 513–526 (1987).
35. Cohen, A. H., Nast, C. C. HIV-associated nephropathy. A unique combined glomerular, tubular, and interstitial lesion. *Mod. Pathol., 1:* 87–97 (1988).
36. D'Agati, V., Suh, J.-I., Carbone, L., Cheng, J.-T., Appel, G. Pathology of HIV-associated nephropathy: a detailed morphologic and comparative study. *Kidney Int., 35:* 1358–1370 (1989).
37. Sidhu, G. S., Stahl, R. E., El-Sadr, W., Cassai, N. D., Forrester, E. M., Zolla-Pazner, S. The acquired immunodeficiency syndrome: an ultrastructural study. *Hum. Pathol., 16:* 377–386 (1985).
38. Kostianovsky, M., Orenstein, J. M., Schaff, Z., Grimley P. M. Cytomembranous inclusions observed in acquired immunodeficiency syndrome: clinical and experimental review. *Arch. Pathol. Lab. Med., 111:* 218–223 (1987).
39. Dolislager, D., Tune, B. The hemolytic-uremic syndrome. Spectrum of severity and significance of prodrome. *Am. J. Dis. Child, 132:* 55–58 (1978).
40. Kaplan, B. S., Cleary, T. G., Obrig, T. G. Recent advances in understanding the pathogenesis of the hemolytic uremic syndromes. *Pediatr. Nephrol., 4:* 276–283 (1990).
41. Kavi, J., Wise, R. Causes of the haemolytic uraemic syndrome. *Br. Med. J., 298:* 65–66 (1989).
42. Martin, D. L., MacDonald, K. L., White, K. E., Soler, J. T., Osterholm, M. T. The epidemiology and clinical aspects of the hemolytic uremic syndrome in Minnesota. *N. Engl. J. Med., 323:* 1161–1167 (1990).
43. Griffin, P. M., Ostroff, S. M., Tauxe, R. V., Greene, K. D., Wells, J. G., Lewis, J. H.,

Blake, P. A. Illnesses associated with *Escherichia coli* 0157:H7 infections. A broad clinical spectrum. *Ann. Intern. Med., 109:* 705–712 (1988).

44. Chart, H., Smith, H. R., Scotland, S. M., Rowe, B., Milford, D. V., Taylor, C. M. Serological identification of *Escherichia coli* 0157:H7 infection in haemolytic uraemic syndrome. *Lancet, 337:* 138–140 (1991).
45. Raghupathy, P., Date, A., Shastry, J.C.M., Sudarsanam, A., Jadhav, M. Haemolytic-uraemic syndrome complicating shigella dysentery in south Indian children. *Br. Med. J., 1:* 1518–1521 (1978).
46. Lian, E.C.-Y. Pathogenesis of thrombotic thrombocytopenic purpura. *Semin. Hematol., 24:* 82–100 (1987).
47. Kirchner, K. A., Smith, R. M., Gockerman, J. P., Luke, R. G. Hereditary thrombotic thrombocytopenic purpura: Microangiopathic hemolytic anemia, thrombocytopenia, and renal insufficiency occurring in consecutive generations. *Nephron, 30:* 28–30 (1982).
48. Yang, C., Nussbaum, M., Park, H. Thrombotic thrombocytopenic purpura in early pregnancy. Remission after plasma exchange. *Acta. Haematol., 62:* 112–116 (1979).
49. Fillastre, J. P., Viotte, G., Morin, J. P., Moulin, B. Nephrotoxicity of antitumoral agents. *Adv. Nephrol., 17:* 175–218 (1988).
50. Lesesne, J. B., Rothschild, N., Erickson, B., Korec, S., Sisk, R., Keller, J., Arbus, M., Woolley, P. V., Chiazze, L., Schein, P. S., Neefe, J. R. Cancer-associated hemolytic-uremic syndrome: Analysis of 85 cases from a national registry. *J. Clin. Oncol., 7:* 781–789 (1989).
51. Giroux, L., Bettez, P., Giroux, L. Mitomycin-C nephrotoxicity: a clinico-pathologic study of 17 cases. *Am. J. Kidney Dis., 6:* 28–39 (1985).
52. Jackson, A. M., Rose, B. D., Graff, L. G., Jacobs, J. B., Schwartz, J. H., Strauss, G. M., Yang, J.P.S., Rudnick, M. R., Elfenbein, I. B., Narins, R. G. Thrombotic microangiopathy and renal failure associated with antineoplastic chemotherapy. *Ann. Intern. Med., 101:* 41–44 (1984).
53. Tumlin, J. A., Sands, J. M., Someren, A. Hemolytic-uremic syndrome following "crack" cocaine inhalation. *Am. J. Med. Sci., 299:* 366–371 (1990).
54. Dixon, A. C., Kwock, D. W., Nakamura, J. M., Yanagihara, E. T., Saiki, S. M., Bodner, A. J., Alexander, S. S. Thrombotic thrombocytopenic purpura and human T-lymphotrophic virus, type 1 (HTLV-1). *Ann. Intern. Med., 110:* 93–94 (1989).
55. Siddiqui, F. A., Lian, E.C.-Y. Novel platelet-agglutinating protein from a thrombotic thrombocytopenic purpura plasma. *J. Clin. Invest., 76:* 1330–1337 (1985).
56. Kelton, J. G., Moore, J., Santos, A., Sheridan, D. Detection of a platelet-agglutinating factor in thrombotic thrombocytopenic purpura. *Ann. Intern. Med., 101:* 589–593 (1984).
57. Monnens, L., van de Meer, W., Langenhuysen, C., van Munster, P., van Oostrom, C. Platelet aggregating factor in the epidemic form of hemolytic-uremic syndrome in childhood. *Clin. Nephrol., 24:* 135–137 (1985).
58. Neame, P. B. Immunologic and other factors in thrombotic thrombocytpenic purpura (TTP). *Sem. Thromb. Hemostasis, 6:* 416–429 (1980).
59. Krupsky, M., Sarel, R., Hurwitz, N., Resnitzky, P. Late appearance of thrombotic thrombocytopenic purpura after autoimmune hemolytic anemia and in the course of chronic autoimmune thrombocytopenic purpura: two case reports. *Acta Haematol., 85:* 139–142 (1991).
60. Moake, J. L. Thrombotic thrombocytopenic purpura and the hemolytic-uremic syndrome. In: *Hematology, Basic Principles and Practice*. (R. Hoffman, E. J. Benz, S. J. Shattil, B. Furie, H. J. Cohen, eds.) Churchill Livingstone, New York. (1991).
61. Moake, J. L., Rudy, C. K., Troll, J. H., Weinstein, M. J., Colannino, N. M., Azocar, J., Seder, R. H., Hong, S. L., Deykin, D. Unusually large plasma factor VIII : von Willebrand factor multimers in chronic relapsing thrombotic thrombocytopenic purpura. *N. Engl. J. Med., 307:* 1432–1435 (1982).

62. Rose, P. E., Enayat, S. M., Sunderland, R., Short, P. E., Williams, C. E. Abnormalities of factor VIII related protein multimers in the haemolytic uraemic syndrome. *Arch. Dis. Child, 59:* 1135–1140 (1984).
63. Moake, J. L., Byrnes, J. J., Troll, J. H., Rudy, C. K., Weinstein, M. J., Colannino, N. M., Hong, S. L. Abnormal VIII : von Willebrand factor patterns in the plasma of patients with the hemolytic-uremic syndrome. *Blood, 64:* 592–598 (1984).
64. Peterson, D. M., Stathopoulos, N. A., Giorgio, T. D., Hellums, J. D., Moake, J. L. Shear-induced platelet aggregation requires von Willebrand factor and platelet membrane glycoproteins Ib and IIb/IIIa. *Blood, 69:* 625–628 (1987).
65. Myers, T. J., Wakem, C. J., Ball, E. D., Tremont, S. J. Thrombotic thrombocytopenic purpura: combined treatment with plasmapheresis and antiplatelet agents. *Ann. Intern. Med., 92*(Pt. 1): 149–155 (1980).
66. Bukowski, R. M., Hewlett, J. S., Reimer, R. R., Groppe, C. W., Weick, J. K., Livingston, R. B. Therapy of thrombotic thrombocytopenic purpura: an overview. *Sem. Thromb. Hemostasis, 7:* 1–8 (1981).
67. Misiani, R., Appiani, A. C., Edefonti, A., Gotti, E., Bettinelli, A., Giani, M., Rossi, E., Remuzzi, G., Mecca, G. Haemolytic uraemic syndrome: therapeutic effect of plasma infusion. *Br. Med. J., 285:* 1304–1306 (1982).
68. Hakim, R. M., Schulman, G., Churchill, W. H., Lazarus, J. M. Successful management of thrombocytopenia, microangiopathic anemia, and acute renal failure by plasmapheresis. *Am. J. Kidney Dis., 5:* 170–176 (1985).
69. Lichtin, A. E., Schreiber, A. D., Hurwitz, S., Willoughby, T. L., Silberstein, L. E. Efficacy of intensive plasmapheresis in thrombotic thrombocytopenic purpura. *Arch. Intern. Med., 147:* 2122–2126 (1987).
70. Loirat, C., Sonsino, E., Hinglais, N., Jais, J. P., Landais, P., Fermanian, J. Treatment of childhood haemolytic uraemic syndrome with plasma. A multicentre randomized controlled trial. *Pediatr. Nephrol., 2:* 279–285 (1988).
71. Pohl, M. A., Lan, S.-P., Berl, T. Plasmapheresis does not increase the risk for infection in immunosuppressed patients with severe lupus nephritis. *Ann. Intern. Med., 114:* 924–929 (1991).
72. Wing, E. J., Bruns, F. J., Fraley, D. S., Segel, D. P., Adler, S. Infectious complications with plasmapheresis in rapidly progressive glomerulonephritis. *J.A.M.A., 244:* 2423–2426 (1980).
73. Gold, J. W. M. Infectious complications in patients with HIV infection. *AIDS, 2:* 327–334 (1988).
74. Mittelman, A., Bertram, J., Henry, D. H., Snyder, H. W., Messerschmidt, G. L., Ciavarella, D., Ainsworth, S., Kiprov, D., Arlin, Z. Treatment of patients with HIV thrombocytopenia and hemolytic uremic syndrome with protein A (Prosorba Column) immunoadsorption. *Semin. Hematol., 26*(suppl 1): 15–18 (1989).
75. Korec, S., Schein, P. S., Smith, F. P., Neefe, J. R., Woolley, P. V., Goldberg, R. M., Phillips, T. M. Treatment of cancer-associated hemolytic uremic syndrome with staphylococcal protein A immunoperfusion. *J. Clin. Oncol., 4:* 210–215 (1986).
76. Rose, M., Eldor, A. High incidence of relapses in thrombotic thrombocytopenic purpura. Clinical study of 38 patients. *Am. J. Med., 83:* 437–444 (1987).
77. Ponticelli, C., Rivolta, E., Imbasciati, E., Rossi, E., Mannucci, P. M. Hemolytic uremic syndrome in adults. *Arch. Intern. Med., 140:* 353–357 (1980).
78. Morel-Maroger, L., Kanfer, A., Solez, K., Sraer, J.-D., Richet, G. Prognostic importance of vascular lesions in acute renal failure with microangiopathic hemolytic anemia (hemolytic-uremic syndrome): Clinicopathologic study in 20 adults. *Kidney Int., 15:* 548–558 (1979).
79. Glassock, R. J. (moderator). Human immunodeficiency virus (HIV) infection and the kidney. *Ann. Intern. Med., 112:* 35–49 (1990).

80. Price, R. W., Brew, B. Management of the neurologic complications of HIV-1 infection and AIDS. In: *The Medical Management of AIDS*. (M. A. Sande, P. A. Volberding, eds.) W. B. Saunders Co., Philadelphia (1990).
81. Poole, G., Stradling, P., Worlledge, S. Potentially serious side effects of high-dose twice-weekly rifampicin. *Br. Med. J., 3:* 343–347 (1971).
82. Mauri, J. M., Fort, J., Bartolome, J., Camps, J., Capdevila, L., Morlans, M., Martin-Vega, C., Piera, L. Antirifampicin antibodies in acute rifampicin-induced renal failure. *Nephron, 31:* 177–179 (1982).
83. Chugh, K. S., Singhal, P. C., Sharma, B. K., Mahakur, A. C., Pal, Y., Datta, B. N., Das, K. C. Acute renal failure due to intravascular hemolysis in the North Indian patients. *Am. J. Med. Sci., 274:* 139–146 (1977).
84. Roth, D., Alarson, F. J., Fernandez, J. A., Preston, R. A., Bourgoignie, J. J. Acute rhabdomyolysis associated with cocaine intoxication. *N. Engl. J. Med., 319:* 673–677 (1988).
85. Citron, B. P., Halpern, M., McCarron, M., Lundberg, G. D., McCormick, R., Pincus, I. J., Tatter, D., Haverback, B. J. Necrotizing angiitis associated with drug use. *N. Engl. J. Med., 283:* 1003–1011 (1970).
86. Cello, J. P. AIDS-associated gastrointestinal disease. In *The Medical Management of AIDS*. (M. A. Sande, P. A. Volberding, eds.) W. B. Saunders Co., Philadelphia. (1990).

V
Pathology

24
Pathology of the Hemolytic Uremic Syndrome

Renée Habib *Hôpital Necker–Enfants Malades, Paris, France*

The term *hemolytic uremic syndrome* (HUS) describes the condition of children and adults who present with abrupt onset of acquired hemolytic anemia, thrombocytopenia, hematuria, proteinuria, and varying degrees of renal failure, together with variable neurological abnormalities. When these characteristic clinical features are associated with the lesions of thrombotic microangiopathy (TMA), it is a well-defined clinicopathological entity. However, as underlined by Kaplan and Drummond (1):

> This constellation of findings may occur in a number of distinctly different situations and in all likelihood is the result of a variety of pathogenetic mechanisms. In this context, an appropriate parallel can be drawn between the hemolytic-uremic syndrome and the nephrotic syndrome in which a host of different injuries, ranging from immune-complex deposition to mercury intoxication, result in glomerular damage that is expressed as massive proteinuria

In other words, limiting the syndrome to HUS with TMA would be like limiting the nephrotic syndrome to idiopathic nephrosis with minimal change disease. On the other hand, overexpanding the concept of the clinical syndrome may lead to the recognition of unreliable pathogenetic mechanisms and, therefore, to the use of inappropriate treatments. Furthermore, the lack of specificity of the arteriolopathy observed in HUS increases the difficulty in delineating the condition. If arteriolar TMA is the central lesion that explains the principal components of the syndrome (increased platelet destruction, microangiopathic hemolytic anemia, and impaired renal function), it must be emphasized that similar lesions may be observed in malignant hypertension, cyclosporine nephrotoxicity, and transplant rejection, for example, without the clinical features of HUS.

Consequently, describing the pathology of HUS is not easy. We will describe the *primary forms* of the syndrome; the *recurrent and the familial subsets;* the forms that are *secondary* to various presumed etiological factors; and HUS superimposed on preexisting conditions.

HISTOLOGICAL REVIEW

To understand the complexity of the problem, we have summarized the history of HUS with special emphasis on the eternal debate on the relationship between HUS and thrombotic thrombocytopenic purpura (TTP). The history of HUS and TTP begins in 1925, with the report by E. Moschcowitz of an "undescribed disease" concerning a 16-year-old girl who presented with "an acute febrile pleiochromic anemia with hyaline thrombosis of the terminal arterioles and capillaries," and who died 4 days after admission (2). About 10 years later Baehr and colleagues (3) reported four similar cases, by which time thrombocytopenia was recognized as a contributing factor to the bleeding problems. In subsequent reports, the emphasis was always on the triad consisting of thrombocytopenic purpura, hemolytic anemia, and varying neurological manifestations; this entity was called TTP a term that, regrettably, does not include hemolytic anemia. For many years, renal involvement did not seem to be an essential component of TTP.

From a pathological viewpoint, the characteristic feature of TTP was described as being the widespread occurrence of "hyaline thrombi" involving arterioles and capillaries. In fact, the vascular lesion of TTP consists of a bland platelet–fibrin mixture in varying stages of organization, occurring chiefly at the level of the arteriolar–capillary junction, and the underlying vessel shows no evidence of vasculitis. Although the individual thrombotic lesion is nonspecific, the florid, disseminated nature of the process is quite distinctive. The most commonly involved organs are heart, brain, kidneys, pancreas, and adrenal glands. In 1952, Symmers proposed the term *thrombotic microangiopathy* to designate this type of vascular lesion (4).

In 1955, Gasser et al. (5) described a clinical syndrome which they called the hemolytic uremic syndrome. They considered that this was a new syndrome and that it was different from TTP. First, the disease affected four infants and a 7-year-old girl, whereas TTP had been reported mainly in adults. Second, the five children presented with acute renal failure, whereas, at that time, renal involvement in TTP was ignored or underestimated. Third, the pathology was reported as being renal cortical necrosis, and only patient 3 (a 6-month-old infant) was mentioned as having Symmer's thrombotic microangiopathy affecting small arteries, arterioles, and capillaries in myocardium, kidneys, brain, lungs, thyroid, and adrenal glands.

In 1957, when we published our first case of TTP in a 10-month-old infant (6), we were surprised by the severity of the glomerular changes which, to our knowledge, had never been mentioned previously. We reviewed the pathology of 60 cases who had died of acute renal failure in the Department of Pediatrics at the Hôpital des Enfants Malades in Paris over a period of 10 years and found 6 similar cases. All 6 had presented with hemolytic anemia and thrombocytopenia, in addition to acute renal failure. But, more interestingly, each had the same specific glomerular pathology, and the arteriolar lesions were limited to the kidneys (7). We called it "maladie thrombotique artériolocapillaire du rein" and described the glomerular lesion in the following way: The glomerular lesion is characterized by a thickening of the capillary walls, with a double-contour appearance caused by a widening of the subendothelial space. The endothelial cells are swollen, and there is no increase in the number of mesangial cells. In the few patent capillary lumina, thrombi having the characteristic staining for fibrin are occasionally present. Thrombotic arteriolar lesions are constant and preferentially involve the afferent arterioles in which the primary lesion seems to concern the endothelium.

Thereafter, we were unhappy about the lack of precision in the term "maladie thrombotique arteriolocapillaire du rein" and asked Symmers if he would allow us to extend to the glomerular capillary the term thrombotic microangiopathy. Thrombotic microangiopathy had been chosen to designate the arteriolar lesion, but we hypothesized that the involvement of the glomeruli was merely the prolongation within the tuft of the endothelial lesions of the arterioles. In 1960, with his agreement, we published a paper in which we called thrombotic microangiopathy both the glomerular and the vascular lesion and proposed a unifying concept for Moschcowitz's disease, Gasser's disease, and our arteriologlomerular disease, the common denominator being the vascular lesion (8).

In the following years, with better knowledge of all the varieties of glomerulopathies, gained from the use of renal biopsy, it appeared that glomerular TMA was a pathognomonic pattern seen exclusively in the setting of a hemolytic uremic syndrome (9). Conversely, patients presenting with idiopathic HUS could show one of three morphological variants of the disease: (a) widespread arteriolar lesions as in TTP; (b) cortical necrosis as in Gasser's disease; and (c) exclusive renal involvement with lesions of glomerular TMA similar to the ones we had reported in 1958, in 1960, and in subsequent publications (10–13).

More recently (14), we have shown that the prognosis of the disease is related to the severity of the vascular changes. We have added a fourth pattern called *arterial TMA*, which is characterized by the predominant involvement of the arterioles and interlobular arteries. In this morphological variant, the changes observed in the glomeruli are of the ischemic type. They are the result of vascular obstruction, therefore, differing from the changes that occur in glomerular TMA. Arterial TMA is usually associated with severe hypertension.

Since renal failure dominates the clinical picture in children the term HUS has always been widely used by pediatricians to designate this condition. By contrast, in adults, neurological involvement often dominates the clinical picture and this accounts for TTP being the predominant diagnosis in this aged group. In the adult literature, the term HUS appeared only in the 1970s (15–21), and until recently, there has been a great confusion concerning the relationship between PTT and HUS.

In fact, in the initial case report by Moschcowitz (2), the urine was noted to have shown "marked traces of albumin with hyaline and granular casts," the kidneys were reported to have "marked parenchymatous degeneration in the tubules and congestion of the parenchyma" and "many of the arterioles and capillaries in the middle zone, in the region of the vasa recta, showed hyaline thrombi of the same morphology as those in the heart." In the subsequent report by Baehr et al. (3), all four cases had signs of renal involvement, and at autopsy, the vascular lesions of their cases were reported as "most common in the cortex of the kidneys and the adrenals, the myocardium and the pancreas," with the renal lesions being "most common in the cortical zone adjacent to the medulla."

Even after the 1966 review on TTP by Amorosi and Ultmann (22), who showed that renal involvement was demonstrable in 88% of the 271 cases reported in the literature, kidney involvement was not considered an important feature of TTP.

During the last decade, two important reviews (23–24) have focused on the importance of renal involvement in TTP, and Eknoyan and Riggs (24) have suggested that renal involvement in TTP could be categorized into three types depending on the severity of TTP. The first type includes cases presenting as an acute devastating illness, in which renal insufficiency is severe and a dominant component of the disease. The second type includes cases that pursue a more protracted course with subsequent acute exacerbations of TTP and in which renal insufficiency is variable and less severe than in the first group. The third group is composed of cases with a mild form of TTP, in which renal involvement consists primarily of an abnormal urine sediment and azotemia that corrects rapidly following fluid replacement. Renal involvement cannot, therefore, be considered as a clinical feature differentiating HUS from TTP.

As far as the vasculopathy is concerned, although the kidney is the main target in HUS, the multiorgan involvement characteristic of TTP can also be observed in HUS as shown in two recent studies (25, 26).

As examples of the overlap between the two conditions, we will quote some interesting observations of the literature. A girl reported by Shumway and Miller (27) as having HUS in one episode, is reported by MacWhinney et al. (28) as having TTP during another one, several years later. Three families in which both diseases occurred have been reported: two HLA identical brothers, one presenting with HUS at 19 years of age, the other one, a 24-year-old, with TTP 6½ years later (29); a 27-year-old mother with TTP and her 24-year-old daughter with HUS (30); and three siblings, two with TTP and one with HUS (31).

In conclusion, it can be said that if a typical case of HUS is quite different from a typical case of TTP, it is now generally accepted that HUS and TTP are two closely related conditions that represent opposite ends of the spectrum of the same disease process (32). Their common denominator is the presence of microangiopathic hemolytic anemia, thrombocytopenia, and arteriolar thrombosis.

PRIMARY HEMOLYTIC UREMIC SYNDROME

Clinical Manifestations

The hemolytic uremic syndrome can be classified into two forms: a *typical form* that occurs principally as summer outbreaks and, for this reason, is often called *epidemic form,* and an *atypical form* that occurs as isolated cases and is sometimes called *sporadic form*. Two other features differentiate these two forms, the existence, or the absence, of a prodromal phase before the occurrence of hemolytic anemia and thrombocytopenia, and the type of renal involvement.

Typical Form of Hemolytic Uremic Syndrome

Most of the infants under aged 2 years, half of the older children and approximately 20% of adults present with this form of the disease. After a short prodromal phase, most often characterized by gastrointestinal symptoms with diarrhea, the patients present abruptly with pallor, petechiae, bleeding, acute renal failure, and sometimes central nervous system (CNS) symptoms. Oliguria is extremely frequent and may last from 2 to 20 days or more. Normal urine output with a decreased glomerular filtration rate (GFR) is seen in mild cases. Proteinuria and hematuria are invariably present, and blood pressure is normal or mildly elevated. This form generally has a good prognosis if standard treatment for acute renal failure is given.

Atypical Form of Hemolytic Uremic Syndrome

As opposed to the typical form, the patients may be classified as having an atypical form when there is no prodromal phase and when they have a more protracted course with normal urine output, at least at onset. Apart from severely impaired renal function, these patients have hematuria and marked proteinuria sometimes leading to a nephrotic syndrome. Hypertension is a hallmark of this form of the disease and may become uncontrollable or be uncontrollable from onset, whereas CNS symptoms are less often observed. This form of HUS is extremely rare in infants, occurs in many older children, and is very frequent in adults. Its prognosis is usually poor, and terminal renal failure occurs after a few days or a few weeks. Hypertension may be severe enough to justify bilateral nephrectomy.

Pathology

Surprisingly, there are few good descriptions of the pathological features of primary HUS (10, 12–15, 19, 33–37). The central lesion of primary HUS is a characteristic arteriolopathy, extending into the glomerular capillaries, called TMA. However, various patterns of involvement of the renal parenchyma may be seen. They can be classified according to the predominant pattern observed. Interestingly, however, the clinical symptoms of HUS may occur in the absence of arteriolar and glomerular lesions, as reported by Courtecuisse et al. (38), Larbre et al. (39), Levy et al. (40), and Bohle et al. (41).

Cortical Necrosis

All degrees of severity may be observed. Cortical necrosis may be patchy (Fig. 1) and involve a group of glomeruli and tubules, or it may diffuse to the whole superficial cortex. Its extent is impossible to evaluate on biopsy specimens. The aspect varies according to the date the specimen is obtained. In late specimens, it is not unusual to find calcifications of the necrotic structures and large amounts of hemosiderin at the periphery of the necrotic zone. In the noninfarcted portions of the cortex and in the deep cortex, lesions of glomerular and arteriolar TMA are always present together with ischemic glomeruli. Interlobular and arcuate arteries are often obstructed by a mixture of fibrous endarteritis and fibrinoid necrosis. Interlobar arteries are always normal.

Glomerular Thrombotic Microangiopathy

The striking feature is the variegated appearance of the glomeruli (Fig. 2). Several patterns of involvement coexist, side by side, in a variable proportion according to the severity of the disease.

The most characteristic lesion is that of glomerular TMA. The glomeruli are enlarged and show a thickening of the capillary walls (Fig. 3), with a double-contour appearance caused by a widening of the subendothelial space, whereas the basement

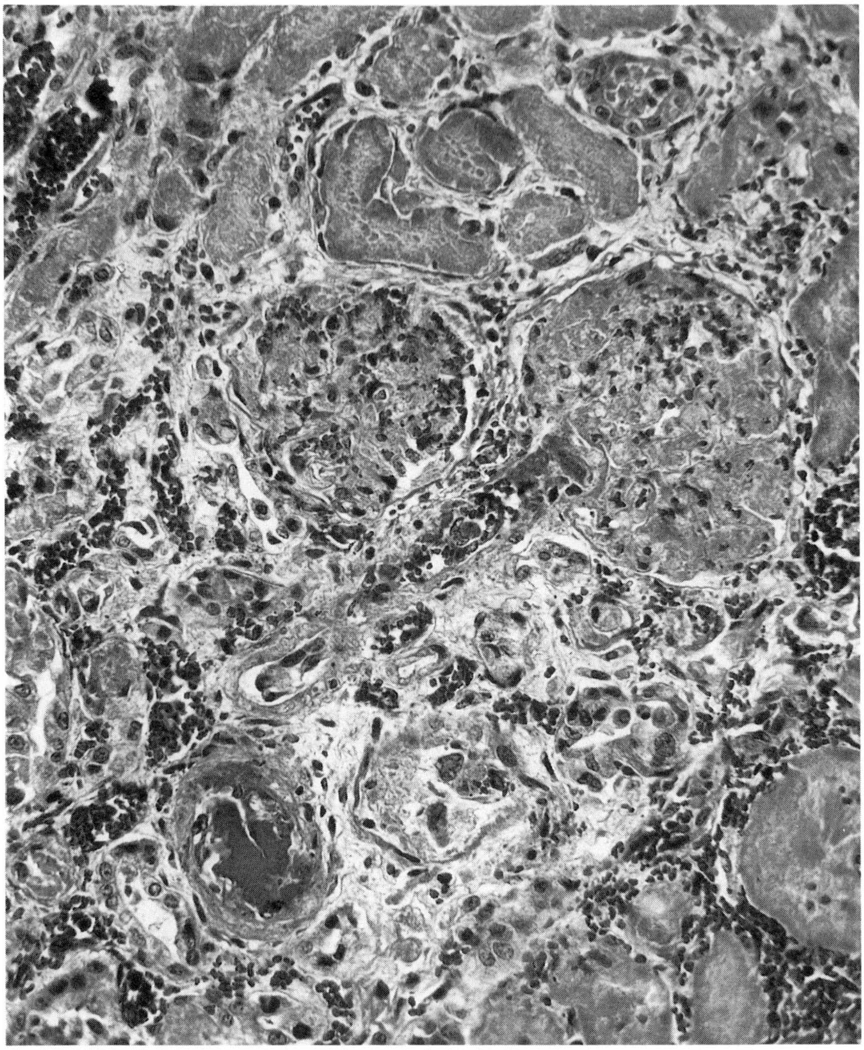

Figure 1 Cortical necrosis × 200. Necrotic glomeruli and tubules close to a thrombosed preglomerular artery.

membrane itself appears unaltered (Fig. 4). The endothelial cells are swollen, and the mesangial cells, although often swollen, are not increased in number. The mesangial matrix has a fibrillar appearance, and an interposition of mesangial matrix along the peripheral capillary walls may be seen; this, together with the widening of the subendothelial space, leads to the narrowing or to the complete obstruction of the capillary lumina (Fig. 5). In the few patent capillary lumina, red blood cells and platelets may be present, whereas thrombi that have the characteristic staining for fibrin are observed occasionally (Fig. 6). Lesions of mesangiolysis (42), are unusual. Podocytes often are swollen and may contain hyalin droplets, but crescents are very rarely seen.

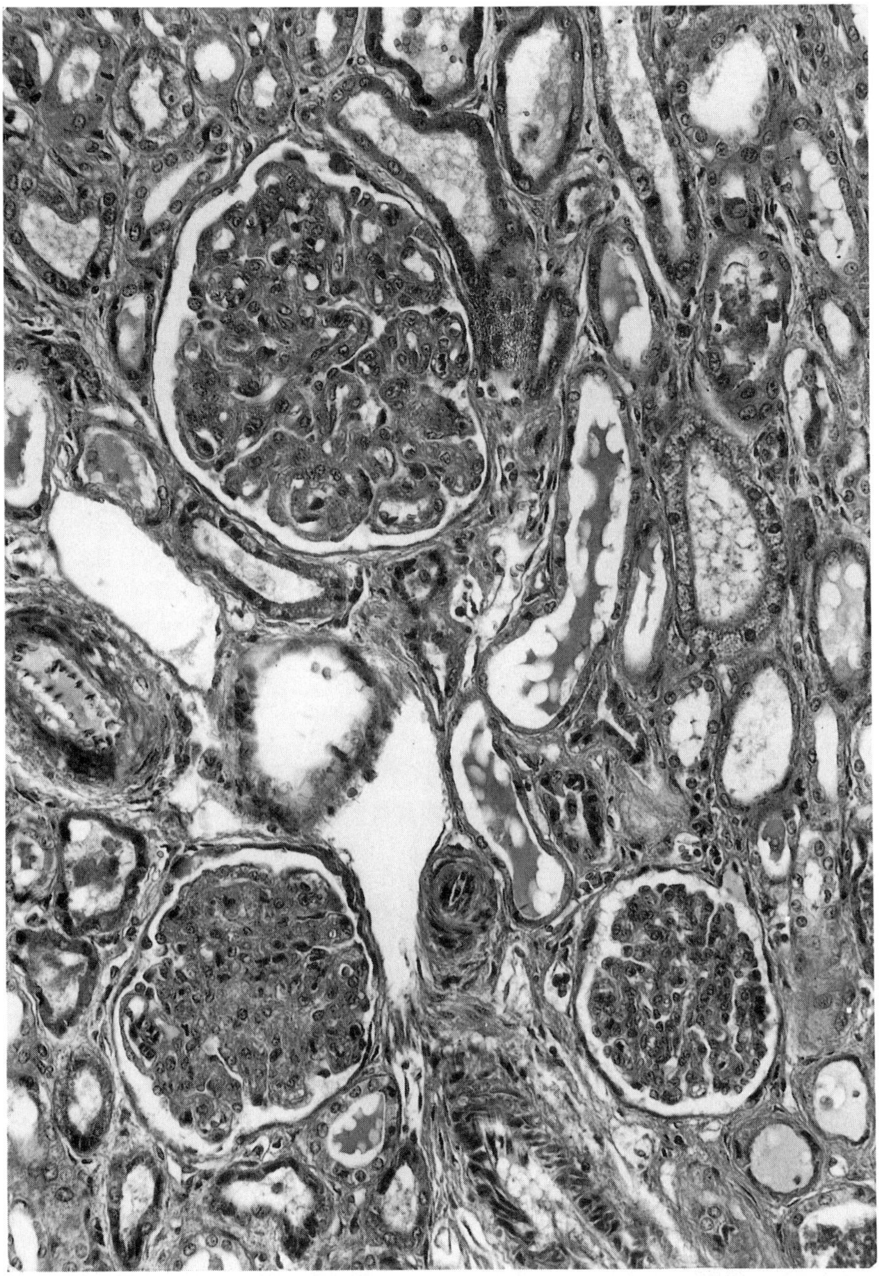

Figure 2 Glomerular thrombotic microangiopathy (TMA) × 200. Note the variegated appearance of the glomeruli and the subendothelial widening of the arteriole.

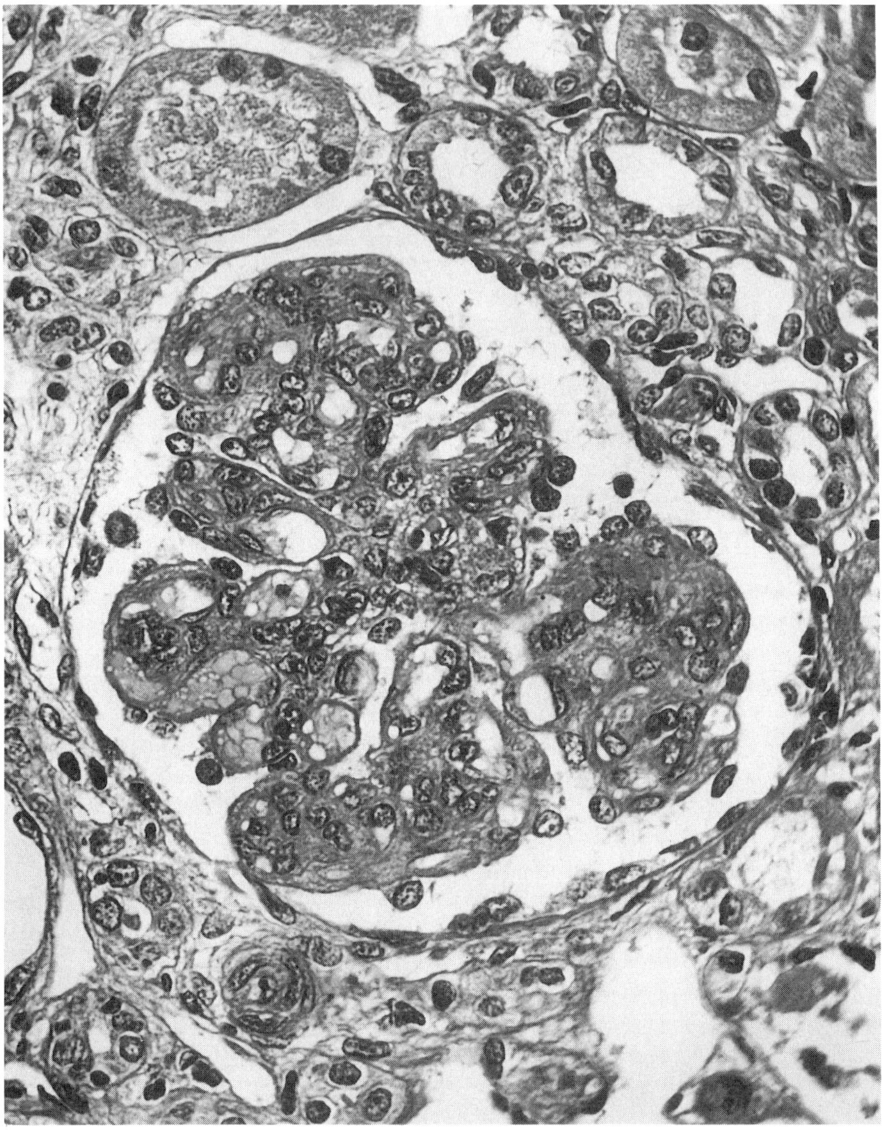

Figure 3 Glomerular TMA × 700. Thickening of the capillary walls with fibrillar appearance of the mesangial matrix. Note the subendothelial widening of the preglomerular arterioles.

A second pattern concerns glomeruli that are also enlarged, have marked dilatation of the capillary lumina, contain numerous red blood cells, and have either normal or split capillary walls. Such "paralytic" glomeruli are most likely related to the obstruction of efferent arterioles.

In a variable proportion of glomeruli, the only change is a fibrillar widening of mesangial areas with occasional double-contours of the peripheral capillary walls.

In other glomeruli, there is a shrinkage of the tuft, with wrinkling of the capillary walls and, sometimes, a widening of Bowman's space, which gives the appearance of

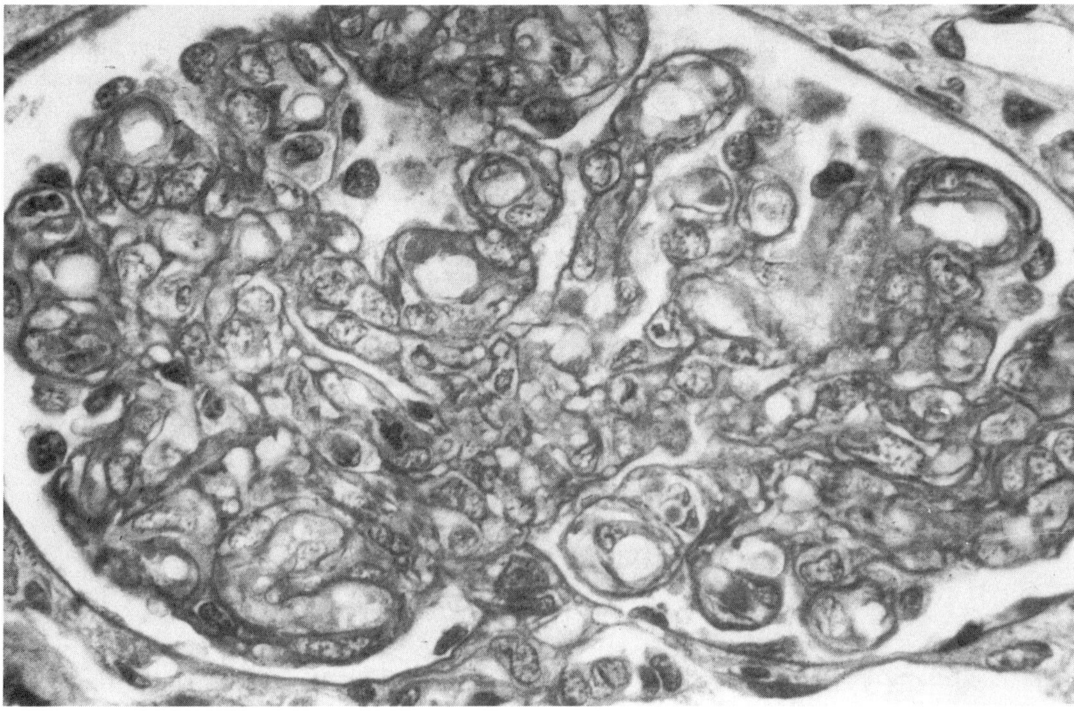

Figure 4 Glomerular TMA × 900. Higher magnification showing the double contour appearance of the capillary walls and the widening of the subendothelial space.

pseudocystic glomeruli. These glomerular cysts are particularly abundant in end-stage kidneys and predominate in the superficial cortex. Some glomeruli may appear normal.

Preglomerular arteriolar changes are always associated with these various glomerular lesions. They are variable both within a single biopsy specimen (Fig. 7) and according to the interval between onset and biopsy. In most infants and in some older children, these changes are discrete and are merely characterized by a widening of the subendothelial space. Sometimes, the lesions are more marked, and the swelling of the endothelial and subendothelial layers may lead to the narrowing of the arteriolar lumen. In some arterioles, fibroelastic intimal thickening imparts an onion-skin appearance to the arteriolar wall. Luminal thrombosis is far from being a constant feature, but fibrinoid intimal necrosis is frequently seen. Necrosis of the myocytes is exceptional. In autopsy specimens, which by definition concern severe cases of HUS, medium-sized arteries, up to arcuates, may be involved by the same process and often show an obstruction by fibrous endarteritis.

Ultrastructural studies confirm these findings and show severe changes of the endothelium and of the mesangial matrix. The lamina densa of the capillary wall is normal, and the double-contoured appearance is caused by separation of the endothelium from the glomerular basement membrane (GBM). The space between the lamina densa and the detached endothelium is filled with pale fluffy material, which may contain cellular debris (Fig. 8). The endothelial cells are swollen and show signs

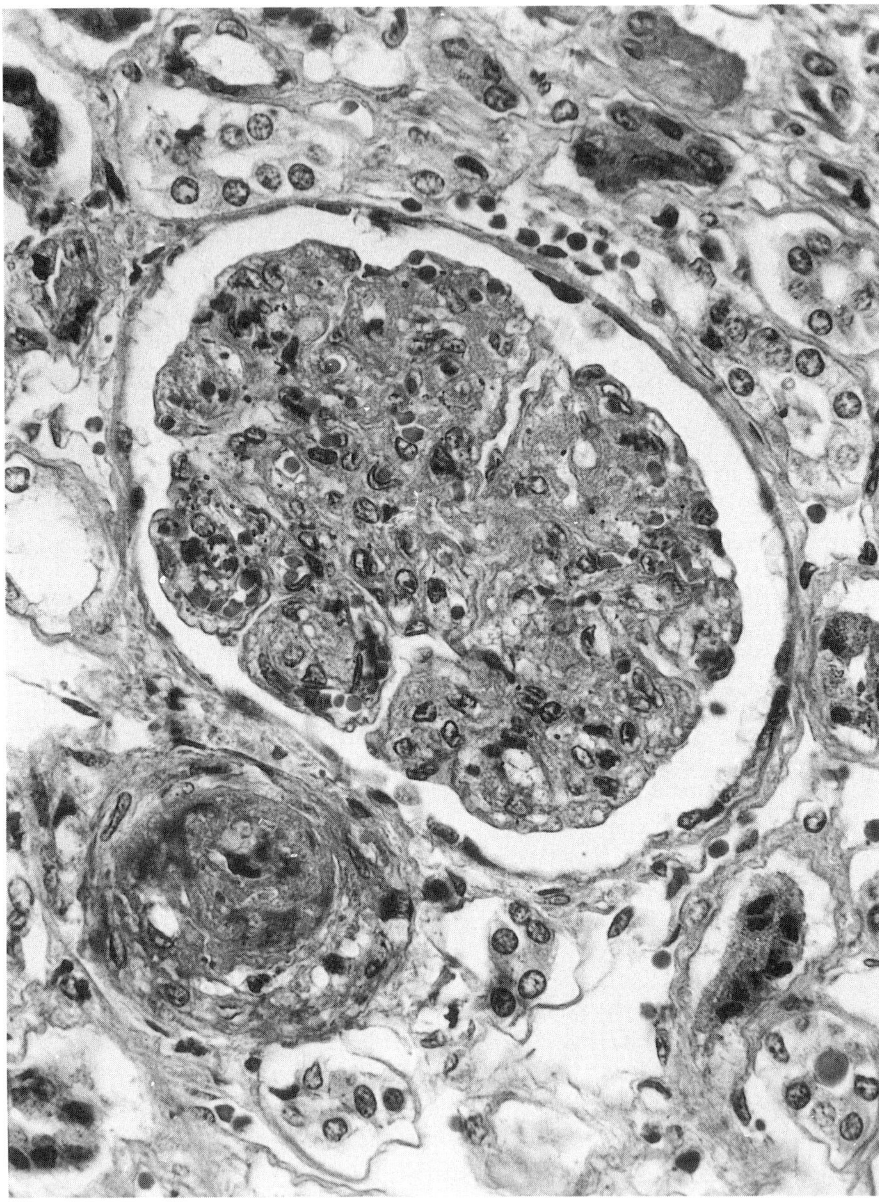

Figure 5 Glomerular TMA × 660. Obstruction of most of the capillary lumens and thrombosis of the preglomerular arteriole.

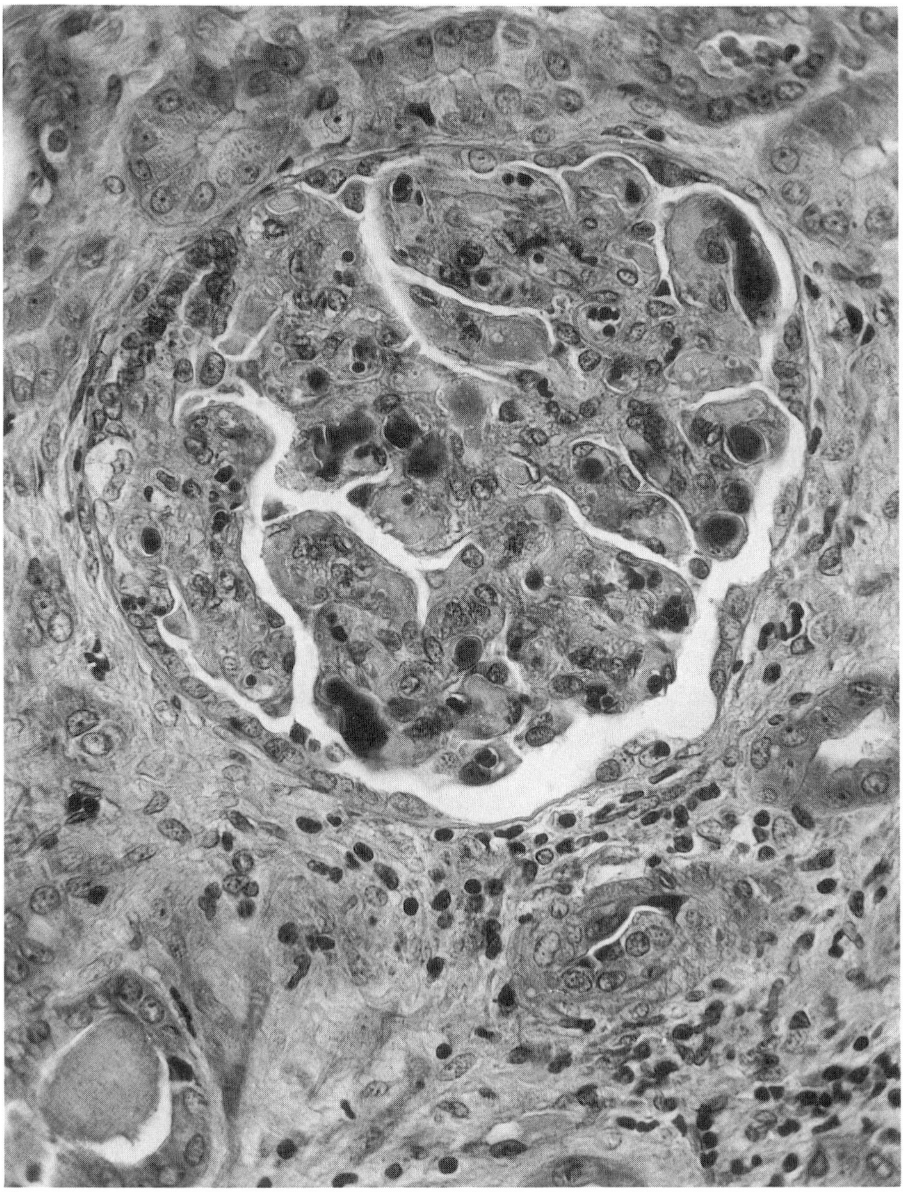

Figure 6 Glomerular TMA × 550. Note the presence of fibrin thrombi in some of the patent capillary lumens and the subendothelial necrosis of the preglomerular arteriole.

of activity, with numerous intracytoplasmic organelles. The mesangial matrix (42) is swollen (Fig. 9) and has the appearance of a meshwork filled with electron-opaque, finely granular or fibrillar material, similar to that observed in the subendothelial space. The mesangial cells are generally hypertrophied and show increased amounts of rough-surfaced endoplasmic reticulum, enlarged cytoplasmic processes, cytolysosomes, and lipid droplets. Peripheral extension of mesangial cell cytoplasm and

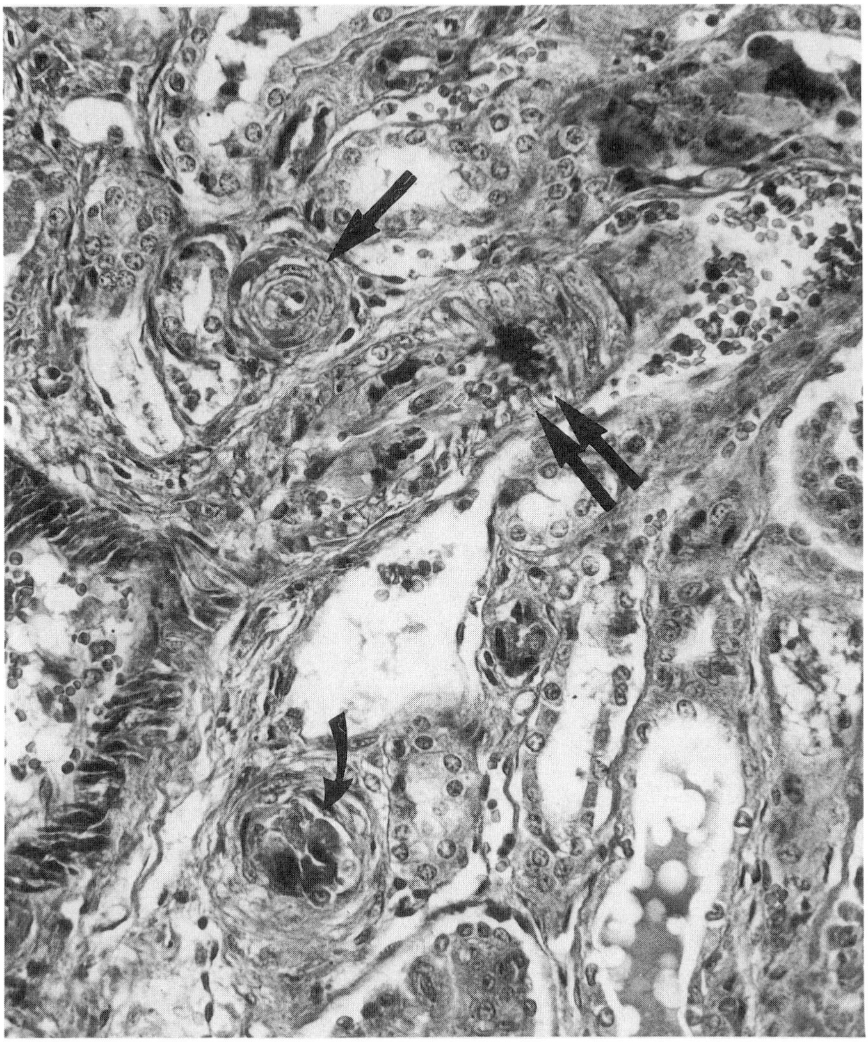

Figure 7 Glomerular TMA × 200. All types of arterial lesions may be seen. Fibroelastric intimal thickening giving the arteriolar wall an onion skin appearance (→). Thrombosis of another arteriole (↷) and subendothelial necrosis of an interlobular artery (⇉).

matrix into the capillary contributes to the narrowing of the capillary lumen (42). We have shown (43) that numerous platelets can be present in the lumen of some glomerular capillaries, sometimes in close contact with the capillary wall, and fragments of platelets may even be present in the GBM.

By immunofluorescence microscopy (IF), there is a strong fixation of antifibrin serum along all the capillary walls and more intensely so on some thrombi in the capillary lumina (Fig. 10). Fibrin may also be present in the lumina of the arterioles (14, 44). Deposits of IgM and C3 are unusual (45, 46) and do not lend support to an immune pathogenesis.

All of these features, taken together, define a very characteristic pattern of involvement. It is obvious that the fundamental lesion of TMA is the endothelial

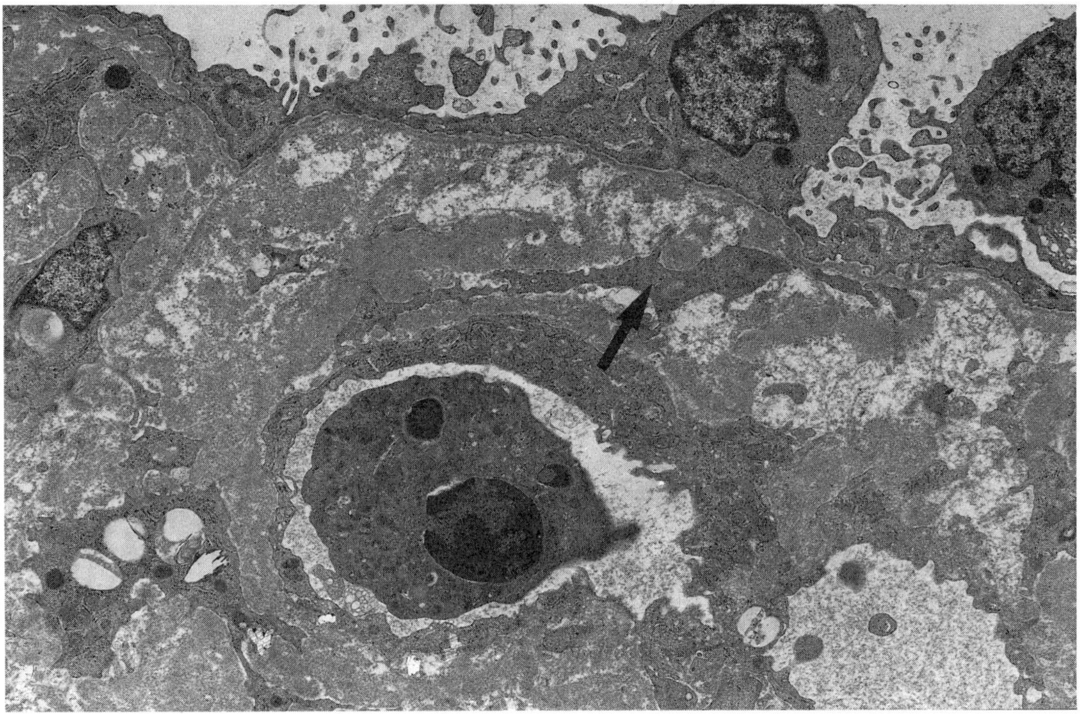

Figure 8 Electron microscopy × 6600. Glomerular TMA. Thickening of the capillary wall. The space between the normal lamina densa and the endothelium is filled with a pale fluffy material together with mesangial expansion (→) (Courtesy MC Gubler).

abnormality and that intravascular thrombosis is a secondary phenomenon. The only glomerular pattern that resembles glomerular TMA is allograft glomerulopathy (47), which is observed in some forms of chronic rejection.

Arterial Thrombotic Microangiopathy

In this form of TMA, arterioles and interlobular arteries are severely involved, but, in association with these widespread vascular lesions, most glomeruli appear "ischemic," showing splitting of the capillary walls, with a widening of the subendothelial space and wrinkling of the GBM (Fig. 11). Mesangial matrix changes are much less conspicuous than in glomerular TMA and, in some capillary loops, segmental lesions of mesangiolysis may be observed. These ischemic glomeruli are seen mainly in the superficial cortex, whereas glomeruli showing the characteristic features of glomerular TMA may be observed in the deep cortex. Electron microscopic studies confirm these findings (14, 15, 33–36) (Fig. 12).

By IF with antifibrin antiserum, there is either no labeling of the glomeruli, or segmental deposits of fibrin are seen along some capillary walls. Deposits of fibrin are present in the widened subendothelial space of arterioles and medium-sized arteries (14).

Arterial TMA is the pattern of involvement that is most frequently seen in adults. It is unusual in infants. It has been observed in specimens obtained later in the disease in children (26) and, in some cases, it might represent a late stage of

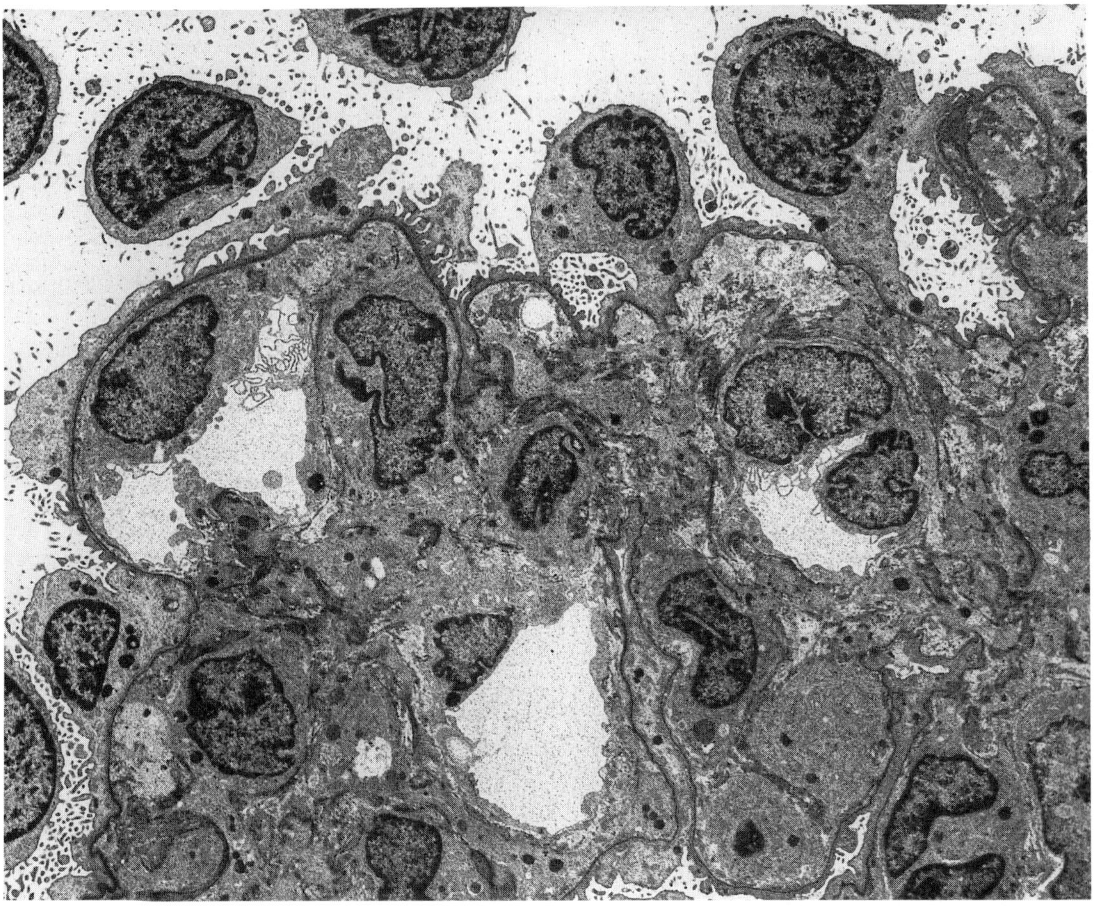

Figure 9 Electron microscopy × 3000. Glomerular TMA. Swelling of the mesangial matrix and hyertrophy of endothelial and mesangial cells leading to a marked reduction of the capillary lumen (Courtesy MC Gubler).

glomerular TMA when there may be associated severe vascular changes. We had the opportunity of examining renal tissue from four patients obtained both early and late in the course of the disease. Arterial TMA was observed in bilateral nephrectomy specimens, whereas glomerular TMA had been present in early biopsy specimens. The similarity of arterial TMA, which is always associated with severe hypertension, with the glomerular and vascular lesions of malignant hypertension, raises a problem of interpretation. Bohle et al. (34), rejecting the term TMA, suggest that this disease be called "primary malignant nephrosclerosis" because, in their opinion, the vascular lesions would induce hypertension, as opposed to "secondary malignant nephrosclerosis" in which hypertension would induce the vascular lesion. This suggestion has not received wide acceptance. The main criticism is that this term does not cover the whole range of renal changes seen in HUS. As an alternative to the term TMA, Thoenes and John (35, 36) have proposed the term "endotheliotropic nephroan-

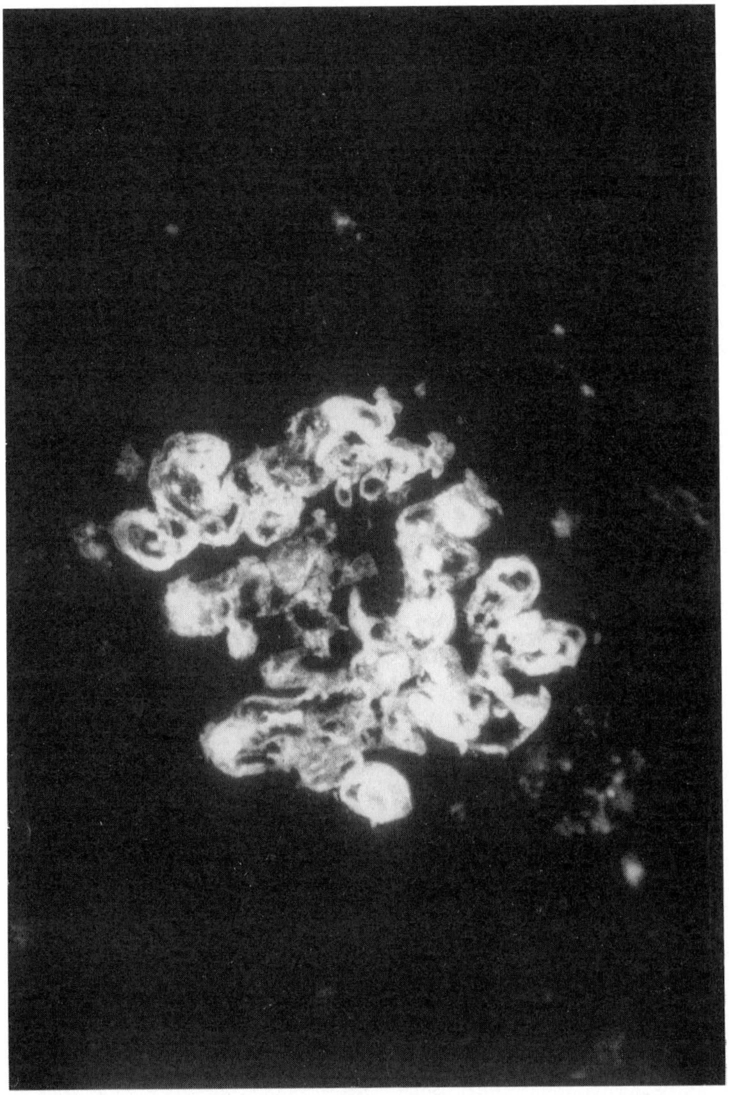

Figure 10 Immunofluorescence microscopy × 400 glomerular TMA. Antifibrin serum. Strong labeling of the capillary walls. Thrombi may be seen in some capillary lumens.

giopathy," which would encompass both the glomerular and arterial forms of the disease.

In conclusion, the distinction between the three patterns of involvement we have described are important because of the prognosis of each of these morphological types. It must be remembered however, that there are no clearcut differences between these different patterns and that a mixture of the three patterns is not unusual in a given specimen. Accordingly, the morphological diagnosis should be based on the predominant pattern of involvement.

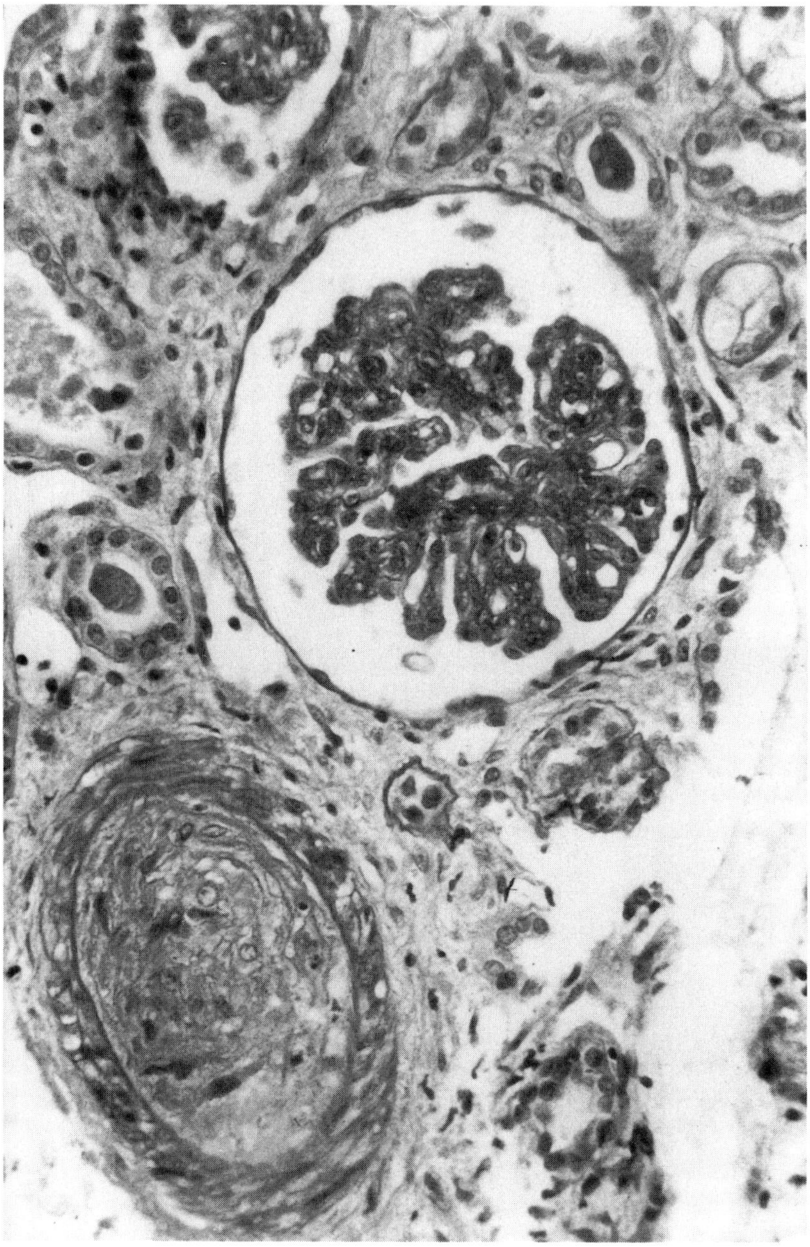

Figure 11 Arterial TMA × 280. Wrinkling of the glomerular capillary walls and obstruction of the interlobular artery lumen by an organized thrombus.

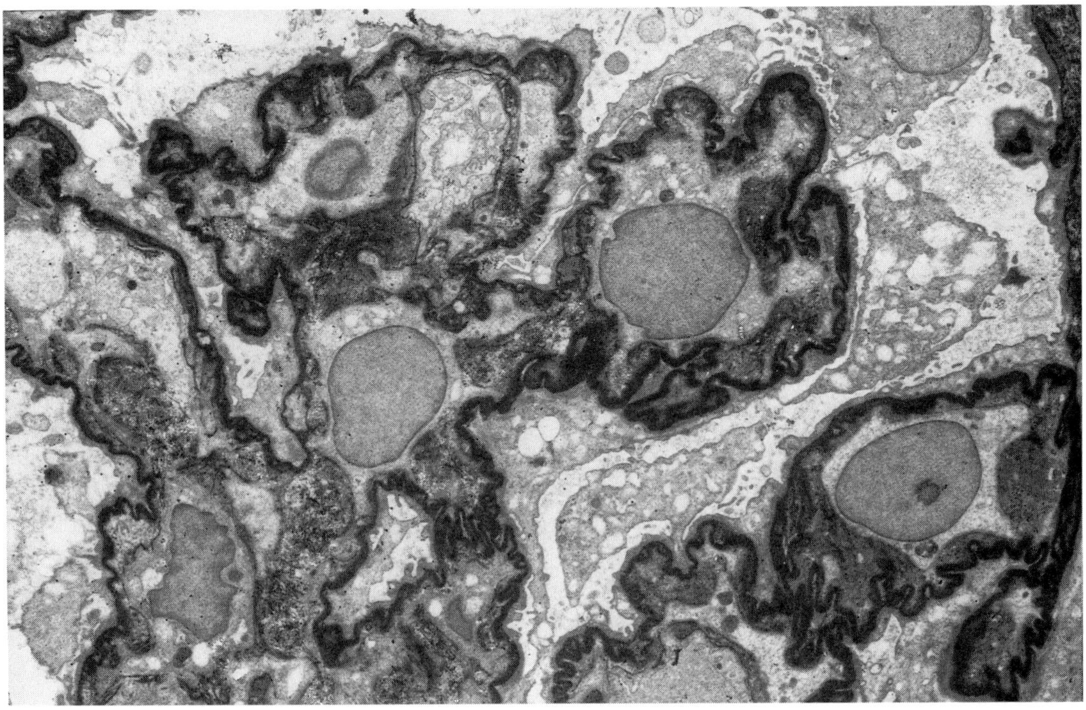

Figure 12 Electron microscopy × 300. Arterial TMA. Wrinkling of the capillary walls with subendothelial widening and collapse of the capillary lumens (Courtesy MC Gubler).

Clinicopathological Correlations

As shown in Figure 13, almost all patients who have *cortical necrosis* are infants. After a prodromal phase, they are usually anuric and the period of anuria is possibly related to the extent of cortical necrosis. They are momotensive or have moderate hypertension. The prognosis of the disease is also related to the extent of cortical necrosis. In our experience, of ten patients in whom cortical necrosis was diagnosed, two progressed to end-stage renal failure (ESRF) whereas three recovered fully, and five had residual renal symptoms (14) (see Figure 14). The two patients who progressed to ESRF improved after the initial episode, but developed hypertension a year later and reached ESRF 13 and 18 months after onset.

Glomerular Thrombotic Microangiopathy

Glomerular TMA with mild arteriolar involvement is also seen mainly in young children. It is characterized by abrupt onset, very often preceded by a diarrheal episode, of acute renal failure with anuria or oliguria, nomotension or mild hypertension, and minimal proteinuria. In our experience, the severity of the disease is well correlated with the proportion of glomeruli showing lesions of glomerular TMA (14). Among the 20 patients who had fewer than 50% of glomeruli involved, 19 recovered, and 1 has mild proteinuria with a follow-up of 4 years. Among the 9 patients who had

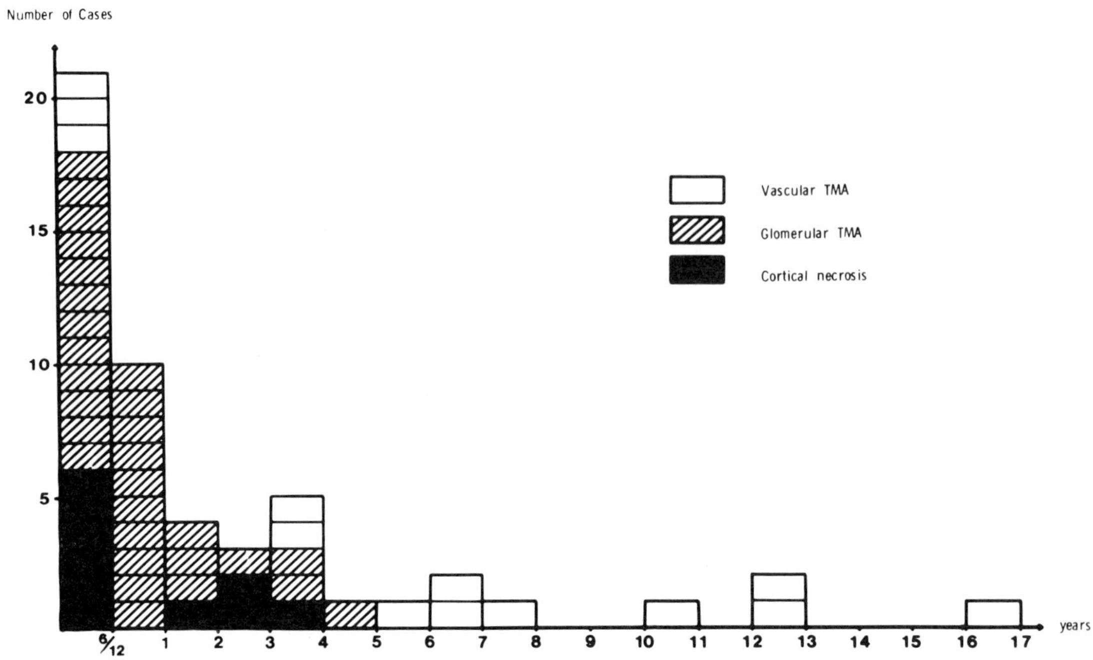

Figure 13 Clinicopathological correlations. In young children glomerular TMA and cortical necrosis are seen predominantly whereas vascular TMA is mainly seen in older children.

more than 50% of glomeruli involved, only 2 recovered. Of the remaining 7, 6 had residual renal symptoms (mild proteinuria in 2, moderate hypertension in 2, mild decrease in GFR in 2), and 1 patient aged 3 months, died suddenly after 5 days of anuria. At autopsy, most of his glomeruli were involved (see Figure 14).

In older children and in adults, the onset of symptoms may be more progressive with no prodromal phase, normal urine output (although oligoanuria may develop later), massive proteinuria, and often hypertension. Marked arteriolar changes are almost constant. In this group of patients, which corresponds to the atypical form of HUS, successive attacks of the disease or of hemolysis may be seen, and as opposed to the anuric form, a high proportion of these patients progress to ESRF.

Arterial Thrombotic Microangiopathy

The clinical features of arterial TMA are also quite different from those observed in the typical form of glomerular TMA with mild arteriolar involvement. The prognosis is related to the severity of the vascular involvement (19). Hypertension and marked proteinuria are constant. In our experience (14), this pattern was observed in 13 patients, 10 of whom were more than 3 years old (see Fig. 13). The 3 infants were, respectively, 2, 4, and 5 months old at onset. The latter 2 were siblings in whom the disease developed 2 years apart. Anuria did not occur in association with this pattern, but heavy proteinuria and hypertension were constant. The outcome was severe for 12 of the 13 patients whether they were oliguric (8 patients) or not (5 patients) (see Figure 14). At onset, 5 patients (3 oliguric and 2 nonoliguric) had uncontrollable hypertension. One of the 2 nonoliguric patients had had, 5 days of anuria, 3 months earlier; he had completely recovered from this. A bilateral nephrectomy was required in 3 of these hypertensive patients 75, 167, and 244 days after onset. Two others died 42 and 188 days after onset. Hypertension was controllable in the remaining 8 patients (5 oliguric and 3 nonoliguric). During the course of the disease, hypertension became uncontrollable in 5 of these 8 patients, requiring bilateral nephrectomy 57, 67, 81, and 119 days after onset in 4 of them. The fifth patient, an infant, died after 66 days of oliguria. Hypertension remained controllable in the remaining 3 patients, but 2 progressed to ESRF within 45 and 153 days. The only survivor in this group of patients, a 12-year-old girl, remains hypertensive.

Prognosis

In the early 1960s, the prognosis of HUS was poor. Two factors have changed the outcome: (a) better management of acute renal failure and (b) better recognition of the milder forms of the disease.

Age at onset, a diarrheal episode in the prodromal phase, presentation in the summer months in miniepidemics, the duration of anuria, and the severity of hypertension are generally recognized as the most reliable prognostic factors (48–54). These clinical features are also closely related to the morphological variants of the disease (14).

In can now be said that HUS has become a benign disease in infants who have diarrheal prodrome, a short period of anuria, and no hypertension. This “typical form” of HUS is usually associated with patchy cortical necrosis or glomerular TMA. In the few patients who progress to ESRF, or who have residual renal symptoms, the outcome may be explained by extensive cortical necrosis or a high proportion of glomeruli showing the pattern of glomerular TMA. The prognosis is much more guarded in older children and in adults who have no prodrome, normal urine output, heavy proteinuria, and severe hypertension. This “atypical or sporadic form of HUS” is usually associated with arterial TMA or with glomerular TMA with marked arteriolar involvement. In a recent study performed in my unit (unpublished data), of 44 children with HUS who were more than 3 years of age, 22 progressed to ESRF. Nineteen presented with the atypical form of the disease with no diarrheal prodrome and the reamining 3 had the typical form with extensive cortical necrosis. In the same study it was clear that the absence of oliguria at onset was a poor prognostic feature, unless it corresponded to mild cases with rapid recovery.

What about the long-term prognosis of HUS, and what will become of those children who recover or have mild residual symptoms after the acute episode of the disease? Three recent studies have given interesting figures, but in none was the pathology taken into account (55–57).

Of 46 patients studied by Van Dyck et al. (55) 10 years after the acute phase of the disease, 14 had late sequelae (11 mild and 3 severe). Of 37 patients studied by O’Regan et al. (57), GFR, measured by plasma slope clearance using ^{99m}Tc-DTPA was below 60 ml/min per 1.73 m^2 in 11 patients, 6 to 11 years after an acute episode of HUS. In a 10-year follow-up study of 73 children, de Jong and Monnens (56) subdivided their patients into three groups, according to the duration of oliguria or anuria. Four out of 38 patients belonging to the first group (oligura for fewer than 7 days) had a slightly increased blood pressure as the only sequelae. Two patients out of 29 in group 2 (oliguria for 7–14 days or anuria for fewer than 7 days) had a diminished GFR and a reduced concentrating capacity, some proteinuria, and mild hypertension. Five other patients had slight proteinuria (<500 mg/24 hr) and 1 had a mild hypertension. All 6 patients belonging to the third group (oliguria for more than 14 days or anuria for more than 7 days) had late sequelae: 2 required hemodialysis more than 10 years after the initial phase; 3 had a decreased GFR and concentrating capacity. The remaining patient had only a decreased concentrating capacity. Their results showed, in addition, that all children with a normal GFR 2 years after the acute episode had a normal GFR 10 years later as shown previously by Trompeter et al. (51).

Our experience is slightly different (58). Of 35 children followed for 10–24 years after the acute episode, 15 had late sequelae, 1 having progressed to ESRF 24 years after onset. Four of these 15 patients had completely recovered from the acute episode with normal renal function at 5 years. It is also of interest that 2 patients who had a low GFR at 5 years were normal at 10 years. We correlated long-term prognosis with the pathologic appearance of the initial biopsy specimen. Ninety percent of the patients with cortical necrosis and 60% of those who had shown more than 50% of glomeruli involved with glomerular TMA, had late sequelae. These results suggest that, in patients with residual renal symptoms, the latter are related to the extent of renal damage during the acute episode and, therefore, to scarring of the renal parenchyma, rather than to a progressive disease, as suggested by Cossio et al. (59).

To confirm this hypothesis we undertook a prospective study including a renal biopsy soon after onset and a second biopsy 1 year later (14). In the 25 cases available for study, we were able to demonstrate that glomeruli affected with lesions of glomerular TMA had progressed to complete sclerosis, as evidenced by the presence in sequential specimens of a proportion of fibrosed glomeruli identical with the proportion of glomeruli showing glomerular TMA on initial biopsy. Stripes of interstitial fibrosis, containing atrophic tubules and a few scattered inflammatory cells, were also present. The vessels were, however, normal. We concluded that the lesions of glomerular TMA are not reversible and are responsible for scarring of the renal parenchyma. This observation includes patients who had completely recovered from the acute episode.

Transplantation

There are contradictory reports about the overall risk of recurrence of HUS in the renal allograft. Three reasons may partially explain these discrepancies: (a) Clinically, HUS may be mimicked in the renal allograft recipient by antilymphoblast globulin reaction, severe acute vascular rejection, malignant hypertension, and by many factors that damage the endothelium. (b) Morphologically, the similarity between the lesions of allograft glomerulopathy and glomerular TMA (47), and the nonspecific character of the vascular lesions of TMA, make the differential diagnosis with rejection difficult and render the interpretation of some grafts hazardous. This is exemplified in 3 of the 11 patients, reported by Hebert et al. (60), who presented with histological features consistent with HUS, but lacked the clinical features of the syndrome. (c) In addition, several cases of de novo HUS have been documented in allografts of patients whose original disease was not HUS (61–67). Some of these were treated with cyclosporine (68–74).

Until 1986, a recurrence of HUS in renal allografts seemed unusual in children (14, 75) and adults (76), and only individual case reports had been published (77–84). In 1986, Hebert et al. (60) described a definite recurrence of HUS in the allografts of

7 of 14 patients who received transplants. All grafts but one were from living-related donors. Except in 3 adults reported by Griño et al. (85), these gloomy results have not been confirmed by others (86–90). In the report by Eijgenraam et al. (88), 24 grafts, mostly cadaver kidneys, were transplanted into 20 patients whose primary disease had been HUS. Recurrence of HUS was suspected, but not proved, to be the cause of first graft failure in 2 patients and impaired graft function in a third. A short interval between HUS and kidney transplantation seemed to adversely affect graft survival.

In our experience (90), the risk of recurrence of HUS in a renal allograft is extremely small, even with living-related donors. However, graft loss, especially from chronic vascular rejection, seems more frequent than in the general transplant population. We reviewed the outcome of 31 transplantations performed in our unit over the past 15 years in 25 children whose original disease was HUS. Each was studied histologically. The patients were aged 2–22 years at time of transplantation. Three grafts were from living-related donors (father), and 28 were cadaver transplants. Among the 28 cadaver kidney grafts, only 12 (44.5%) are currently functioning. One child died 2 months posttransplantation from hypertension, possibly because of his native kidney. Four grafts were lost within the first 10 days from acute vascular rejection (1 case) and vascular thrombosis in small children (3 cases). Ten patients lost their graft within 4–8 years from chronic vascular rejection, with an allograft glomerulopathy in 3. Only one clinical and pathological recurrence of HUS was observed 3 weeks posttransplantation in a girl who received a transplant 6 months after the onset of HUS. A second transplantation functioned for 12 years. No recurrence was observed in the remaining 30 grafts, the delay between transplantation and HUS being 1–12 years. The actuarial survival rate of the 28 cadaver kidney grafts was 66% at 1 year, 59% at 2 years, and 37% at 5 years, whereas it was 80, 75, and 69%, respectively, in our general transplantation population up to 1985. By contrast, the 3 paternal grafts were successful, with a follow-up of 8, 18, and 48 months.

Because of the possible occurrence of HUS following the administration of cyclosporine, some physicians are reluctant to use this drug in patients receiving transplants whose original disease was HUS. In our use of cyclosporine from 1985, no patient who has received a transplant has ever developed HUS. This includes the 17 whose original disease was HUS.

In conclusion, so many factors are present in patients following renal transplantation that a diagnosis of recurrence of HUS should be made only after other causes of renal failure have been excluded.

RECURRENT AND FAMILIAL FORMS OF HEMOLYTIC UREMIC SYNDROME

Recurrent Forms of Hemolytic Uremic Syndrome

Relapses during the course of the illness can occur in primary HUS and are often associated with a poor prognosis but a true recurrence after full recovery is unusual (see Chap. 13). Of a total of 200 cases we have studied, all histologically documented, only 1 child had a recurrence of typical HUS. This 6½-year-old girl presented after a prodromal phase with a typical form of HUS, characterized by 6 days of anuria and a mild glomerular TMA. She progressively recovered from this acute episode, and 3 months later she developed a new episode of hemolysis, with normal urine output, heavy proteinuria, and uncontrollable hypertension that required bilateral nephrectomy 75 days after onset. Similarly, only 1 of 67 patients reported by another French group (52) had a recurrence of HUS. Among the 30 patients with more than one episode of HUS previously published and reviewed by Kaplan in 1977 (91), only 5 lived in areas in which HUS is said to be endemic. We agree with Kaplan that these patients, together with the few patients reported subsequently (92–104), belong to a different subset, although they present with the characteristic clinical features of HUS. In addition, the heterogeneity of this subset is striking.

Recurrent episodes tend to occur in familial cases. In Kaplan's review (91), six patients with recurrences had affected siblings. Two of the siblings had recurrent episodes and two patients with recurrent HUS were cousins (38). Recurrent episodes have been reported since then in two additional families (98, 104).

In several cases, recurrent HUS occurred in patients in association with hypocomplementemia (92, 93, 97, 98, 102, 103). The abnormalities of the complement system appeared to be a primary familial or hereditary defect that acted as the factor predisposing to recurrence in some (97, 98, 102, 103), whereas, in others, the levels of C3 were depressed only during the acute phase of the recurrence (92, 93). It must be emphasized that the complement system is usually normal in HUS and TTP (105).

The outcome of the patients belonging to this subset is very variable. Approximately half of them have a poor outcome, and each recurrence seems to aggravate renal function. By contrast, in the other half, the disease seems remarkably benign and, in several reports, each recurrence is characterized by mild oliguric acute renal failure followed by rapid and complete recovery (38, 39, 92, 94, 95). I have had the opportunity of reviewing the renal biopsies of most of the patients of the second group as well as several unpublished ones. None of them showed the typical lesions of HUS, and the renal parenchyma was normal.

Finally, a case report of recurrent TTP after viral infection (96) is obviously a HUS superimposed on a "chronic glomerular disease" as recently reported by our group (106).

Familial Forms of Hemolytic Uremic Syndrome

The heterogeneity of the familial forms of HUS (see Chap. 18) is even greater than that of the recurrent forms, with which there is some overlap (91, 98, 104). In 1975, Kaplan et al. (107) in a review of 83 siblings belonging to 41 families, distinguished two groups of families on the basis of (a) the interval between the onset of disease in affected sibs, (b) geographic location (endemic versus nonendemic) of the families, and (c) severity of the syndrome, as indicated by mortality. The authors speculated that the milder disease occurring simultaneously in sibs in families living in endemic areas could be attributed to environmental agents, whereas genetic factors may have played an important role in the severe form of the disease, occurring in sibs after longer intervals, in families living in nonendemic areas. Subsequent studies have confirmed these findings and show that the stronger the genetic evidence, the worse the prognosis (29–31, 44, 98, 104, 108–120). However, two modes of inheritance have been reported. In one, a recessive inheritance is suggested. This group comprises either children or adult siblings, often affected at a similar age, but years apart (29, 31, 44, 104, 108–113). The disease is classified as being TTP or HUS, and sometimes both may occur in the same family (29, 31). In the second, a dominant inheritance seems likely. This group comprises patients with both juvenile- and adult-onset, who belong to different generations, and in whom the disease occurs years apart (30, 98, 114–118). In only one report, the disease occurred simultaneously in a mother and her child (120). It has been suggested that some inherited cases might be related to a familial deficiency of a plasma factor stimulating vascular prostacyclin activity (121, 122).

In fact, if the number of familial cases of simultaneous occurrence and good prognosis, which are probably more common than is generally realized (123), are excluded, familial forms of HUS are relatively rare. Of the 200 cases we have observed, we have seen only two pairs of sibs in two families who developed the disease years apart. The four patients, all infants, had predominantly arterial TMA and progressed to ESRF. The prognosis of the hereditary forms is usually bad, but it is not easy to conclude from the pathological reports if they are all true examples of HUS with TMA. It is not unlikely that some cases may represent a superimposed HUS on hereditary preexisting disease (98). In a recent study by our group of eight patients with a "nail–patella-like" syndrome, with numerous bundles of fibrillar collagen within the extracellular glomerular matrix, but without extrarenal symptoms, two siblings had developed a fatal HUS (106).

SECONDARY HEMOLYTIC UREMIC SYNDROME

The hemolytic uremic syndrome may occur as a complication of a variety of conditions, including infection, drug toxicity, transplantation, cancer, or pregnancy. It may also occur as a superimposed feature on a preexisting condition. These various types of secondary HUS raise a problem of pathogenesis, since HUS is a rare complication of these disorders. In addition, if a likely causative agent of endothelial damage can be identified in most instances, such as bacterial toxin in infection-associated HUS or chemotherapeutic drug toxicity in mitomycin-associated HUS, the pathology, and especially the glomerular lesion, is often distinct from that observed in the classic forms of HUS. The secondary forms illustrate, in our opinion, the crucial role of the vasculopathy in determining the clinical features of the syndrome.

Infection-Associated Hemolytic Uremic Syndrome

Most of the infectious agents suggested as causes, and listed in a recent review by Kwaan (124), may have no causal role, and we will discuss only three in which the pathological features have been documented.

Shigellosis

Observations that episodes of HUS occurred in clusters and were frequently preceded by bloody diarrhea suggested that endotoxin, derived from the intestinal tract, produced a Shwartzman-like reaction in the renal microvasculature. However, clinical studies failed to identify circulating endotoxin or a consistent infectious agent. Enthusiasm was, therefore, raised by the publication, by Koster et al. (125), of a series of children in Bangladesh in whom this occurred in association with shigellosis and severe colitis. *Shigella dysenteriae* serotype 1 was, subsequently, considered as a causative agent of HUS. However, Koster et al. published another paper in 1984 (126) recognizing that HUS following dysentery caused by *S. dysenteriae* type 1 is clinically similar to, but not identical with, idiopathic HUS. Moreover, the study of renal necropsy specimens of nine children, who died of HUS following shigellosis, showed extensive glomerular thrombosis or cortical necrosis, but these authors never found the characteristic and mesangial lesions of idiopathic HUS. It is likely that these patients showed features of diffuse intravascular coagulation (DIC), which is a well-known complication of severe sepsis.

Verocytotoxin-Producing Escherichia coli *Infections*

In contrast to shigellosis, there are many reasons to believe that some cases of typical HUS may be related to verocytotoxin-producing *E. coli* (VTEC). After the publication by Karmali et al. (127) showing that 75% of children with HUS observed in Toronto had been found to have an infection with VTEC of different serotypes, including the most commonly recognized one O157:H7, several reports have confirmed this finding. This issue has been extensively reviewed by Kaplan et al. (128). Moreover, a recent report from the Toronto group shows that the histopathology of VTEC-associated HUS is identical with the one observed in typical HUS (129). In this context the classic form of HUS may in the future be considered postinfectious.

Acquired Immunodeficiency Syndrome

Several cases of HUS or TTP have been reported in patients with acquired immunodeficiency syndrome (AIDS) or in human immunodeficiency virus (HIV) seropositive patients (130–136). Boccia et al. (130) reported the occurrence of HUS and the presence of fibrin thrombi in most interlobular arteries and in some glomerular capillaries, but their patient had also received chemotherapeutic agents. The only other report mentioning pathological results is that of Jokela et al. (131), whose patient showed the classic features of TTP, including histological evidence of fibrin thrombi in small blood vessels in the bone marrow (See Chap. 23).

Drug-Associated Hemolytic Uremic Syndrome

Many drugs and toxins have been implicated in the development of HUS (124). The most common group of drugs are the *chemotherapeutic agents* used in the treatment of malignancies, of which *mitomycin* seems the most frequently involved. This problem has recently been reviewed by Murgo (137), who states that, in the various published cases of mitomycin-related HUS: "the characteristic features of thrombotic microangiopathy are present in every case and are similar to those seen in HUS from other causes." A careful study of the pathological reports published, however, shows that this interpretation is erroneous. In fact, in almost every case in which a good description of the morphological changes was given, including the first three cases reported by Liu et al. (138), more or less extensive lesions of mesangiolysis with atypical nuclei were present (139–141). These distinctive features were also observed in the 23 cases gathered in a multicenter study in France by Cordonnier et al. (142), who emphasized that this complication occurred usually several months after the onset of the treatment by mitomycin. If focal and segmental lesions of mesangiolysis may very occasionally be observed in primary HUS, such extensive lesions of mesangiolysis may be considered as very suggestive of mitomycin-associated HUS.

Delayed HUS or TTP has also been reported following the administration of chemotherapeutic agents other than mitomycin (13, 140–150). In all these instances, when pathologic evaluation was available, the lesions observed in the kidneys were described as typical of glomerular TMA, and no lesions of mesangiolysis were mentioned. We have recently observed such a case. However, when abdominal irradiation was associated with chemotherapeutic agents, lesions of mesangiolysis were present, although not always recognized as such (151–157). In these reports, HUS was considered to be related to radiation nephritis (see following section on transplantation-associated HUS).

Cyclosporine is often mentioned as a possible cause of HUS. This complication concerns mainly patients receiving transplants in whom a causal relationship is not always easy to establish. As already discussed in a previous paragraph (see earlier section on transplantation), HUS may occur in renal allograft recipients either as a recurrence or as de novo HUS in patients with transplants who are receiving cyclosporine. A few cases have been reported in liver allograft recipients and in bone marrow transplantation (see following section on transplantation-associated HUS). In patients without transplants, cyclosporine is currently being widely administered for autoimmune diseases. To my knowledge, this complication has occurred in only 2 patients with Behçet's disease (158). Both had an arterial TMA.

Transplantation-Associated Hemolytic Uremic Syndrome

The hemolytic uremic syndrome has been reported in renal, liver, and bone marrow transplant recipients (see Chap. 15). We have already mentioned the problem of de novo HUS occurring in renal transplantation patients whose original disease was not HUS, including those who received cyclosporine (61–74). One case of HUS and one case of TTP have been reported in liver allograft recipients (159, 160), but no pathological studies were done. Both were receiving cyclosporine. However, in one case there was unequivocal evidence of disseminated intravascular coagulation (159).

Apart from renal and liver transplantation-associated HUS, almost all cases have been reported in bone marrow transplant (BMT) recipients (162–177). In several instances, this complication was related to the use of cyclosporine which was administered to prevent graft-versus-host disease (161–166). In the two histologically documented reports (162–163), HUS occurred early in the transplantation course, and the renal involvement was characterized by the presence of a few arteriolar and glomerular capillary thromboses. By contrast, 10 of the 66 allogeneic marrow graft recipients, reported by Holler et al. (166), suffered from severe microangiopathy that resembled TTP, but the authors concluded that their patients showed "generalized endothelial damage distinct from isolated nephrotoxicity," and their data do not allow interpretation of the miroangiopathy as a consequence of cyclosporine nephrotoxicity. Similarly, the arteriolar lesions classified as "a type of TMA" reported in bone marrow transplant recipients by Nizze et al. (167) and considered to be related to cyclosporine (CsA arteriolopathy), might be due to other causes, since in BMT recipients, several factors may play a role in the development of a HUS or of arteriolar lesions similar to TMA.

We described seven patients who developed acute renal failure several months after BMT and total-body irradiation (168). In four of them, renal failure was associated with hemolytic anemia and thrombocytopenia. In all of the patients, renal biopsy specimens showed a uniform pattern of severe glomerular involvement, characterized by extensive lesions of mesangiolysis associated with severe arteriolonecrosis (Fig. 15). We reviewed the literature and found several similar cases (169–174), and others have been published since (175–177). Because of the similarity

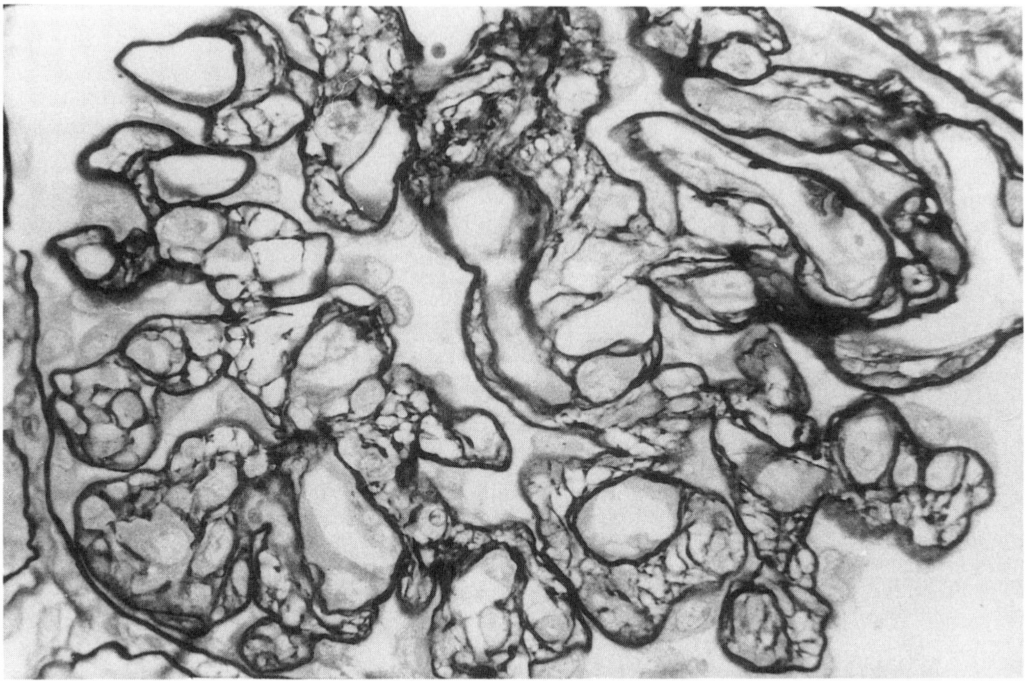

Figure 14 Radiation nephritis in a child with HUS secondary to total body irradiation before bone marrow transplantation. Most glomeruli showed extensive lesions of mesangiolysis.

of the lesions observed in our patients with those seen in radiation nephritis (152–157, 178–184) we concluded that the nephropathy was related to total-body irradiation enhanced by chemotherapy, rather than to chemotherapy alone. As stated earlier (see section on drug-associated HUS), extensive lesions of mesangiolysis are seen only in mitomycin-associated HUS, a drug that none of the patients ever received, as well as in radiation nephritis. Radiation nephritis and mitomycin-associated nephropathy are, therefore, two examples of the occurrence of HUS without the typical lesions of glomerular TMA.

Carcinoma-Associated Microangiopathic Hemolytic Anemia

In an extensive review of the literature, Murgo (137) found that patients with cancer who develop microangiopathic hemolytic anemia (MAHA) usually have widely metastatic carcinomas, 75% of which are derived from gastric, breast, and lung primaries. In addition, unlike chemotherapy-related HUS, renal failure is an uncommon feature in patients with carcinoma-associated MAHA. The most characteristic pathological feature is the presence of extensive involvement of blood and lymphatic vessels; pulmonary vessels are most frequently involved. Tumor emboli are frequently seen within small vessels, including the small pulmonary arteries and arterioles, together with fibrin microthrombi. Other common sites of microthrombi include the myocardium and kidneys (185–186). In addition, intimal proliferation may be seen in the pulmonary vessels in association with tumor emboli. These microvascular changes may explain the hemolysis. However, neither the localization of the vascular lesions nor their pattern of involvement are similar to those seen in TTP or HUS.

Hemolytic Uremic Syndrome of Young Women

In a high proportion of adults with HUS, the syndrome occurs in the postpartum period or in women taking oral contraceptives (187). The term HUS of young women has been proposed in a *Lancet* editorial (187) to encompass these two etiological circumstances. However, according to Hayslett (188), postpartum HUS, should be limited to cases who develop microangiopathic hemolytic anemia and clinical signs of renal insufficiency several days to approximately 10 weeks after a normal pregnancy and delivery. If pregnancy or delivery is complicated by any of the usual causes of acute renal failure in late pregnancy, the diagnosis is less certain, because most of causes of acute renal failure in the third trimester may be associated with disseminated intravascular coagulation. Of 57 cases of acute renal failure in pregnant women, Grünfeld et al. (189) found only 5 cases of postpartum renal failure with TMA. Postpartum HUS represents, therefore, a small part of acute renal failure related to pregnancy. It was not until the 1970s that the term HUS was used in this setting, partly because of the ignorance by "adult" pathologists and nephrologists of the pediatric literature and also because of the specific clinical and pathological features presented by this type of patient. A characteristic feature of postpartum HUS is both the severity of hypertension and the predominant vascular involvement. It is not, therefore, surprising that the early reports called the disease "malignant nephrosclerosis" (193) or "accelerated nephrosclerosis" (194). However, glomerular TMA (195), as well as cortical necrosis (189), has also been observed. Another feature of postpartum HUS is its poor prognosis. The initial reports stressed the invariably fatal outcome of the disease (196). In a 1979 literature review of postpartum HUS, 49 cases were listed (197). There was a fatal outcome in 61% of the reported cases, a complete recovery in 9.5%, and persistent renal symptoms in the remaining patients. A lupus anticoagulant associated with renal TMA has been found in patients with pregnancy-related renal failure (198) (see Chap. 20).

The syndrome that follows after a variable period on an oral contraceptive regimen is clinically indistinguishable from that following pregnancy. It was first described by Tobon (199) and Brown et al. (200) and confirmed in several other reports (81). Renal histopathological changes in postpill HUS were considered compatible with the diagnosis of malignant nephrosclerosis (201) or with that of TMA (199) (see Chap. 19).

Hemolytic Uremic Syndrome Superimposed on Preexisting Conditions

Microangiopathic hemolysis with thrombocytopenia can occur as a secondary phenomenon complicating preexisting conditions, such as malignant hypertension. This occurrence may be more frequent than usually thought, and it is possible that some children and many adults with HUS may be examples of this complication. These patients were known to be hypertensive and abruptly developed malignant hypertension with HUS (19). The similarity of the vascular lesions of nephroangiosclerosis and of arterial TMA, and their consequences on the pattern of glomerular involvement, as stressed by Bohle et al. (34), make the differential diagnosis very difficult. Therefore, only the clinical data can allow the distinction between a patient with primary HUS who develops severe hypertension and one with HUS complicating malignant hypertension. We have observed the occurrence of HUS in patients followed for various renal diseases (14): one with segmental hypoplasia (reflux nephropathy), one with Schonlein–Henoch purpura nephritis, one with congenital nephrotic syndrome, one with idiopathic nephrosis (202), one with a nail–patella-like syndrome (106), and a girl with IgA nephropathy who was taking oral contraceptives (203). In all of them, the symptoms of HUS occurred in association with uncontrollable hypertension, and all showed severe arterial TMA. A similar patient has been reported by Dumas et al. (204). Hemolytic uremic syndrome has also been reported in patients with various glomerular diseases and apparently no hypertension at presentation: acute glomerulonephritis (205, 206), membranous nephropathy (207), membranoproliferative glomerulonephritis (208), nephrosis (208, 209), and anti-glomerular basement membrane glomerulonephritis (210). The common denominator of all these observations is the presence of arteriolar changes mimicking TMA, but none had the characteristic changes of glomerular TMA. Finally, HUS may complicate systemic diseases such as scleroderma (211) and systemic lupus erythematosus (105).

This group of patients is extremely interesting. It emphasizes the fundamental role of the arteriolopathy, whatever its pathogenesis, in determining the clinical features of HUS.

CONCLUSION

Hemolytic uremic syndrome and TTP are *clinical syndromes*, the characteristic features of which can be reached by different pathways, whereas TMA is a *lesion* that affects arterioles and the glomerular capillaries. As opposed to the arteriolopathy that is nonspecific, glomerular TMA may be considered pathognomonic, because this glomerular lesion is always associated with HUS. When HUS is associated with glomerular TMA, it is definitely a clinicopathological entity. However, a patient may develop the clinical symptoms of HUS without showing the characteristic changes of glomerular TMA. By contrast, the arteriolopathy may be associated with either primary or secondary HUS, but it may also be observed without any of the clinical features of HUS. For the sake of clarity, *the term arteriolar TMA should be used exclusively when associated with HUS or TTP*. Better definitions, both clinical and pathological, would permit a more accurate delineation of this heterogeneous condition called HUS.

REFERENCES

1. Kaplan, B. S., Drummond, K. N., The hemolytic uremic syndrome is a syndrome. *N. Engl. J. Med.*, *298*: 964–966 (1978).
2. Moschcowitz, E., An acute febrile pleiochromic anemia with hyalin thrombosis of the terminal arterioles and capillaries. An undescribed disease. *Arch. Intern. Med.*, *36*: 89 (1925).

3. Baehr, G., Klemperer, P., Schifrin, A., An acute febrile anemia and thrombocytopenic purpura with diffuse platelet thromboses of capillaries and arterioles. *Trans. Assoc. Am. Physicians, 51*: 43–58 (1936).
4. Symmers, W. S. C., Thrombotic microangiopathic haemolytic anaemia (thrombotic microangiopathy). *Br. Med. J., 2*: 897–903 (1952).
5. Gasser, V. C., Gautier, E., Steck, A., Seibenmann, E. E., Oeschlin, R., Hämolytisch-urämische Syndrome: Bilaterale Nierenindennekrosen bei akuten erworbenen hämolytischen Anämien. *Schweiz. Med. Wochenschr., 85*: 905–909 (1955).
6. Clement, R., Bernard, J., Papaioannou, A., Mathé, G., Habib, R., Designolle, M., Purpura thrombotique thrombocytopénique (Maladie de Moschcovitz) chez une enfant de 10 mois. *Presse Med., 94*: 2144–2146 (1957).
7. Habib, R., Mathieu, H., Royer, P., Maladie thrombotique artériolo-capillaire du rein chez l'enfant. *Rev. Fr. Et. Clin. Biol. 3*: 891–895 (1958).
8. Royer, P., Habib, R., Mathieu, H., La microangiopathie thrombotique du rein chez l'enfant. *Ann. Pediatr. (Paris), 36*: 572–587 (1960).
9. Habib, R., Classification anatomique des néphropathies glomérulaires. *Pediatr. Fortbildungskurse, Praxis 28*: 3–47 (1970).
10. Habib, R., Mathieu, H., Royer, P., Le syndrome hémolytique et urémique de l'enfant. Aspects cliniques et anatomiques dans 27 observations. *Nephron, 4*: 139–172 (1967).
11. Mathieu, H., Leclerc, F., Habib, R., Royer, P., Etude clinique et biologique de 37 observations de syndrome hémolytique et urémique. *Arch. Fr. Pediatr., 26*: 369–390 (1969).
12. Habib, R., Courtecuisse, V., Leclerc, F., Mathieu, H., Royer, P., Etude anatomopathologique de 35 observations de syndrome hémolytique et urémique de l'enfant. *Arch. Fr. Pediatr., 26*: 391–416 (1969).
13. Habib, R., Leclerc, F., Mathieu, H., Royer, P. Comparaison clinique et anatomopathologique entre les formes mortelles et curables du syndrome hémolytique et urémique. *Arch. Fr. Pediatr. 26*: 417–432 (1969).
14. Habib, R., Levy, M., Gagnadoux, M. F., Broyer, M., Prognosis of the hemolytic uremic syndrome in children. *Adv. Nephrol., 11*: 99–128 (1982).
15. Vitsky, B. H., Suzuki, Y., Strauss, L., Churg, J., The hemolytic-uremic syndrome: A study of renal pathologic alterations. *Am. J. Pathol., 57*: 627–647 (1969).
16. Clarkson, A. R., Lawrence, J. R., Meadows, R., Seymour, A. E., The hemolytic–uremic syndrome in adults. *Q. J. Med, 39*: 227–239 (1970).
17. Mery, J. P., Grünfeld, J. P., Berry, J. P., Le syndrome hémolytique et urémique de l'adulte. *Journ. Réanim. Hôp. Claude-Bernard, Paris*, pp. 27–40 (1970).
18. Goldstein, M. H., Churg, J., Strauss, L., Gribetz, D., Hemolytic–uremic syndrome. *Nephron*, 23: 263–272 (1979).
19. Morel-Maroger, L., Kanfer, A., Solez, K., Sraer, J. D., Richet, G., Prognostic importance of vascular lesions in acute renal failure with microangiopathic hemolytic anemia (hemolytic uremic syndrome): Clinicopathologic study in 20 adults. *Kidney Int., 15*: 548–558 (1979).
20. Morel-Maroger, L. Adult hemolytic uremic syndrome. *Kidney Int., 18*: 125–134 (1980).
21. Ponticelli, C., Rivolta, E., Imbasciati, E., Rossi, E., Manucci, P. M., Hemolytic uremic syndrome in adults. *Arch. Intern. Med., 140*: 353–357 (1980).
22. Amorosi, E. L., Ultmann, J. E., Thrombotic thrombocytopenic purpura: Report of 16 cases and review of the literature. *Medicine, 45*: 139–159 (1966).
23. Ridolfi, R. L., Bell, W. R., Thrombotic thrombocytopenic purpura. Report of 25 cases and review of the literature. *Medicine, 60*: 413–428 (1981).
24. Eknoyan, G., Riggs, S. A., Renal involvement in patients with thrombotic thrombocytopenic purpura. *Am. J. Nephrol., 6*: 117–131 (1986).
25. Upadhyaya, K., Barwick, K., Fishaut, M., Kashgarian, M., Siegel, N. J., The im-

portance of non renal involvement in hemolytic uremic syndrome. *Pediatrics, 65*: 115–120 (1980).

26. Argyle, J. C., Hogg, R. J., Pysher, T. J., Silva, F. G., Siegler, R. L., A clinicopathological study of 24 children with hemolytic uremic syndrome. A report of the Southwest Pediatric Nephrology Study Group. *Pediatr. Nephrol. 4*: 52–58 (1990).
27. Shumway, C. N., Jr, Miller, G., An unusual syndrome of hemolytic anemia, thrombocytopenic purpura and renal disease. *Blood, 12*: 1045–1060 (1957).
28. MacWhinney, J. B., Packer, J. T., Miller, G., Greendyke, R. M., Thrombotic thrombocytopenic purpura in childhood. *Blood, 19*: 181–199 (1962).
29. Hellman, R. M., Jackson, D. V., Buss, D. H., Thrombotic thrombocytopenic purpura and hemolytic uremic syndrome in HLA-identical siblings. *Ann. Intern. Med., 93*: 283–284 (1980).
30. Kirchner, K. A., Smith, R. M., Gockerman, J. P., Luke, R. G., Hereditary thrombotic thrombocytopenic purpura, microangiopathic hemolytic anemia, thrombocytopenia and renal insufficiency occurring in consecutive generations. *Nephron, 30*: 28–30 (1982).
31. Elias, M., Horovitz, J., Tal, I., Kohn, D., Flatau, E., Thrombotic thrombocytopenic purpura and haemolytic uraemic syndrome in three siblings. *Arch. Dis. Child., 63*: 644–646 (1988).
32. Remuzzi, G., Hemolytic uremic syndrome and thrombotic thrombocytopenic purpura: Variable expression of a single entity. *Kidney Int. 32*: 292–308 (1987).
33. Mery, J. P., Grünfeld, J. P., Watchi, J. M., de Montera, H., Insuffisance rénale aiguë avec microangiopathie thrombotique chez l'adulte. In *Actual. Nephrol. Hôp. Necker*, Paris, Flammarion Med. Sc., pp. 449–484 (1967).
34. Böhle, A., Helmchen, Grund, K. E., Gartner, H. V., Meyer, D., Bock, K. D., Bulla, M., Bunger, P., Diekmann, L., Fortscher, U., Haydu, K. K., Koster, S. W., Strauch, M., Scheler, F., Christ, H., Malignant nephrosclerosis in patients with hemolytic uremic syndrome (primary malignant nephrosclerosis). *Curr. Top. Pathol.*, 65: 81–113 (1977).
35. Thoenes, W., John, H. D., Endotheliotropic (hemolytic) nephroangiopathy and its various manifestation forms (thrombotic microangiopathy, primary malignant nephrosclerosis, hemolytic uremic syndrome). *Klin. Wochenschr., 58*: 173–184 (1980).
36. John, H. D., Thoenes, W., The glomerular lesions in endotheliotropic hemolytic nephroangiopathy (hemolytic–uremic syndrome, malignant nephrosclerosis, post-partum renal insufficiency). *Pathol. Res. Pract., 173*: 236–259) (1982).
37. Churg, J., Strauss, L., Renal involvement in thrombotic microangiopathies. *Semin. Nephrol., 5*: 46–56 (1985).
38. Courtecuisse, V., Dommergues, J. P., Rivron, J., Chaon, P., Syndrome hémolytique et urémique familial avec biopsie rénale normale. *Arch. Fr. Pediatr, 32*: 749–755 (1975).
39. Larbre, F., Dechelette, E., Sellem, C., Parchoux, B., Marchal, A., Le syndrome hémolytique et urémique récidivant. A propos de 6 observations recueillies dans la région Rhone-Alpes. *Pédiatrie, 24*: 433–441 (1979).
40. Levy, M., Gagnadoux, M. F., Habib, R., Pathology of hemolytic uremic syndrome in children. In *Hemostasis, Prostaglandins and Renal disease* (G. Remuzzi, G. Mecca, G. de Gaetano, eds.), Raven Press, New York, pp. 383–397 (1980).
41. Böhle, A., Grabensee, B., Fischer, R., Berg, E., Klust, H., On four cases of hemolytic–uremic syndrome without microangiopathy. *Clin. Nephrol., 24*: 88–92 (1985).
42. Shigematsu, H., Dikman, S. H., Churg, J., Grishman, E., Duffy, J. L., Mesangial involvement in hemolytic–uremic syndrome. *Am. J. Pathol., 85*: 349–362 (1976).
43. Courtecuisse, V., Habib, R., Monnier, C., Non lethal hemolytic and uremic syndrome in children: An electron microscope study of renal biopsies from 6 cases. *Exp. Mol. Pathol., 7*: 327–347 (1967).
44. Gervais, M., Richardson, J. B., Chiu, J., Drummond, K. N., Immunofluorescent and histologic findings in the hemolytic uremic syndrome *Pediatrics, 47*: 352–359 (1971).

45. McCoy, R. C., Abramowski, C. R., Krueger, R., The hemolytic uremic syndrome, with positive immunofluorescence studies. *J. Pediatr., 85*: 170–174 (1974).
46. Gonzalo, A., Mampaso, F., Gallego, N., Bellas, C., Segui, J., Ortuño, J., Hemolytic uremic syndrome with hypocomplementemia and deposits of IgM and C3 in the involved renal tissue. *Clin. Nephrol., 16*: 193–199 (1981).
47. Habib, R., Antignac, C., Hinglais, N., Gagnadoux, M. F., Broyer, M., Glomerular lesions in the transplanted kidney in children. *Am. J. Kidney Dis., 10*: 198–207 (1987).
48. Gianantonio, C. A., Vitacco, M., Mendilaharzu, F., Gallo, G., The hemolytic–uremic syndrome. Renal status of 76 patients at long-term follow-up. *J. Pediatr., 72*: 757–765 (1968).
49. Gianantonio, C. A., Vitacco, M., Mendilaharzu, F., Gallo, G. E., Sojo, E. T., The hemolytic–uremic syndrome. *Nephron, 11*: 174–192 (1973).
50. Janssen, F., Potvliege, P. R., Vainsel, M., Vis, H. L., Le pronostic à court terme et à long terme du syndrome hémolytique et urémique. *Arch. Fr. Pediatr., 31*: 59–69 (1974).
51. Trompeter, R. S., Schwartz, R., Chantler, C., Dillon, M. J., Haycok, G. B., Kay, R., Barratt, T. M., Haemolytic–uraemic syndrome: An analysis of prognostic features. *Arch. Dis. Child., 58*: 101–105 (1983).
52. Loirat, C., Sonsino, E., Varga Moreno, A., Pillion, G., Mercier, J. C., Beaufils, F., Mathieu, H., Hemolytic–uremic syndrome: An analysis of the natural history and prognostic features. *Acta Paediatr. Scand., 73*: 505–514 (1984).
53. Guyot, C., Daniel, M. D., Roze, J. C., Renoult, E., Dubigeon, P., Buzelin, F., Pronostic du syndrome hémolytique et urémique chez l'enfant. Importance de l'atteinte extra-rénale. *Arch. Fr. Pediatr., 43*: 253–258 (1986).
54. Sieniawska, M., Korniszewska, J., Gura, C., Welc-Dobies, J., Lewicki, Z., Prognostic significance of certain factors in the haemolytic–uraemic syndrome. *Pediatr. Nephrol., 4*: 213–218 (1990).
55. Van Dyck, M., Proesmans, W., Depraetere, M., Hemolytic uremic syndrome in childhood: Renal function ten years later. *Clin Nephrol., 29*: 109–112 (1988).
56. DeJong, M., Monnens, L., Haemolytic–uraemic syndrome: A 10–year follow-up study of 73 patients. *Nephrol. Dial. Transplant., 3*: 379–382 (1988).
57. O'Regan, S., Blais, N., Russo, P., Pison, C. F., Rousseau, L., Hemolytic uremic syndrome: Glomerular filtration rate, 6 to 11 years later measured by ^{99m}Tc DTPA plasma slope clearance. *Clin. Nephrol., 32*: 217–220 (1989).
58. Gagnadoux, M. F., Habib, R., Broyer, M., Royer, P. Pronostic à long terme du syndrome hémolytique et urémique de l'enfant [abstract]. *Clin. Invest. Med., 10*: A 67 (1987).
59. Cossio, P. M., Laguens, R. P., De Bracco, M. M. E., Molinas, F., Voyer, L. E., Arana, R. M., Persistent glomerulonephritis following the hemolytic uremic syndrome: Immunopathological and morphological studies. *Clin. Exp. Immunol., 29*: 361–368 (1977).
60. Hebert, D., Sibley, R. K., Mauer, S. M., Recurrence of hemolytic uremic syndrome in renal transplant recipients. *Kidney Int., 30*: S51–S58 (1986).
61. Lichtman, M. A., Hoyer, L. W., Sears, D. A., Erythrocyte deformation and hemolytic anemia coincident with the microvascular disease of rejecting renal homotransplants. *Am. J. Med. Sci., 256*: 239–246 (1968).
62. Hutton, M. M., Prentice, C. R. M., Allison, M. E. M., Duguid, W. P., Kennedy, A. C., Struthers, N. W., McNicol, G. P., Renal homotransplant rejection associated with microangiopthic hemolytic anemia. *Br. Med. J., 3*: 87–88 (1970).
63. Petersen, P. V., Olsen, S. T., Late renal transplant failure due to the hemolytic uremic syndrome. *Acta Med. Scand., 189*: 377–382 (1971).
64. Pillay, V. K. G., Kurtzman, N. A., Manaligod, J. R., Jonasson, A., Selective thrombocytopenia due to localised microangipathy of renal allografts. *Lancet, 2*: 988–991 (1973).

65. Magalhaes, R. L., Braun, W. E., Straffon, R. A., Hoffman, G. C., Shainoff, J. R., Osborne, G., Deodhar, S. D., Microangiopathic hemolytic anemia in renal allotransplantation: Report of a successfully treated case and review of the literature. *Am. J. Med.*, *58*: 862–868 (1975).
66. Kohler, T. R., Tilney, N. L., Microangiopathic hemolytic anemia associated with hyperacute rejection of a kidney allograft. *Transplant. Proc.*, *14*: 444–446 (1982).
67. Chavers, B. M., Wells, T. G., Burke, B. A., Mauer, S. M., De novo hemolytic uremic syndrome following renal transplantation. *Pediatr. Nephrol.*, *4*: 62–64 (1990).
68. Van Buren, D., Van Buren, C. T., Flechner, S. M., Maddox, A. M., Verani, R., Kahan, B. D., De novo hemolytic uremic syndrome in renal transplant recipients immunosuppressed with cyclosporine. *Surgery*, *98*: 54–62 (1985).
69. Sommer, B. G., Innes, J. T., Whitehurst, R. M., Sharma, H. M., Ferguson, R. M., Cyclosporine-associated renal arteriopathy resulting in loss of allograft function. *Am. J. Surg.*, *149*: 756–764 (1985).
70. Kirste, G., Wilms, H., Steinhauer, H. B., Hörl, W., Hemolytic anemia in a patient with cyclosporine therapy after kidney transplantation. *Transplant. Proc.*, *17*: 2648–2650 (1985).
71. Wolfe, J. A., McCann, R. L., Sanfilippo, F., Cyclosporine associated microangiopathy in renal transplantation: A severe but potentially reversible form of early graft injury. *Transplantation*, *41*: 541–544 (1986).
72. Dyck, R. F., Kappel, J. E., Sheridan, D., Card, R. D., Reversible cyclosporine-associated hemolytic uremic syndrome in a renal transplant recipient: A role for a platelet aggregating factor? *Transplant. Proc.*, *18*: 228–229 (1986).
73. Giroux, L., Smeesters, C., Corman, J., Paquin, F., Allaire, G., St. Louis, G., Daloze, P., Hemolytic uremic syndrome in renal allografted patients treated with cyclosporin. *Can. J. Physiol. Pharmacol.*, *65*: 1125–1131 (1987).
74. Verpooten, G. A., Paulus, G. J., Roels, F., De Broe, M. E., De novo occurrence of hemolytic uremic syndrome in a cyclosporine-treated renal allograft patient. *Transplant. Proc.*, *19*: 2943–2945 (1987).
75. Cerilli, G. J., Nelsen, C., Dorfman, L., Renal homotransplantation in infants and children with hemolytic uremic syndrome. *Surgery*, *71*: 66–71 (1972).
76. Arias-Rodriguez, M., Sraer, J. D., Kourilsky, O., Smith, M. D., Renal transplantation and immunological abnormalities in thrombotic microangiopathy of adults: Reports of 5 cases. *Transplantation*, *23*: 360–365 (1977).
77. Howard, R. J., Mauer, S. M., Miller, K., Simmons, R. L., Najarian, J. S., Biopsy proven recurrence of hemolytic uremic syndrome early after kidney transplantation with a favorable outcome [abstract]. *Kidney Int.*, *10*: 544 (1976).
78. Folman, R. Arbus, G. S., Churchill, B., Gaum, L., Huber, J., Recurrence of the hemolytic uremic syndrome in a 3½ year old child, 4 months after renal transplantation. *Clin. Nephrol.*, *10*: 121–127 (1978).
79. Williams, C., Anderton, J. L., Yates, P. A., Microangiopathic haemolytic anaemia before and after renal transplantation. *Scot. Med. J.*, *25*: 323–326 (1980).
80. Stevenson, J. A., Dumke, A., Glassock, R. J., Rajfer, J., Cohen, A. H., Thrombotic microangiopathy: Recurrence following renal transplant and response to plasma infusion. *Am. J. Nephrol.*, *2*: 227–231 (1981).
81. Hauglustaine, D., van Damme, B., Vanreterghem, Y., Michielsen, P., Recurrent hemolytic uremic syndrome during oral contraception. *Clin. Nephrol.*, *15*: 148–153 (1981).
82. Leithner, C., Sinzinger, H., Pohauka, E., Schwarz, M., Kretschmer, G., Syré, G., Occurrence of hemolytic uremic syndrome under cyclosporine treatment: Accident or possible side effect mediated by a lack of prostacyclin-stimulating plasma factor? *Transplant. Proc.*, *15*: 2787–2789 (1983).

83. Bonsib, S. M., Ercolani, L., Ngheim, D., Hamilton, H. E., Recurrent thrombotic microangipathy in a renal allograft. Case report and review of the literature. *Am. J. Med., 79*: 520–529 (1985).
84. Case records of the Massachusetts General Hospital (case 15-1986). *N. Engl. J. Med., 314*: 1032–1040 (1986).
85. Griño, J. M., Caralps, A., Carreras, L., Nogues, R., Castelao, A. M., Romero, R., Carreras, M., Alsina, J., Apparent recurrence of hemolytic uremic syndrome in azathioprine-treated allograft recipients. *Nephron, 49*: 301 (1988).
86. Pirson, Y., Leclerq, B., Squifflet, J. P., Alexandre, G. P. J., Van Ypersele de Strihou C., Good prognosis of the hemolytic uremic syndrome after renal transplantation [abstract]. *Nephrol. Dial. Transplant. 1*: 134 (1986).
87. van den Berg-Wolf, M. G., Koote, A. M. M., Weening, J. J., Paul, L. C., Recurrent hemolytic uremic syndrome in a renal transplant recipient and review of the Leiden experience. *Transplantation, 45*: 248–251 (1988).
88. Eijgenraam, F. J., Donckerwolcke, R. A., Monnens, A. H., Proesmans, W., Wolff, E. D., van Damme, B., Renal transplantation in 20 children with hemolytic uremic syndrome. *Clin. Nephrol., 33*: 87–93 (1990).
89. Repetto, H. A., Vasquez, L. A., Calvo, P., Patti, G., Renal transplantation in children with idiopathic "classic" hemolytic uremic syndrome [abstract]. *Pediatr. Nephrol., 3*: C185 (1989).
90. Gagnadoux, M. F., Broyer, M., Habib, R., Renal transplantation in hemolytic uremic syndrome. Report of 31 cases [abstract]. *Pediatr. Nephrol., 3*: C184 (1989).
91. Kaplan, B. S., Hemolytic uremic syndrome with recurrent episodes: An important subset. *Clin. Nephrol., 8*: 495–498 (1977).
92. Drukker, A., Winterborn, M., Bennett, B., Churg, J., Spitzer, A., Greifer, I., Recurrent hemolytic-uremic syndrome: A case report. *Clin. Nephrol., 4*: 68–72 (1975).
93. Barré, P., Kaplan, B. S., de Chadarevian, J. P., Drummond, K. N., Hemolytic uremic syndrome with hypocomplementemia, serum C3 NeF and glomerular deposits of C3. *Arch. Pathol. Lab. Med., 101*: 357–361 (1977).
94. Spirer, Z., Knobel, B., Earon, J., Heyman, I., Bogair, N., Recurrent hemolytic–uremic syndrome. A report of two cases. *Helv. Paediat. Acta, 32*: 165–172 (1977).
95. Devictor, D., Nathanson, M., Perelman, R., Syndrome hemolytique à rechute. A propos d'un cas à biopsie rénale non caractéristique. *Med. Infant., 85*: 895–900 (1978).
96. Wasserstein, A., Hill, G., Goldfarb, S., Goldberg, M., Recurrent thrombotic thrombocytopenic purpura after viral infection. *Arch. Intern. Med., 141*: 685–687 (1981).
97. Thompson, R. A., Winterborn, M. H., Hypocomplementemia due to a genetic deficiency of β1H globulin. *Clin. Exp. Immunol., 46*: 110–119 (1981).
98. Carreras, L., Romero, R., Requesens, C., Oliver, A. J., Carrera, M., Clavo, M. Alsina, J., Familial hypocomplementemic hemolytic uremic syndrome with HLA-A3B7 haplotype. *JAMA, 245*: 602–604 (1981).
99. Beattie, T. J., Murphy, A. V., Willoughby, M. L. N., Machin, S. J., Defreyn, G., Plasmapheresis in the hemolytic–uremic syndrome in children. *Br. Med. J., 282*: 1667–1668 (1981).
100. Sweny, P., Winning, A., Gross, M. P., Moorehead, J. F., Plasmapheresis in the haemolytic–uremic syndrome in children [letter]. *Br. Med. J., 282*: 2137 (1981).
101. Feldhoff, C. M., Luboldt, N., Bussman, K., Schrör, K. Plasma exchanges in frequently recurrent hemolytic–uremic syndrome in a child. *Int. J. Pediatr. Nephrol. 4*: 239–242 (1983).
102. Wyatt, R. J., Jones, D., Stapelton, F. B., Roy, S., Odom, T. W., McLean, R. H., Recurrent hemolytic–uremic syndrome with the hypomorphic fast allele of the third component of complement. *J. Pediatr. 107*: 564–566 (1985).

103. Bogdanovic, R., Cvoric, A., Nikolic, V., Sindjic, M., Recurrent haemolytic–uraemic syndrome with hypocomplementaemia: A case report. *Pediatr. Nephrol., 2*: 236–238 (1988).
104. Mattoo, T. K., Mahmood, M. A., Al-Harbi, M. S., Mikail, I., Familial, recurrent hemolytic-uremic syndrome. *J. Pediatr., 114*: 814–816 (1989).
105. Neame, P. D., Immunologic and other factors in thrombotic thrombocytopenic purpura (TTP). *Semin. Thromb. Hemost., 6*: 416–429 (1980).
106. Gubler, M. C., Dommergues, J. P., Furioli, J., Foulard, M., Bensman, A., Boccon-Gibod, L., Broyer, M., Habib, R., Syndrome de "nail-patella" sans atteinte extra-rénale. Une nouvelle néphropathie héréditaire. *Ann. Pediatr. (Paris), 37*: 78–82 (1990).
107. Kaplan, B. S., Chesney, R. W., Drummond, K. N., Hemolytic uremic syndrome in families. *N. Engl. J. Med., 292*: 1090–1093 (1975).
108. Bergstein, J., Michael, A., Kjellstrand, C., Simmons, R., Najarian, J., Hemolytic uremic syndrome in adult sisters. *Transplantation, 17*: 487–490 (1974).
109. Blattler, W., Wegmann, W., Herold, H., Straub, P. W., Familiäre hämolytisch-uramisches syndrom. *Schweiz. Med. Wochenschr., 105*: 1773–1774 (1975).
110. Wallace, D. C., Lovric, A., Clubb, J. S., Carseldine, D. B., Thrombotic thrombocytopenic purpura in 4 siblings. *Am. J. Med., 58*: 724–734 (1975).
111. Fuchs, W. E., George, J. N., Dotin, L. N., Sears, D. A., Thrombotic thrombocytopenic purpura occurrence 2 years apart during late pregnancy in two sisters. *JAMA, 235*: 2126–2127 (1976).
112. Quazi, Q. H., Schutta, E. J., Hemolytic uremic syndrome in sibs. *Arch. Dis. Child., 52*: 337–338 (1977).
113. Edelsten, A. D., Tuck, S. Familial haemolytic uraemic syndrome. *Arch. Dis. Child, 53*: 255–256 (1978).
114. Feldhoff, C., Pistor, K., Bachmann, H., Horacek, U., Olbing, H., Hemolytic uremic syndrome in 3 siblings. *Clin. Nephrol., 22*: 44–46 (1984).
115. Farr, M. J., Roberts, S., Morley, A. R., Dewar, J. J., Roberts, B. F., Uldall, P. R. The hemolytic–uremic syndrome: A family study. *Q. J. Med., 44*: 161–188 (1975).
116. Karlsberg, R. P., Lacher, J. W., Bartecchi, C. E., Adult hemolytic–uremic syndrome. Familial variant. *Arch. Intern. Med., 137*: 1155–1157 (1977).
117. Perret, B., Gaze, H., Zimmermann, A., Oetliker, O., Syndrome hémolytique urémique familial non endémique: néphrectomie et transplantation. *Helv. Paediatr. Acta, 34*: 167–176 (1977).
118. Hogewind, B. L., Brutel de la Rivière, G., Van Es, L. A., Veltkamp, J. J., Familial occurrence of the haemolytic uraemic syndrome. *Acta Med. Scand., 207*: 73–77 (1980).
119. Merrill, R. H., Knupp, C. L., Jennette, J. C., Familial thrombotic microangiopathy. *Q. J. Med., 57*: 749–759 (1985).
120. Siegler, C. L., Bond, R. E., Simultaneous microangiopathic hemolytic anemia, thrombocytopenia an acute nephropathy in a mother and a child. *Am. J. Dis. Child., 134*: 991–992 (1980).
121. Remuzzi, G., Marchesi, D., Misiani, R., Mecca, G., de Gaetano, G., Donati, M. B., Familial deficiency of a plasma factor stimulating vascular prostacyclin activity. *Thromb. Res., 16*: 517–525 (1973).
122. Jorgensen, K. A., Pedersen, R. S., Familial deficiency of prostacyclin production stimulating factor in the hemolytic uremic syndrome of children. *Thromb. Res., 21*: 311–315 (1981).
123. Tune, B. M., Groshon, G. T., Plumer, L. B., Mendoza, S. A., The hemolytic–uremic syndrome in siblings: A prospective survey. *J. Pediatr., 84*: 682–683 (1974).
124. Kwaan, H. C., Miscellaneous secondary thrombotic microangiopathy. *Semin. Hematol., 24*: 141–147 (1987).
125. Koster, F. T., Levin, J., Walker, L., Tung, K. S. K., Gilman, R. H., Rahaman, M. M.,

Majid, M. A., Islam, S., Williams, R. C., Hemolytic uremic syndrome after shigellosis. Relation to endotoxemia and circulating immune complexes. *N. Engl. J. Med.*, *298*: 927–933 (1978).

126. Koster, F. T., Boonpucknavig, V., Sujaho, S., Gilman, R. H., Rahaman, M. M., Renal histopathology in the hemolytic uremic syndrome following shigellosis. *Clin. Nephrol.*, *21*: 126–133 (1984).
127. Karmali, M. A., Steele, B. T., Petric, M., Lim, C., Sporadic cases of haemolytic–uraemic syndrome associated with faecal cytotoxin and cytotoxin-producing *Escherichia coli* in stools. *Lancet*, *1*: 619–620 (1983).
128. Kaplan, B. S., Cleary, T. G., Obrig, T. G., Recent advances in understanding the pathogenesis of the hemolytic uremic syndromes. *Pediatr. Nephrol.*, *4*: 276–283 (1990).
129. Richardson, S. E., Karmali, M. A., Becker, L. E., Smith, C. R., The histopathology of the hemolytic–uremic syndrome associated with verocytotoxin-producing *Escherichia coli* infections. *Hum. Pathol.*, *19*: 1102–1108 (1988).
130. Boccia, R. V., Gelmann, E. P., Baker, C. C., Marti, G., Longo, D. L., A hemolytic uremic syndrome with the acquired immunodeficiency syndrome. *Ann. Intern. Med.*, *101*: 716–717 (1984).
131. Jokela, J., Flynn, T., Henry, K., Thrombotic thrombocytopenic purpura in a human immunodeficiency virus sero-positive homosexual male. *Am. J. Hematol.*, *25*: 341–343 (1987).
132. Botti, C. B., Hyde, P., Dipillo, F., Thrombotic thrombocytopenic purpura in a patient who subsequently developed the acquired immunodeficiency syndrome. *Ann. Intern. Med.*, *109*: 242–243 (1988).
133. Leaf, A. N., Laubenstein, L. J., Raphael, B., Hochester, H., Baez, L., Karpatkin, S., Thrombotic thrombocytopenic purpura associated with human immunodeficiency virus type I infection. *Ann. Intern. Med.*, *109*: 194–197 (1988).
134. Nair, J. M. G., Bellevue, R., Bertoni, M., Dosik, H., Thrombotic thrombocytopenic purpura in patients with the acquired immunodeficiency syndrome related complex. *Ann. Intern. Med.*, *109*: 209–212 (1988).
135. Platanias, L. C., Paiusco, D., Bernstein, S., Murali, M. R., Thrombotic thrombocytopenic purpura as the first manifestation of human immunodeficiency virus infection. *Am. J. Med.*, *87*: 699–700 (1989).
136. Dixon, A. C., Kwock, D. W., Nakamura, J. M., Yanagihara, E. T., Saiki, S. M., Bodner, A. J., Alexander, S. S., Thrombotic thrombocytopenic purpura and human T-lymphotropic virus, type 1 (HTLV-1). *Ann. Intern. Med.*, *110*: 93–94 (1989).
137. Murgo, A. J. Thrombotic microangiopathy in the cancer patient including those induced by chemotherapeutic agents. *Semin. Hematol.*, *24*: 161–177 (1987).
138. Liu, K., Mittelman, A., Sproul, E. E., Elias, E. G., Renal toxicity in man treated with mitomycin C. *Cancer*, *28*: 1314–1320 (1971).
139. Hanna, N. T., Krauss, S., Regester, R. F., Murphy, W. M., Renal disease after mitomycin C therapy. *Cancer*, *48*: 2583–2588 (1981).
140. Mazzuco, G., Fornari, G., Monga, G., Severe glomerular mesangiolysis in a patient with rectal adenocarcinoma treated with cytotoxic drugs. *Virchows Arch. [A]*, *398*: 197–203 (1982).
141. Simon, P., Hervé, J. P., Ramée, M. P., Leroy, J. P., Ang, K. S., Leguy, P., Vignoud, J., Cledes, J., La néphropathie de la mitomycine C. Trois nouvelles observations et revue de la littérature. *Néphrologie*, *3*: 152–157 (1982).
142. Cordonnier, D., Vert-Pré, F. C., Bayle, F., Alix, J. L., Couderc, P., La néphrotoxicité de la mitomycine C (à propos de 25 observations). Résultats d'une étude multicentrique organisée par la Société de Néphrologie. *Néphrologie*, *6*: 19–26 (1985).
143. Laffay, D. L., Tubbs, R. R., Valenzuela, R., Hall, P. M., McCormack, L. J., Chronic glomerular microangiopathy and metastatic carcinoma. *Hum. Pathol.*, *10*: 433–438 (1972).

144. Kressel, B. R., Ryan, K. P., Duong, A. G., Berenber, G. J., Schein, P. S., Microangiopathic hemolytic anaemia, thrombocytopenia and renal failure in patients treated for adenocarcinoma. *Cancer, 48*: 1738–1745 (1981).
145. Jackson, A. M., Burton, D. R., Graff, L. G., Jacobs, J. B., Schwartz, J. H., Strauss, G. M., Yang, J. P. S., Rudnick, M. R., Elfinbein, B., Narins, R. G., Thrombotic microangiopathy and renal failure associated with antineoplastic chemotherapy. *Ann. Intern. Med., 101*: 41–44 (1984).
146. Desablens, B., Fievet, P., Pruna, A., Claisse, J. F., Westeel, P. F., Tolani, M., Fournier, A., Hemolytic–uremic syndrome after cancer chemotherapy without mitomycin C. *Nephron, 42*: 343–344 (1986).
147. Byrnes, J. J., Baquerizo, H., Gonzalez, M., Hensely, G. T., Thrombocytopenic purpura subsequent to acute myelogeous leukemia chemotherapy. *Am. J. Hematol., 21*: 299–304 (1986).
148. Ries, F., Klastersky, J., Nephrotoxicity induced by cancer chemotherapy with special emphasis on cisplatin therapy. *Am. J. Kidney Dis., 8*: 368–378 (1986).
149. Hostetter, A. L., Tubbs, R. R., Ziegler, T., Gephardt, G. N., McMahon, J. T., Schreiber, M. J., Chronic glomerular microangiopathy complicating metastasic carcinoma. *Hum. Pathol., 18*: 342–348 (1987).
150. Weinblatt, M. E., Kahn, E., Scimeca, P. G., Kochen, J. A., Hemolytic uremic syndrome associated with cisplastin therapy. *Am. J. Pediatr. Hematol. Oncol., 9*: 295–298 (1987).
151. Arneil, G. C., Emmanuel, I. G., Flatman, G. E., Harris, F., Young, D. G., Zachary, R. B., Nephritis in 2 children after irradiation and chemotherapy for nephroblastomea. *Lancet, 1*: 960–963 (1974).
152. Kapur, S., Chandra, R., Antonovych, T., Acute radiation nephritis. *Arch. Pathol. Lab. Med., 101*: 469–473 (1977).
153. Cogan, M. G., Arieff, A. J., Radiation nephritis and intravascular coagulation. *Clin. Nephrol., 10*: 74–78 (1978).
154. Churchill, D. N., Hong, K., Gault, M. H., Radiation nephritis following combined abdominal radiation and chemotherapy (bleomycin–vinblastine). *Cancer, 41*: 2162–2164 (1978).
155. Steele, B. T., Lierenman, D. S., Acute radiation nephritis and the hemolytic uremic syndrome. *Clin. Nephrol., 11*: 272–274 (1979).
156. Harrell, R. M., Sibley, R., Vogelzang, N. J., Renal vascular lesions after chemotherapy with vinblastine, bleomycin and cisplatin. *Am. J. Med., 73*: 429–433 (1982).
157. Ironside, J. A. D., Davey, P. G., Scott, J. S., Radiation nephritis in a case of a spindle cell neoplasm in remission after combination treatment with abdominal radiotherapy and chemotherapy. *Clin. Oncol., 9*: 153–158 (1983).
158. Beaufils, H., de Groc, F., Gubler, M. C., Wechsler, B., Le Hoang, P., Baumelou, A., Chomette, G., Jacobs, C., Hemolytic uremic syndrome in patients with Behçet's disease treated with cyclosporin A: Report of 2 cases. *Clin. Nephrol., 34*: 157–162 (1990).
159. Bonser, R. S., Adu, D., Franklin, I., McMaster, P., Cyclosporin-induced hemolytic uremic syndrome in liver allograft recipient [letter]. *Lancet, 2*: 1337 (1984).
160. Dzik, W. H., Georgi, B. A. Khettry, U., Jenkins, R. L., Cyclosporine-associated thrombotic thrombocytopenic purpura following liver transplantation. Successful treatment with plasma exchange. *Transplantation, 44*: 570–572 (1987).
161. Powles, R. L., Clink, H. M., Spence, D., Morgenstern, G., Watson, J. C., Selby, P. J., Woods, M., Barret, A., Jameson, B., Sloane, J., Lawler, S. D. Kay, H. E. M., Lawson, D., McElwain, T. J., Alexander, P., Cyclosporin A to prevent graft-versus host disease in man after allogeneic bone-marrow transplantation. *Lancet, 1*: 327–329 (1980).
162. Shulman, H., Striker, G., Deeg, H. J., Kennedy, M., Storb, R., Thomas, E. D.,

Nephrotoxicity of cyclosporin A after allogeneic marrow transplantation. Glomerular thromboses and tubular injury. *N. Engl. J. Med., 305*: 1392–1395 (1981).

163. Atkinson, K., Briggs, J. C., Hayes, H., Ralston, M., Dodds, A. J., Concannon, A. J., Naidoo, D., Cyclosporin A associated nephrotoxicity in the first 100 days after allogeneic bone marrow transplantation: 3 distinct syndromes. *Br. J. Haematol., 54*: 59–67 (1983).
164. Hows, J. M., Smith, J. M., Baughan, A., Gordon Smith, E. C., Nephrotoxicity in marrow graft recipients treated with cyclosporine. *Transplant. Proc., 155* (Suppl. 1): 2708–2711 (1983).
165. Textor, S. C., Forman, S. J., Bravo, E. L., Carlson, J., De novo accelerated hypertension during sequential cyclosporine and prednisolone therapy in normotensive bone marrow transplant recipients. *Transplant. Proc., 20*: 480–486 (1988).
166. Holler, E., Kolb, H. J., Hiller, E., Mraz, W., Lehmacher, B., Gleixner, C., Seeber, U., Jehn, H. H., Gerhatz, G., Brehm, G., Wilmanns, N., Microangiopathy in patients on cyclosporine prophylaxis who developed acute graft-versus-host disease after HLA identical bone marrow transplantation. *Blood, 73*: 2018–2024 (1989).
167. Nizze, H., Mihatsch, M. J., Zollinger, H. U., Brocheriou, C., Gokel, J. M., Henry, K., Sloane, J. P., Stovin, P. G., Cyclosporine associated nephropathy in patients with heart and bone marrow transplants. *Clin. Nephrol., 30*: 248–260 (1988).
168. Antignac, C., Gubler, M. C., Leverger, G., Broyer, M., Habib, R., Delayed renal failure with extensive mesangiolysis following bone marrow transplantation. *Kidney Int., 35*: 1336–1344 (1989).
169. Spruce, W. E., Forman, S. J., Blume, K. G., Bearman, R. M., Bixby, H., Ching, A., Drinkard, J., San Marco, A., Hemolytic uremic syndrome after bone marrow transplantation. *Acta Haematol. (Basel), 67*: 206–210 (1982).
170. Rozenbaum, A., Colin, J. P., Flesh, M., Hory, B., Saint-Hillier, Y., Leconte des Floris, R., Pérol, C., Syndrome hémolytique et urémique (SHU) après chimiothérapie et greffe autologue de moelle osseuse: à propos de 2 observations [abstract]. *Néphrologie, 5*: 48 (1984).
171. Bergstein, J., Andreoli, S. P., Provisor, A. J., Yum, M., Radiation nephritis following total-body irradiation and cyclophosphamide in preparation for bone marrow transplantation. *Transplantation, 41*: 63–66 (1986).
172. Craig, J. I. O., Sheehan, T., Bell, K., The haemolytic uraemic syndrome and bone marrow transplantation [letter]. *Br. Med. J., 295*: 887 (1987).
173. Marshall, R. J., Sweny, P., HUS in recipients of bone marrow transplants not treated with CSA. *Histopathology, 10*: 953–962 (1986).
174. Guinan, E., Tarbell, N., Niemeyer, C., Sallan, S., Weinstein, H., Intravascular hemolysis and renal insufficiency after bone marrow transplantation. *Blood, 72*: 451–455 (1988).
175. Chappell, M. E., Keeling, D. M., Prentice, H. G., Sweny, P., Haemolytic uraemic syndrome after bone marrow transplantation: An adverse effect of total body irradiation? *Bone Marrow Transplant, 3*: 339–347 (1988).
176. Loomis, L. J., Aronson, A. J., Rudinsky, R., Spargo, B. H., Hemolytic uremic syndrome following bone marrow transplantation: A case report and review of the literature. *Am. J. Kidney Dis., 14*: 324–328 (1989).
177. Tschuchnigg, M., Bradstock, K. F., Koutts, J., Stewart, J., Enno, A., Seldon, M., A case of thrombotic thrombocytopenic purpura following allogeneic bone marrow transplantation. *Bone Marrow Transplant., 5*: 61–63 (1990).
178. Zuelzer, W. W., Palmer, H. D., Newton, W. A., Jr., Unusual GN in young children, probably radiation nephritis. *Am. J. Pathol., 26*: 1019–1039 (1950).
179. Cogan, S. R., Ritter, I., Radiation nephritis. A clinicopathologic correlation of 3 surviving cases. *Am. J. Med., 24*: 530–534 (1958).

180. Rosen, S., Swerdlow, M. A., Muehrcke, R. C., Pirani, C. L., Radiation nephritis. Light and electron microscopic observations. *Am. J. Clin. Pathol., 41*: 482–502 (1964).
181. Mostofi, M. K., Radiation effects on the kidney. In *The Kidney* (M. K. Mostofi, D. E. Smith, eds.), Williams & Wilkins, Baltimore, pp. 338–386 (1966).
182. Madrazo, A., Suzuki, Y., Churg, J., Radiation nephritis. II. Chronic changes after high doses of radiation. *Am. J. Pathol., 61*: 37–44 (1970).
183. Keane, W. F., Crosson, J. T., Staley, N. A., Anderson, W. R., Shapiro, F. L., Radiation-induced renal disease. *Am. J. Med., 60*: 127–137 (1976).
184. Birembaut, P., Parjoie, R., Ploton, D., Rebaiz, K., Wolf, C., Atteinte rénale après irradiation et chimiothérapie par l'Adriamycine, la vincristine et le 5-fluorouracile. *Nephrologie, 2*: 11–14 (1981).
185. Lohrman, H. P., Adam, W., Heymer, B., Kubanek, B., Microangiopathic hemolytic anemia in metastatic carcinoma. Report of eight cases. *Ann. Intern. Med., 79*: 368–375 (1973).
186. Antman, K. H., Skarin, A. T., Mayor, R. J., Hargreaves, H. K., Canellos, G. P., Microangiopathic hemolytic anemia and cancer. A review. *Medicine, 58*: 377–384 (1979).
187. Editorial: Haemolytic uraemic syndrome of young women. *Lancet, 1*: 943–944 (1976).
188. Hayslett, J. P., Postpartum renal failure. *N. Engl. J. Med., 312*: 1556–1559 (1985).
189. Grünfeld, J. P., Ganeval, D., Bournerias, F., Acute renal failure in pregnancy. *Kidney Int., 18*: 179–191 (1980).
190. Churg, J., Loffer, D., Paronetto, F., Ronat, E., Barnett, R. N., Hemolytic uremic syndrome as a cause of postpartum renal failure. *Am. J. Obstet. Gynecol., 108*: 253–261 (1970).
191. Ponticelli, C., Imbasciati, E., Tarantino, A., Graziani, G., Redaelli, B., Postpartum renal failure with microangiopathic haemolytic anaemia. *Nephron, 9*: 27–41 (1972).
192. Beller, F. K., Intorp, H. W., Losse, H., Loew, H., Moenninghoff, W., Schmidt, E. H., Grundmann, E., Malignant nephrosclerosis during pregnancy and in the postpartum period (the uremic hemolytic syndrome). *Am. J. Obstet. Gynecol., 125*: 633–639 (1976).
193. Scheer, R. L., Jones, D. B., Malignant nephrosclerosis in women post partum. *JAMA, 201*: 600–604 (1967).
194. Wagoner, R. D., Holley, D. E., Johnson, W. J., Accelerated nephrosclerosis and post partum acute renal failure in normotensive patients. *Ann. Intern. Med., 69*: 237–248 (1968).
195. Rosenmann, E., Kanter, A., Bacani, R. A., Pirani, C. L., Pollak, V. E., Fatal late post partum intravascular coagulation with acute renal failure. *Am. J. Med. Sci., 257*: 269–273 (1969).
196. Robson, J. S., Martin, A. M., Rickley, F. A., MacDonald, M. K., Irreversible post partum renal failure. *Q. J. Med., 37*: 423–435 (1968).
197. Segonds, A., Louradour, N., Suc, J. M., Orfila, C., Post partum hemolytic uremic syndrome: A study of 3 cases with a review of the literature. *Clin. Nephrol., 12*: 229–242 (1979).
198. Kincaid-Smith, P., Fairley, K. F., Kloss, M., Lupus anticoagulant associated with renal microangiopathy and pregnancy-related renal failure. Q. *J. Med., 258*: 795–815 (1988).
199. Tobon, H., Malignant hypertension, uremia and hemolytic anemia in a patient on oral contraceptives. *Obstet. Gynecol., 40*: 681–685 (1972).
200. Brown, C. B., Clarkson, A. R., Robson, J. K., Cameron, J. S., Thomson, D., Ogg, C. S., Haemolytic uraemic syndrome in women taking oral contraceptives. *Lancet, 1*: 1479–1481 (1973).
201. Schoolwerth, A. C., Sandler, R. S., Klahr, S., Kissane, J. M., Nephrosclerosis postpartum and in women taking oral contraceptives. *Arch. Intern. Med., 136*: 178–185 (1976).

202. Levêque, B., Habib, R., Courtecuisse, V., Desbois, J. C., Desbauchez, C., Marie, J., Syndrome hémolytique et urémique et syndrome néphrotique idiopathique. Association chez une enfant de 7 ans [abstract]. *Arch. Fr. Pediatr., 24*: 1078 (1967).
203. Levy, M., Antignac, C., Habib, R., Niaudet, P., Gagnadoux, M. F., Hemolytic uremic syndrome in a girl with a Turner's syndrome receiving oestroprogestative treatment and presenting Berger's disease [abstract]. *Int. J. Pediatr. Nephrol., 3*: (1982).
204. Dumas, R., Baldet, P., Rolin, B., Hypertension and segmental renal hypoplasia causing a syndrome of haemolysis and uraemia. *Arch. Dis. Child., 56*: 403–404 (1981).
205. de Chadarevian, J. P., Goodyer, P. R., Kaplan, B. S., Acute glomerulonephritis and hemolytic uremic syndrome. *Can. Med. Assoc. J., 123*: 391–394 (1980).
206. Medani, C. R., Pearl, P. L., Hall-Craggs, M., Acute renal failure, hemolytic anemia and thrombocytopenia in post streptococcal glomerulonephritis. *South. Med. J., 80*: 370–373 (1987).
207. Dische, F. E., Culliford, E. J., Parsons, V., Haemolytic uremic syndrome and idiopathic membranous glomerulonephritis. *Br. Med. J., 1*: 1112–1113 (1978).
208. Siegler, R. L., Brewer, E. D., Pysher, T. J., Hemolytic uremic syndrome associated with glomerular disease. *Am. J. Kidney Dis., 13*: 144–147 (1989).
209. Krensky, A. M., Ingelfinger, J. R., Grupe, W. E., Rosen, E., Hemolytic uremic syndrome and crescentic glomerulonephritis complicating childhood nephrosis. *Clin. Nephrol., 19*: 99–106 (1983).
210. Stave, G. M., Croker, B. P., Thrombotic microangiopathy in antiglomerular basement membrane glomerulonephritis. *Arch. Pathol. Lab. Med., 108*: 747–751 (1984).
211. Salyer, W. R., Salyer, D. C., Heptinstall, R. H., Scleroderma and microangiopathic hemolytic anemia. *Ann. Intern. Med., 78*: 895–897 (1973).

VI
Pathogenesis

25
Oxygen-Derived Free Radicals in the Pathogenesis of the Hemolytic Uremic Syndrome

C. M. Taylor *The Children's Hospital, Birmingham, England* **H. R. Powell** *The Royal Children's Hospital, Melbourne, Australia*

The hemolytic uremic syndromes comprise a wide range of different disorders. At one end of the spectrum is the disease that is now common in North America and parts of Europe, which follows a prodrome of diarrhea that is usually bloody and is associated with infection by verocytotoxin-producing *Escherichia coli* (VTEC) (1–3). There are several similarities between this disorder and the form of hemolytic uremic syndrome (HUS) associated with *Shigella dysenteriae* type 1 infection in the tropics (4, 5). These disorders can be considered together as an *extrinsic* form of the syndrome in which environmental agents play a major role. Although uncommon, HUS related to radiation, drugs, such a mitomycin; or other toxins, such as neuraminidase, can be regarded as discrete etiologies within the extrinsic group. By contrast, there is a heterogeneous group of diseases that give rise to the syndrome without any obvious prodrome. These *intrinsic* forms are rare in comparison with the diarrhea-associated types, and within this group are patients with relapsing or familial diseases, primary complement abnormalities, and an adverse prognosis.

Endothelial injury is widely accepted as being a central event in all forms of HUS and, given the multiplicity of causes of the syndrome, it is reasonable to explore the possibility that common final pathogenetic pathways may be involved. Endothelial injury by oxygen-derived radicals has been considered for this role, but the evidence supporting a phlogistic hypothesis is fragmentary. The purpose of this chapter is to give an overview of the action of oxygen metabolites in relevant pathological mechanisms and critically review the present evidence for free radical injury in HUS.

OXYGEN-DERIVED FREE RADICALS

Figure 1 shows the stepwise reduction of molecular oxygen to form the stable hydroxyl ion. In this process, electrons are donated to oxygen and, when the product

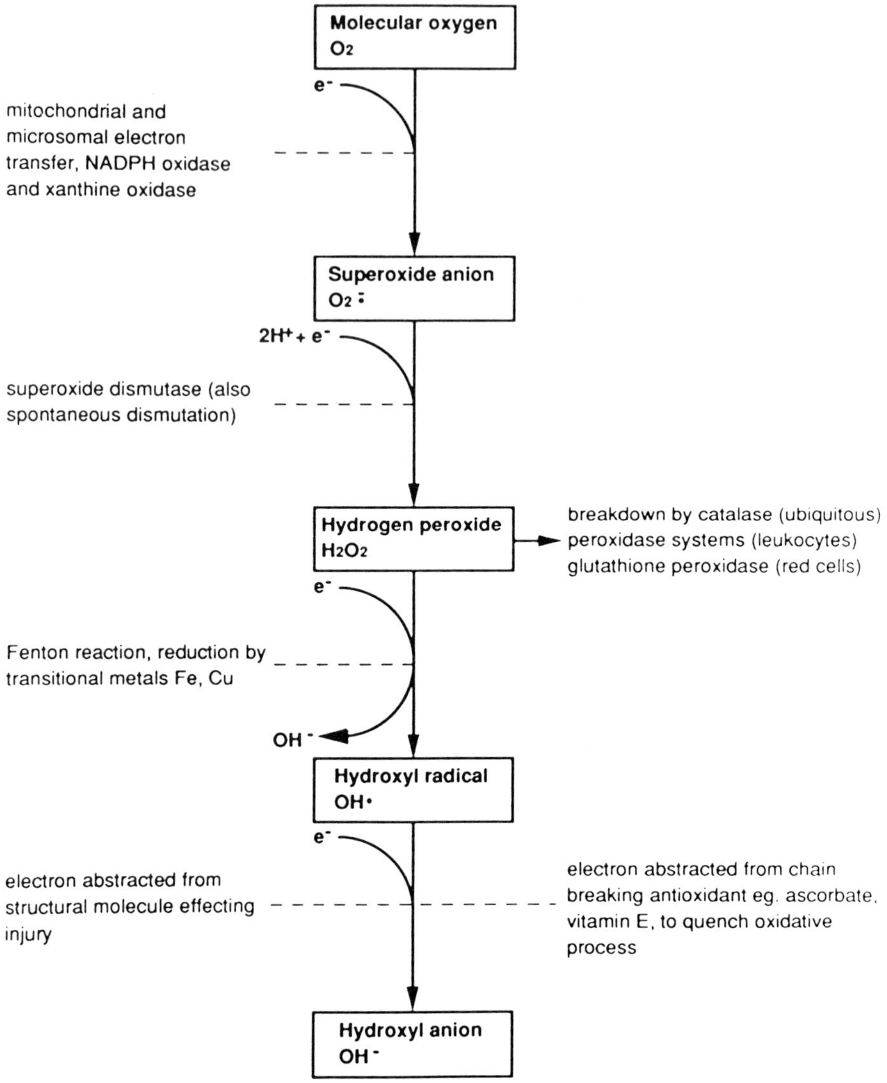

Figure 1 The reduction of molecular oxygen.

has an unpaired electron in the outer electron shell, an oxygen-derived free radical (ODFR) is formed. In standard chemical formulas these radicals are denoted by a dot. These species are highly reactive and, in certain circumstances, will abstract a further electron from complex macromolecules, such as lipids, proteins, or DNA, thereby oxidizing them and completing the reduction of oxygen to a stable end product. Oxygen-derived free radicals can be produced enzymatically or nonenzymatically. An example of the latter is the production of hydroxyl radicals in water by ionizing radiation. Much of the cytotoxicity of radiation results from free radical generation, and the sensitivity of certain tumors to radiotherapy reflects a reduced antioxidant potential in susceptible cells.

Enzyme-induced generation of ODFRs is an essential biological process, and it has been estimated that 5% of the molecular oxygen used by mitochondria undergoes single electron reduction (6). Production of ODFR also occurs in microsomal electron transfer chain reactions and prostaglandin (PG) synthesis. Germane to the following discussion is the enzymatic generation of radicals both by activated neutrophils, as part of the microbicidal response toward invading organisms, and as a result of xanthine oxidase activity following ischemia. Certain drugs metabolized by cytochrome-P450 undergo redox cycling in which an electron is removed from the xenobiote and transferred to oxygen. The ODFR so formed then reoxidizes the drug and the process is repeated. This process has the potential to generate large numbers of ODFRs and is the likely mechanism of hepatotoxicity by acetaminophen (paracetamol) and carbon tetrachloride, the pulmonary toxicity of paraquat, and the cardiotoxicity of daunorubicin and doxorubicin.

In an aerobic environment, polyunsaturated fatty acids are especially vulnerable to oxidation and, once oxidized, may themselves behave as free radicals to propagate molecular damage. A scheme for the autooxidation of lipid peroxides is shown in Figure 2. Given the theoretical ability of ODFRs to propagate and inflict structural damage on cell components, the role of antioxidants in limiting this process is crucial. Superoxide is rapidly removed by superoxide dismutase, and hydrogen peroxide and lipid hydroperoxides are removed by both catalase and the glutathione peroxidase systems. However, it appears that containment of both the hydroxyl radical and lipid peroxides depends not on enzymatic systems, but on chain-breaking antioxidants that readily and sacrifically donate electrons. In the lipid layer of cell membranes, vitamin E is of prime importance, being arranged in intimate contact with the 2-esterified unsaturated fatty acids of phospholipids (7). At other sites the containment of free radicals is provided by different scavengers such as ascorbic acid or β-carotene.

Oxygen-Derived Free Radicals and the Neutrophil

Current concepts of the neutrophil's ability to discharge oxidizing species and the mechanisms for focusing and limiting chemical attack have been reviewed recently (8, 9). Following stimulation, neutrophils exhibit an abrupt increase in oxygen uptake known as the *respiratory burst*. This is intimately linked to the enzymatic reduction of molecular oxygen by the plasma membrane-associated NADPH oxidase system and results in the generation of superoxide radicals.

Dismutation of superoxide radicals occurs spontaneously and rapidly at pH 7 to form hydrogen peroxide, although the process can be accelerated a thousand times by superoxide dismutase. Hydrogen peroxide, unlike the superoxide radical, is able to diffuse freely across cell membranes and, in turn, is converted to another oxidant, hypohalous acid, by the catalytic action of neutrophil-derived myeloperoxidase. Chloride is the most prevalent extracellular halide ion, and it is widely accepted that hypochlorous acid is the main product of the superoxide generated by activated neutrophils. This oxidant is an unparalleled bactericidal agent and capable of attacking a wide range of important macromolecules, including proteins, nucleotides, and unsaturated fatty acids. It can also react with primary or secondary amines to produce a further generation of weaker oxidants, the chloramines.

There is debate over whether the highly reactive hydroxyl radical or singlet oxygen can be produced by neutrophils. There is only indirect evidence that neu-

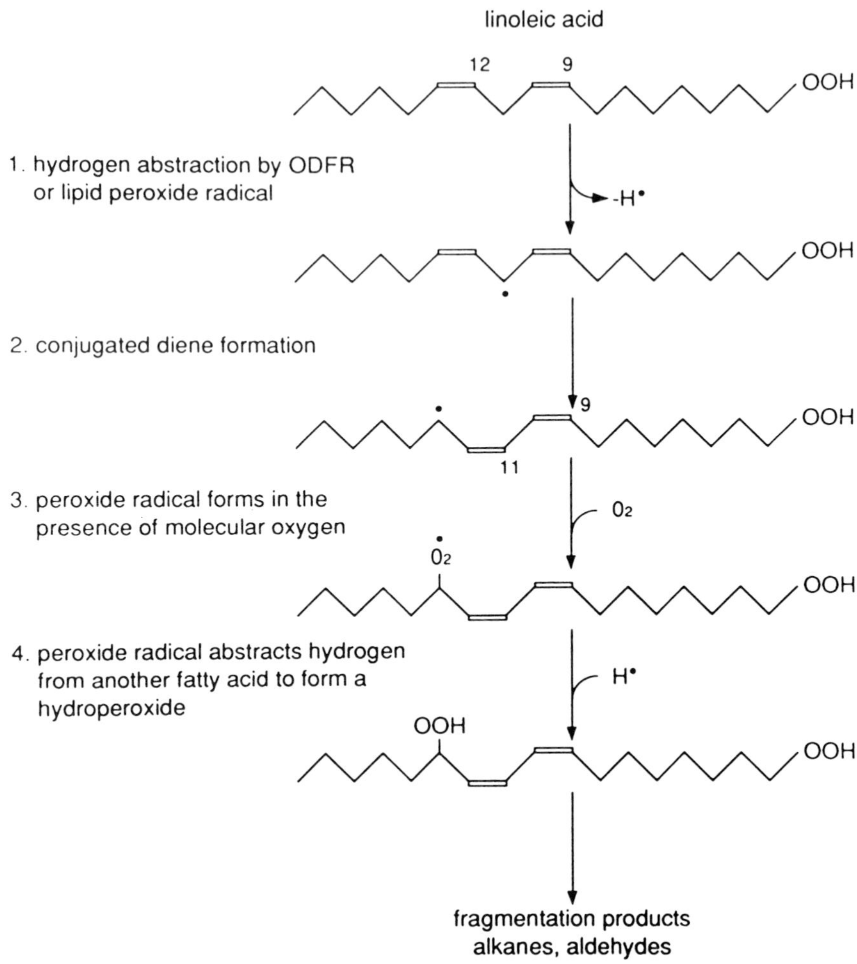

Figure 2 A scheme for the autooxidation of unsaturated fatty acids by lipid peroxide radicals.

trophils and monocytes can generate $OH^{\bullet}$ (10, 11) in that they can release ethylene from the substrate methional. This process is thought to implicate the $OH^{\bullet}$ radical, and was inhibited by scavengers known to interact with hydroxyl. The Fenton reaction, shown below, by which hydroxyl generation would occur, demands the availability of iron in a suitable catalytic form (12).

$$Fe^{3+} + O_2^{\bullet -} \rightarrow Fe^{2+} + O_2$$

$$Fe^{2+} + H_2O_2 \rightarrow Fe^{3+} + OH^- + OH^{\bullet}$$

Neutrophils liberate lactoferrin during activation, which serves to bind avidly to any available iron. This would have the effect of preventing production of $OH^{\bullet}$ and led Britigen et al. (13) to doubt the role of this radical. However, one may question whether there is such security over catalytic iron when there is widespread intravascular hemolysis and intimate red cell–neutrophil interaction, such as that seen in HUS (14) (Fig. 3). Together hemoglobin and hydrogen peroxide can form a potent radical (15, 16). This hemoprotein-associated oxidant is active over a prolonged period, which rules out a role for the hydroxyl radical itself, and it is capable of attacking polyunsaturated membrane fatty acids and phospholipds, certain carbohydrates, and proteins. Moreover, these observations may go some way toward explaining the acute oliguric renal failure provoked by myoglobin or free hemoglobin, which appears to involve oxygen metabolites (17).

Oxygen-Derived Free Radicals and Reperfusion Injury

In the kidney, the main site of metabolic work, and thus oxygen demand, is the tubular epithelium, the blood supply of which is derived from the glomerular efferent artery. Glomerular obstruction from endothelial detachment and swelling, or from a capillary thrombus, gives rise to ischemia of the whole nephron. In patients who die in the acute illness of HUS, postmortem examination typically reveals multiple infarcts in the renal cortex, accompanied by focal hemorrhage. Similarly, renal histological observations in survivors may show areas of acute cortical necrosis. Over the last 2 decades, studies of tissue ischemia have shown that cellular injury may be accentuated during the phase of post ischemic reperfusion and that ODFRs are responsible for this effect (18). Most of this work has been performed with gut, heart, or brain, but the principles seem to be universal, and parallel observations have been made on the kidney.

During hypoxia, there is failure to maintain normal intracellular concentrations of ATP and, consequently, reduced active transport of ions out of the cell (Fig. 4). As a result, there is accumulation of the catabolic products of ATP and an influx of ions, notably calcium. Xanthine dehydrogenase itself does not participate in the generation of ODFRs, but it is readily converted to xanthine oxidase by a protease that is induced by the calcium influx. Once molecular oxygen is again supplied to the cell, the stage is set for the production of superoxide by the following reaction:

$$\text{xanthine} + 2O_2 + H_2O \xrightarrow[\text{xanthine oxidase}]{} \text{uric acid} + 2H^+ + O_2^{\bullet}$$

Support for this concept comes from many studies in which the pathway is interrupted by either xanthine oxidase inhibition or the antioxidant effect of superoxide dismutase, catalase, and other scavengers. For example, treatment with allopurinol reduced the reperfusion damage to transplanted canine, rat, and pig hearts (19–21), and similar observations have been made in brain (22) and skin (23). In models of necrotizing enterocolitis, superoxide dismutase and catalase were consistently protective (15), whereas allopurinol alone was not (24). This led to the suggestion that xanthine oxidase is not the sole source of ODFRs in that model, and the involvement of neutrophils in reperfusion injury was suggested (15). After investigating a canine model of acute myocardial ischemia, Engler et al. (25) drew attention to the importance of leukocytes that are trapped in capillaries and adhere to endothelium. A similar observation was made in rabbits exposed to the ischemia–reperfusion of hemorrhagic shock, in which blockade of the neutrophil adherence antigen CD18 with a monoclonal antibody attenuated injury to the gut (26).

These reports suggest that in ischemia there might be synergism between the production of cytotoxic ODFRs from within the endothelial cell by xanthine oxidase

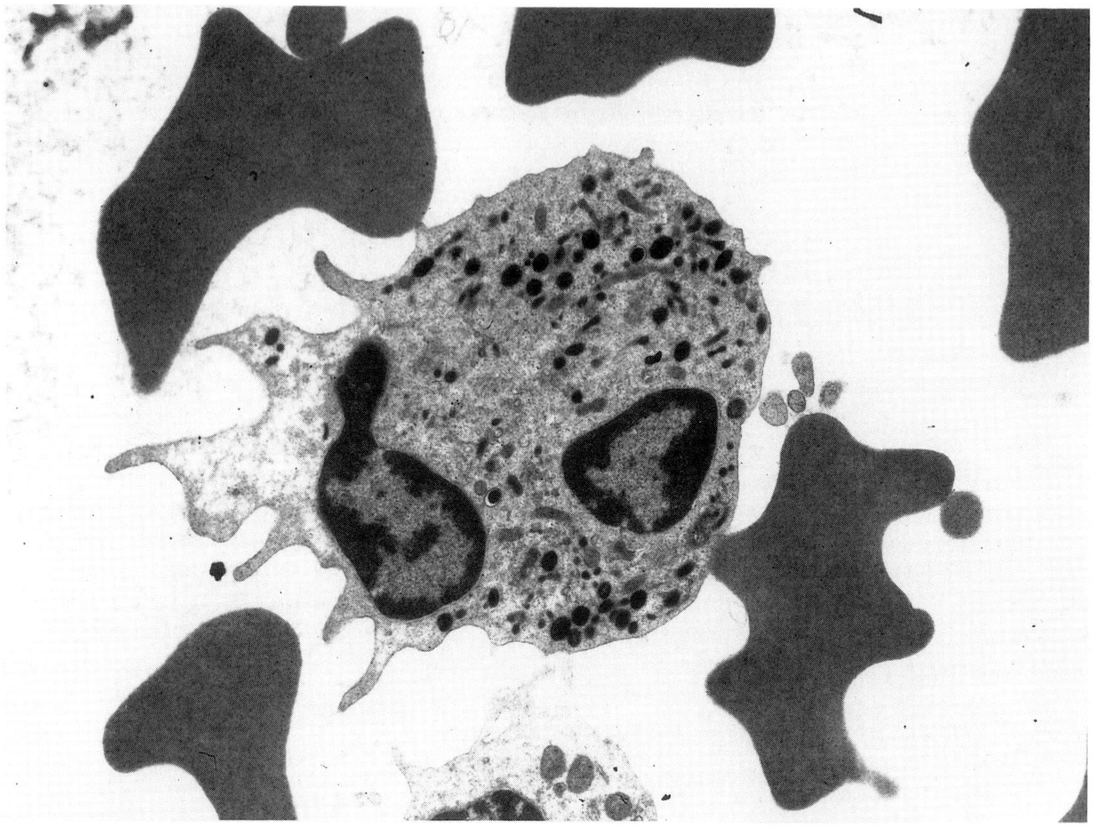

a

Figure 3 Intimate contact between neutrophil and red cell (a) 15,000 magnification (b) 40,000 magnifications.

and attack from without by activated neutrophils. Although incomplete, this view is supported by the observations that xanthine oxidase, presumably by the release of superoxide, increases the susceptibility of endothelium to damage by neutrophil-derived elastase (27). It is necessary to explain why neutrophil–endothelial adhesion occurs in reperfusion. Superoxide induces a neutrophil chemotactic factor in plasma, possibly an oxidized fatty acid bound to albumin (28). Arachidonic acid has also been oxidized to yield a neutrophil attractant, both by a xanthine-oxidase system (29) and by heme proteins and hydrogen peroxide (30, 31).

Xanthine oxidase is not present in all organs, but has been located in gut, liver, heart, lung, and kidney. Enzyme concentrations vary among mammalian species, and humans have lower levels than the usual experimental animals: rat, rabbit, and dog (32). Interestingly, it is found predominantly in the endothelial cells of capillaries, including the vasa rectae of the kidney and is not found in large arteries (33). In the cat, however, the enzyme has more recently been found in epithelial cells in the gut.

As far as the kidney is concerned, in rats, the ODFR scavenger dimethylthiourea was protective against the acute renal failure that followed short periods of ischemia

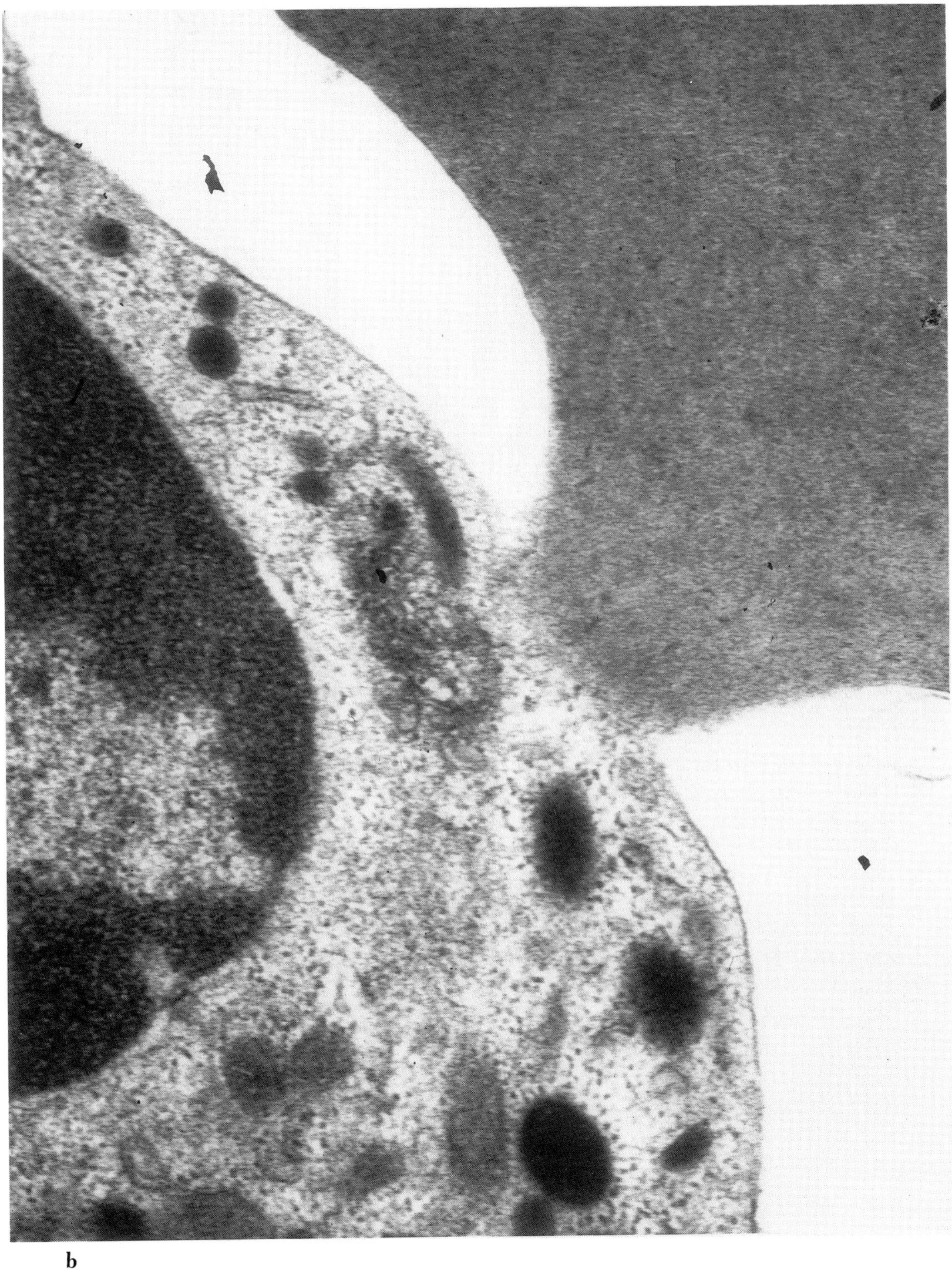

b

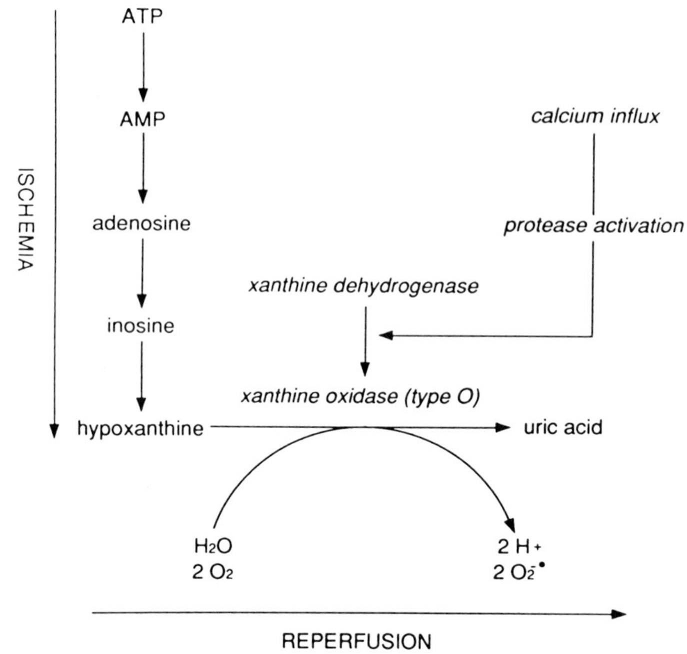

Figure 4 The role of xanthine oxidase in reperfusion injury.

(34). Moreover, perfusion of isolated kidneys with either hydrogen peroxide, or glucose oxidase, which generates oxygen metabolites, caused a reduction in glomerular filtration rate, perfusate flow, and sodium reabsorption. These events occurred in parallel with consumption of antioxidants and, again, could be prevented by administration of catalase or dimethylthiourea (35). Similarly, superoxide dismutase and catalase reduced warm ischemic injury in autografted pig kidneys (36). Allopurinol was able to reduce ischemic renal injury in dogs (37, 38) and rabbits (39), but, when added to the perfusate of human kidneys for transplantation, no benefit was seen (40). The latter was a controlled study, but may not have been a fair trial, as numbers were small and good operative technique minimized warm ischemia time in both treated and control kidneys. An overview of the role of oxygen metabolites in renal disease, although somewhat speculative in parts, has been provided by Canavese and coauthors (41, 42).

METHODS OF IDENTIFYING OXIDANT INJURY

Free radicals, because of their reactivity with organic molecules, exist only for brief periods, and their involvement in biological systems can be deduced only from a combination of peripheral observations. The subject has been well reviewed by Dormandy (43), and for further reading see the *CRC Handbook of Methods for Oxygen Radical Research* (44).

In whole-animal experiments, the ameliorating effect of interrupting ODFR synthesis or the use of antioxidants provides supportive data. However, in the clinical setting, it is far less easy to ascribe a beneficial pharmacologic effect to antioxidants, and some of the more promosing agents, such as superoxide dismutase, are not available for human treatment trials. Measurements of oxidation end products have provided several laboratory tests. A popular example is to measure malondialdehyde, a breakdown product of fatty acid peroxidation, which is detectable in biological tissues by using the thiobarbituric acid reaction (45). We found increased concentrations on malondialdehyde in HUS plasma (unpublished data), but this may reflect the increased prostaglandin turnover of platelet activation and cannot be used as a reliable marker of lipid peroxidation in HUS.

An attractive method that can be applied in vivo, and that has not been applied to HUS, is the measurement of expired ethane and pentane. These gases are produced by peroxidation of ω-3- and ω-6-unsaturated fatty acids, respectively (46). Further support for oxidative injury may be sought in the loss of normal antioxidants or, better, a disturbed ratio between the intact antioxidant and its oxidized product (e.g., ascorbate and dehydroascorbate, or tocopherol and hydroquinone). Interest has been shown in trap assays that test the total antioxidant capacity of a biological sample when exposed to a standard oxidant (47). Although tests for oxidative damage have focused on lipids because of their special vulnerability, other structures are denatured by ODFRs to distinctive products and may prove useful markers. An example of this is hydroxylation of the aromatic amino acids that give IgG a fluorescent property (48).

EVIDENCE FOR LIPID PEROXIDATION IN HEMOLYTIC UREMIC SYNDROME

Wolman (49) first considered a role for lipid peroxides in HUS, drawing attention to the similarity with the renal cortical necrosis and hemolysis induced by feeding laboratory animals with rancid lipids or diets deficient in vitamin E. Since then, the injurious nature of lipid peroxides in experimental circumstances has been studied further. Lipid peroxides inhibit antithrombin III (50) and have procoagulant properties (51). Arachidonic or linoleic acid hydroperoxides injected into rabbits cause direct endothelial damage (52, 53), and the former blocks endothelial prostacyclin production in human tissues (54). Prostacyclin abnormalities in HUS are variable and include both reduced plasma stimulatory activity and the presence of inhibitors (55). Levin et al. (56) found that plasma from children with HUS contained an inhibitor of prostacyclin production that initially appeared to be confined to patients with the intrinsic, nonprodromal form of the syndrome, but later it was shown in some with the postenteropathic type of HUS (Walters, personal communication). The inhibitor was not firmly identified, but was extractable in a mixture of cyclohexane and ethyl acetate, suggesting that it was a polar lipid.

O'Reagan et al. (57) demonstrated depletion of phosphoethanolamine in the red cell membrane of HUS patients. The same authors comment that the plasma concentration of total tocopherol was subnormal in some cases, but unfortunately, the tocopherol levels were not related to plasma lipid concentrations, which would have made the result more meaningful. Later, depletion of arachidonic acid was found in red cell membranes (58), which is also compatible with the concept that oxidative damage had occurred. As phospholipid-derived arachidonate is the source for prostaglandin synthesis, it is possible that the loss of this substrate is linked to the prostacyclin abnormality of HUS.

More direct evidence of lipid peroxidation was provided by Situnayake et al. (59). During the process of hydrogen abstraction from unsaturated fatty acids, the diene bonds become rearranged. The conjugated diene isomer so formed cannot be regarded as an end product, but it may be used as a marker of traffic on this pathway (60), and most of the observed diene conjugation relates to the conversion of linoleic acid from the parent, 9,12- to the 9,11- form. In children with the postenteropathic type of HUS, these markers in plasma lipid fractions were increased, compared with those of patients with chronic renal failure or recent urinary infection who acted as controls. The patients with HUS demonstrated the expected hypertrigylceridemia found in the syndrome (61). However, the normal relationship between vitamin E and plasma lipid concentration was disturbed and was remarkably low in some patients. In two children who had the nonprodromal, intrinsic type of HUS, diene conjugates were found to be normal. As one of the differences between the extrinsic and intrinsic forms of HUS is that neutrophilia is not a feature of the latter, it was suggested that the diene conjugation marker may reflect neutrophil activity.

NEUTROPHIL ACTIVATION IN POSTENTEROPATHIC HEMOLYTIC UREMIC SYNDROME

In recent years, there has been an accumulation of human and experimental evidence that neutrophils play a central role in the pathogenesis of HUS induced by both *S. dysenteriae* type 1 and verocytotoxin-producing *E. coli*. These observations have not been linked directly to cytotoxicity by ODFRs. Although neutrophil-derived oxygen metabolites are themselves capable of attacking host cells, an important action is to remove antiproteinase cover so that locally released enzymes can make an uninterrupted attack on target tissues (8). In an elegant rat model, Johnson et al. (62) demonstrated the necessary synergism of myeloperoxidase and hydrogen peroxide in causing glomerular capillary damage. Whether it is the action of ODFRs or enzymes, such as elastase, that predominate in this intricate system is the subject of debate. For example, in one model, complement-activated neutrophils appeared to injure endothelial cells through oxygen metabolites (63), whereas in other experiments, elastase took precedence (64). Some of the discrepancy may depend on the stimulus to the neutrophil, the type of endothelium used, and the proximity between leukocyte and target. In vivo it is conceivable that these experimental differences may be artificial.

Shiga toxin is identical with verocytotoxin-1 (VT1) and similar to verocytotoxin-2 (VT2), and it is not surprising that there are parallels between shigella and VTEC-associated HUS (3). In shigellosis neutrophilia, endotoxemia and complement activation correlate with the development of HUS (5). In the United Kingdom where most of the diarrhea-associated HUS is related to VTEC infection, there is a strong correlation between the peripheral blood neutrophil count at onset and poor outcome (2, 3, 65); about half the variance of outcome being explained by this variable alone (66). It is unlikely that the leukocytosis is a passive marker, as plasma concentrations of elastase are also elevated and correlate positively with an adverse clinical course (67). Moreover, neutrophils harvested from children during the acute stage of HUS exhibit increased adhesion to human umbilical vein endothelial cells

(HUVEC) in vitro (68) and, on examination of their ultrastructure, appear to have released their granules (Milford, D. V., and Raafat, F., personal communication).

Verocytotoxin is directly injurious to proliferating HUVEC (69, 70), but as yet, there is no hypothesis linking this endotoxin to the neutrophil response seen in HUS. Lipopolysaccharide endotoxin, however, is known to stimulate monocytes to release cytokines, notably interleukin-1 and tumor necrosis factor (71), and these mediators, in turn, coordinate the neutrophil–endothelial interaction of acute inflammation. Interestingly, the plasma concentration of factor VIII-related antigen, widely regarded as a marker of endothelial injury, although elevated in patients with both intrinsic and extrinsic HUS, does not correlate with outcome (72). A possible explanation for this is that endothelial injury is consistent in the disorder, but is reversible, to a large extent, whereas organ destruction depends more on the inflammatory response and parenchymal ischemia.

Experiments inducing vascular injury with endotoxin have a long history and give broadly consistent results. In rabbits, the generalized Shwartzman reaction includes intravascular fibrin deposition in renal vessels and acute cortical necrosis, and it resembles human HUS. Although lipopolysaccharide (LPS) may be directly toxic to human glomerular endothelium in culture (73), in intact systems, leukocyte involvement is crucial (74–76). Leukocyte infiltration in glomeruli was present within 1 hr of starting an infusion of LPS and preceded fibrin deposition (77). Moreover, it appears that the increased procoagulant activity in glomeruli is explained by the presence of leukocytes (78). Vedanarayanan et al. (79) showed that peripheral blood neutrophils were activated, releasing their β-glucuronidase into plasma and demonstrating depressed chemotaxis. They also claimed evidence for lipid peroxidation in renal cortical tissues of endotoxin treated animals, but their method is criticizable in that they used malondialdehyde as a marker, and this may reflect only exaggerated prostanoid catabolism.

Although involvement of neutrophils is confirmed in these models, there is a lack of direct evidence that they induce damage by ODFR release. However, in a study of the effect of LPS on HUVEC cultures, generation of tissue factor was increased markedly in the presence of hydrogen peroxide (80). In other examples of leukocyte-dependent renal inflammation, such as acute interstitial infection by *E. coli* in primates, superoxide dismutase (81) or allopurinol (82) reduced tissue damage, supporting the concept that oxidative processes are at work. Clearly similar experiments need to be undertaken in endotoxin models of HUS.

DRUGS, RADICALS, AND HEMOLYTIC UREMIC SYNDROME

Several drugs have been associated with the development of HUS, and some of these are known to behave as free radicals or are involved in the generation of ODFRs. Mitomycin as a well-recorded example (83–85) and has been developed into an interesting animal model of the disease (86). The metabolism of mitomycin has been extensively studied (87). The molecule is reduced within the cell by a NADPH-dependent quinone reductase, and an incompletely reduced semiquinone radical appears to be the reactive moiety. The drug is also thought to undergo redox cycling. The mechanism of DNA cleavage by mitomycin is related to ODFR action in that it is inhibited by free radical scavengers or superoxide dismutase and catalase (88, 89).

Metronidazole, under anaerobic conditions, is reduced to a nitro anion radical, but, in the presence of oxygen, it donates an electron to generate superoxide. It is likely that the ability of metronidazole to augment the cytotoxic effect of radiation in hypoxic tumors is explained by this. Powell et al. (90) reported an association between metronidazole and HUS in six children who also had diarrhea, four of them having recently undergone bowel surgery. Three of the patients were shown to have low proportions of arachidonic acid in erythrocyte membranes, a finding compatible with oxidative stress. More recently, we identified another three patients at the Children's Hospital, Birmingham, who received metronidazole during the diarrheal prodrome before disclosing HUS, all of whom had an unexpectedly poor outcome (unpublished data). Although it is attractive to consider oxygen radicals as an explanation, these observations do not provide proof, and alternatives include the possibility that metronidazole was given because these patients were sicker, or that the drug changed gut flora unfavorably.

Finally, cyclosporine has been linked to the syndrome (91, 92). Phair et al. (93) found reduced proportions of arachidonic acid in red cells of renal transplant patients treated with cyclosporine compared with those receiving prednisone and azathioprine alone. This reduction parallels that seen in children with diarrhea-associated HUS, but only hints at a common pathogenesis.

THE HYPOTHESIS

A scheme for the hypothesis is given in Figure 5, in which solid arrows indicate the better-established pathogenic pathways and interrupted ones more circumstantial links. In both VTEC- and *S. dysenteriae* type 1-induced HUS, the exotoxins and endotoxin are discussed separately. Although verocytotoxin is able to kill endothelial

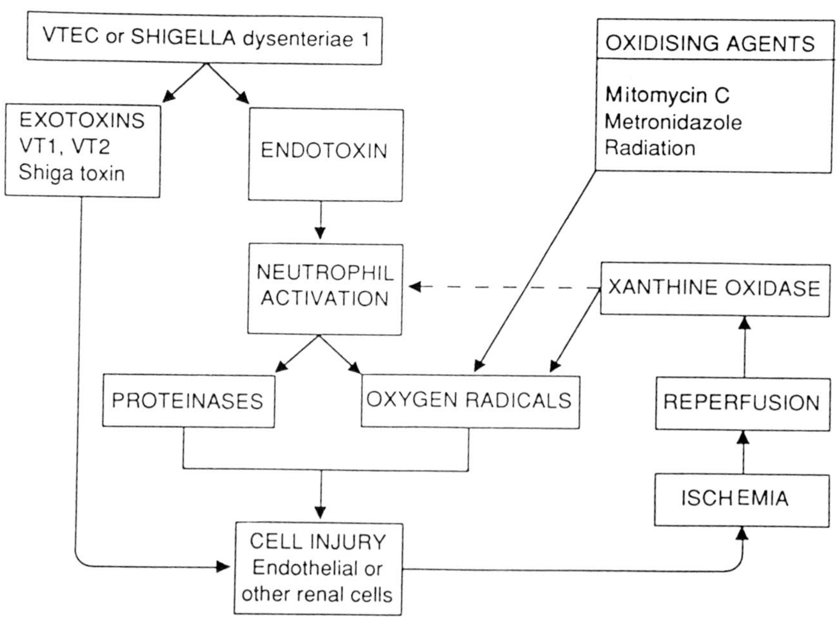

Figure 5 A scheme for the hypothesis that oxygen-derived free radicals are involved in the pathogenesis of HUS.

cells in culture and epidemiologically these exotoxins are of great importance, there is no evidence connecting their action to oxygen radicals. On the other hand, it has been clearly shown that endotoxin promotes the neutrophil–endothelial interaction seen in both these extrinsic forms of HUS in humans and in the Shwartman reaction in laboratory animals. Furthermore, it is the aspect of neutrophil activation that correlates positively with irreversible renal damage. Oxygen-derived free radicals are part of the neutrophils' armamentarium, and they are capable of potentiating the action of proteinases as well as directly targeting membrane constituents. There is evidence of lipid peroxidation in the syndrome, necessarily indirect, and it is reasonable to think that leukocytes are a source of oxygen radicals in the diarrhea-associated disease.

Drugs, some of which are known to promote the release of ODFRs, are associated with HUS. Antioxidant deficiency, which in animals may give rise to vascular injury, has not been convincingly shown in humans. If the hypothesis is substantiated, one would expect to find consumption of antioxidants and an increase in their degradation products as a secondary phenomenon. Reperfusion injury is an attractive adjunct to the theory, especially since synergism appears to exist between this and neutrophil–endothelial interaction. However, it has not been tested in models resembling HUS, and this deserves to be pursued. Likewise the concept that erythocyte abnormalities or the acute renal failure itself may be caused by oxidants remains to be investigated.

THERAPEUTIC IMPLICATIONS

If oxidant damage to tissues becomes established as an important pathogenetic mechanism in the HUS, various antioxidants or ODFR scavengers could be used in management. Oral vitamin E has been tried in two pilot studies (94, 95). However, the enteric absorption of vitamin E is relatively slow, and this may be a drawback. Other substances available for trial include allopurinol, (deferoxamine), and superoxide dismutase. Vasodilatory prostaglandins (96) or intravenous arachidonic acid (96) may also have a role either alone, or in combination with the former, if they can be shown to reduce ischemia. The heterogeneity of HUS and the good prognosis for patients with the diarrhea-associated form pose logistic problems on treatment trials. Further investigations in this area are necessary and may have implications for other toxic or ischemic diseases in which oxidant injury is suspected.

ACKNOWLEDGMENT

The authors are grateful to Dr. F. Raafat, and Eva Halloran, Department of Histopathology, for the electron micrographs, to Kathleen Snow and Harry Buglass, Department of Medical Illustration for figures, and to Veronica Penny and Karen Day for secretarial help.

REFERENCES

1. Karmali, M. A., Petrie, M., Lim, C., Flemming, P. C., Arbus, G. S., Lior, H., The association between idiopathic haemolytic uremic syndrome and infection by verotoxin-producing *Escherichia coli*. *J. Infect. Dis.*, *151*: 775–782 (1985).

2. Milford, D. V., Taylor, C. M., Guttridge, B., Hall, S., Rowe, B., Kleanthous, H., Haemolytic uraemic syndrome in the British Isles, 1985–1988; association with verocytoxin-producing *Escherichia coli*. Part 1, Clinical and epidemiological aspects. *Arch. Dis. Child.*, *65*: 716–721 (1990).
3. Milford, D. V., Taylor, C. M., New insights into haemolytic uraemic syndromes. *Arch. Dis. Child.*, *65*: 713–715 (1990).
4. Butler, T., Islam, M. R., Asad, M. A. K., Jones, P. K., Risk factors for the development of hemolytic uremic syndrome during shigellosis. *J. Pediatr.*, *110*: 894–897 (1987).
5. Koster, K., Levin, J., Walker, L., Tong, K. S. K., Gilman, R. H., Ragaman, M. M., Majid, M. A., Islam, S., Williams, R. C., Hemolytic-uremic syndrome after shigellosis: Relation to endotoxemia and circulating immune complexes. *N. Engl. J. Med.*, *298*: 927 (1978).
6. Boveris, A., Cadenas, E., Production of superoxide radical and hydrogen peroxide in mitochondria. In *Superoxide and Superoxide Dismutase*," Vol. 2 L. W. Oberly, (ed); CRC Press, Boca Raton, pp. 15–30 (1982).
7. Diplock, A. T., The role of vitamin E in biological membranes. *Ciba Found. Symp. 101*: 45–55 (1983).
8. Weiss, S. J., Tissue destruction by neutrophils. *N. Engl. J. Med.*, *320*: 365–376. (1989).
9. Malech, H. L., Gallin, J. I., Neutrophils in human disease. *N. Engl. J. Med.*, *317*: 687–694 (1987).
10. Tauber, A. I., Babior, B. M., Evidence for hydroxyl radical production by human neutrophils. *J. Clin. Invest.*, *60*: 374–379 (1977).
11. Weiss, S. J., King, G. W., Lobuglio, A. F., Evidence of hydroxyl radical generation by human monocytes. *J. Clin. Invest.*, *60*: 370–373 (1977).
12. Halliwell, B., Gutteridge, J. M. C., The importance of free radicals and catalytic metals in human diseases. *Mol. Aspects Med.*, *8*: 89–193 (1985).
13. Britigan, B. E., Cohen, M. S., Rosen, G. M., Hydroxyl radical formation in neutrophils. *N. Engl. J. Med.*, *318*: 858–859 (1988).
14. Bolande, R. P., Kaplan, B. S., Experimental studies on the hemolytic uremic syndrome. *Nephron*, *39*: 228–236 (1985).
15. Grisham, M. B., Granger, D. N., Neutrophil-mediated mucosal injury; role of reactive oxygen metabolites. *Dig. Dis. Sci.*, *33*(Suppl.): 6s–15s (1988).
16. Grisham, M. B., Everse, J., Pro-oxidant activity of hemoglobin and myoglobin. In *Peroxidases in Chemistry and Biology* (J. Everse, M. B. Grisham, eds.), CRC Press, Boca Raton (1990).
17. Paller, M. S., Hemoglobin and myoglobin-induced acute renal failure in rats: Role of iron in nephrotoxicity. *Am. J. Physiol.*, *255*: F539 (1988).
18. McCord, J. M., Oxygen-derived free radicals in post ischaemic tissue injury. *N. Engl. J. Med. 312*: 159–163 (1985).
19. Hearse, D., Manning, A. S., Downey, J. M., Yellon, D. M., Xanthine oxidase: A critical mediator of myocardial injury during ischemia and reperfusion? *Acta Physiol. Scand. Suppl.*, *548*: 65–78 (1986).
20. Bando, K., Tago, M., Teramoto, S., Prevention of free radical-induced myocardial injury by allopurinol. *J. Thorac. Cardiovasc. Surg.*, *95*: 465–473 (1988).
21. Jurmann, M. J., Schaefers, H.-J., Dammenhayn, L., Haverich, A., Oxygen-derived free radical scavengers for amelioration of reperfused damage in heart transplantation. *J. Thorac. Cardiovasc. Surg.*, *95*: 368–377 (1988).
22. Taylor, M. D., Mellert, T. K., Parmentier, J. L., Eddy, L. J., Pharmacological protection of re-oxygenation damage in in-vitro brain slice tissue. *Brain Res.*, *347*: 268–273 (1985).
23. Im, M. J., Shen, W.-H., Pak, C. J., Manson, P. N., Bulkley, G. B., Hoopes, J. E., Effect of allopurinol on the survival of hyperemic island skin flaps. *Plast. Reconstruct. Surg.*, *73*: 276–278 (1989).

24. Clarke, D. A., Fornabaio, D. M., McNeill, H., Mullane, K. M., Caravella, S. J., Miller, M. J. S., Contribution of oxygen-derived free radicals to experimental necrotizing enterocolitis. *Am. J. Pathol., 130*: 537–542 (1988).
25. Engler, R. L., Dahlgren, M. D., Morris, D. D., Peterson, M. A., Schmid-Schonbein, G. W., Role of leukocytes in response to acute myocardial ischemia and reflow in dogs. *Am. J. Physiol., 251*: H314–323 (1986).
26. Vedder, N. B., Winn, R. K., Rice, C. L., Chi, E. Y., Arfors, K.-E., Harlan, J. M., A monoclonal antibody to the adherence-promoting leukocyte glycoprotein CD18, reduces organ injury and improves survival from haemorrhagic shock and resuscitation in rabbits. *J. Clin. Invest., 81*: 939–944 (1988).
27. Rodell, T. C., Cheronis, J. C., Ohnemus, C. L., Piermattei, D. J., Repine, J. E., Xanthine oxidase mediates elastase induced injury to isolated lungs and endothelium. *J. Appl. Physiol., 63*: 2159–2163 (1987).
28. Petrone, W. F., English, D. K., Wong, K., McCord, J. M., Free radicals and inflammation: Superoxide-dependent activation of a neutrophil chemotactic factor in plasma. *Proc. Natl. Acad. Sci. USA, 77*: 1159–1163 (1980).
29. Perez, H. D., Weksler, B. B., Goldstein, I. M., Generation of a chemotactic lipid from arachidonic acid by exposure to a superoxide-generation system. *Inflammation, 4*: 313–328 (1980).
30. Grisham, M. B., Grainger, D. N., Free radicals: Reactive metabolites of oxygen as mediators of post ischaemic reperfusion injury. In *Splanchnic Ischaemia and Multiple Organ Failure* (A. Marston, G. B. Bulkley, R. G. Fiddian-Green, U. H. Haglund, eds.), Edward Arnold, London, pp. 135–144 (1989).
31. Grisham, M. B., Myoglobulin-catalysed hydrogen peroxide dependent arachidonic acid peroxidation. *J. Free Radical Biol. Med., 1*: 227–232 (1985).
32. Parks, D. A., Granger, D. N., Xanthine oxidase: Biochemistry, distribution and physiology. *Acta Physiol. Scand. Suppl., 548*: 87–99 (1986).
33. Jarasch, E. D., Bruder, G., Heid, H. W., Significance of xanthine oxidase in capillary endothelial cells. *Acta Physiol. Scand. Suppl., 548*: 39–46 (1986).
34. Linas, S. L., Whittenburg, D., Repine, J. E., O_2 metabolites cause reperfusion injury after short but not prolonged renal ischaemia. *Am. J. Physiol., 253*: F685–691 (1987).
35. Linas, S. L., Shanley, P. F., White, C. W., Parker, N. P., Repine, J. E., O_2 metabolite-mediated injury in perfused kidneys is reflected by consumption of DTMU and glutathione. *Am. J. Physiol., 253*: F692–701 (1987).
36. Bosco, P. J., Schweizer, R. T., Use of oxygen radical scavengers on autografted pig kidneys after warm ischaemia and 48-hour perfusion preservation. *Arch. Surg., 123*: 601–604 (1988).
37. Vasko, K. A., Delwall, R. A., Riley, A. M., Effect of allopurinol in renal ischemia. *Surgery, 71*: 787–790 (1972).
38. Toledo-Pereyra, L. H., Simmons, R. L., Najarian, J. S., Effect of allopurinol on the preservatiaon of ischemic kidneys perfused with plasma or plasma substitutes. *Ann. Surg., 180*: 780–782 (1974).
39. Hansson, R., Gustafsson, B., Jonsson, O., Lundstaus, S., Pettersson, S., Schersten, T., Waldenstrom, J., Effects on xanthine oxidase inhibition on renal circulation after ischaemia. *Transplant. Proc., 14*: 51–58 (1982).
40. Toledo-Pereyra, L. H., Simmons, R. L., Olson, L. C., Najarian, J. S., Clinical effect of allopurinol on preserved kidneys. A randomised double-blind study. *Ann. Surg., 185*: 128–131 (1977).
41. Canavese, C., Stratta, P., Vercellone, A., Oxygen free radicals in nephrology. *Int. J. Artif. Organs, 10*: 379–389 (1987).
42. Canavese, C., Stratta, P., Vercellone, A., The case for oxygen free radicals in the pathogenesis of ischaemic acute renal failure. *Nephron, 49*: 9–15 (1988).
43. Dormandy, T. L., An approach to free radicals. *Lancet, 2*: 1010–1014 (1983).

44. Greenwald, R. A., *CRC Handbook of Methods for Oxygen Radical Research,* CRC Press, Boca Raton (1985).
45. Yagi, K., Assay for serum lipid peroxide level and its clinical significance. In *Lipid Peroxides in Biology and Medicine* (K. Yagi, ed.), Academic Press, New York, pp. 223–242 (1982).
46. Tappel, A., Measurement of in vivo lipid peroxidation via exhaled pentane and protection by vitamin E. In *Lipid Peroxides in Biology and Medicine* (K. Yagi, ed.), Academic Press, New York (1982).
47. Wayner, D. D. M., Burton, G. W., Ingold, K. U., Locke, S., Quantitative measurement of the total, peroxyl radical-trapping antioxidant capability of human blood plasma by controlled peroxidation. *FEBS Lett., 187*: 33–37 (1985).
48. Wickens, D. G., Norden, A. G., Lunec, J., Dormandy, T. L., Fluorescent changes in human gamma-globulin induced by free radical activity. *Biochim. Biophys. Acta, 742*: 607–616 (1983).
49. Wolman, M., Etiology and pathogenesis of the haemolytic–uremic syndrome. A hypothesis. *Isr. J. Med. Sci., 8*: 984–986 (1972).
50. Gray, E., Barrowcliffe, T. W., Inhibition of anti-thrombin III by lipid peroxides. *Thromb. Res. 37*: 241–250 (1985).
51. Barrowcliffe, T. W., Gutteridge, J. M., Gray, E., Oxygen radicals, lipid peroxidation and the coagulation system. *Agents Actions, 22*: 347–348 (1987).
52. Hirai, S., Koichi, O., Mitsunori, M., Lipid peroxide in the aging process. In *Lipid Peroxides in Biology and Medicine* (K. Yagi, ed.), Academic Press, New York, pp. 305–315 (1982).
53. Yagi, K., Ohkawa, H., Ohishi, N., Yamashita, M., Nakashima, T., Lesions of aortic intima caused by intravenous administration of linoleic acid hydroperoxide. *J. Appl. Biochem., 3*: 58–65 (1981).
54. Moncada, S., Higgs, E. A., Vane, J. R., Human arterial and venous tissues generate prostacyclin (prostaglandin X), a potent inhibitor of platelet aggregation. *Lancet, 1*: 18–21 (1977).
55. Turi, S., Beattie, T. J., Belch, J. J. F., Murphy, A. V., Disturbances of prostacyclin metabolism in children with hemolytic–uremic syndrome and in first degree relatives. *Clin. Nephrol. 25*: 193–198 (1986).
56. Levin, M., Elkon, K. B., Nokes, T. J. C., Buckle, A. M., Dillon, M. S., Hardisty, R. M., Barratt, T. M., Inhibitor of prostacyclin production in sporadic haemolytic uraemic syndrome. *Arch. Dis. Child., 58*: 703–708 (1983).
57. O'Reagan, S., Chesney, R. W., Kaplan, B. S., Drummond, K. N., Red cell membrane phospholipid abnormalities in the hemolytic uremic syndrome. *Clin. Nephrol., 15*: 14–17 (1981).
58. Powell, H. R., Groves, V., McCredie, D. A., Low red cell arachidonic acid in hemolytic uremic syndrome. *Clin. Nephrol., 27*: 8–10 (1987).
59. Situnayake, R. D., Crump, P. J., Thurnam D. J., Taylor, C. M., Further evidence of lipid peroxidation in post-enteropathic haemolytic-uraemic syndrome. *Pediatr Nephol* 5: 387–392 (1991).
60. Inverson, S. A., Cawood, P., Dormandy, T. L., A method for the determination of the diene conjugated derivative of linoleic acid 18:2 (9,11) in serum phospholipid and possible origins. *Ann. Clin. Biochem., 22*: 137–140 (1985).
61. Kaplan, B. S., Gale, D., Ipp, T., Hyperlipidemia in the hemolytic–uremic syndrome. *Pediatrics, 47*: 777–779 (1971).
62. Johnson, R. J., Couser, W. G., Chi, E. Y., Adler, S., Klebanoff, S. J., New mechanism for glomerular injury. Myeloperoxidase–hydrogen peroxide–halide system. *J. Clin. Invest., 61*: 1379–1387 (1978).
63. Sacks, T., Moldrow, C. F., Craddock, P. R., Bowers, T. K., *J. Clin. Invest., 62*: 1161–1167 (1978).

64. Smedley, L. A., Tonnesen, M. G., Sandhaus, R. A., Haslett, C., Guthrie, L. A., Johnston, R. B., Henson, P. M., Worthen, G. S., Neutrophil-mediated injury to endothelial cells. Enhancement by endotoxin and essential role of neutrophil elastase. *J. Clin. Invest.*, *77*: 1233–1243 (1986).
65. Walters, M. D. S., Matthei, I. U., Kay, R., Dillon, M. S., Barratt, T. M., The polymorphonuclear leucocyte count in childhood haemolytic uraemic syndrome. *Paediatr. Nephrol.*, *3*: 130–134 (1989).
66. Coad, N. A. G., Marshall, T., Rowe, B., Taylor, C. M., Changes in the post-enteropathic form of the haemolytic uremic syndrome in children. *Clin. Nephrol.*, *35*: 10–16 (1991).
67. Milford, D. V., Taylor, C. M., Rafaat, F., Halloran, E., Neutrophil elastase and haemolytic uraemic syndrome. *Lancet*, *2*: 1153 (1989).
68. Forsyth, K. D., Simpson, A. C., Fitzpatrick, M. M., Barratt, T. M., Levinsky, R. J., Neutrophil-mediated endothelial injury in haemolytic uraemic syndrome. *Lancet*, *2*: 411–414 (1989).
69. Obrig, T. G., Del Vecchio, P. J., Karmali, M. A., Petric, M., Moran, T. P., Judge, T. K., Pathogenesis of haemolytic uraemic syndrome. *Lancet*, *2*: 687 (1987).
70. Kavi, J., Chant, I., Maris, M., Rose, P. E., Cytopathic effect of verotoxin on endothelial cells. *Lancet*, *2*: 1035 (1987).
71. Mathison, J. C., Wolfson, E., Ulevitch, R. J., Participation of tumour necrosis factor in the mediation of gram negative bacterial lipopolysaccharide-induced injury in rabbits. *J. Clin. Invest.*, *81*: 1925–1927 (1988).
72. Milford, D. V., Stater, J., MacGreggor, I., Dawes, J., Taylor, C. M., Hill, F. G., Prognostic markers in diarrhoea-associated haemolytic uraemic syndrome: Initial neutrophil count, human neutrophil elastase and von Willebrand factor antigen. (submitted for publication).
73. Raghu, G., Striker, L. J., Striker, G. E., Lipopolysaccharide-mediated injury to cultured human glomerular endothelial cells. *Clin. Immunol. Immunopathol.*, *38*: 275–281 (1986).
74. Butler, T., Rahaman, H., Al-Mahmua, K. A., Islam, M., Bardham, P., Kabir, I., Rahman, M. M., An animal model of haemolytic–uremic syndrome in shigellosis: Lipopolysaccharides of *Shigella dysenteriae* I and *S. flexeri* produce leucocyte-mediated renal cortical necrosis in rabbits. *Br. J. Exp. Pathol.*, *66*: 7–15 (1985).
75. Bohn, E., Muller-Berghaus, G., The effect of leukocyte and platelet transfusion on the activation of intravascular coagulation by endotoxin in granulocytopenia and thrombocytopenic rabbits. *Am. J. Pathol.* *84*: 239–258 (1976).
76. Niemetz, J., Fari, K., Thrombogenic activity of leukocytes. *Blood*, *42*: 47–59 (1973).
77. Bertani, T., Abbate, M., Zoja, C., Corna, D., Remuzzi, G., Sequence of glomerular changes in experimental endotoxemia: A possible model of haemolytic uremic syndrome. *Nephron*, *53*: 330–337 (1989).
78. Brukman, J., Wiggins, R. C., Procoagulant activity in kidneys of normal and bacterial lipopolysaccharide-treated rabbits. *Kidney Int.*, *32*: 31–38 (1987).
79. Vedanarayanan, V. V., Kaplan, B. S., Fong, J. S. C., Neutrophil function in an experimental model of hemolytic uremic syndrome. *Pediatr. Res.*, *21*: 252–256 (1987).
80. Schorer, A. E., Rick, P. D., Swam, W. R., Moldow, C. F., Structural features of endotoxin required for stimulation of endothelial cell tissue factor production; exposure of preformed tissue factor after oxidant-mediated endothelial cell injury. *J. Lab. Clin. Med.*, *106*: 38–42 (1985).
81. Roberts, J. A., Roth, J. K., Dominque, G., Lewis, R. W., Kaack, B., Baskin, B., Immunology of pyelo-nephritis in the primate model V. Effect of superoxide dismutase. *J. Urol.*, *128*: 1394 (1982).
82. Roberts, J. A., Kaack, M. B., Fussell, E. N., Baskin, G., Immunology of pyelonephritis. VII. Effect of allopurinol. *J. Urol.*, *136*: 960–963 (1986).

83. Crocker, J., Jones, E. L., Haemolytic–uraemic syndrome complicating long term mitomycin C–5-fluorouracil therapy for gastric carcinoma. *J. Clin. Pathol., 36*: 24–29 (1983).
84. Lesesne, J. B., Rothchild, N., Erickson, B., Korec, S., Sisk, R., Keller, J., Arbus, M., Wooley, P. V., Chiazze, L., Schein, P. S., Neefe, J. R., Cancer-associated hemolytic–uremic syndrome: Analysis of 85 cases from a national registry. *J. Clin. Oncol. 7*: 781–789 (1989).
85. Giroux, L., Bettes, P., Giroux, L., Mitomycin-C nephrotoxity: A clinico-pathological study of 17 cases. *Am. J. Kidney Dis., 6*: 28–34 (1985).
86. Cattell, V., Mitomycin-induced haemolytic uraemic syndrome (rat model). *Am. J. Pathol., 121*: 88–95 (1985).
87. Pratt, W. B., Ruddon, R. W., *The Anticancer Drugs*. Oxford University Press, Oxford, pp. 174–194 (1979).
88. Tomasz, M., H_20_2 generation during the redox cycle of mitomycin C and DNA-bound mitomycin C. *Chem. Biol. Interact., 13*: 89–97 (1976).
89. Lown, J. W., Begleiter, A., Johnson, D., Morgan, R., Studies related to anti tumour antibiotics. Part V. Reactions of mitomycin C with DNA examined by ethidium fluorescence assay. *Can. J. Biochem., 54*: 110–119 (1976).
90. Powell, H. R., Davidson, P. M., McCredie, D. A., Phair, P., Walker, R. G., Haemolytic–uraemic syndrome after treatment with metronidazole. *Med. J. Aust., 49*: 222–223 (1988).
91. Leither, C., Sinzinger, H., Pohanka, E., Schwarz, M., Krotschmer, G., Syre, G., Recurrence of haemolytic uraemic syndrome triggered by cyclosporin A after renal transplantation. *Lancet, 1*: 1470 (1982).
92. Bonser, R. S., Adu, D., Franklin, I., McMaster, P., Cyclosporin-induced haemolytic uraemic syndrome in liver allograft recipient. *Lancet, 2*: 1337 (1984).
93. Phair, P. G., Powell, H. R., McCredie, D. A., Walker, R. G., D'Apice, A. J. F., Low red cell arachidonic acid in cyclosporin treated patients. *Clin. Nephrol., 32*: 57–61 (1989).
94. Powell, H. R., McCredie, D. A., Taylor, C. M., Burke, J. R., Walker, R. G., Vitamin E in the haemolytic uraemic syndrome. *Arch. Dis. Child., 59*: 401–404 (1984).
95. Thomson, P. D., Milner, L. S., A randomly selected trial of vitamin E in the haemolytic uraemic syndrome. *Proc. Int. Congr. Nephrol.* p. 98 (1988).
96. Beattie, T. J., Murphy, A. V., Willoughby, M. L. N., Prostacyclin infusion in haemolytic uraemic syndrome of children. *Br. Med. J., 283*: 470 (1981).
97. Defreyn, G., Proesmans, W., Machin, S. J., Lemmens, F., Vermylen, J., Abnormal prostacyclin metabolism in the hemolytic uremic syndrome: Equivocal effect of prostacyclin infusions. *Clin. Nephrol., 18*: 43–49 (1982).
98. Powell, H. R., McCredie, D. A., Essential fatty acid therapy in haemolytic uraemic syndrome. *Aust. N.Z.J. Med., 10*: 483 (1980).

26
Hemolytic Uremic Syndrome, Thrombotic Thrombocytopenic Purpura, the Generalized Shwartzman Reaction, Coagulation, and Fibrinolysis

Jerry Michael Bergstein *Indiana University School of Medicine, Indianapolis, Indiana*

In both the hemolytic uremic syndrome (HUS) and thrombotic thrombocytopenic purpura (TTP), fibrin thrombi may be detected in several organs, including the glomerular capillaries of the kidneys. Such deposits appear to play a major role in the development of the clinical manifestations of the disease process. The factors leading to fibrin formation are not clearly understood. Evaluation of the coagulation and fibrinolytic systems in these diseases and the study of animal models of intravascular fibrin deposition may ultimately reveal the precise pathogenesis of the microvascular thrombi.

THE COAGULATION AND FIBRINOLYTIC SYSTEMS

The formation of fibrin results from the activation of coagulation factor X. Activation (Fig. 1) may be effected by an *intrinsic* pathway that contains all the coagulation factors, in solution in the blood, necessary to activate factor X, or by an *extrinsic* pathway that requires the participation of tissue factor (thromboplastin). Once activated, factor X initiates a final common pathway, resulting in the conversion of prothrombin to thrombin, a proteolytic enzyme that converts circulating fibrinogen to fibrin. The coagulation system can also be activated secondarily through pathways developed after complement or kinin activation (1).

In conjunction with fibrin formation, the fibrinolytic system is activated to remove vascular thrombi (2). The fibrinolytic system is composed of a circulating inactive proenzyme, plasminogen, which is converted to the fibrinolytic enzyme, plasmin, by agents called plasminogen activators (see Fig. 1). Two types of plasminogen activator have been defined in humans, tissue plasminogen activator (t-PA) and urokinase (u-PA) (3). Both types of activator have been detected in several

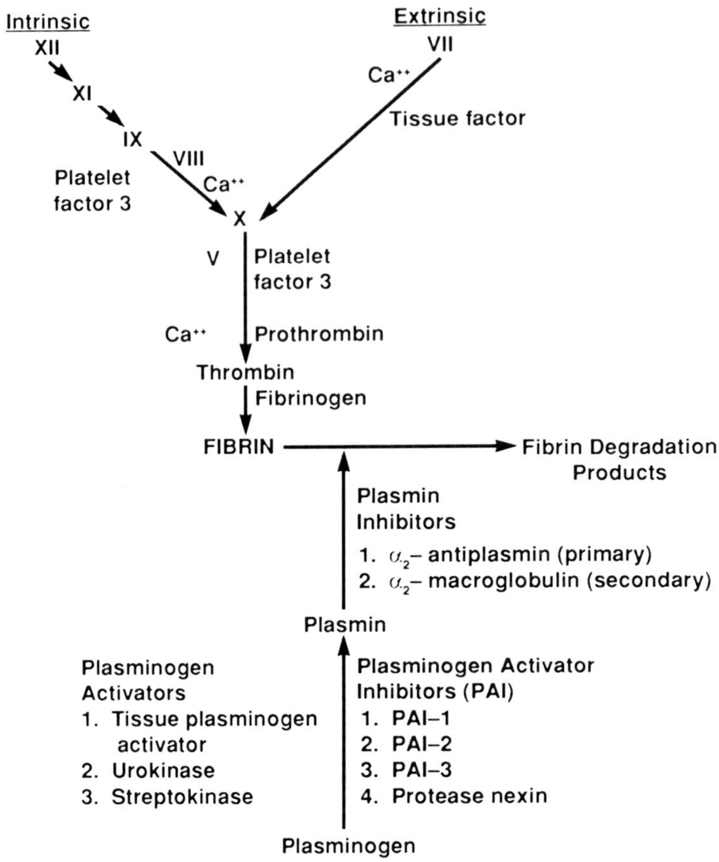

Figure 1 Pathways of the coagulation and fibrinolytic systems.

locations throughout the body, including endothelial cells (4) and glomeruli (5, 6). Inhibitors of both plasminogen activators have been described (3). Plasminogen activator inhibitor-1 (PAI-1), produced by endothelial cells and platelets, is the primary inhibitor of both t-PA and u-PA in the plasma. Plasminogen activator inhibitor-2, plasminogen activator inhibitor-3, and protease nexin appear to be only minor inhibitors of the plasminogen activators. A third type of plasminogen activator, streptokinase, is produced by group C streptococci.

THE GENERALIZED SHWARTZMAN REACTION

Although the generalized Shwartzman reaction (gSr) is typically produced in rabbits (7), a similar reaction will develop after a single intravenous injection of endotoxin in pregnant rats (8, 9). This predisposition to the gSr may result, at least in part, from decreased fibrinolytic capacity (10, 11).

In rabbits, the gSr is produced by two intravenous injections of appropriate amounts (12) of endotoxin (lipopolysaccharide derived from the cell wall of gram-negative bacteria) approximately 24 hr apart (7). After the second (provoking) injection of endotoxin, disseminated intravascular coagulation occurs in association with the development of generalized vascular thrombosis.

The renal lesion is characterized by massive intracapillary glomerular fibrin deposition, as proved by immunohistological (Fig. 2) and electron microscopic techniques (13–15). Glomerular fibrin deposition can be prevented by anticoagulants, such as sodium warfarin (16) and heparin (17), and by the production of severe hypofibrinogenemia with ancrod (Arvin; a venom protease enzyme derived from *Agkistrodon rhodostoma;* (18), confirming that glomerular thrombosis is associated with activation of the coagulation system. The development of the glomerular fibrin deposits seems to occur in two phases (19–21). Initially, the coagulation system is activated, generating thrombin, which results in the formation of circulating soluble fibrin complexes. In the second phase, these complexes are deposited in the glomerular capillaries. Although the first phase can be prevented by anticoagulants, the second phase seems independent of the coagulation process.

The Pathogenesis of the Generalized Shwartzman Reaction

Initiation of the gSr requires activation of the coagulation process. Several mechanisms may be involved in the processes whereby endotoxin activates coagulation (22).

Endotoxin may stimulate coagulation by activating the complement (23) and kinin (24) systems. It may stimulate clotting by activating or damaging vascular

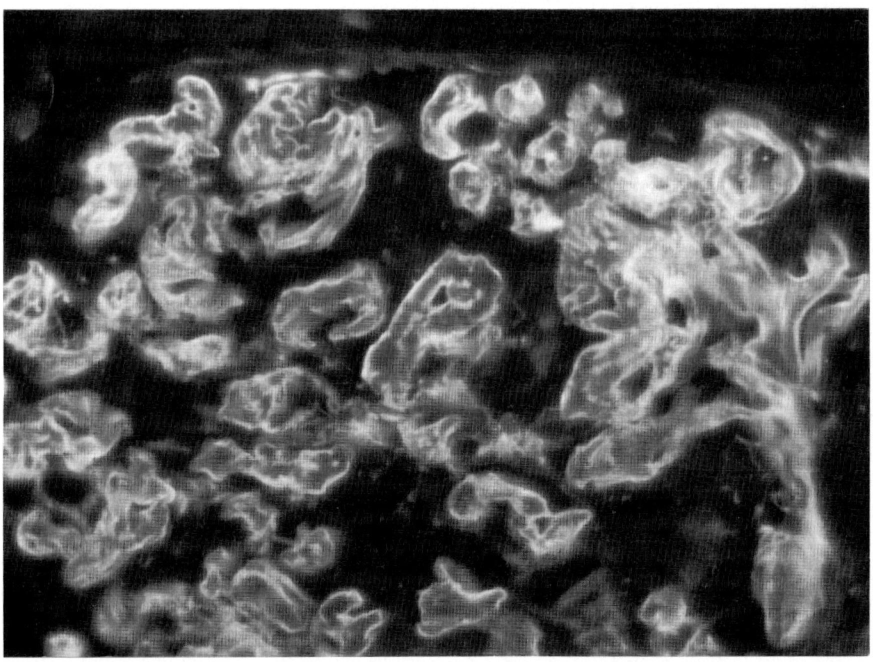

Figure 2 Immunofluorescence microscopy of a glomerulus from a rabbit with the generalized Shwartzman reaction, demonstrating massive intracapillary fibrin deposition (fluorescein-labeled goat antirabbit fibrinogen serum, original magnification × 480). (From Ref. 13.)

endothelial cells (25–27). That endotoxin may be directly toxic to endothelial cells is suggested by the observations that endotoxin may be detected within vascular endothelial cells after intravenous infusion (28), that endotoxin injury occurs despite granulocyte depletion (29) or anticoagulation with heparin (25), that endotoxin damages endothelial cells in tissue culture (30, 31), and by the development of a unilateral Shwartzman reaction in kidneys prepared with an infusion of endotoxin through the renal artery (32). Direct endothelial cell injury could activate clotting by exposing the glomerular basement membrane, which can aggregate platelets (33–35), and the thrombogenic subendothelium, which contains the procoagulant tissue factor (36), or by stimulating endothelial cell synthesis of tissue factor (37). Increased levels of procoagulant activity have been detected in glomeruli of rabbits treated with endotoxin (38).

The synthesis of tissue factor by endothelial cells may be enhanced by endotoxin-induced release of tumor necrosis factor and interleukin-1 from leukocytes, endothelial cells, and mesangial cells (39–42). Indeed, the intravenous infusion of tumor necrosis factor in rabbits produces a generalized Shwartzman-like reaction, strongly supporting the idea that tumor necrosis factor is an important mediator of endotoxin-induced glomerular injury (43).

Endotoxin, tumor necrosis factor, and interleukin-1 may also stimulate intravascular coagulation by (a) decreasing endothelial cell expression of thrombomodulin (44), a promoter of proteins C and S, which inhibit thrombin formation and inactivate plasminogen activator inhibitor (45); (b) stimulating endothelial cell production of plasminogen activator inhibitor (46–48); (c) enhancing leukocyte and endothelial cell production of platelet-activating factor (49), a mediator of inflammation and vascular injury; and (d) stimulating endothelial cell release of large multimers of von Willebrand factor (50), which promote the attachment of platelets to areas of endothelial injury.

In addition, other factors may play important roles in the pathogenesis of the gSr. Granulocytes are required for the development of the reaction (7, 51–55). Following reaction with endotoxin, granulocytes can promote clotting by releasing tissue factor (56–58) or by producing neutral proteases and toxic oxygen radicals (59–61) that injure endothelial cells. Platelets may be necessary for development of the gSr (62, 63), although their exact role (vide infra) remains to be determined (51, 55, 64–69). The sympathetic nervous system appears to be involved in the production of the reaction, as infusion of norepinephrine promotes the reaction (70), whereas surgical (71) and chemical (72) sympathectomy and alpha-adrenergic blockade (70) prevent the reaction. Prostaglandins may also be involved in production of gSr, as its development is suppressed by aspirin, indomethacin, and intravenous infusions of prostaglandins E_1 or I_2 (73–77).

Cortisone (78, 79), Thorotrast (a colloidal suspension of thorium dioxide; 80, 81), trypan blue (80), and colloidal carbon (82) may be substituted for the first (preparatory) injection of endotoxin in the production of the gSr. Although blockade of the reticuloendothelial system was initially postulated as the mechanism whereby these agents substitute for endotoxin (83), subsequent studies have indicated that cortisone, Thorotrast, and trypan blue prepare for the gSr by inhibiting fibrinolysis (84–88).

The importance of inhibition of fibrinolysis in the pathogenesis of the gSr was confirmed by the observations that ϵ-aminocaproic acid, a potent inhibitor of fibrinolysis, can substitute for either the preparatory (89) or provoking (83) injection of endotoxin. Later studies revealed that activation of fibrinolysis with streptokinase will both prevent and reduce glomerular fibrin deposition (90–92) and that treatment with intravenous t-PA effectively removes glomerular fibrin deposits (93).

Although endotoxin inhibits glomerular as well as circulating fibrinolytic activity (94), the mechanism is unknown. That high concentrations of endotoxin in saline fail to inhibit glomerular fibrinolytic activity in vitro (94) suggests that endotoxin inhibits fibrinolysis through other mediators; platelets and endothelial cells may be involved. The complement system is not involved in the mechanism of fibrinolysis inhibition (95).

Platelets contain inhibitors of fibrinolysis such as PAI-1 and α-antiplasmin (96–99), which may be released following direct interaction with endotoxin (100–102). Interestingly, antiplatelet antibody can be substituted for the preparatory injection of endotoxin in the gSr. Animals prepared with either antiplatelet antibody or endotoxin develop thrombocytopenia and decreased glomerular fibrinolytic activity in association with an inhibitor of glomerular fibrinolysis in the circulation (103). In addition, fibrinolysis of normal glomeruli is inhibited in vitro by an agent that diffuses from washed normal platelets (103). This suggests that platelet destruction, mediated by antibody or endotoxin, releases an inhibitor of fibrinolysis that plays an important role in the development of the gSr.

Decreased fibrinolytic activity could also result from diminished plasminogen activator production by endothelial cells following endotoxin-induced injury. In addition, endotoxin (46, 64, 104, 105), thrombin (105, 106), tumor necrosis factor (45, 48, 107), and interleukin-1 (45, 47) can stimulate endothelial cells to produce plasminogen activator inhibitors (108–110).

The important role of the fibrinolytic system in the development and subsequent fate of intravascular glomerular fibrin deposits is also supported by observations in the rat model of the gSr. In the rabbit, glomerular plasminogen activator activity is lost following endotoxin-induced glomerular fibrin deposition, resulting in cortical necrosis (94). In the pregnant rat, however, glomerular plasminogen activator activity is retained after endotoxin-induced glomerular fibrin deposition, with subsequent clearing of the fibrin deposits (111). This confirms that glomerular plasminogen activator activity plays an important role in the removal of intravascular glomerular fibrin.

Because the precise pathogenesis of HUS is unknown, the validity of the gSr as an experimental model of HUS is unclear. However, it seems likely that mechanisms observed in studying the gSr, such as localized activation of intravascular coagulation, the effects of endothelial cell and platelet activation or damage, and the role of inhibition of fibrinolysis, will apply to the development of HUS.

HEMOLYTIC UREMIC SYNDROME, COAGULATION, AND FIBRINOLYSIS

Levels of coagulation factors are typically normal (112–116) in HUS, although diminished levels of factors II, V, VII, VIII, IX, and XI have been described (116–118). The relationship between occasionally diminished levels of the vitamin K-dependent clotting factors (II, VII, IX, X) and a clinical deficiency of vitamin K in these patients is unclear.

Fibrinogen levels and fibrinogen turnover studies are generally normal (112, 113, 116, 119–121), suggesting that fibrinogen is no longer being consumed, and that fibrin deposition has ceased by the time the patient is initially seen. The detection of elevated levels of fibrin breakdown products in the blood and urine of patients with HUS (112, 122–128) indicates activation of the fibrinolytic system.

Thrombocytopenia and decreased platelet survival are typical in HUS (121) and may result from platelet adherence to intravascular thrombi or injured endothelium and to damge acquired during passage through the thrombosed microvasculature, with subsequent removal from the circulation by the reticuloendothelial system. Adherent platelets may undergo the release reaction, inducing further platelet aggregation and vasoconstriction through the release of thromboxanes. In vitro, platelet aggregation is reduced during the acute phase of HUS (129–132), suggesting that the remaining circulating platelets may have already undergone the release reaction. The presence of elevated plasma levels of β-thromboglobulin (133), platelet factor 4 (133), serotonin (132), factors that aggregate platelets (132, 134, 135), and platelet-derived growth factors (136), in certain patients, supports the hypothesis of intravascular platelet activation in HUS. Whether these platelet abnormalities are involved in the pathogenesis of the disease, or whether they result from the development of the disease, remains to be determined. The treatment of patients, who have HUS, with antiplatelet agents (137–140) has failed to clarify this dilemma.

Abnormalities in prostacyclin (PGI_2) production may play a role in the pathogenesis of HUS. Produced primarily by vascular endothelial cells, prostacyclin is a potent vasodilator and inhibitor of platelet aggregation (141). Some patients with HUS demonstrate decreased vascular prostaglandin production and diminished plasma levels of prostacyclin metabolites (132, 142–146), sometimes in association with the absence of a plasma factor that stimulates endothelial cell prostacyclin release (143, 145, 147–149) or the presence of an inhibitor of vascular prostacyclin regeneration (142). However, other patients have normal or elevated plasma levels of prostacyclin metabolites (145, 150, 151) and show no evidence for an inhibitor of vascular prostacyclin production (152). The irregularities in prostacyclin metabolism have led to the treatment of HUS with plasma infusion (153–156) or by plasmapheresis (156–164) in the hope of replacing the missing prostacyclin-stimulation factor or of removing potential circulating inhibitors of prostacyclin production. The value of such therapy is unclear, and one study (165) suggests that plasma therapy may have a harmful effect.

Inhibition of glomerular fibrinolytic activity may play a central role in the pathogenesis and outcome of HUS. Patients with HUS have a circulating inhibitor of glomerular fibrinolysis (166), which has recently been shown to be PAI-1 (167), probably the same inhibitor as detected in rabbits with the gSr (168). Persistence of the inhibitor in the plasma beyond 2 weeks after hospitalization results in incomplete recovery. However, the inhibitor may be removed from the plasma by peritoneal dialysis (166).

THROMBOTIC THROMBOCYTOPENIC PURPURA AND COAGULATION

Generally, coagulation profiles and fibrinogen levels are normal in TTP, the platelet count is diminished, levels of fibrin breakdown products in the plasma are elevated, and fibrinolytic activity is reduced (169–173). Prostacyclin levels have not been adequately studied in TTP, although accelerated prostacyclin degradation, (174) caused by diminished binding to plasma proteins (which may protect prostacyclin from hydrolysis), has been described (175).

Plasma from some patients with TTP contains antiendothelial cell antibody (176), whereas plasma from others contains a platelet-aggregating factor (177–181), sometimes in association with large multimers of von Willebrand factor (182, 183). Some studies suggest that the platelet-aggregating factor can be inhibited by IgG from normal adult plasma, but, interestingly, not by IgG purified from an infant (184, 185); other investigators dispute this finding (182).

These observations have led to the treatment of TTP with inhibitors of platelet aggregation and plasma infusion or exchange. Such therapy seems effective in many patients (186, 187).

REFERENCES

1. Sundsmo, J. S., Fair, D. S., Relationships among the complement, kinin, coagulation, and fibrinolytic systems. *Springer Semin. Immunopathol.*, *6*: 231–258 (1983).
2. Bachmann, F., Fibrinolysis. In *Thrombosis and Haemostasis* (M. Verstraete, J. Vermylen, H. R. Lijnen, J. Arnout, eds.), International Society on Thrombosis and Haemostasis, Leuven University Press, Leuven, pp. 227–265 (1987).
3. Hekman, C. M., Loskutoff, D. J., Fibrinolytic pathways and the endothelium. *Semin. Thromb. Hemost.*, *13*: 514–527 (1987).
4. Luskutoff, D. J., Mussoni, L., Interactions between fibrin and plasminogen activators produced by cultured endothelial cells. *Blood, 62*: 62–68 (1983).
5. Bergstein, J. M., Riley, M., Bang, N. U., Analysis of the plasminogen activator activity of the human glomerulus. *Kidney Int.*, *33*: 868–874 (1988).
6. Angles-Cano, E., Rondeau, E., Delarue, F., Hagege, J., Sultan, Y., Sraer, J. D., Indentification and cellular localization of plasminogen activators from human glomeruli. *Thromb. Haemost.*, *54*: 688–692 (1985).
7. Thomas, L., Good, R. A., Studies on the generalized Shwartzman reaction. I. General observations concerning the phenomenon. *J. Exp. Med.*, *96*: 605–624 (1952).
8. Muller-Berghaus, G., Schmidt-Ehry, B., The role of pregnancy in the induction of the generalized Shwartzman reaction. *Am. J. Obstet. Gynecol.*, *114*: 847–849 (1972).
9. Wong, T. C., A study on the generalized Shwartzman reaction in pregnant rats induced by bacterial endotoxin. *Am. J. Obstet. Gynecol.*, *84*: 786–797 (1962).
10. Epstein, M. D., Beller, F. K., Douglas, G. W., Kidney tissue activator of fibrinolysis in relation to pregnancy. *Obstet. Gynecol.*, *32*: 494–504 (1968).
11. Gans, H., Krivit, W., Effect of endotoxin on the clotting mechanism. II. On the variation in response in different species of animals. *Ann. Surg.*, *153*: 453–458 (1961).
12. Corrigan, J. J., Abildgaard, C. F., Vanderheiden, J. F., Shulman, I., Quantitative aspects of blood coagulation in the generalized Shwartzman reaction. *Pediatr. Res.*, *1*: 39–49 (1967).
13. Bergstein, J. M., Michael, A. F., Jr., Generalized Shwartzman reaction in the rabbit. Immunopathologic findings in the kidney. *Arch. Pathol.*, 97: 230–231 (1974).
14. McKay, D. G., Gitlin, D., Craig, J. M., Immunochemical demonstration of fibrin in the generalized Shwartzman reaction. *Arch. Pathol.* *67*: 270–273 (1959).
15. Watanabe, T., Tanaka, K., Electron microscopic observations of the kidney in the generalized Shwartzman reaction. *Virchows Arch. [A]*, *374*: 183–196 (1977).
16. Shapiro, S. S., McKay, D. G., The prevention of the generalized Shwartzman reaction with sodium warfarin. *J. Exp. Med.*, *107*: 377–381 (1958).
17. Corrigan, J. J., Jr., Effect of anticoagulating and nonanticoagulating concentrations of heparin on the generalized Shwartzman reaction. *Thromb. Diath. Haemorrh.*, *24*: 136–145 (1970).
18. Bell, W. R., Miller, R. E., Levin, J., Inhibition of the generalized Shwartzman reaction by hypofibrinogenemia. *Blood, 40*: 697–708 (1972).

19. Lipinski, B., Gurewich, V., Nowak, A., Wetmore, R., The effect of heparin and dipyridamole on the deposition of fibrin-like material in rabbits infused with soluble fibrin monomer or fibrinogen. *Thromb. Res.*, *5*: 343–358 (1974).
20. Muller-Berghaus, G., Hocke, M., Production of the generalized Shwartzman reaction in rabbits by Ancrod (Arvin) infusion and endotoxin injection. *Br. J. Haematol.*, *25*: 111–112 (1973).
21. Muller-Berghaus, G., Roka, L., Lasch, H. G., Induction of a glomerular microclot formation by fibrin monomer infusion. *Thromb. Diath. Haemorrh.*, *29*: 375–383 (1973).
22. Morrison, D. C., Ulevitch, R. J., The effects of bacterial endotoxins on host mediation systems. *Am. J. Pathol.*, *93*: 527–618 (1978).
23. Kane, M. A., May, J. E., Frank, M. M., Interactions of the classical and alternate complement pathway with endotoxin lipopolysaccharide. *J. Clin. Invest.*, *52*: 370–376 (1973).
24. Kimball, H. R., Melmon, K. L., Wolff, S. M., Endotoxin-induced kinin production in man. *Proc. Soc. Exp. Biol. Med.*, *139*: 1078–1082 (1972).
25. Gaynor, E., Bouvier, C., Spaet, T. H., Vascular lesions: Possible pathogenic basis of the generalized Shwartzman reaction. *Science*, *170*: 986–988 (1970).
26. Gaynor, E., Increased mitotic activity in rabbit endothelium after endotoxin. *Lab. Invest.*, *24*: 318–320 (1971).
27. McGrath, J. M., Stewart, G. J., The effect of endotoxin on vascular endothelium. *J. Exp. Med.*, *129*: 833–839 (1969).
28. Rubenstein, J. S., Fine, J., Coons, A. H., Localization of endotoxin in the walls of the peripheral vascular system during lethal endotoxemia. *Proc. Soc. Exp. Biol. Med.*, *111*: 458–467 (1962).
29. Gaynor, E., The role of granulocytes in endotoxin-induced vascular injury. *Blood*, *41*: 797–808 (1973).
30. Harlan, J. M., Harker, L. A., Reidy, M. A., Gadjusek, C. M., Schwartz, S. M., Striker, G. E., Lipopolysaccharide-mediated bovine endothelial cell injury in vitro. *Lab. Invest.*, *48*: 269–274 (1983).
31. Harlan, J. M., Harker, L. A., Striker, G. E., Weaver, L. J., Effects of lipopolysaccharide on human endothelial cells in culture. *Thromb. Res.*, *29*: 15–26 (1983).
32. Raij, L., Keane, W. F., Michael, A. F., Unilateral Shwartzman reaction: Cortical necrosis in one kidney following in vivo perfusion with endotoxin. *Kidney Int.*, *12*: 91–95 (1977).
33. Freytag, J. W., Dalrymple, P. N., Maguire, M. H., Strickland, D. K., Carraway, K. L., Hudson, B. G., Glomerular basement membrane. Studies on its structure and interaction with platelets. *J. Biol. Chem.*, *253*: 9069–9074 (1978).
34. Hughes, J., Mahieu, P., Platelet aggregation induced by basement membranes. *Thromb. Diath. Haemorrh.*, *24*: 395–408 (1970).
35. Ts'ao, C.-H., In vitro platelet reaction with isolated glomerular basement membrane. *Thromb. Diath. Haemorrh.*, *25*: 507–516 (1971).
36. Weiss, H. J., Turitto, V. T., Baumgartner, H. R., Nemerson, Y., Hoffman, T., Evidence for the presence of tissue factor activity on subendothelium. *Blood*, *73*: 968–975 (1989).
37. Schorer, A. E., Rick, P. D., Swaim, W. R., Moldow, C. F., Structural features of endotoxin required for stimulation of endothelial cell tissue factor production; exposure of preformed tissue factor after oxidant-mediated endothelial cell injury. *J. Lab. Clin. Med.*, *106*: 38–42 (1985).
38. Brukman, J., Wiggins, R. C., Procoagulant activity in kidneys of normal and bacterial lipopolysaccharide-treated rabbits. *Kidney Int.*, *32*: 31–38 (1987).
39. Baud, L., Oudinet, J.-P., Bens, M., Noe, L., Peraldi, M.-N., Rondeau, E., Etienne, J., Ardaillou, R., Production of tumor necrosis factor by rat mesangial cells in response to bacterial lipopolysaccharide. *Kidney Int.*, *35*: 1111–1118 (1989).

40. Bevilacqua, M. P., Pober, J. S., Majeau, G. R., Fiers, W., Cotran, R. S., Gimbrome, M. A., Jr., Recombinant tumor necrosis factor induces procoagulant activity in cultured human vascular endothelium: Characterization and comparison with the actions of interleukin 1. *Proc. Natl. Acad. Sci. USA, 83*: 4533–4537 (1986).
41. Bevilacqua, M. P., Pober, J. S., Wheeler, M. E., Cotran, R. S., Gimbrone, M. A., Jr., Interleukin-1 activator of vascular endothelium. *Am. J. Pathol., 121*: 393–403 (1985).
42. Libby, P., Ordovas, J. M., Auger, K. R., Robbins, A. H., Birinyi, L. K., Dinarello, C. A., Endotoxin and tumor necrosis factor induce interleukin-1 gene expression in adult human vascular endothelial cells. *Am. J. Pathol., 124*: 179–185 (1986).
43. Bertani, T., Abbate, M., Zoja, C., Corna, D., Perico, N., Ghezzi, P., Remuzzi, G., Tumor necrosis factor induces glomerular damage in the rabbit. *Am. J. Pathol., 134*: 419–430 (1989).
44. Moore, K. L., Esmon, C. T., Esmon, N. L. Tumor necrosis factor leads to internalization and degradation of thrombomodulin from the surface of bovine aortic endothelial cells in culture. *Blood, 73*: 159–165 (1989).
45. Schleef, R. R., Loskutoff, D. J., Fibrinolytic system of vascular endothelial cells. *Haemostasis, 18*: 328–341 (1988).
46. Colucci, M., Paramo, J. A., Collen, D., Generation in plasma of a fast-acting inhibitor of plasminogen activator in response to endotoxin stimulation. *J. Clin. Invest., 75*: 818–824 (1985).
47. Emeis, J. J., Kooistra, T., Interleukin-1 and lipopolysaccharide induce an inhibitor of tissue-type plasminogen activator in vivo and in cultured endothelial cells. *J. Exp. Med., 163*: 1260–1266 (1986).
48. Van Hinsbergh, V. W. M., Kooistra, T., Van Den Berg, E. A., Princen, H. M. G., Fiers, W., Emeis, J. J., Tumor necrosis factor increases the production of plasminogen activator inhibitor in human endothelial cells in vitro and in rats in vivo. *Blood, 72*: 1467–1473 (1988).
49. Bussolino, F., Camussi, G., Baglioni, C., Synthesis and release of platelet-activating factor by human vascular endothelial cells treated with tumor necrosis factor or interleukin 1. *J. Biol. Chem., 263*: 11856–11861 (1988).
50. Gralnick, H., McKeown, L. P., Wilson, O. M., Williams, S. B., Klein, R. J., von Willebrand factor release induced by endotoxin. *J. Lab. Clin. Med., 113*: 118–122 (1989).
51. Bohn, E., Muller-Berghaus, G., The effect of leukocyte and platelet transfusion on the activation of intravascular coagulation by endotoxin in granulocytopenic and thrombocytopenic rabbits. *Am. J. Pathol., 84*: 239–258 (1976).
52. Foreman, E. N., Abildgaard, C. F., Bolger, J. F., Johnson, C. A., Schulman, I., Generalized Shwartzman reaction: Role of the granulocyte in intravascular coagulation and renal cortical necrosis. *Br. J. Haematol., 16*: 507–515 (1969).
53. Horn, R. G., Collins, R. D., Studies on the pathogenesis of the generalized Shwartzman reaction. The role of granulocytes. *Lab. Invest., 18*: 101–107 (1968).
54. Lerner, R. G., Rapaport, S. I., Spitzer, J. M., Endotoxin-induced intravascular clotting: The need for granulocytes. *Thromb. Diath. Haemorrh., 20*: 430–443 (1968).
55. Lipinski, B., Gurewich, V., The effect of leukopenia versus thrombocytopenia on endotoxin induced intravascular coagulation. *Thromb. Res., 8*: 403–411 (1976).
56. Kociba, G. J., Griesemer, R. A., Disseminated intravascular coagulation induced with leukocyte procoagulant. *Am. J. Pathol., 69*: 407–420 (1972).
57. Lerner, R. G., Goldstein, R., Cummings, G., Endotoxin induced disseminated intravascular coagulation: Evidence that it is mediated by neutrophil production of tissue factor. *Thromb. Res., 11*: 253–261 (1977).
58. Niemetz, J., Coagulant activity of leukocytes. *J. Clin. Invest., 51*: 307–313 (1972).
59. Harlan, J. M., Killen, P. D., Harker, L. A., Striker, G. E., Wright, D., Neutrophil-mediated endothelial injury in vitro. *J. Clin. Invest., 68*: 1394–1403 (1981).

60. Rehan, A., Johnson, K. J., Kunkel, R. G., Wiggins, R. C., Role of oxygen radicals in phorbol myristate induced glomerular injury. *Kidney Int.*, *27*: 503–511 (1985).
61. Vadanarayanan, V. V., Kaplan, B. S., Fong, J. S. C., Neutrophil function in an experimental model of hemolytic uremic syndrome. *Pediatr. Res.*, *21*: 252–256 (1987).
62. Margaretten, W., McKay, D. G., The role of the platelet and leukocyte in disseminated intravascular coagulation caused by bacterial endotoxin. *Thromb. Diath. Haemorrh.*, *36*(Suppl.): 151–157 (1969).
63. Margaretten, W., McKay, D. G., The role of the platelet in the generalized Shwartzman reaction. *J. Exp. Med.*, *129*: 585–590 (1969).
64. Eckhardt, T., Muller-Berghaus, G., The role of blood platelets in the precipitation of soluble fibrin by endotoxin. *Scand. J. Haematol.*, *14*: 181–189 (1975).
65. Kramer, W., Muller-Berghaus, G., Effect of platelet antiserum on the activation of intravascular coagulation by endotoxin. *Thromb. Res.*, *10*: 47–70 (1977).
66. Muller-Berghaus, G., Goldfinger, D., Margaretten, W., McKay, D. G., Platelet factor 3 and the generalized Schwartzman reaction. *Thromb. Diath. Haemorrh.*, *18*: 726–735 (1967).
67. Muller-Berghaus, G., Kramer, W., Effect of platelet antiserum on the precipitation of soluble fibrin by endotoxin. *Thromb. Haemost.*, *35*: 237–248 (1976).
68. Niemetz, J., Marcus, A., The stimulatory effect of platelets and platelet membranes on the procoagulant activity of leukocytes. *J. Clin. Invest.*, *54*: 1437–1443 (1974).
69. Semeraro, N., Fumarola, D., Mertens, F., Vermylen, J., Evidence that endotoxins enhance the factor X activator activity of washed human platelets. *Br. J. Haematol.*, *38*: 243–249 (1978).
70. McKay, D. G., Muller-Berghaus, G., Cruse, V., Activation of Hageman factor by ellagic acid and the generalized Shwartzman reaction. *Am. J. Pathol.*, *43*: 393–420 (1969).
71. Palmerio, C., Ming, S. C., Frank, E., Fine, J., The role of the sympathetic nervous system in the generalized Shwartzman reaction. *J. Exp. Med.*, *115*: 609–612.
72. Bolton, W. K., Atuk, N. O., Study of chemical sympathectomy in endotoxin-induced lethality and fibrin deposition. *Kidney Int.*, *13*: 263–270 (1978).
73. Campos, A., Kim, Y., Azar, S., Vernier, R. L., Michael, A. F., Prevention of the generalized Shwartzman reaction in pregnant rats by prostacyclin infusion. *Lab. Invest.*, *48*: 705–710.
74. Howes, E. L., Jr., Kwok, M. T., McKay, D. G., The effects of indomethacin on the generalized Schartzman reaction. *Am. J. Pathol.*, *91*: 7–22 (1978).
75. Latour, J.-G., Bernard, F., Prevention by aspirin of the classic generalized Shwartzman reaction. *Am. J. Pathol.*, *91*: 595–606 (1978).
76. Latour, J.-G., Leger-Gauthier, C., Prostaglandins in the pathogenesis of the generalized Shwartzman reaction. *Am. J. Obstet. Gynecol.*, *135*: 577–580 (1979).
77. Szczepanski, M., Lucer, C., Staff-Zielinska, E., Inhibitory effect of I.V. acetylsalicylic acid on the generalized Shwartzman reaction in the rabbit. *Thromb. Res.*, *29*: 85–90 (1983).
78. Thomas, L., Good, R. A., The effect of cortisone on the Shwartzman reaction. *J. Exp. Med.*, *95*: 409–427 (1952).
79. Latour, J.-G., Prejean, J. B., Margaretten, W., Corticosteroids and the generalized Shwartzman reaction. *Am. J. Pathol.*, *65*: 189–200 (1971).
80. Good, R. A., Thomas, L., Studies on the generalized Shwartzman reaction. II. The production of bilateral cortical necrosis of the kidneys by a single injection of bacterial toxin in rabbits previously treated with Thorotrast or trypan blue. *J. Exp. Med.*, *96*: 625–641 (1952).
81. Muller-Berghaus, G., Schneberger, R., Hageman factor activation in the generalized Shwartzman reaction. *Br. J. Haematol.*, *21*: 513–527 (1971).
82. Smith, R. T., Thomas, L., Good, R. A., Generalized Shwartzman reaction. V. In-

travenous injection of colloidal iron or carbon on response to rabbits to meningococcal toxin. *Proc. Soc. Exp. Biol. Med.*, *82*: 712–715 (1953).
83. Lee, L., Reticuloendothelial clearance of circulating fibrin in the pathogenesis of the generalized Shwartzman reaction. *J. Exp. Med.*, *115*: 1065–1982 (1962).
84. Bergstein, J. M., Michael, A. F., Jr., The effect of Thorotrast and cortisone on renal cortical fibrinolytic activity in the rabbit. *Am. J. Pathol.*, *71*: 113–118 (1973).
85. Dano, K., Reich, E., Plasminogen activator from cells transformed by an oncogenic virus. *Biochim. Biophys. Acta*, *566*: 138–151 (1979).
86. Laug, W. E. Glucocorticoids inhibit plasminogen activator production by endothelial cells. *Thromb. Haemostas.*, *50*: 888–892 (1983).
87. Moroz, L., Inhibition of fibrinolytic activity of plasmin by suramin (Antrypol) and trypan blue. *Thromb. Res.*, *10*: 605–611 (1977).
88. Szczepanski, M., Lucer, C., The influence of large doses of hydrocortisone on the generalized Shwartzman reactions in the rabbit. *Thromb. Res.*, *8*: 71–81 (1976).
89. Lipinski, B., Worowski, K., Jeljaszewica, J., Niewiarowski, S., Rejniak, L., Participation of soluble fibrin monomer complexes and platelet factor 4 in the generalized Shwartzman reaction. *Thromb. Diath. Haemorrh.*, *20*: 285–295 (1968).
90. Condie, R. M., Hong, C. Y., Good, R. A., Reversal of the lesions of the generalized Shwartzman phenomenon by treatment of rabbits with streptokinase. *J. Lab. Clin. Med.*, *50*: 803–804 (1957).
91. Kliman, A., McKay, D. G., The prevention of the generalized Shwartzman reaction by fibrinolytic activity. *Arch. Pathol.*, *66*: 715–719 (1958).
92. Rodrigues-Erdmann, F., Studies on the pathogenesis of the generalized Schwartzman reaction. II. Role played by experimentally induced fibrinolysis. *Thromb. Diath. Haemorrh.*, *12*: 462–470 (1964).
93. Bergstein, J. M., Tissue plasminogen activator therapy of glomerular thrombi in the Shwartzman reaction. *Kidney Int.*, *35*: 14–18 (1989).
94. Bergstein, J. M., Michael, A. F., Jr., Renal cortical fibrinolytic activity in the rabbit following one or two doses of endotoxin. *Thromb. Diath. Haemorrh.*, *29*: 27–31 (1973).
95. Bergstein, J. M., Michael, A. F., Jr., Failure of cobra venom factor to prevent the generalized Shwartzman reaction and loss of renal cortical fibrinolytic activity. *Am. J. Pathol.*, *74*: 19–30 (1974).
96. Booth, N. A., Anderson, J. A., Bennett, B., Platelet release protein which inhibits plasminogen activators. *J. Clin. Pathol.*, *38*: 825–830 (1985).
97. Erickson, L. A., Ginsberg, M. H., Loskutoff, D. J., Detection and partial characterization of an inhibitor of plasminogen activator in human platelets. *J. Clin. Invest.*, *74*: 1465–1472 (1984).
98. Joist, J. H., Nierwiarowski, S., Nath, N., Mustard, J. F., Platelet antiplasmin: Its extrusion during the release action, subcellular localization, characterization, and relationship to antiheparin in pig platelets. *J. Lab. Clin. Med.*, *87*: 659–669 (1976).
99. Plow, E. F., Collen, D., The presence and release of alpha$_2$-antiplasmin from human platelets. *Blood*, *58*: 1069–1074 (1981).
100. Ausprunk, D. H., Das, J., Endotoxin-induced changes in human platelet membranes: Morphologic evidence. *Blood*, *51*: 487–495 (1978).
101. Horowitz, H. I., Des Pres, R. M., Hook, E. W., Effects of bacterial endotoxin on rabbit platelets. *J. Exp. Med.*, *116*: 619–633 (1962).
102. Nagayama, M., Zucker, M. B., Beller, F. K., Effects of a variety of endotoxins on human and rabbit platelet function. *Thromb. Diath. Haemorrh.*, *26*: 467–473 (1971).
103. Bergstein, J. M., Platelet inhibition of renal cortical fibrinolytic activity in the rabbit. *Lab. Invest.*, *35*: 171–178 (1976).

104. Crutchley, D. J., Conanan, L. B., Endotoxin induction of an inhibitor of plasminogen activator in bovine pulmonary artery endothelial cells. *J. Biol. Chem.*, *261*: 154–159 (1986).
105. Hanss, M., Collen, D., Secretion of tissue-type plasminogen activator and plasminogen activator inhibitor by cultured human endothelial cells: Modulation by thrombin, endotoxin, and histamine. *J. Lab. Clin. Med.*, *109*: 97–104 (1987).
106. Loskutoff, D. J., Effect of thrombin on the fibrinolytic activity of cultured bovine endothelial cells. *J. Clin. Invest.*, *64*: 329–332 (1979).
107. Dosne, A. M., Dubor, F., Lutcher, F., Parant, M., Chedid, L., Tumor necrosis factor (TNF) stimulates plasminogen activator inhibitor (PAI) production by endothelial cells and decreases blood fibrinolytic activity in the rat. *Thromb. Res.*, *8*(Suppl): 115–122 (1988).
108. Loskutoff, D. J., Edgington, T. S., An inhibitor of plasminogen activator in rabbit endothelial cells. *J. Biol. Chem.*, *256*: 4142–4145 (1981).
109. Loskutoff, D. J., Van Mourik, J. A., Erickson, L. A., Lawrence, D., Detection of an unusually stable fibrinolytic inhibitor produced by bovine endothelial cells. *Proc. Natl. Acad. Sci. USA*, *80*: 2956–2960 (1983).
110. Philips, M., Juul, A., Thorsen, S., Human endothelial cells produce a plasminogen activator inhibitor and a tissue-type plasminogen activator-inhibitor complex. *Biochim. Biophys. Acta*, *802*: 99–110 (1984).
111. Bergstein, J. M., Hoyer, J. R., Michael, A. F., Jr., Glomerular fibrinolytic activity following endotoxin-induced glomerular fibrin deposition in the pregnant rat. *Am. J. Pathol.*, *75*: 195–202 (1974).
112. Katz, J., Lurie, A., Kaplan, B. S., Krawitz, S., Metz, J., Coagulation findings in the hemolytic–uremic syndrome of infancy: Similarity to hyperacute renal allograft rejection. *J. Pediatr.*, *78*: 426–434. (1971).
113. Kisker, C. T., Rush, R. A., Absence of intravascular coagulation in the hemolytic–uremic syndrome. *Am. J. Dis. Child.*, *129*: 223–226 (1975).
114. Morel-Maroger, L., Kanfer, A., Solez, K., Sraer, J.-D., Richet, G., Prognostic importance of vascular lesions in acute renal failure with microangiopathic hemolytic anemia (hemolytic–uremic syndrome): Clinicopathologic study in 20 adults. *Kidney Int.*, *15*: 548–558 (1979).
115. Sorrenti, L. Y., Lewy, P. R., The hemolytic–uremic syndrome. Experience at a center in the Midwest. *Am. J. Dis. Child.*, *132*: 59–62 (1978).
116. Monnens, L., Kleynen, F., Van Munster, P., Schretlen, E., Bonnerman, A., Coagulation studies and streptokinase therapy in the haemolytic–uraemic syndrome. *Helv. Paediatr. Acta*, *27*: 45–54 (1972).
117. Gianantonio, C. A., Vitacco, M., Mendilaharzu, F., Gallo, G. E., Sojo, E. T., The hemolytic–uremic syndrome. *Nephron*, *11*: 174–192 (1973).
118. Willougby, M. L. N., Murphy, A. V., McMorris, S., Jewell, F. G., Coagulation studies in haemolytic uraemic syndrome. *Arch. Dis. Child.*, *47*: 766–771 (1972).
119. Riella, M. C., George, C. R. P., Hickman, R. O., Striker, G. E., Slichter, S. J., Harker, L., Quadracci, L. J., Renal microangiopathy of the hemolytic–uremic syndrome. *Nephron*, *17*: 188–203 (1976).
120. Katz, J., Krawitz, S., Sacks, P. V., Levin, S. E., Thomson, P., Levin, J., Metz, J., Platelet, erythrocyte, and fibrinogen kinetics in the hemolytic–uremic syndrome of infancy. *J. Pediatr.*, *83*: 739–748 (1973).
121. Harker, L. A., Slichter, S. J., Platelet and fibrinogen consumption in man. *N. Engl. J. Med.*, *287*: 999–1005 (1972).
122. Ambrus, J. L., Baliah, T., Ambrus, C. L., Mink, I. B., Murphy, G. P., Fibrin–fibrinogen degradation products in children with renal disease. *N. Y. State J. Med.*, *1*: 1396–1402 (1974).

123. Avalos, J. S., Vitacco, M., Molinas, F., Penalver, J., Gianantonio, C., Coagulation studies in the hemolytic–uremic syndrome. *J. Pediatr., 76*: 538–548 (1970).
124. Ekert, H., Barratt, T. M., Chantler, C., Turner, M. W., Immunologically active equivalents of fibrinogen in sera and urine of children with renal disease. *Arch. Dis. Child., 47*: 90–96 (1972).
125. Hedner, U., Nilsson, I. M., Renal disease and fibrinogen degradation products. *Adv. Nephrol., 3*: 241–271 (1974).
126. Steihm, E. R., Trygstad, C. W., Split products of fibrin in human renal disease. *Am. J. Med., 46*: 774–786 (1969).
127. Taira, K., Matsunaga, T., Kawahara, S., Sakamoto, S., Kamitsuji, H., Fragments of urinary fibrin/fibrinogen degradation products and cross-linked fibrin degradation products in various renal diseases. *Thromb. Res., 53*: 367–377 (1989).
128. Uttley, W. S., Serum levels of fibrin/fibrinogen degradation products in the haemolytic–uraemic syndrome. *Arch. Dis. Child., 45*: 587–589 (1970).
129. Fong, J. S. C., Kaplan, B. S., Impairment of platelet aggregation in hemolytic–uremic syndrome: Evidence for platelet "exhaustion." *Blood, 60*: 564–569 (1982).
130. Kaplan, B. S., Fong, J. S. C., Reduced platelet aggregation in hemolytic–uremic syndrome. *Thromb. Haemost., 43*: 154–157 (1980).
131. Pareti, F. I., Capitanio, A., Mannucci, L., Ponticelli, C., Mannucci, P. M., Acquired dysfunction due to the circulation of "exhausted" platelets. *Am. J. Med., 69*: 235–240 (1980).
132. Walters, M. D. S., Levin, M., Smith, C., Nokes, T. J. C., Hardisty, R. M., Dillon, M. J., Barratt, T. M., Intravascular platelet activation in the hemolytic–uremic syndrome. *Kidney Int., 33*: 107–115 (1988).
133. Appiani, A. C., Edefonti, A., Bettininelli, A., Cossu, M. M., Paracchini, M. L., Rossi, E., The relationship between plasma levels of the factor VIII complex and platelet release products (beta-thromboglobulin and platelet factor 4) in children with the hemolytic–uremic syndrome. *Clin. Nephrol., 17*: 195–199 (1982).
134. Moake, J. L., Byrnes, J. J., Troll, J. H., Rudy, C. K., Weinstein, M. J., Colannino, N. M., Hong, S. L., Abnormal VIII: von Willebrand factor patterns in the plasma of patients with the hemolytic–uremic syndrome. *Blood, 64*: 592–598 (1984).
135. Monnens, L., Van De Meer, W., Langenhuysen, C., Van Munster, P., Van Oostrom, C., Platelet aggregating factor in the epidemic form of hemolytic–uremic syndrome in childhood. *Clin. Nephrol., 24*: 135–137 (1985).
136. Levin, M., Stroobant, P., Walters, M. D. S., Cheng, D. J., Waterford, M. D., Barratt, T. M., Platelet-derived growth factors as possible mediators of vascular proliferation in the sporadic haemolytic uraemic syndrome. *Lancet, 2*: 830–833 (1986).
137. Arenson, E. B., Jr., August, C. S., Preliminary report: Treatment of the hemolytic–uremic syndrome with aspirin and dipyridamole. *J. Pediatr., 86*: 957–961 (1975).
138. Thorsen, C. A., Rossi, E. C., Green, D., Carone, F. A., The treatment of the hemolytic–uremic syndrome with inhbitors of platelet function. *Am. J. Med., 66*: 711–716 (1979).
139. O'Regan, S., Chesney, R. W., Mongeau, J.-G., Robitaille, P., Aspirin and dipyridamole therapy in the hemolytic–uremic syndrome. *J. Pediatr., 97*: 473–476 (1980).
140. Van Damme-Lombaerts, R., Proesmans, W., Van Damme, B., Eeckels, R., Binda ki Muaka, P., Mercieca, V., Vlietinck, R., Vermylen, J., Heparin plus dipyridamole in childhood hemolytic–uremic syndrome: A prospective, randomized study. *J. Pediatr., 113*: 913–918 (1988).
141. Moncada, S., Vane, J. R., Prostacyclin and blood coagulation. *Drugs, 21*: 430–437 (1981).
142. Stuart, M. J., Spitzer, R. E., Coppe, D., Abnormal platelet and vascular prostaglandin synthesis in an infant with hemolytic uremic syndrome. *Pediatrics, 71*: 120–124 (1983).

143. Defreyn, G., Proesmans, W., Machin, S. J., Lemmens, F., Vermylen, J., Abnormal prostacyclin metabolism in the hemolytic uremic syndrome: Equivocal effect of prostacyclin infusions. *Clin. Nephrol., 18*: 43–49 (1982).
144. Webster, J., Rees, A. J., Lewis, P. J., Hensby, C. N., Prostacyclin deficiency in haemolytic–uraemic syndrome. *Br. Med. J., 281*: 271 (1980).
145. Turi, S., Beattie, T. J., Belch, J. J. F., Murphy, A. V., Disturbances of prostacyclin metabolism in children with hemolytic–uremic syndrome and in first degree relatives. *Clin. Nephrol., 25*: 193–198 (1986).
146. Deckmyn, H., Proesmans, W., Vermylen, J., Prostacyclin production by whole blood from children: Impairment in the hemolytic uremic syndrome and excessive formation in chronic renal failure. *Thromb. Res., 30*: 13–18 (1983).
147. Chamone, D. A., Proesmans, W. C., Monnens, L. A., Binda ki Muaka, P., Vermylen, J. G., Reversible deficient prostacyclin release in childhood hemolytic uremic syndrome. *Int. J. Pediatr. Nephrol., 3*: 13–16 (1982).
148. Jorgensen, K. A., Pedersen, R. S., Familial deficiency of prostacyclin production stimulating factor in the hemolytic uremic syndrome of childhood. *Thromb. Res., 21*: 311–315 (1981).
149. Levin, M., Elkon, K. B., Nokes, T. J. C., Buckle, A. M., Dillon, M. J., Hardisty, R. M., Barratt, T. M., Inhibitor of prostacylcin production in sporadic haemolytic uraemic syndrome. *Arch. Dis. Child., 58*: 703–708 (1983).
150. Hautekeete, M. L., Nagler, J. M., Cuykens, J. J., Parizel, G., Laekeman, G. M., Herman, A. G., 6-Keto-PGF1-alpha levels and prostacyclin therapy in 2 adult patients with hemolytic uremic syndrome. *Clin. Nephrol., 26*: 157–159 (1986).
151. Stuart, M. J., Spitzer, R. E., Walenga, R. W., Boone, S., Prostanoids in hemolytic uremic syndrome. *J. Pediatr., 106*: 936–939 (1985).
152. Schlegel, N., Maclouf, J., Loirat, C., Drouet, L., Marotte, R., Scarabin, P. Y., Mathieu, H., Absence of plasma prostacyclin stimulating activity deficiency in hemolytic uremic syndrome. *J. Pediatr., 11*: 71–77 (1987).
153. Loirat, C., Sonsino, E., Hinglais, N., Jais, I. P., Landais, P., Fermanian, J., Treatment of the childhood haemolytic uraemic syndrome with plasma. *Pediatr. Nephrol., 2*: 279–285 (1988).
154. Rizzoni, G., Claris-Appiani, A., Edefonti, A., Facchin, P., Franchini, F., Gusmano, R., Imbasciatti, E., Pavanello, L., Perfumo, F., Remuzzi, G., Plasma infusion for hemolytic–uremic syndrome in children: Results of a multicenter controlled trial. *J. Pediatr., 112*: 284–290 (1988).
155. Sheth, K. J., Gill, J. C., Hanna, J., Leichter, H. E., Failure of fresh frozen plasma infusions to alter the course of hemolytic uremic syndrome. *Child. Nephrol. Urol., 9*: 38–41 (1988).
156. Thysell, H., Oxelius, V.-A., Norlin, M., Successful treatment of hemolytic uremic syndrome and thrombotic thrombocytopenia purpura with fresh frozen plasma and plasma exchange. *Acta Med. Scand., 212*: 285–288 (1982).
157. Bambauer, R., Jutzler, G. A., Hartmann, H. G., Stolz, D., Schmengler, K., Koehler, M., Wahlen, M., In *Plasmapheresis* (Y. Nose, P. S. Malchesky, J. W. Smith, R. S. Kraukauer, eds.), Raven Press, New York, pp. 379–386 (1983).
158. Beattie, T. J., Murphy, A. V., Willoughby, M. L. N., Machin, S. J., Defreyn, G., Plasmapheresis in the haemolytic–uraemic syndrome in children. *Br. Med. J., 282*: 1667–1668 (1981).
159. Bergada, E., Torras, A., Puig, L., Arrizabalaga, P., Revet, L., Plasmapheresis-dependent recovery from recurrent hemolytic uremic syndrome. *Int. J. Artif. Organs, 6*: 79–80 (1982).
160. Cathran, D. C., Adult hemolytic–uremic syndrome: Successful treatment with plasmapheresis. *Am. J. Kidney Dis., 3*: 275–279 (1984).

161. Feldhoff, C. M., Lubolt, W., Bussmann, K., Schror, K., Plasma exchanges in frequently recurrent hemolytic–uremic syndrome in a child. *Int. J. Pediatr. Nephrol., 4*: 239–242 (1983).
162. Gillor, A., Bulla, M., Roth, B., Bussman, K., Schror, K., Tekook, A., Gladtke, E., Plasmapheresis as a therapeutic measure in hemolytic–uremic syndrome in children. *Klin. Wochenschr., 61*: 363–367 (1983).
163. Remuzzi, G., Misiani, R., Marchesi, D., Livio, M., Mecca, G., de Gaetano, G., Donati, M. B., Treatment of the hemolytic uremic syndrome with plasma. *Clin. Nephrol., 12*: 279–284 (1979).
164. Spencer, C. D., Crane, F. M., Kumar, J. R., Alving, B. M., Treatment of postpartum hemolytic uremic syndrome with plasma exchange. *JAMA, 247*: 2808–2809 (1982).
165. Eddy, A. A., Geary, D. F., Balfe, J. W., Clark, W. F., Baumal, R., Prolongation of acute renal failure in two patients with hemolytic–uremic syndrome due to excessive plasma infusion therapy. *Pediatr. Nephrol., 3*: 420–423 (1989).
166. Bergstein, J. M., Kuederli, U., Bang, N. U., Plasma inhibitor of glomerular fibrinolysis in the hemolytic–uremic syndrome. *Am. J. Med., 73*: 322–327 (1982).
167. Bergstein, J. M., Bang, N. U., Plasminogen activator inhibitor-1 (PAI-1) is the circulating inhibitor of fibrinolysis (PAI-HUS) in the hemolytic syndrome (HUS) [abstract]. *Kidney Int., 37*: 254 (1989).
168. Krishnamurti, C., Barr, C. F., Hassett, M. A., Young, G. D., Alving, B. M., Plasminogen activator inhibitor: A regulator of ancrod-induced fibrin deposition in rabbits. *Blood, 69*: 798–803 (1987).
169. Rosove, M. H., Ho, W. G., Goldfinger, D., Ineffectiveness of aspirin and dipyridamole in the treatment of thrombotic thrombocytopenic purpura. *Ann. Intern. Med., 96*: 27–33 (1982).
170. Myers, T. J., Wakem, C. J., Ball, E. D., Tremont, J., Thrombotic thrombocytopenic purpura: Combined treatment with plasmapheresis and antiplatelet agents. *Ann. Intern. Med., 92*: 149–155 (1980).
171. Jaffe, E. A., Nachman, R. L., Merskey, C., Thrombotic thrombocytopenic purpura—coagulation parameters in twelve patients. *Blood, 42*: 499–507 (1973).
172. Berberich, F. R., Cuene, S. A., Chard, R. L., Jr., Hartmann, J. R., Thrombotic thrombocytopenic purpura. Three cases with platelet and fibrinogen survival studies. *J. Pediatr., 84*: 503–509 (1974).
173. Glas-Greenwalt, P., Hall, J. M., Panke, T. W., Kant, K. S., Allen, C. M., Pollak, V. E., Fibronolysis in health and disease: Abnormal levels of plasminogen activator, plasminogen activator inhibitor and protein C in thrombotic thrombocytopenic purpura. *J. Lab. Clin. Med., 108*: 415–422 (1986).
174. Wu, K. K., Hall, E. R., Rossi, E. C., Papp, A. C., Serum prostacyclin binding defects in thrombotic thrombocytopenic purpura. *J. Clin. Invest., 75*: 168–174 (1985).
175. Tsai, A., Manner, C. E., Rudersdorf, T., Wu, K. K., Quantitation of serum prostacyclin-binding in thrombotic thrombocytopenic purpura. *Thromb. Res., 51*: 583–592 (1988).
176. Burns, E. R., Zucker-Franklin, D., Pathologic effects of plasma from patients with thrombotic thrombocytopenic purpura on platelets and cultured vascular endothelial cells. *Blood, 60*: 1030–1037 (1982).
177. Lian, E. C.-Y., Savaraj, N., Effects of platelet inhibitors on the platelet aggregation induced by plasma from patients with thrombotic thrombocytopenic purpura. *Blood, 58*: 354–359 (1981).
178. Kelton, J.-G., Moore, J., Santos, A., Sheridan, D., Detection of a platelet-agglutinating factor in thrombotic thrombocytopenic purpura. *Ann. Intern. Med., 101*: 589–593 (1984).
179. Hussey, C. V., Hause, L. L., Gottschall, J. L., Anderson, T., A platelet aggregating

factor in thrombotic thrombocytopenic purpura: Initial activity, fluctuations, and removal by plasma exchange. *Thromb. Res.*, *44*: 355–364 (1986).
180. Siddiqui, F. A., Lian, E. C.-Y., Novel platelet-agglutinating protein from a thrombotic thrombocytopenic plasma. *J. Clin. Invest.*, *76*: 1330–1337 (1985).
181. Lian, E. C.-Y., Pathogenesis of thrombotic thrombocytopenic purpura. *Semin. Hematol.*, *24*: 82–100 (1987).
182. Kelton, J.-G., Moore, J. C., Murphy, W. G., Studies investigating platelet aggregation and release initiated by sera from patients with thrombotic thrombocytopenic purpura. *Blood*, *69*: 924–928 (1987).
183. Moake, J. L., Rudy, C. K., Troll, J. H., Weinstein, M. J., Colannino, N. M., Azocar, J., Seder, R. H., Hong, S. L., Deykin, D., Unusually large plasma factor VIII: von Willebrand factor multimers in chronic relapsing thrombotic thrombocytopenic purpura. *N. Engl. H. Med.*, *307*: 1432–1435 (1982).
184. Lian, E. C.-Y., Mui, P. T. K., Siddiqui, F. A., Chui, A. Y. Y., Chiu, L. L. S., Inhibition of platelet-aggregating activity in thrombotic thrombocytopenic purpura plasma by normal adult immunoglobulin G. *J. Clin. Invest.*, *73*: 548–555 (1984).
185. Siddiqui, F. A., Lian, E. C.-Y., Platelet-agglutinating protein P37 from a thrombotic thrombocytopenic purpura plasma forms a complex with human immunoglobulin G. *Blood*, *71*: 299–304 (1988).
186. Schmidt, J. L., Thrombotic thrombocytopenic purpura: Successful treatment unlocks etiologic secrets. *Mayo Clin. Proc.*, *64*: 956–961 (1989).
187. Shepard, K. V., Bukowski, R. M., The treatment of thrombotic thrombocytopenic purpura with exchange transfusions, plasma infusions, and plasma exchange. *Semin. Hematol.*, *24*: 178–193. (1987).

27
The Pivotal Role of the Endothelial Cell in the Pathogenesis of HUS

Carla Zoja and Giuseppe Remuzzi *Mario Negri Institute for Pharmacological Research, Bergamo, Italy*

The hemolytic uremic syndrome (HUS) (1–4) which may have platelet thrombi in the microcirculation, shares many similarities with thrombotic thrombocytopenic purpura (TTP) (5–8). Although attempts have been made to differentiate HUS from TTP (7, 9), none of the proposed criteria clearly separate the two syndromes (7, 9, 10). Evaluations of reported cases may indicate that in clinical practice distinction between multiorgan involvement in TTP and renal involvement in HUS (9) is not always apparent. The fundamental pathological lesion, thrombotic microangiopathy (TMA) (11, 12), is identical in HUS and TTP, although it can involve different organs (3, 13). The concept that HUS and TTP could be distinguished on the basis of response to treatment with heparin (9) was challenged by a study from Proesmans et al. (14) who showed that HUS also does not respond to anticoagulants. Even the most widely utilized classic criteria for distinguishing HUS from TTP—the presence of renal failure in HUS and of neurological symptoms in TTP—may fail to separate the two syndromes. In fact, neurological involvement has been observed in HUS (1, 2, 15), and a high percentage of patients classified as having TTP have renal failure (5, 6, 16, 17). Identical etiological agents and pathogenetic mechanisms have been proposed for both syndromes (10).

Morphologic evidence suggests that endothelial damage represents a key step in the development of microangiopathic lesions. It is of interest in this context that all the proposed causative agents of HUS and TTP are, in fact, "toxic" to vascular endothelium. In this context, bacterial endotoxin, verotoxins, and neuraminidase; circulating antibodies directed against endothelial cells; and drugs, such as cyclosporine and mitomycin (18), may all induce endothelial injury. The properties of normal endothelium then become altered after the initial insult. It is possible that abnormalities in hemostatic mediators of endothelial cell origin, including prostacyclin (PGI_2), von Willebrand factor (vWF), and tissue plasminogen activator (t-PA), are part of the reactive process that follows endothelial cell perturbation or damage (10, 18). Conceivably, such complex abnormalities then contribute to the development of microangiopathic lesions.

In this chapter the available evidence for a crucial role of vascular endothelium in the pathogenesis of HUS/TTP will be discussed.

MORPHOLOGICAL EVIDENCE OF ENDOTHELIAL DAMAGE IN HEMOLYTIC UREMIC SYNDROME

The typical pathological lesion of HUS involves microvessels, especially of the kidney, which is the main target organ (12, 19–21). In young children, changes are mainly confined to the glomeruli and are characterized by endothelial cell swelling and degeneration, thickening of capillary walls with formation of "double contours," fragmentation of erythrocytes, and intraluminal thrombi. As a result of the insult, the endothelial cell is detached from the underlying basement membrane (Fig. 1), and a subendothelial space, filled with fluffy materials that include lipids, products of

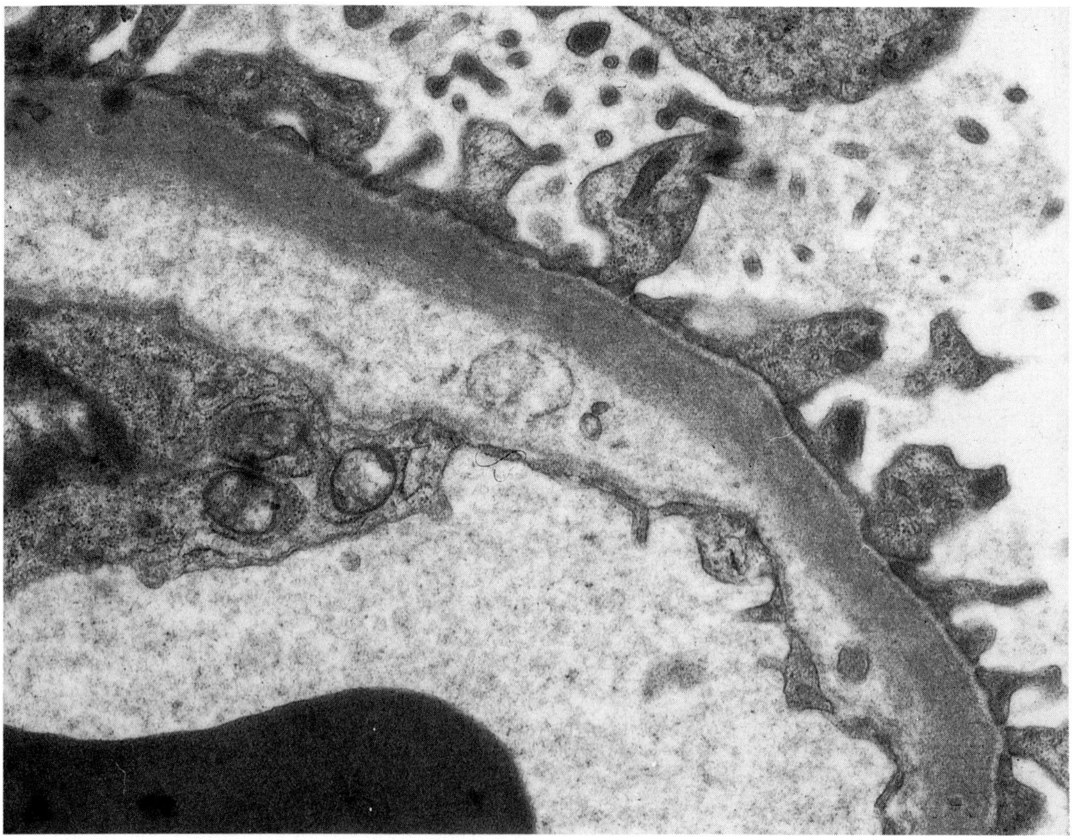

Figure 1 Electron micrograph of glomerular capillary wall from a patient with HUS. Note the marked widening of the subendothelial space resulting from detachment of endothelium from the glomerular basement membrane (× 30,000).

erythrocyte fragmentation, platelets, and fibrin strands is formed (21, 22). As a result of these changes, and occasional thrombi, the glomerular capillary lumina may become occluded. Glomerular thrombi consist of fibrin and platelets, with platelets being preponderant in the early lesions. Even in severe cases glomerular thrombi may completely resolve, and the capillary structure may recover perfectly. In older children and adults, the process mainly involves arteries and arterioles, and the prognosis is poorer than in young children (21, 23). The main findings are edema and proliferation of the intima, necrosis of the arterial wall, and some vessels are thrombosed. In some cases, a "glomeruloid" structure of the small arteries is observed. This is probably the result of endothelial and myointimal proliferation of small arteries adjacent to the glomeruli (24). Glomerular ischemia, thickening and wrinkling of the glomerular basement membrane, atrophy of glomerular tufts, and thickening of Bowman's capsule can also be seen. In a few patients, the histologic appearance is that of cortical or tubular necrosis. Extrarenal lesions have been found at autopsy in 35 of 62 HUS cases; these included microthrombotic lesions in the colon, heart, brain, and pancreas (25). Intracranial hemorrhages and microthrombi, mainly in the choroid plexus, have also been described (25).

EVIDENCE THAT CAUSATIVE AGENTS FOR HEMOLYTIC UREMIC SYNDROME MAY INDUCE ENDOTHELIAL DAMAGE

Experimental evidence indicates that all the factors known to cause HUS may damage vascular endothelium. Bacterial endotoxin has been suggested as one of the causative agents, as documented in cases of HUS associated with endotoxin-producing bacteria (*Shigella* and *Salmonella* species) (26, 27). A lipopolysaccharide derived from *Escherichia coli*, *Salmonella minnesota*, and *Salmonella typhosa* directly injured cultured bovine endothelial cells, induced cell detachment, and caused cell lysis (28). In human endothelial cells in culture, however, the lipopolysaccharide produced the same cytotoxic effect only in the presence of a protein synthesis inhibitor (29). In other in vitro systems, endotoxin-induced endothelial injury required the presence of granulocytes (30). Therefore, the cytotoxic activity of endotoxin was attributed, in part, to its capability to promote granulocyte adhesion to endothelium and to stimulation of granulocyte production of toxic oxygen radicals (30). Two intravenous injections of endotoxin from gram-negative bacteria, spaced 18–24 hr apart, produced a generalized Shwartzman reaction, characterized by disseminated intravascular coagulation and bilateral cortical necrosis of the kidneys in rabbits (31). The earliest histological lesion was the deposition of a homogeneous, eosinophilic material, which stained for fibrin, within the lumina of glomerular capillaries. Disseminated intravascular coagulation is believed to be responsible for fibrin deposition in glomerular capillaries and is the result of a complicated series of events, including platelet aggregation, activation of complement, inhibition of fibrinolysis, stimulation of leukocytes, and endothelial damage. However, this process is rare in human HUS. Infusion of endotoxin over a 5-hr period induces a syndrome in the rabbit that more closely resembles human HUS (32). In this model the sequence of glomerular pathological changes have been analyzed by light and electron microscopy at various time intervals from the onset of endotoxin infusion (33). Focal irregularities of endothelial fenestrae, with areas of endothelial swelling, are detected a few minutes after the beginning of the infusion, followed by leukocyte and, subsequently, platelet adhesion and accumulation within glomerular capillaries. One hour after the beginning of the infusion a marked polymorphonuclear cell infiltration was observed in the glomerular capillary lumina; at 5 hours, numerous platelets were found, with loss of endothelial fenestrae and diffuse swelling of endothelial cells. Fibrinlike material was detected as free strands in the lumina or as large clumps along the luminal surface of the endothelial layer (Figs. 2 and 3). In these animals the damage was completely reversible; by 48 hours after the end of the infusion, only mild endothelial changes and occasional polymorphs, but no fibrin deposits were detected in the glomeruli. The favorable outcome of HUS in many young children (12) strongly suggests spontaneous resolution of the microangiopathic process and active removal of fibrin. This may occur in the so-called glomerular type of HUS (21).

An association has been found between HUS and enteric infections with verocytotoxin-producing *E. coli* (VTEC) (34–37). Verocytotoxin is also produced by *Shigella dysenteriae* type 1 (38) so that epidemic cases of HUS reported during infection with *S. dysenteriae* might share the same pathogenetic mechanism as the

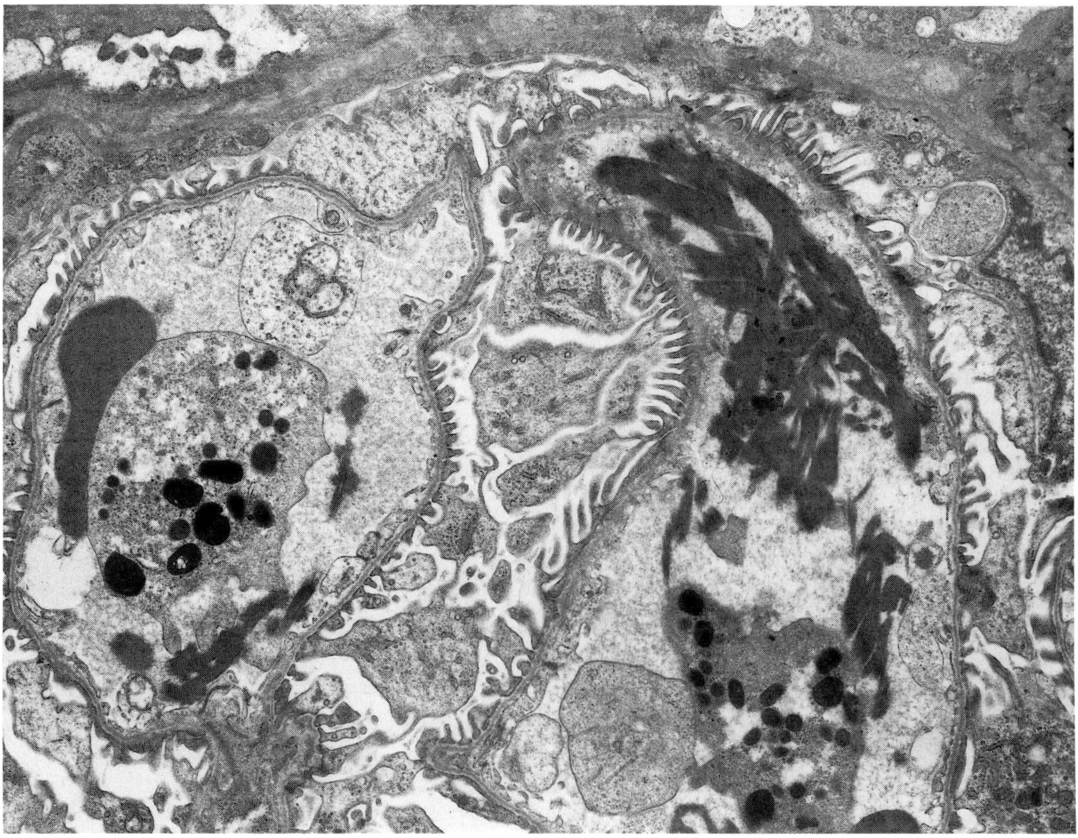

Figure 2 Electron micrograph of glomerular capillary loops in a rabbit infused with endotoxin for 5 hr. Glomerular endothelium shows areas of cellular swelling. Fibrin strands and polymorphonuclear leukocytes are present in the glomerular capillary lumina (× 3000).

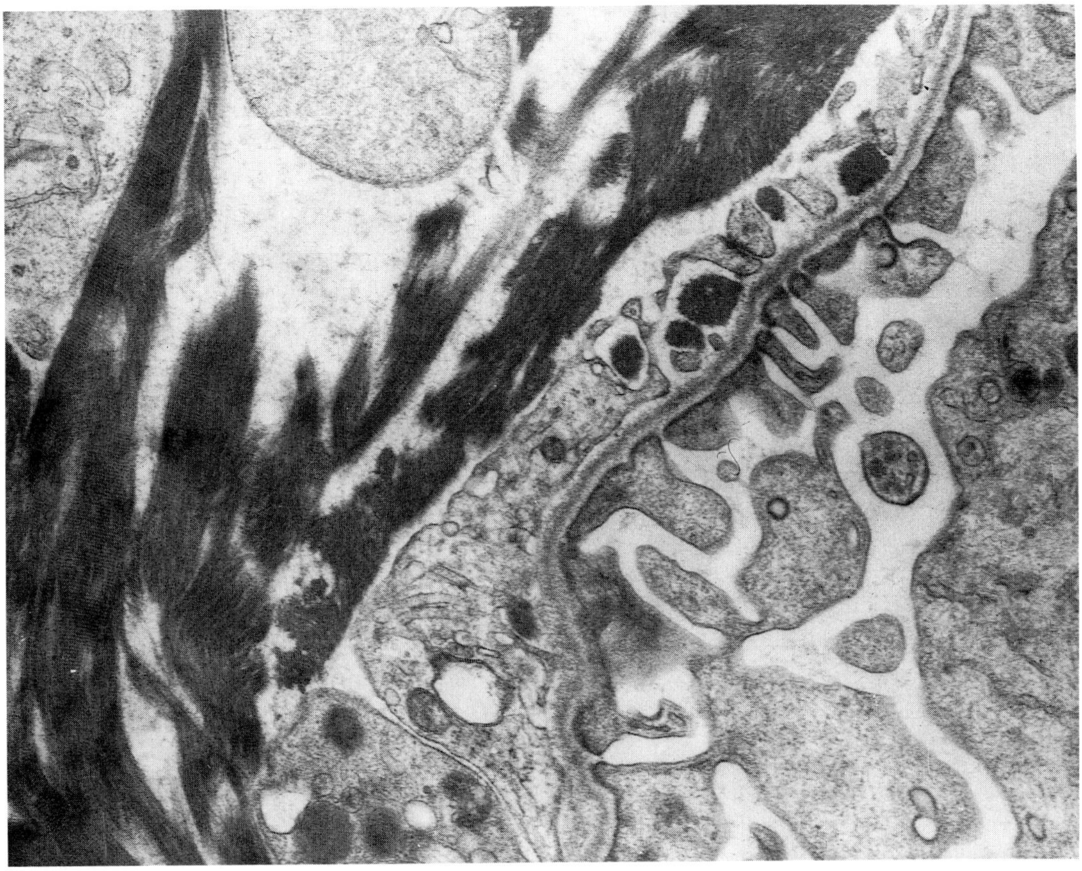

Figure 3 Electron micrograph of a glomerular capillary loop in a rabbit infused with endotoxin for 5 hr. Note the presence of fibrin deposits in the subendothelial space (× 12,000).

VTEC-associated HUS. The VTEC consists of a biologically active subunit A and a number of B subunits (39) which allow binding of the toxin to a specific receptor, the glycolipid, globotriaosyl ceramide (Gb_3) (40). Binding is followed by internalization of the A subunit, which then inhibits protein synthesis by inactivating 60S ribosomal subunits, thereby leading to cell death (39). Shiga toxin and VTEC are directly cytotoxic to cultured human endothelial cells (41–43). The cytopathic effect of VTEC on vascular endothelium was accompanied by release of factor VIII (42) and by reduced synthesis of PGI_2 in rat aortic tissue (44). After intravenous infusion of VTEC into rabbits, endothelial swelling of the brain, gastrointestinal tract capillary, and arterioles, and occasional fibrin microthrombi were found (45). We and Lingwood have shown that rabbits injected with verotoxin 1 purified from *E. coli* O157:H7 had microvascular damage confined to brain, cerebellum, lungs, and caecum, whereas no kidney lesions were documented (personal communication). This can be explained by the finding in the rabbit (Lingwood, personal communication) of Gb_3 receptors in all of the foregoing organs, except the kidney. Bacterial neuraminidase also has been implicated as an etiological factor in HUS (46) and is capable of exposing the Thomsen–Friedenreich receptors on glomerular capillaries, red blood cells, and platelets. The generation of an anti-Thomsen–Friedenreich IgM antibody promotes the agglutination of red blood cells and platelets, and they are subsequently deposited in the microcirculation.

Endothelial damage in HUS might also be immunologically mediated: sera from 13 of 14 children with acute HUS contained complement-fixing IgG and IgM antibodies that lysed cultured human umbilical vein endothelial cells (47).

Forsyth et al. (48) studied children with the diarrhea-associated form of HUS, which is accompanied by neutrophil leukocytosis, and found increased adherence of the patients' neutrophils to endothelial cells in culture in comparison with control neutrophils. Patients' neutrophils induced endothelial injury, as assessed by degradation of endothelial cell fibronectin. When the hyperadhesive neutrophils were incubated with a CD18 antibody directed against the common β-chain of the leukocyte integrin molecules that allow neutrophil adhesion to endothelium, endothelial damage was abrogated in four of ten subjects. They suggested that neutrophils release proteases that attack the surface of endothelium and, therefore, are an important component in the pathogenesis of HUS. The view that neutrophil activation may be central to the process has been supported by the demonstration of increased concentrations of neutrophil elastase in plasma from children with the diarrhea-associated form of HUS in comparison with uninfected children with chronic renal failure (49a, 49b). Children with a poor outcome (chronic renal failure, hypertension, or death) had higher concentrations than those who did well (49b).

Cyclosporine (formerly Cyclosporin A; CyA) and mitomycin—the drugs most frequently associated with the development of an HUS-type of microangiopathic lesions—also induce endothelial damage (50–56). Exposure of cultured bovine aortic endothelial cells to CyA-induced time-and dose-dependent cell injury, with cell detachment and lysis (57) (Fig. 4). Moreover, in cultured rat microvascular endothelial cells, CyA induced dose-dependent inhibition of cell replication (58). It was suggested that through its direct inhibition of endothelial cell replication, CyA could potentiate glomerular endothelial injury in vivo by impairing the regenerative response of endothelium to injury. Extended administration of CyA to rats induced glomerular endothelial damage, with swelling of endothelium, focal loss of fenestrae, doubling of glomerular basement membrane, and a mononuclear cell infiltration and platelet accumulation (59). Perfusion of the rat renal artery with mitomycin also induced the ultrastructural changes of HUS. The initial lesions were confined to vascular endothelium; this was followed by platelet deposition and obliteration of capillary lumina, with the formation of lucent subendothelial expansions (60).

ENDOTHELIAL CELL PERTURBATION OR INJURY AS THE TRIGGER FOR INTRAVASCULAR PLATELET AGGREGATION

Endothelial cells synthesize PGI_2 and von Willebrand factor (vWF), which have a major modulatory role on platelet vessel wall interaction in both normal conditions and in disease. Prostacyclin is a vasodilator and a potent endogenous inhibitor of platelet aggregation (61). Circulating PGI_2 levels are very low and are not sufficient to inhibit platelet function (62). However, at the site of endothelial cell injury, PGI_2 achieves higher concentrations and, thereby, limits thrombus formation. von Willebrand factor, a protein composed of protomeric subunits arranged in a series of

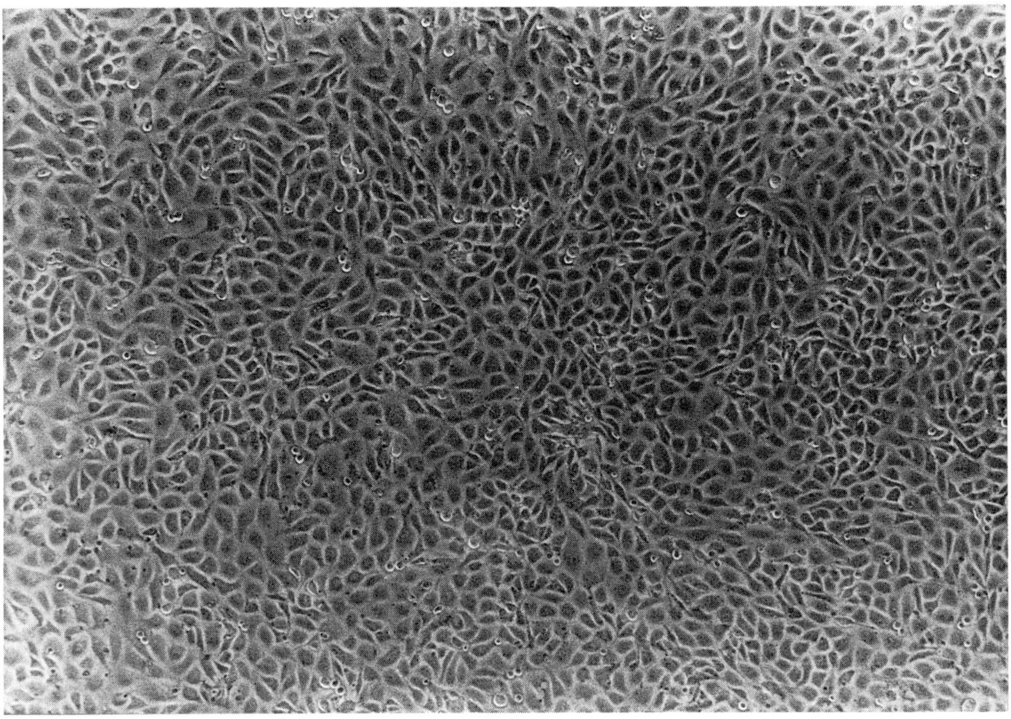

a

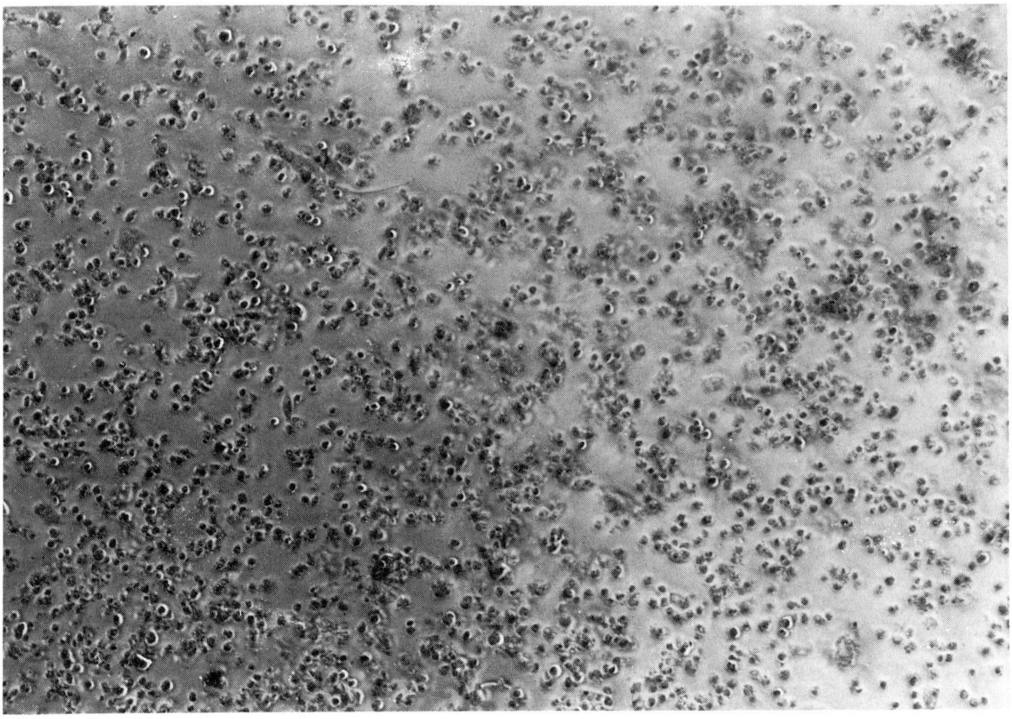

b

Figure 4 Morphological changes of bovine aortic endothelial cells exposed to cyclosporine. (a) Cells incubated for 24 hr with the cyclosporine vehicle (ethanol). (b) Cells incubated with 10 μM cyclosporine for 24 hr (phase-contrast microscopy, $\times$ 250).

complex multimers, has an important role in primary hemostasis because it is required for platelet adhesion to subendothelial collagen (63, 64).

Defective bioavailability of PGI_2 and complex abnormalities in the multimeric structure of vWF have been described in HUS patients (65, 66). Vascular specimens from adult patients with HUS were found to have a reduced capacity to generate PGI_2 (67), which has subsequently, been confirmed in adults and children (68–70). Defective vascular PGI_2 synthesis might favor platelet activation and deposition at the site of vascular injury. However, experimental evidence indicates that endothelial damage stimulates, rather than suppresses, PGI_2 synthesis (71) and, therefore, the reason for reduced vascular PGI_2 synthesis in HUS is unclear. One explanation is that the repeated stimulation of endothelial cells by endotoxin might "exhaust" their capacity to produce PGI_2 (72). Therefore, it is possible that PGI_2 synthesis is stimulated in the early phase of HUS, but is later depressed when more pronounced vascular damage occurs. Inhibition of PGI_2 synthetase by lipid peroxides, formed during the activation of the arachidonic acid cascade that follows extensive endothelial injury, may be another factor that inhibits PGI_2 biosynthesis (73). The causes of reduced bioavailability of vascular PGI_2 in HUS have not been established, and several mechanisms may be involved. One of these may be deficiency of a plasma factor that stimulates PGI_2 synthesis (67). This factor is present in normal plasma, and it stimulates PGI_2 generation by cultured endothelial cells (74). It has been partially purified and characterized in plasma from human volunteers (75) and is a stable, highly polar substance, with a relative molecular mass (*M*r) of 300–400 Da that protects the vascular PGI_2-forming system from inactivation during persistent endothelial injury. Deficiency of this factor may explain the occurrence of remissions in some adults after infusion of fresh-frozen plasma (76, 77). The significance of abnormal plasma PGI_2-stimulating activity in HUS seems to be a feature of adult and atypical childhood forms of the HUS, whereas most children with typical HUS have normal PGI_2-stimulating activity (65). Changes in PGI_2-stimulating activity may be related to the different phases of the disease. In patients with HUS, the deficiency of a plasma factor found in the acute phase of the disease may persist long after clinical remission (70, 78). A similar deficiency has been documented in family members of HUS patients who had no history of microangiopathy (78, 79). However, not all the methods used to evaluate PGI_2-stimulating activity of plasma from HUS patients measure the PGI_2 produced by the endothelial cells actually involved in the microangiopathic process (80). Therefore, although plasma from HUS patients often has a decreased capability to stimulate PGI_2 generation by endothelium, its relationship to the pathogenesis of the disease remains difficult to establish. Other mechanisms implicated in the reduced bioavailability of vascular PGI_2 in HUS include defective serum PGI_2 binding (81) and accelerated PGI_2 degradation (82). Decreased PGI_2-stimulating activity in the sporadic form of HUS was ascribed to the presence of an inhibitor of PGI_2 production, rather than to a deficiency of stimulating factors (83). These findings suggest that a primary or secondary defect in PGI_2 bioavailability is present in HUS. Recent studies (84) in children, during the acute phase of the disease, have measured in vivo formation of PGI_2 in parallel with that of thromboxane-A_2 (TxA_2). The latter is a potent vasoconstrictor and platelet-aggregating prostanoid that is synthesized mainly by platelets. A highly specific, noninvasive method demonstrated a marked increase in the urinary TxA_2 metabolites—11-dehydro-TxB_2 and 2,3-dinor-TxB_2, which are index metabolites of TxA_2 activation in the systemic circulation (85, 86)—and TxB_2, primarily reflecting renal TxA_2 formation (87). The increased TxA_2 formation was apparently associated with an enhanced endogenous biosynthesis of PGI_2, as assessed by measuring urinary excretion of 2-3-dinor-6-keto $PGF_{1\alpha}$ and 6-keto $PGF_{1\alpha}$, which are possible indexes of extrarenal and renal synthesis of PGI_2, respectively (88, 89). However, when considering the relative increase in urinary excretion of TxA_2 and PGI_2 metabolites, the enormous increase in TxA_2 (up to 160 times the basal value) was accompanied by a modest increase of PGI_2 (up to 40 times the basal value). Therefore, the normal "balance" between the two eicosanoids was shifted toward the proaggregatory TxA_2 in HUS because of a relative deficiency in PGI_2 synthesis. This is the best evidence yet of a relative deficiency of PGI_2 synthesis in HUS. The finding that TXA_2 biosynthesis is increased during the acute phase of the HUS is not surprising in view of the process of concomitant platelet activation.

Vascular damage can also alter mechanisms governing endothelial cell release of vWF in HUS. Unusually large vWF multimers were found in plasma samples from four patients with chronic relapsing forms of TTP (90). These large vWF multimers were similar to the very large vWF multimers synthesized and secreted by human endothelial cells in culture and were most apparent in plasma obtained during remission. Relapses were characterized by intravascular platelet agglutination, thrombocytopenia, symptoms of vascular ischemia, and decreased plasma levels of the unusually large vWF multimers (presumably because they were binding to and agglutinating platelets in vivo). It was suggested (90) that these patients had a defect in the processing of the large vWF multimers after synthesis and secretion by endothelial cells and that, because these multimers persisted in the circulation, they predisposed patients to microvascular thrombosis and relapses. Abnormalities in vWF were found only during the acute episodes in the plasma of patients with HUS (66). However, the type of vWF abnormality was distinct from that observed in the plasma of patients with chronic relapsing TTP. In the seven patients studied, the largest vWF forms were relatively decreased. Plasma vWF multimer patterns returned to normal as the patients recovered. It was suggested that the largest vWF multimer forms could have been selectively deposited onto the exposed subendothelial surfaces of injured renal vessels, thereby increasing platelet–subendothelial attachment (66). Alternatively, selective interactions between the largest plasma vWF forms and platelets could have occurred during the acute HUS episode, so that these largest plasma vWF multimer forms were then relatively diminished in peripheral venous samples. Unusually large vWF multimer forms derived from endothelial cells were not found in the plasma of any of the seven patients, either during or after their HUS episodes. In contrast to patients with chronic relapsing TTP, there was no evidence that the HUS patients had a defect in the conversion of unusually large vWF multimers derived from endothelial cells to the vWF forms normally present in the circulation. Rose et al. (91) observed an increase in the concentration of high molecular mass vWF multimers during the acute phase of HUS in children. It seems that changes in vWF multimeric structure occur often in TTP and HUS; however, whether they are the cause or a consequence of endothelial injury is a matter of speculation.

In an attempt to interpret all these findings it must be recognized that artifacts caused by in vitro proteolysis may have influenced the data, because most studies did not use protease inhibitors during sampling. This issue of enhanced proteolysis of vWF occurring in vivo has been studied in eight patients with acute HUS or TTP whose blood samples were collected into an anticoagulant that contained a cocktail of protease inhibitors to inhibit in vitro proteolysis (92). Enhanced proteolytic degradation of vWF was found in all. This was expressed as a relative decrease in the intact 225-kd subunit of vWF and a relative increase in the 176-kd fragment in comparison with normal subjects or plasma from HUS or TTP patients during remission. However, enhanced vWF proteolysis was not accompanied by the loss of larger vWF multimers, as previously reported (66), but seven of the eight patients had a supranormal multimeric structure (i.e., a subset of multimers larger than the large forms present in normal plasma). In five patients (three with HUS and two with chronic relapsing TTP) who survived the acute disease and underwent plasma exchange, subunits and fragments returned to normal values and supranormal multimers disappeared. Consequently, it was suggested (92) that during acute disease, supranormal multimers leak from damaged endothelial cells, and that plasma exchange, by removing substances injurious to endothelial cells, stops endothelial damage. Supranormal multimers reappear in plasma during remission only in patients with the chronic relapsing form of TTP, in which a pathological process that maintains endothelial damage is active (90).

Plasma from patients with TTP can induce agglutination of autologous and homologous platelets (93). This is consistent with the isolation from the plasma of some TTP patients of an IgG antibody that specifically binds to endothelial cells, causing cell damage and inducing platelet aggregation (94). It has been hypothesized that these mechanisms could also operate in vivo to produce endothelial destruction and thrombotic vascular occlusions. Moreover, the isolation and purification from TTP plasma of an 37,000-Da protein that is a potent agglutinator of normal platelets (95) supports the hypothesis that complex abnormalities in circulating factors promote thrombus formation in the microcirculation by interacting with platelets, vWF and vascular endothelium.

IMPAIRMENT OF ENDOTHELIAL CELL FIBRINOLYTIC ACTIVITY IN THE HEMOLYTIC UREMIC SYNDROME

In addition to PGI_2 and vWF other substances of endothelial origin are involved in the antithrombotic process of normal endothelium and may be produced abnormally in HUS and TTP (96). Endothelial cells synthesize and release tissue plasminogen activator (t-PA), which has an important role in the fibrinolytic system (97, 98). Inhibitors of fibrinolysis acting against t-PA are also produced by endothelial cells (98). Absence of t-PA activity has been found in the vessels occluded by thrombi of TTP patients (98, 99). This abnormality predominated in capillaries in which, under normal conditions, fibrinolytic activity is most active. It was suggested that the absence of local fibrinolytic activity at the site of the lesion could be the result of primary endothelial damage or, alternatively, of the secretion by platelets of plasminogen activator and plasmin inhibitors.

Bergstein et al. (100), using a fibrin slide technique, demonstrated the presence of a circulating inhibitor of glomerular fibrinolysis in plasma from children with HUS and suggested that the inhibitor could play an important role in the pathogenesis and persistence of glomerular fibrin deposition. An impaired fibrinolytic activity in HUS and TTP was further documented by Glas-Greenwalt et al. (101), who measured the t-PA and inhibitors of fibrinolysis in the peripheral blood of patients with TTP. They found that in 11 of 12 patients t-PA activity was low or unmeasurable, whereas t-PA inhibitors were significantly elevated in all of the patients. It was hypothesized that t-PA inhibitors could originate from profusely proliferating endothelial cells in the HUS or TTP lesion and by forming complexes with t-PA, render the circulating t-PA inactive (101).

CONCLUSIONS

There is increasing recognition that endothelial cells have a pivotal role in the pathogenesis of HUS and TTP. The microvascular lesion is central to the pathogenesis in this syndrome (102). Morphological studies performed in the best available model of HUS indicates that the endothelial damage precedes the deposition of polymorphonuclear leukocytes and platelets within the glomerular capillary lumen (33). Toxins, drugs, or stimuli of different origins have been suggested as causative agents of HUS and TTP. Such agents may induce endothelial damage, thereby triggering the sequence of events leading to the deposition and formation of platelet thrombi in microvessels. Changes in mediators of endothelial origin, such as PGI_2, vWF, and t-PA, may be crucial in determining the severity of the lesions and the duration and outcome of the syndrome. Although, in recent years, many attempts have been made to identify the different factors possibly involved in the pathogenesis of HUS and TTP, further studies that will enable us to better understand the disease and improve the present therapeutic strategies are still needed.

REFERENCES

1. Gasser, C., Gautier, E., Steck, A., Siebenmann, R. E., Oechslin, R., Hamolytisch–uramische syndrome: Bilaterale nierenrindennekrosen bei akuten erworbenen hamolytischen anamien. *Schweiz. Med. Wochenschr.*, *85*: 905–909 (1955).
2. Gianantonio, C. A., Vitacco, M., Mendilarzu, F., Gallo, G. E., Sojo, E. T., The hemolytic–uremic syndrome. *Nephron, 11*: 174–192 (1973).
3. Fong, J. S. L., de Chadarevian, J. P., Kaplan, B. S., Hemolytic–uremic syndrome. Current concepts and management. *Pediatr. Clin. North Am.*, *29*: 835–856 (1982).
4. Kaplan, B. S., Remuzzi, G., The haemolytic uraemic syndrome. In *Haemostasis and the Kidney*, Vol. 6 (G. Remuzzi, E. C. Rossi, eds.), Butterworths, London, pp. 201–236 (1989).
5. Moschcowitz, E., Acute febrile pleiochromic anemia with hyaline thrombosis of the terminal arterioles and capillaries: An undescribed disease. *Arch. Intern. Med.*, *36*: 89–93 (1925).
6. Amorosi, E. L., Ultmann, J. E., Thrombotic thrombocytopenic purpura: Report of 16 cases and review of the literature. *Medicine, 45*: 139–159 (1966).
7. Bukowski, R. M., Thrombotic thrombocytopenic purpura: A review. In *Progress in Hemostasis and Thrombosis* (T. H. Spaet, ed.), Grune & Stratton, New York, pp. 287–336 (1982).
8. Rossi, E. C., Thrombotic thrombocytopenic purpura: A disseminated form of thrombotic microangiopathy. In *Haemostasis and the Kidney* (G. Remuzzi, E. C. Rossi, eds.), Butterworths, London, pp. 237–258 (1989).
9. Nalbandian, R. M., Henry, R. L., Bick, R. L., Thrombotic thrombocytopenic purpura. An extended editorial. *Semin. Thromb. Hemost.*, *5*: 216–240 (1979).
10. Remuzzi, G., HUS and TTP: Variable expression of a single entity. *Kidney Int.*, *32*: 292–308 (1987).
11. Symmers, W. S. C., Thrombotic microangiopathic haemolytic anaemia (thrombotic microangiopathy). *Br. Med. J.*, *2*: 897–903 (1952).

12. Habib, R., Mathieu, H., Royer, P., Le syndrome hemolitique et uremique de l'enfant. *Nephron, 4*: 139–172 (1967).
13. Gore, I., Disseminated arteriolar and capillary platelet thrombosis; a morphologic study of its histogenesis. *Am. J. Pathol., 26*: 155–175 (1950).
14. Proesmans, W., Muaka, K. I., Van Damme, B., Eeckels, R., The use of heparin in childhood hemolytic–uremic syndrome. In *Hemostasis, Prostaglandins and Renal Disease* (G. Remuzzi, G. Mecca, and G. de Gaetano, eds.), Raven Press, New York, pp. 407–411 (1980).
15. Sheth, K. J., Swich, H. M., Haworth, N., Neurological involvement in hemolytic–uremic syndrome. *Ann. Neurol., 19*: 90–93 (1986).
16. Dunea, G., Muehrcke, R. C., Nakamoto, S., Schwartz, F. D., Thrombotic thrombocytopenic purpura with acute anuric renal failure. *Am. J. Med., 41*: 1000–1006 (1966).
17. Eknoyan, G., Riggs, S. A., Renal involvement in patients with thrombotic thrombocytopenic purpura. *Am. J. Nephrol., 6*: 117–131 (1986).
18. Remuzzi, G., Thrombotic thrombocytopenic purpura and allied disorders. In *Thrombosis and Haemostasis* (M. Verstraete, J. Vermylen, H. R., Lijnen, J., Arnout, eds.), Leuven University Press, Leuven, pp. 673–708 (1987).
19. Vitsky, B. H., Suzuki, Y., Strauss, L., Churg, J., The hemolytic–uremic syndrome: A study of renal pathologic alterations. *Am. J. Pathol., 57*: 627–647 (1969).
20. Habib, R., Courtecuisse, V., Leclerc, F., Mathieu, H., Royer, P., Etude anatomopathologique de 35 observations de syndrome hémolytique et urémique de l'enfant. *Arch. Fr. Pediatr., 26*: 391–416 (1969).
21. Levy, M., Gagnadoux, M. F., Habib, R., Pathology of hemolytic–uremic syndrome in children. In *Hemostasis, Prostaglandins and Renal Disease* (G. Remuzzi, G. Mecca, G. De Gaetano, eds.), Raven Press, New York, pp. 383–397 (1980).
22. Churg, J., Goldstein, M. H., Bernstein, J., Thrombotic microangiopathy including hemolytic–uremic syndrome, thrombotic thrombocytopenic purpura, and postpartum renal failure. In *Renal Pathology with Clinical and Functional Correlations*, Vol. 2. (C. C. Tisher, B. M., Brenner, eds.), J. B. Lippincott, Philadelphia, pp. 1081–1113 (1989).
23. Kanfer, A., Morel-Maroger, L., Solez, K., Sraer, J. D., Richet, G., The value of renal biopsy in hemolytic uremic syndrome in adults. In *Hemostasis, Prostaglandins and Renal Disease* (G. Remuzzi, G. Mecca, G. de Gaetano, eds.), Raven Press, New York, pp. 399–406 (1980).
24. Pirani, C. L., Coagulation and renal disease. In *Glomerular Injury 300 Years After Morgagni* (T. Bertani, G. Remuzzi, eds.), Wichtig Editore, Milan, pp. 119–138 (1983).
25. Gianantonio, C. A., Extrarenal manifestations of the hemolytic uremic syndrome. In *Acute Renal Disorders and Renal Emergencies* (J. Strauss, ed.), J. Martinus Nijhoff, Boston, pp. 43–50 (1984).
26. Koster, F., Levin, J., Walker, L., Tung, K. S. K., Gilman, R. H., Rahaman, M. M., Majid, M. A., Islam, S., Williams, R C., Hemolytic–uremic syndrome after shigellosis: Relation to endotoxemia and circulating immune complexes. *N. Engl. J. Med., 298*: 927–933 (1978).
27. Baker, N. M., Millis, A. E., Rachman, I., Thomas, J. E. P., Haemolytic–uraemic syndrome in typhoid fever. *Br. Med. J., 2*: 84–87 (1974).
28. Harlan, J. M., Harker, L. A., Reidy, M. A., Gajdusek, C. M., Schwartz, S. M., Striker, G. E., Lipopolysaccharide-mediated bovine endothelial cell injury in vitro. *Lab. Invest., 48*: 269–274 (1983).
29. Harlan, J. M., Harker, L. A., Striker, G. E., Weaver, L. J., Effects of lipopolysaccharide on human endothelial cell in culture. *Thromb. Res., 29*: 15–26 (1983).
30. Yamada, O., Moldow, C. F., Sacks, T., Craddock, P. R., Boogaerts, M. A., Jacob, H. S., Deleterious effect of endotoxin on cultured endothelial cells: An in vitro model of vascular injury. *Inflammation, 5*: 115–126 (1981).

31. Thomas, L., Good, R. A., Studies on the generalized Shwartzman reaction. I. General observations concerning the phenomenon. *J. Exp. Med.*, *96*: 605–613 (1952).
32. Vedanarayanan, V. V., Kaplan, B. S., Fong, J. S. C., Neutrophil function in an experimental model of hemolytic uremic syndrome. *Pediatar. Res.*, *21*: 252–256 (1987).
33. Bertani, T., Abbate, M., Zoja, C., Corna, D., Remuzzi, G., Sequence of glomerular changes in experimental endotoxemia: A possible model of hemolytic uremic syndrome. *Nephron*, *53*: 330–337 (1989).
34. Karmali, M. A., Steele, B. T., Petric, M., Lim, C., Sporadic cases of haemolytic–uraemic syndrome associated with faecal cytotoxin and cytotoxin-producing *Escherichia coli* in stools. *Lancet*, *1*: 619–620 (1983).
35. Karmali, M. A., Petric, M., Lim, C., Fleming, P. C., Arbus, G. S., Lior, M., The association between idiopathic hemolytic uremic syndrome and infection by verotoxin-producing *Escherichia coli*. *J. Infect. Dis.*, *151*: 775–782 (1985).
36. Editorial, Unravelling HUS. *Lancet*, *2*: 1437–1439 (1987).
37. Kavi, J., Wise, R., Causes of the haemolytic uraemic syndrome. It might be verocytotoxin produced by *Escherichia coli*. *Br. Med. J.*, *298*: 65–66 (1989).
38. O'Brien, A. D., Lively, T. A., Chen, M. E., Rothman, S. W., Formal, S. B., *Escherichia coli* O157:H7 strains associated with haemorrhagic colitis in the United States produce a *Shigella dysenteriae* 1 (Shiga) like cytotoxin. *Lancet*, *1*: 702 (1983).
39. O'Brien, A. D., Holmes, R. K., Shiga and Shiga-like toxins. *Microbiol. Rev.*, *51*: 206–220 (1987).
40. Lingwood, C. A., Law, H., Richardson, S., Petric, M., Brunton, J. L., de Grandis, S., Karmali, M., Glycolipid binding of purified and recombinant *E. coli* produced verotoxin in vitro. *J. Biol. Chem.*, *262*: 8834–8839 (1987).
41. Obrig, T. G., Del Vecchio, P. J., Karmali, M. A., Petric, M., Moran, T. P., Judge, T. K., Pathogenesis of haemolytic uraemic syndrome (letter). *Lancet*, *2*: 687 (1987).
42. Kavi, J., Chant, I., Maris, M., Rose, P. E., Cytopathic effect of verotoxin on endothelial cells. *Lancet*, *2*: 1035 (1987).
43. Obrig, T. G., Del Vecchio, P. J., Brown, J. E., Moran, T. P., Rowland, B. M., Judge, T. K., Rothman, S. W., Direct cytotoxic action of Shiga toxin on human vascular endothelial cells. *Infect. Immun.*, *56*: 2373–2378 (1988).
44. Karch, H., Bitzan, M., Pietsch, R., Stenger, K.-O., von Wulffen, H., Heesemann, J., Dusing, R., Purified verotoxins of *Escherichia coli* 0157:H7 decrease prostacyclin synthesis by endothelial cells. *Microb. Pathogen.*, *5*: 215–221 (1988).
45. Richardson, S. E., Jagadha, V., Smith, C. R., Becker, L. E., Petric, M., Karmali, M. A., Pathological effects on injected H.30 verotoxin (VT) in rabbits. *Abstr. Annu. Meet. Am. Soc. Microbiol.*, p. 42 (1987).
46. Klein, P. J., Bulla, M., Newman, R. A., Muller, P., Uhlenbruck, G., Schaefer, H. E., Kruger, G., Fisher, R., Thomsen–Friedenreich antigen in haemolytic uraemic syndrome (letter). *Lancet*, *2*: 1024–1025 (1977).
47. Leung, D. Y. M., Moake, J. L., Havens, P. L., Kim, M., Pober, J. S., Lytic anti-endothelial cell antibodies in haemolytic–uraemic syndrome. *Lancet*, *2*: 183–186. (1988).
48. Forsyth, K. D., Simpson, A. C., Fitzpatrick, M. M., Barratt, T. M., Levinsky, R. J., Neutrophil-mediated endothelial injury in haemolytic uraemic syndrome. *Lancet*, *2*: 411–414 (1989).
49a. Kaplan, B. S., Mills, M., Elevated serum elastase and alpha-1-antitrypsin levels in hemolytic uremic syndrome. *Clin. Nephrol.*, *30*: 193–196 (1988).
49b. Milford, D., Taylor, C. M., Rafaat, F., Halloran, E., Neutrophil elastases and haemolytic uraemic syndrome. *Lancet*, *2*: 1153 (1989).
50. Mihatsch, M. J., Thiel, G., Spichtin, H. P., Oberholzer, M., Brunner, F. P., Harder, F., Olivieri, V., Bremer, B., Stocklin, E., Torhorst, Y., Gudat, F., Zollinger, H. U., Morphological findings in kidney transplants after treatment with cyclosporine. *Transplant. Proc.*, *15*: 2821–2835 (1983).

51. Shulmann, H., Striker, G., Deeg, H. J., Kennedy, M., Storb, R., Thomas, E. D., Nephrotoxicity of cyclosporin A after allogeneic marrow transplantation: Glomerular thromboses and tubular injury. *N. Engl. J. Med.*, *305*: 1392–1395 (1981).
52. Bonser, R. S., Adu, D., Franklin, I., McMaster, P., Cyclosporin-induced haemolytic uraemic syndrome in liver allograft recipient. *Lancet*, *2*: 1337–1339 (1984).
53. Leithner, C., Sinzinger, H., Pohanka, E., Schwarz, M., Kretschmer, G., Syre, G., Recurrence of haemolytic uraemic syndrome triggered by cyclosporin A after renal transplantation. *Lancet*, *2*: 1470 (1982).
54. Remuzzi, G., Bertani, T., Renal vascular and thrombotic effects of cyclosporine. *Am. J. Kidney Dis.*, *4*: 261–272 (1989).
55. Lyman, N. W., Michaelson, R., Viscuso, R. L., Winn, R., Mulgaonaker, S., Jacobs, M. G., Mitomycin-induced hemolytic uremic syndrome. Successful treatment with corticosteroids and intense plasma exchange. *Arch. Intern. Med.*, *143*: 1617–1618 (1983).
56. Giroux, L., Bettez, P., Giroux, L., Mitomycin-C nephrotoxicity: A clinico-pathologic study of 17 cases. *Am. J. Kidney Dis.*, *6*: 28–39 (1985).
57. Zoja, C., Furci, L., Ghilardi, F., Zilio, P., Benigni, A., Remuzzi, G., Cyclosporin-induced endothelial cell injury. *Lab. Invest.*, *55*: 455–462 (1986).
58. Lau, D. C. W., Wong, K.-L., Hwang, W. S., Cyclosporine toxicity on cultured rat microvascular endothelial cells. *Kidney Int.*, *35*: 604–613 (1989).
59. Bertani, T., Perico, N., Abbate, M., Battaglia, C., Remuzzi, G., Renal injury induced by long-term administration of cyclosporin A to rats. *Am. J. Pathol.*, *127*: 569–579 (1987).
60. Cattell, V., Mitomycin-induced hemolytic uremic kidney. An experimental model in the rat. *Am. J. Pathol.*, *121*: 88–95 (1985).
61. Moncada, S., Prostacyclin and thromboxane A_2 in the regulation of platelet–vascular interactions. In *Hemostasis, prostaglandins and Renal Disease* (G. Remuzzi, G. Mecca, and G. de Gaetano, eds.,), Raven Press, New York, pp. 175–188 (1980).
62. FitzGerald, G. A., Brash, A. R., Falardeau, P., Oates, J. A., Estimated rate of prostacyclin secretion into the circulation of normal man. *J. Clin. Invest.*, *68*: 1272–1276 (1981).
63. Jaffe, E. A., Nachman, R. L., Subunit structure of factor VIII antigen synthesized by cultured human endothelial cells. *J. Clin. Invest.*, *56*: 698–702 (1975).
64. Sixma, J. J., Role of blood vessel, platelet and coagulation interactions in haemostasis. In *Haemostasis and Thrombosis* (A. L. Bloom, D. P. Thomas, eds.), Churchill-Livingston, Edinburgh, pp. 252–267 (1981).
65. Remuzzi, G., Zoja, C., Rossi, E. C., Prostacyclin in thrombotic microangiopathy. *Semin. Hematol.*, *24*: 110–118 (1987).
66. Moake, J. L., Byrness, J. J., Troll, J. H., Rudy, C. K., Weistein, M. J., Colannino, N. M., Hong, S. L., Abnormal fVIII–von Willebrand factor patterns in the plasma of patients with the hemolytic uremic syndrome. *Blood*, *64*: 592–598 (1984).
67. Remuzzi, G., Misiani, R., Marchesi, D., Livio, M., Mecca, G., de Gaetano, G., Donati, M. B., Haemolytic uraemic syndrome deficiency of plasma factor(s) regulating prostacyclin activity? *Lancet*, *2*: 871–872 (1978).
68. Defreyn, G., Proesmans, W., Machin, S. J., Lemmens, F., Vermylen, J., Abnormal prostacyclin metabolism in the hemolytic uremic syndrome: Equivocal effect of prostacyclin infusion. *Clin. Nephrol.*, *18*: 43–49 (1982).
69. Stuart, M. J., Spitzer, R. E., Coppe, D., Abnormal platelet and vascular prostaglandin synthesis in an infant with hemolytic uremic syndrome. *Pediatrics*, *71*: 120–124 (1983).
70. Turi, S., Beattie, T. J., Belch, J. J. F., Murphy, A. V., Disturbances of prostacyclin metabolism in children with hemolytic–uremic syndrome and in first degree relatives. *Clin. Nephrol.*, *25*: 193–198 (1986).
71. Goldsmith, J. C., Contribution of the subendothelium to prostacyclin release after vascular injury. *J. Lab. Clin. Med.*, *100*: 574–584 (1982).

72. Kent, R. S., Diedrich, S. L., Whorton, A. R., Regulation of vascular prostaglandin synthesis by metabolites of arachidonic acid in perfused rabbit aorta. *J. Clin. Invest.*, *72*: 455–456 (1983).
73. Ham, E. A., Egan, R. W., Soderman, D. D., Gale, P. H., Kuehl, F. A., Jr., Peroxidase-dependent deactivation of prostacyclin synthetase. *J. Biol. Chem.*, *254*: 2191–2194 (1979).
74. MacIntyre, D. E., Pearson, J. D., Gordon, J. L., Localisation and stimulation of prostacyclin production in vascular cells. *Nature*, *271*: 549–551 (1978).
75. Deckmyn, H., Zoja, C., Arnout, J., Todisco, A., Vanden Bulcke, F., D'Hondt, L., Hendrickx, N., Gresele, P., Vermylen, J., Partial isolation and function of the prostacyclin regulating plasma factor. *Clin. Sci.*, *69*: 383–393 (1985).
76. Remuzzi, G., Misiani, R., Marchesi, D., Livio, M., Mecca, G., de Gaetano, G., Donati, M. B., Treatment of the hemolytic–uremic syndrome with plasma. *Clin. Nephrol.*, *12*: 279–284 (1979).
77. Misiani, R., Appiani, A. C., Edefonti, A., Gotti, E., Bettinelli, A., Giani, M., Rossi, E., Remuzzi, G., Mecca, G., Haemolytic uraemic syndrome: Therapeutic effect of plasma infusion. *Br. Med. J.*, *285*: 1304–1306 (1982).
78. Remuzzi, G., Marchesi, D., Misiani, R., Mecca, G., de Gaetano, G., Donati, M. B., Familial deficiency of a plasma factor stimulating prostacyclin activity. *Thromb. Res.*, *16*: 517–525 (1979).
79. Jorgensen, K. A., Pedersen, R. S., Familial deficiency of prostacyclin production stimulating factor in the hemolytic uremic syndrome of childhood. *Thromb. Res.*, *21*: 311–315 (1981).
80. Siegler, R. L., Smith, J. B., Linch, M. B., Mohammad, S. F., In vitro prostacyclin production in the hemolytic uremic syndrome. *West. J. Med.*, *144*: 165–168 (1986).
81. Wu, K. K., Hall, R. R., Rossi, E. C., Papp, A. C., Serum prostacyclin binding defects in thrombotic thrombocytopenic purpura. *J. Clin. Invest.*, *75*: 168–174 (1985).
82. Chen, Y. C., McLeod, B., Hall, E. R., Wu, K. K., Accelerated prostacyclin degradation in thrombotic thrombocytopenic purpura. *Lancet*, *2*: 267–269. (1981).
83. Levin, M., Elkon, K. B., Nokes, T. J. C., Bucle, A. M., Dillon, M. J., Hardisty, R. M., Barratt, T. M., Inhibitor of prostacyclin production in sporadic haemolytic uraemic syndrome. *Arch. Dis. Child.*, *58*: 703–708 (1983).
84. Tonshoff, B., Momper, R., Kuhl, P. G., Schweer, H., Scharer, K., Seyberth, H. W., Increased thromboxane biosynthesis in childhood hemolytic uremic syndrome. *Kidney Int.*, *37*: 1134–1141 (1990).
85. Reillly, I. A., Doran, J. B., Smith, B., FitzGerald, G. A., Increased thromboxane biosynthesis in a human model of platelet activation: Biochemical and functional consequences of selective inhibition of thromboxane synthase. *Circulation*, *73*: 1300–1309 (1986).
86. Catella, F., FitzGerald, G. A., Paired analysis of urinary thromboxane B_2 metabolites in humans. *Thromb. Res.*, *47*: 647–656 (1987).
87. Patrono, C., Ciabattoni, G., Remuzzi, G., Gotti, E., Bombardieri, S., Di Munno, O., Tartarelli, G., Cinotti, G. A., Simonetti, B. M., Pierucci, A., Functional significance of renal prostacyclin and thromboxane A_2 production in patients with systemic lupus erythematosus. *J. Clin. Invest.*, *76*: 1011–1018 (1985).
88. FitzGerald, G. A., Brash, A. R., Falardeau, P., Oates, J. A., Estimated rate of prostacyclin secretion into the circulation in normal man. *J. Clin. Invest.*, *68*: 1272–1276 (1981).
89. Catella, F., Nowak, J., FitzGerald, G. A., Measurement of renal and non-renal eicosanoid synthesis. *Am. J. Med.*, *81*: 23–29 (1986).
90. Moake, J. L., Rudy, C. K., Troll, J. H., Weinstein, M. J., Colannino, N. M., Azokar, J., Seder, R. H., Hong, S. L., Deykin, D., Unusually large plasma factor VIII:

von Willebrand factor multimers in chronic relapsing thrombotic thrombocytopenic purpura. *N. Engl. J. Med., 307*: 1432–1435 (1982).

91. Rose, P. E., Enayat, S. M., Sunderland, R., Short, P. E., Williams, C. E., Hill, F. G., Abnormalities of factor VIII related protein multimers in the haemolytic uraemic syndrome. *Arch. Dis. Child., 59*: 1135–1140 (1984).
92. Mannucci, P. M., Lombardi, R., Lattuada, A., Ruggenenti, P., Viganò, G. L., Barbui, T., Remuzzi, G., Enhanced proteolysis of plasma von Willebrand factor (vWF) in thrombotic thrombocytopenic purpura (TTP) and the hemolytic uremic syndrome. *Blood, 74*: 978–983 (1989).
93. Lian, E. C.-Y., Harkeness, D. R., Byrnes, J. J., Wallach, H., Nunez, R., The presence of platelet aggregating factor in the plasma of patients with thrombotic thrombocytopenic purpura and its inhibition by normal plasma. *Blood, 53*: 333–338 (1979).
94. Burns, E. R., Zucker-Franklin, D., Pathologic effects of plasma from patients with thrombotic thrombocytopenic purpura on platelets and cultured vascular endothelial cells. *Blood, 60*: 1030–1037 (1982).
95. Siddiqui, F. A., Lian, E.-Y., Novel platelet-agglutinating protein from a thrombotic thrombocytopenic purpura plasma. *J. Clin. Invest., 76*: 1330–1337 (1985).
96. Remuzzi, G., Bertani, T., Thrombotic thrombocytopenic purpura, hemolytic uremic syndrome, and acute cortical necrosis. In *Disease of the Kidney*, Vol. 2, 4th ed. (R. W. Schner, & C, W. Gottschalk, eds.), Little, Brown & Co., Boston, pp. 2301–2333 (1988).
97. Collen, D., On the regulation and control of fibrinolysis [Edward Kowalsky Memorial Lecture]. *Thromb. Haemost., 43*: 77–89 (1980).
98. Kwaan, H. C., Role of fibrinolysis in thrombotic thrombocytopenic purpura. *Semin. Hematol., 24*: 101–109 (1987).
99. Kwaan, H. C., Astrup, T., Demonstration of cellular fibrinolytic activity by the histochemical fibrin slide technique. *Lab. Invest., 17*: 140–145 (1969).
100. Bergstein, J. M., Kuederli, U., Bang, N. U., Plasma inhibitor of glomerular fibrinolysis in the hemolytic–uremic syndrome. *Am. J. Med., 73*: 322–327 (1982).
101. Glas-Greenwalt, P., Hall, J. M., Panke, T. W., Kant, K. S., Allen, C. M., Pollak, V. E., Fibrinolysis in health and disease: Abnormal levels of plasminogen activator, plasminogen activator inhibitor, and protein C in thrombotic thrombocytopenic purpura. *J. Lab. Clin. Med., 108*: 415–422 (1986).
102. Heptinstall, R. H., Hemolytic uremic syndrome thrombotic thrombocytopenic purpura, and systemic scleroderma (progressive systemic sclerosis). In *Pathology of the Kidney* (R. H. Heptinstall, ed.), Little, Brown & Co., Boston, pp. 907–961 (1983).

28
Pathogenesis of Shiga Toxin (Verotoxin)-Induced Endothelial Cell Injury

Tom G. Obrig *University of Rochester Medical Center, Rochester, New York*

During the past decade we have focused on the mode of action of natural protein toxins. Foremost in this group are the Shiga toxins, a series of closely related multipeptide toxins that are produced by several species of gram-negative bacteria pathogenic to humans. Karmali et al. (1, 2) and others (3–7) noticed the association of Shiga toxin (verotoxin)-producing dysentery bacteria with the development of the hemolytic uremic syndrome (HUS). Our research efforts were directed at defining the subcellular biochemical mode of action of the Shiga toxins, but when we became aware of the Shiga toxin–HUS relationship, we tested the idea that vascular endothelial cells may be sensitive to the toxin. This could help explain the observation that the renal endothelium is damaged in HUS. The positive results of these initial experiments set the stage for further studies. Since then, others have repeated these in vitro endothelial cytotoxicity studies with bacterial *(Escherichia coli)* extracts (8) and with purified Shiga-like toxin (Barrett, T. J., personal communication). Human renal endothelial cells express receptors for, and are very sensitive to, Shiga toxin (9). In addition, new data, discussed in the following and in other chapters of this book, continue to support the hypothesis that Shiga toxins may be capable of eliciting some of the physiological responses required for the development of the typical form of HUS.

This chapter includes a more detailed description of how the Shiga toxins interact with human vascular endothelial cells. In addition, some of the more salient features of the Shiga toxins are reviewed, particularly relative to structure, molecular genetics, and the subcellular action of these agents. Where possible, new information will be presented on data obtained from isolated endothelial cells of human umbilical and renal glomerular origin. These latter cells are the most sensitive to the Shiga toxins that we have tested to date. Finally, possible mechanisms of coagulation will be briefly described because our recent efforts have been directed toward elucidating how the Shiga toxins may cause endothelial cells to become more procoagulant. This will include our hypothesis on the roles of bacterial endotoxin/lipopolysaccharide (LPS) and cytokines (IL-1 β and TNF-α), which interact individually with endothelial cells. In addition, together with Shiga toxins, they may elicit synergistic negative physiological responses by endothelial cells that lead to HUS.

Throughout the chapter we will treat all members of the Shiga toxin family as being equipollent toward human endothelial cells in vitro. This has been our general experience, although the individual toxins differ in other respects (antigenicity, amino acid substitutions, and such), as noted elsewhere in this book.

SHIGA TOXINS: CHARACTERISTICS AND CYTOTOXIC MECHANISMS

Shiga toxin, purified from *Shigella dystenteriae* 1, is a 68,000-kD multisubunit complex that comprises a single 32-kd α-subunit and five 7.7-kD β-subunits (10–13). A generic structure of the Shiga toxins is shown in Figure 1. Shiga-like toxins (SLT-1, SLT-2, and SLT-2v) have also been purified from *E. coli* and, in many respects, appear similar to Shiga toxin (14, 15). These toxins have been the subject of a comprehensive review article (16). More recent work has shown the high degree of nucleotide (NT) sequence homology among Shiga toxin, SLT-1, and SLT-2 (17). It is generally accepted that Shiga toxin and SLT-1 are virtually identical, whereas SLT-2 is more antigenically distinct; all three bind to the same glycolipid receptor, Gb_3. The pig edema factor, SLT-2v, is not only more antigenically distant from the other three toxins, but appears to bind to a different glycolipid (i.e., Gb_4) than do these toxins (18).

Shiga toxin protein is encoded on the chromosome of *Shigella* bacteria, whereas the genes for the Shiga-like toxin produced by *E. coli* are carried by bacteriophages (viruses) that are resident in these bacteria (16). In both cases, the DNA structural genes for α- and β-subunit proteins are tandemly associated (Fig. 2). Therefore, transcription of these genes results in a messenger RNA that is dicistronic (i.e., an mRNA containing a single structural gene for the α-subunit is directly followed by a single copy of the β-subunit gene). Translation of this dicistronic mRNA to yield one α- and five β-proteins is most likely accomplished by more efficient initiation of translation of the β than of the α mRNAs.

The β-subunits of Shiga toxin facilitate binding of holotoxin to galactotriosylceramide (Gb_3), high-affinity (*K*d 10^{-10} M) cell surface receptors containing the unusual

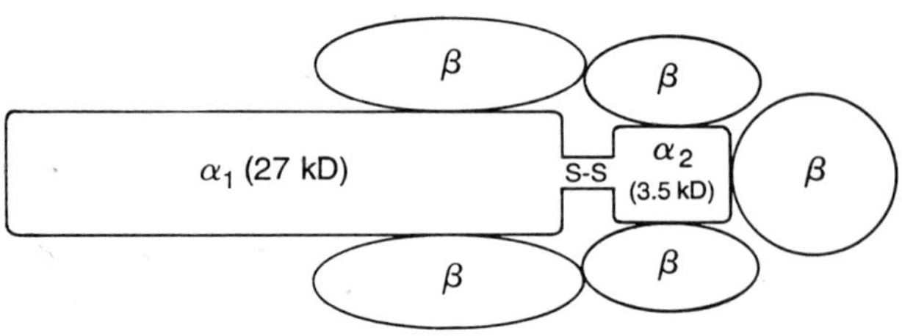

Figure 1 Generic structure of the Shiga toxins: Composition of the holotoxin depicting α- and β-subunits. The α-subunit is processed in target cells by trypsinlike enzyme activity and reduction of a disulfide bond to yield the fully active 27-kd glycosidase described in the text.

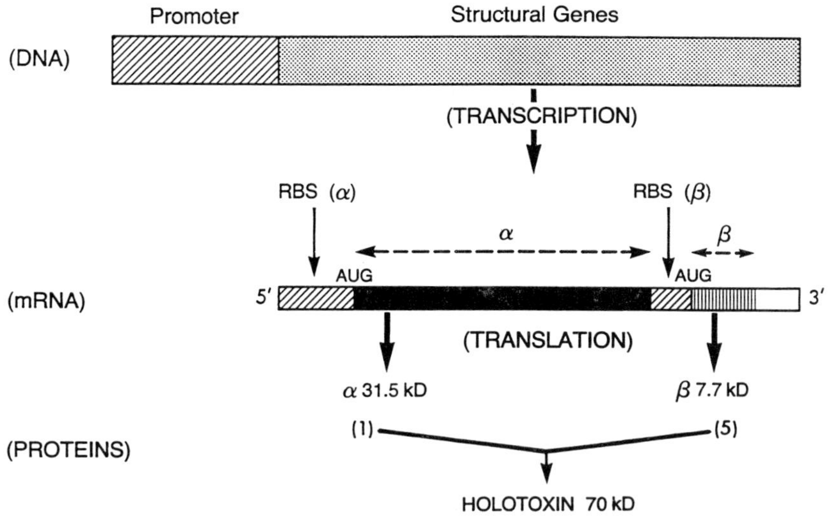

Figure 2 Transcription and translation of a Shiga toxin gene: Depicted are the regulatory and structural genes for SLT-1 and the general scheme for expression of the α- and β-subunit structural genes in *E. coli*. RBS is the ribosomal binding site for translation initiation.

carbohydrate linkage, galα1,4-gal (19). The structure of Gb_3, with its terminal disaccharide, is shown in Figure 3. It is important to recognize that binding of the toxins to Gb_3 has much in common with the binding of lectins to their receptors. More exactly, each of the five β-subunits of Shiga toxin can bind a Gb_3 molecule, which adds to the stability of toxin–receptor complex.

Entry of the holotoxin into "sensitive" cells is facilitated by a process generally recognized as receptor-mediated endocytosis (20–22). Most cell lines sensitive to Shiga toxin are derived from primates (20). Therefore, in vitro studies with the Shiga toxins frequently have been performed with human HeLa cells or monkey kidney

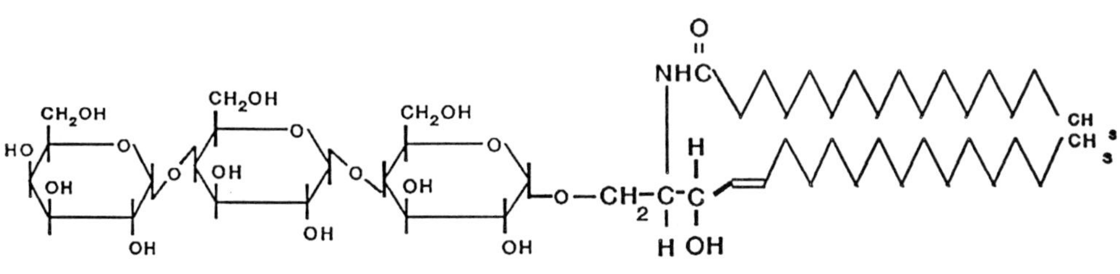

Gal α1→4Gal β1→4Glc β1→1Cer

Figure 3 Structure of the receptor for Shiga toxins: Globotriosyl ceramide (Gb_3) is a glycolipid located in plasma membranes of some eukaryotic cells that respond to Shiga toxin. Shiga toxins specifically recognize the terminal disaccharide and bind with high affinity to this receptor. Only SLT-2v (pig edema toxin) preferentially binds to a different receptor, Gb_4.

Vero cells. The term *verotoxin* is derived from the fact that the toxin from *E. coli* O157:H7 is cytotoxic to Vero cells (3). Other cells that are insensitive to Shiga toxin usually lack the high-affinity receptor, whereas a few may bind, but be unable to internalize the toxin (20, 23). During normal internalization, the α-subunit becomes separated from the β-subunits, and the α-subunit is processed further. Approximately 10% of the α-subunit protein is removed in a trypsinlike process, resulting in a maximally active 27-kD α-subunit enzyme. The specificity of Shiga toxin α-subunit *N*-glycohydrolase is one of the more interesting aspects of the toxin and is discussed in more detail later. Shiga toxin entry into HeLa cells (sensitive) requires energy, a pH of ≥ 6.5, <0.2 M KCl, and a temperature of $>20°C$ (20). Lysomotropic agents, such as chloroquine or NH_4Cl, which inhibit the entry of other toxins (e.g., diphtheria) by raising the internal pH of lysosomes, have no protective effect against Shiga toxin. Other agents (e.g., monensin) protect HeLa cells against Shiga toxin cytotoxic action by preventing fusion of endosomes and lysosomes, steps in the processing of Shiga toxin within the cytoplasm (20, 24).

Shiga toxin enters cells within 1 hr to affect protein synthesis (20). This is the primary process inhibited after exposure of cells to the toxin (25, 26). It is clear, from cell-free (27, 28) and whole-cell (26) protein synthesis data, that the α-subunit of Shiga toxin is responsible for the cytotoxic action, as it is a direct inhibitor of protein synthesis. Another mechanism of cytotoxicity has been proposed based on increased adenylate cyclase activity in cells treated with Shiga toxin (29). Although this is an attractive possibility, no further data have been forthcoming to support this hypothesis. It is equally possible that the toxin may act through signal transduction mechanisms when the agent can bind to, but cannot be internalized by, quiescent vascular endothelial cells. Currently, it is generally accepted that Shiga toxins are cytotoxic because of the catalytic and protein synthesis inhibitory nature of the α-subunit protein.

Whereas the holotoxin is required for inhibition of protein synthesis in whole cells, the 32-kD α-subunit protein alone does this in eukaryotic cell-free systems (13, 30). It has been established that Shiga toxin selectively catalytically inactivates 60S ribosomal subunits (30). That is, one toxin molecule is capable of inactivating 40+ ribosomes per minute at 37°C. A major breakthrough has been made in understanding the mechanism of action of Shiga toxin and other ribosome-inhibiting toxins (e.g., ricin). It is now clear that the physiologically relevant mode of action of these toxins is their *N*-glycohydrolase activity that depurinates (removes) one nucleotide in the 28S ribosomal RNA in a nucleotide-specific manner. Endo and co-workers (31, 32) detected a missing base within the 28S RNA of toxin-treated rat liver ribosomes. This was accomplished by comparison of the sequence of a 400+ NT fragment generated from the 3' terminus of 28S RNA by a contaminating RNase present in control as well as toxin-treated rat liver ribosomes. The sequencing of this fragment revealed that it contained the depurination site. Removal of a single adenine from within this RNA fragment was toxin-dependent, making the adjacent 3'-5'-phosphodiester bond labile to aniline, the cleavage reagent utilized in Maxam–Gilbert chemical sequencing reactions. These experiments have been repeated successfully by using frog oocytes injected with Shiga toxin (33). The *N*-glycohydrolase of these ribosome-inactivating proteins was shown to involve an active site that has amino acid sequence homology among other members of the class of ribosome-inactivating proteins, including ricin, a product of higher plants (34). Remarkably, removal by toxin of a single purine base from a ribosome that is more than 10,000 times larger than the base, renders this ribosome inactive for protein synthesis. Our results suggested that Shiga toxin may have been a ribonuclease, but this activity was demonstrable only when the toxin and free 28S ribosomal RNA were incubated in near equal molar quantity and, then, only in the absence of magnesium ions (35). This result, although consistent with the nature of other ribonuclease-active toxins (36) does not appear to be the functional mechanism of Shiga toxin under physiological conditions.

The corresponding functional lesion caused by Shiga toxin inactivation of ribosomes is at the level of peptide elongation. The primary step that is inhibited is eukaryotic elongation factor-1 (eEF-1)-dependent binding of aminoacyl (aa)-tRNA to ribosomes (37) (Fig. 4). However, the toxin-modified site on 60S ribosomes appears to involve the binding sites for both eEF-1 and eEF-2, which were previously shown to overlap on bacterial and eukaryotic ribosomes. Therefore, Shiga toxin secondarily inhibits eEF-2-dependent translocation of aa-tRNA from the ribosomal *A* to the *P* site (37).

PATHOGENESIS OF *SHIGELLA DYSENTERIAE* 1 AND ENTEROHEMORRHAGIC *ESCHERICHIA COLI*

Our working hypothesis is that *S. dysenteriae* 1 and Shiga toxin-producing *E. coli* are responsible for the vascular disease associated with infection of humans by these organisms. Furthermore, this characteristic is primarily due to the Shiga toxin made by such bacteria. If this is true, then Shiga toxin may not be required for shigellae to successfully colonize and invade colonic epithelial cells, but only for subsequent action at the vascular level. Similarly, Shiga-like toxin produced by enterohemorrhagic *E. coli* (EHEC) may not be necessary for colonizing the intestine or for production of the earlier diarrheal phase of this disease. Both of these pathogens produce at least one form of Shiga toxin, and both cause hemorrhagic colitis (HC) and perhaps HUS (38–44). This is not to say that Shiga toxin can cause HUS without the assistance of other factors, but that it is the primary agent that

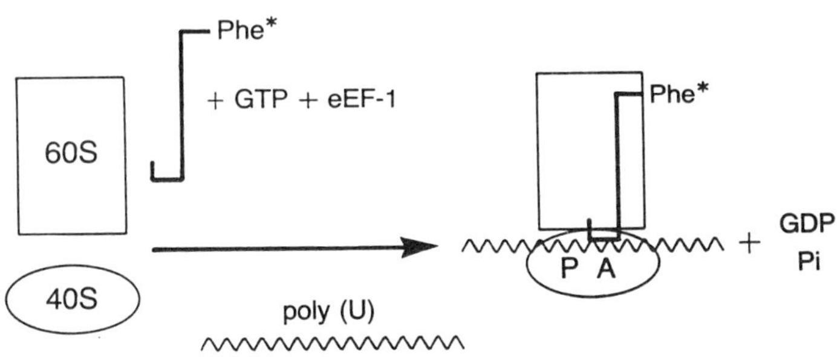

Figure 4 Shiga toxin inhibition of protein synthesis: The primary step of peptide elongation inhibited on Shiga toxin-inactivated ribosomes is presented. Eukaryotic elongation factor 1 (eEF-1) is required for binding of aminoacyl-RNAs (aa-tRNAs) to the ribosomal "acceptor" (A) site in a mRNA codon-dependent manner. Phenylalanyl-tRNA (Phe-tRNA) is used as an example of an aa-tRNA in this figure.

makes the development of HUS possible. Moreover, we have proposed that bacterial endotoxin (LPS) elaborated by the gram-negative Shiga toxin-producing pathogens, and the cytokines elicited by LPS, are necessary for the initiation of HUS.

The role of Shiga toxin in shigella-related dysentery has been a major topic of debate for many years. New data indicate a role for Shiga toxin as a vascular-acting factor, and these data are best viewed in the overall scheme of the infectious process for *S. dysenteriae* 1. The steps include: (a) localization of bacteria on the colonic mucosa; (b) invasion of colonic epithelial cells and multiplication of bacteria within these cells; (c) killing of the colonic cells; (d) ensuing damage to the underlying tissue, resulting in hemorrhage (i.e., bloody dysentery); and (e) in some cases, development of the renal or systemic vascular complication, HUS. This suggests that Shiga toxin is *not* required for steps *a* through *c*. Instead, the results indicate that Shiga toxin is responsible for the vascular aspects of this complicated disease process.

A somewhat recent report has provided important evidence that the Shiga toxins are required for the vascular conditions of hemorrhagic colitis associated with shigella and EHEC infections (45). In this study, a *tox–*, isogenic strain of *S. dysenteriae* 1 was created by modification of the wild-type strain. Inactivation of the Shiga toxin gene was accomplished by insertion of foreign genetic information into the gene for the α-subunit of Shiga toxin. Therefore, only defective α-subunit protein was produced, whereas this newly created isogenic strain remained identical with the wild-type parent in all other respects. Monkeys were then challenged orally with the wild-type or *tox–* isogenic strains. The response of the animals was similar in that both bacterial strains caused gastrointestinal distress other than bloody dysentery. However, only the wild-type *Shigella* was capable of generating gastrointestinal vascular damage (45). This study provides powerful evidence that the primary role of Shiga toxin may be at the vascular level, and that the toxin has nothing to do with other aspects of the pathogenesis of shigella dysentery, and this is probably true for EHEC bacteria as well. A key genetic element that could be added to the Koch's postulate would be to repeat the challenge after reintroducing the α-subunit gene into the *tox–* strain.

SHIGA TOXIN INTERACTION WITH HUMAN ENDOTHELIAL CELLS

Because it is believed that endothelial cells represent the primary site of initiation of HUS, we have focused our attention on the role of endothelial cells in exploration of a relation between the Shiga toxins and vascular disease. Clinical observations were largely responsible for the concept that endothelium could be the site of primary damage in HUS. Histopathological examination of samples from HUS patients revealed glomerular vascular capillaries with swollen endothelial cells (46, 47). Microvascular angiopathy was present in all patients with HUS who were infected with verotoxin-producing *E. coli* (46) and endothelial cells were the putative primary target cells of the verocytotoxin. Different workers concluded that shigella toxin probably acted by damaging endothelial cells (48, 49). Although these investigators were referring to Shiga toxin as a neurotoxin, it has been demonstrated that the Shiga holotoxin exhibits cytotoxic, neurotoxic and enterotoxic activities (50, 51). Moreover, the neurotoxic activity was believed to be secondary to effects on brain vascular endothelium (48, 49, 52).

The endothelial cell may be the most dynamic cell in the human body. Virtually every component of the circulatory system comes into contact with the endothelium. It has a hemostatic role in coagulation and thrombosis (53), and it participates in inflammation (54). The endothelium bars circulating solutes and solvents from entering the underling tissue. It also has a key role in the maintenance of vascular tone. These and other functions of the endothelium are, in large part, due to its ability to recognize signals from outside and respond to these signals through a series of different and complicated biochemical pathways. Occasionally, the response may serve to enhance the biological effect of the original eliciting agent, whereas in other instances, the reverse is true. These events involve expression of receptors on the surface of endothelial cells for various ligands, or synthesis and secretion of different factors by the cells. Therefore, the endothelium has a central role in the development of HUS. It is possible that fibrin deposition and platelet adhesion in glomeruli of HUS patients are directly or indirectly related to changes in endothelial cell physiology. Because it is unclear which of these abnormalities constitutes an early event in HUS, we have chosen to explore the various possibilities in vitro.

We have used human endothelial cells of umbilical origin for this purpose, as they are readily obtained and have been the source of much information in defining the role of endothelium in coagulation. As this has led to the biochemical definition of individual steps in the overall coagulation process, we also anticipate that the in vitro endothelial system will serve as a useful model in HUS research.

Which of the many procoagulative factors or processes would one choose to study? The reader is referred to Chapter 26 for a concise review of the role of coagulation and its numerous facets in the pathogenesis of HUS. As applied to our in vitro endothelial system, there is good reason to explore the increased expression of tissue factor (TF) on the surface of endothelial cells in response to Shiga toxin, LPS, IL-1β and TNF-α (55–61). Tissue factor is a rate-limiting protein in formation of a procoagulative state on endothelial cells. The list of candidates for increased coagulation can be extended to include individual factors or pairs of factors, synthesized by endothelial cells, that have opposing actions in coagulation. For example, reduction in t-PA or an increase in t-PA inhibitor could tilt the environment in the vicinity of endothelial cells toward procoagulation (62–64). As an aside, human renal endothelial cells produce more urokinase than t-PA (65).

A key determinant of susceptibility to Shiga toxin for individual cells, including endothelial cells, is the presence of high-affinity receptors for the toxin. This has been demonstrated by Lingwood and co-workers using Daudi B lymphoma cells, which simultaneously lost their Gb_3 receptors for Shiga toxin and sensitivity to the toxins (66). Sensitivity was regained upon reintroduction of the receptors into the plasma membrane of the Daudi cells by fusion with Gb_3-containing liposomes. Other studies have shown that a population of HeLa cells in vitro consist of a heterogeneous mixture, with individual cells having a defined sensitivity to Shiga toxin (23). This sensitivity appears to be directly correlated with the type of receptor for the toxin expressed by the cells (19, 44, 67). We have seen a similar phenomenon in human endothelial cells, in vitro. Others have extended this concept to whole animals, for which it was concluded that rabbits probably did not develop renal lesions to Shiga toxins because their kidneys were toxin receptor-deficient (68–70). An animal model for HUS has yet to be developed. However, mice infected with toxin-producing *E. coli* develop renal lesions of tubular, rather than of glomerular, origin (71). It has been demonstrated that human kidney contains receptor Gb_3 for Shiga toxin, as would be expected to account for HUS (72). This agrees with our experience that human endothelial cells obtained from glomerular remnants express copious quantities of Gb_3 and are very sensitive to Shiga toxin. Recently, Daniel and co-workers reported that SLT-1 is a potent inhibitor of protein synthesis in human renal microvascular endothelial cells in vitro (9).

Most of the experiments conducted in our laboratory have utilized purified Shiga toxin and human umbilical vein endothelial cells (HUVEC) in vitro. Purified Shiga toxin is directly cytotoxic to human vascular endothelial cells in culture (Fig. 5). Before these studies (73–76), only indirect evidence existed for an effect of purified Shiga toxins on vascular endothelium. We now know that members of the Shiga toxin group, including SLT-1 and SLT-2, are cytotoxic to human umbilical vein endothelial cells in a dose-dependent (70-fg/ml to 7-μg/ml range) and time-dependent manner. In addition, it has been reported that a crude lysate from enterohemorrhagic *E. coli* contained cytotoxic activity toward porcine aortic endothelial cells in vitro (8). Despite a lack of evidence that the toxic agent was a Shiga toxin, these data are consistent with results (see Fig. 5) that showed that actively dividing endothelial cells were more sensitive to the purified Shiga toxins than were nondividing, confluent cells (73).

Our laboratory has now generated a considerable amount of additional data from the Shiga toxin–HUVEC in vitro system. It has been established that Shiga toxin binds to the high-affinity glycolipid receptor present on these cells and that this Gb_3 is a functional receptor for the toxin on HUVECs (74, 75).

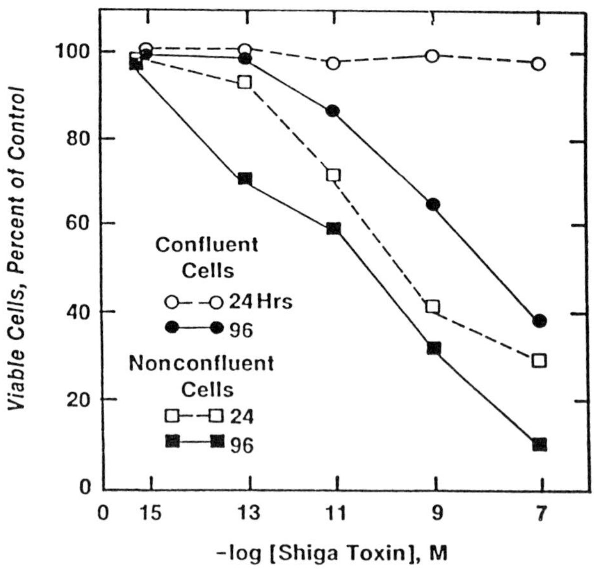

Figure 5 Cytotoxic activity of Shiga toxin on human endothelial cells: A comparison of the effect of Shiga toxin on confluent and nonconfluent HUVEC. The concentrations of Shiga toxin were added to cell cultures at time zero, and the number of viable attached cells remaining was measured at either 24 or 96 hr. (Data from Ref. 74.)

Radiolabeled Shiga toxin-binding studies have revealed the toxin binds in a stable manner (K_d 0.1 nM) to a portion of the approximately 10^6 receptors available on each endothelial cell and becomes internalized within 2 hr (75). Following internalization, protein synthesis is inhibited maximally within 30 min (Fig. 6). That these phenomena are due to Shiga toxin, per se, and not to contaminating factors, was indicated by inhibition of toxin binding and neutralization of cytotoxicity by monoclonal antibodies reactive with the β-subunit of Shiga toxin.

In future studies, we hope to use to advantage the unique features that human endothelial cell cultures offer for the study of HUS. This includes the ability to determine what changes LPS, TNF, IL-1, or others provoke in the normally nonthrombotic surface of endothelial cells when Shiga toxin is present. As endothelial cells from glomerular capillaries of humans are now becoming available, such in vitro studies involving Shiga toxins, cytokines, human platelets, and leukocytes should yield new information pertinent to the mechanisms of Shiga toxin-induced HUS.

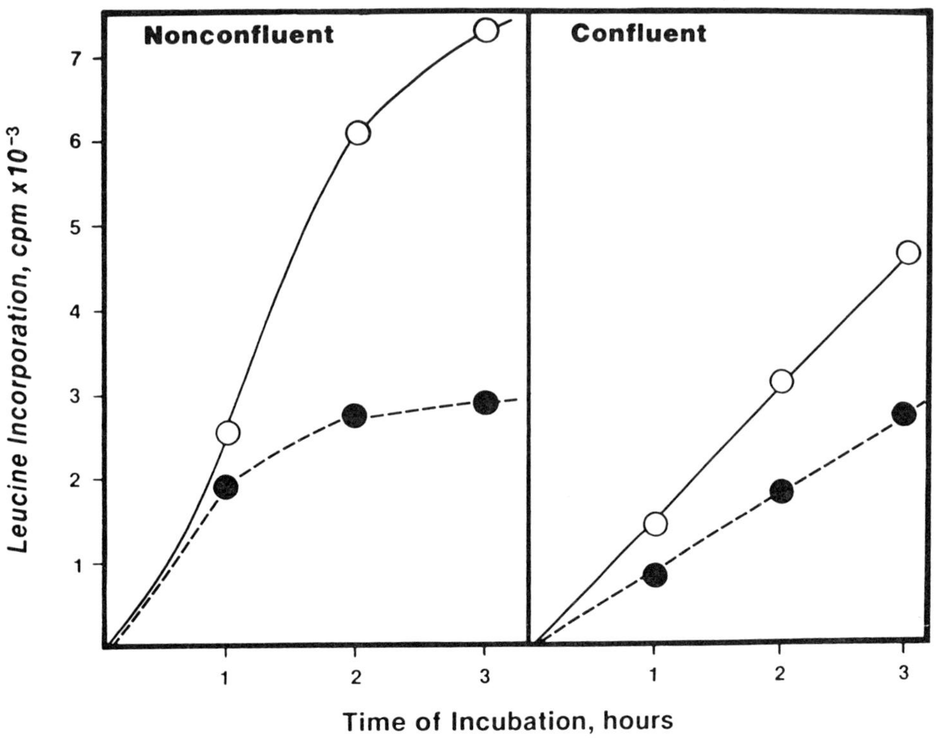

Figure 6 Shiga toxin inhibition of human endothelial cell protein synthesis: Incorporation of [^{3}H]leucine into total cellular protein was performed in the absence (○) or presence (●) of 10 nM Shiga toxin. Cells were preincubated with toxin for 1 hr, followed by addition of [^{3}H]leucine at time zero. At the times indicated, cells were harvested and processed to determine the relative amount of radioactive acid-insoluble protein. (Data from Ref. 74.)

DO ENDOTOXIN AND CYTOKINES COMBINE WITH SHIGA TOXIN TO CAUSE HEMOLYTIC UREMIC SYNDROME?

This appears to be an obvious question of primary importance. Contributions from many different laboratories have pointed to the direct action of LPS, IL-1, and TNF on endothelial cells. Cytokines (LPS, IL-1, TNF) individually exert their effects on endothelial cells (54–60, 77–88) yielding a general increase in the procoagulant state (54, 80). Therefore, one should question whether or not the Shiga toxins act in combination with one or more of the cytokines to enhance their procoagulant properties at the endothelial cell level. Although whole-animal studies indicate that any one of these agents is incapable of mimicking the exact vascular changes of HUS, we have proposed that Shiga toxin represents the additional influence necessary for LPS or the cytokines to create the HUS disease state. During the past decade, the literature has become replete with accounts of LPS and monocyte–macrophage-derived cytokines acting on different cell types of the vasculature, including endothelial cells (77–80).

The many reports of LPS, IL-1, and TNF interaction with endothelial cells provide a basis for future studies which emphasize the use of purified *E. coli* O157:H7 LPS, human recombinant IL-1 β and TNF-α. It is attractive to view Shiga toxins as inhibitors of protein synthesis which, similarly to cycloheximide, may enhance the *direct* effects of LPS and cytokines on endothelial cells (81). These studies realized the importance of low concentrations of LPS ($\leq$10 ng/ml), which alone were without effect on endothelial cells, but which together with cycloheximide, yielded a potent cytotoxic combination. Indeed, in our hands, IL-1 (0.01–10 ng/ml) alone has little or no cytotoxic effect on umbilical vein endothelial cells. However, we have observed that, together with 1 pM Shiga toxin (approximately 20% cytotoxic alone), the combination yielded an enhanced cytotoxicity at concentrations of 1–10 ng/ml of IL-1. More frequently, we have observed synergistic cytotoxicity using combinations of 1–10 ng/ml of TNF (nil cytotoxic activity alone) with 1 pM Shiga toxin.

As mentioned earlier, if Shiga toxins enter the circulation following bloody dysentery, then bacterial LPS would be expected to gain access to the underlying vasculature as well. Therein lies the realization that LPS would stimulate mononuclear cells to produce TNF and IL-1 following infection of humans with *S. dysenteriae* 1 or the enterohemorrhagic *E. coli*. If the hypothesis is correct, then why do only 5–20% of the people afflicted with bacterial bloody dysentery go on to develop HUS? One of the many possibilities is that the biochemical identity of endothelial cells is distinct within each individual, and a part of this identity is the ability of endothelial cells to recognize and respond simultaneously to Shiga toxins and the cytokines. Our preliminary results suggest that this could be a determinant because in vitro each HUVEC cell line (each derived from a separate umbilical cord) presents a defined biochemical response identity for Shiga toxin, LPS, IL-1, and TNF. That is, most of our HUVEC lines are either weakly or nonresponsive to Shiga toxin in a cytotoxic sense. Those that are responsive exhibit an established degree of sensitivity and remain so through at least six and occasionally up to 20 passages. Most of the HUVEC lines are responsive to TNF-α, but may or may not react to IL-1β in a cytotoxic manner.

What then will be the future direction of Shiga toxin–endothelial cell studies in HUS? We hope that the current hypothetical roles in developing HUS of prostacyclin (89), von Willebrand factor complexes (90), induction of procoagulation by Shiga toxin and cytokines, and the effect of shear stress on glomerular capillary function will eventually be tested in both in vitro and in vivo systems. By necessity, these studies will likely focus on the endothelium and its alteration to the procoagulant state. As a by-product of such investigations, researchers should also gain more knowledge of how the human renal vasculature functions and is regulated.

REFERENCES

1. Karmali, M. A., Steele, B. T., Petric, M., Lim, C., Sporadic cases of haemolytic–uraemic syndrome associated with faecal cytotoxin and cytotoxin-producing *Escherichia coli* in stools. *Lancet, 1*: 619–620 (1983).
2. Karmali, M. A., Petric, M., Lim, C., Fleming, P. C., Arbus, G. S., Lior, H., The association between idiopathic hemolytic uremic syndrome and infection by verotoxin-producing *Escherichia coli*. *J. Infect. Dis., 151*: 775–782 (1985).
3. Kononwalchuk, J., Speirs, J. I., Stavric, S., Vero cell response to a cytotoxin of *Escherichia coli*. *Infect. Immun., 18*: 775–779 (1977).
4. Gianantonio, C., Vitacco, M., Mendilaharzu, F., Rutty, A., Mendilanharzu, J., The hemolytic–uremic syndrome. *J. Pediatr., 64*: 478–491 (1964).
5. Koster, F., Levin, J., Walker, L., Tung, K. S. K., Gilman, R. H., Rahaman, M. M., Majid, M. A., Islam, S., Williams, R. C., Jr., Hemolytic uremic syndrome after shigellosis. Relation to endotoxemia and circulating immune complexes. *N. Engl. J. Med., 298*: 927–933 (1978).
6. Johnson, W. M., Lior, H., Bezanson, G. S., Cytotoxic *Escherichia coli* O157:H7 associated with haemorrhagic colitis in Canada. *Lancet, 1*: 76 (1983).
7. Riley, L. W., Remis, R. S., Helgerson, S. D., et al., Hemorrhagic colitis associated with a rare *Escherichia coli* serotype. *N. Engl. J. Med., 308*: 681–685 (1983).
8. Kavi, J., Chaut, J., Maris, M., Rose, P. E., Cytotoxic effect of verotoxin on endothelial cells. *Lancet, 1*: 1035 (1987).
9. Barley-Maloney, L., Obrig, T., Daniel, T., Human renal microvascular endothelial cells (HRMEC) are targets for hemolytic uremic syndrome (HUS)-associated verotoxin (VT) [abstract]. *J. Am. Soc. Nephrol., 1*: 515 (1990).
10. Brown, J. E., Griffin, D. E., Rothman, S. W., Doctor, B. P., Purification and biological characterization of Shiga toxin from *S. dysenteriae* 1. *Infect. Immun., 36*: 996–1005 (1982).
11. O'Brien, A. D., LaVeck, G. D., Griffin, D. E., Thompson, M. R., Characterization of *Shigella dysenteriae* 1 (Shiga) toxin purified by anti-Shiga toxin affinity chromatography. *Infect. Immun., 30*: 170–179 (1980).
12. Olsnes, S., Eiklid, K., Isolation and characterization of *Shigella shigae* cytotoxin. *J. Biol. Chem., 255*: 284–289 (1980).
13. Olsnes, S., Reisbig, R., Eiklid, K., Subunit structure of shigella cytotoxin. *J. Biol. Chem., 256*: 8732–8738 (1981).
14. O'Brien, A. D., LaVeck, G. D., Thompson, M. R., Formal, S. B., Production of *Shigella dysenteriae* type 1-like cytotoxin by *Escherichia coli*. *J. Infect. Dis., 146*: 763 (1982).
15. O'Brien, A. D., LaVeck, G. D., Purification and characterization of a *Shigella dysenteriae* 1-like toxin produced by *Escherichia coli*. *Infect. Immun., 40*: 675–683 (1983).
16. O'Brien, A. D., Holmes, R. K., Shiga and Shiga-like toxins. *Microbiol. Rev., 51*: 206–220 (1987).
17. Strockbine, N. A., Jackson, M. P., Sung, L. M., Holmes, R. K., O'Brien, A. D., Cloning and sequencing of the genes for Shiga toxin from *Shigella dysenteriae* type 1. *J. Bacteriol., 170*: 1116–1121 (1988).

18. Weinstein, D. L., Jackson, M. P., Samuel, J. E., Holmes, R. K., O'Brien, A. D., Cloning and sequencing of a Shiga-like toxin type II variant from an *Escherichia coli* strain responsible for edema disease of swine. *J. Bacteriol., 170*: 4223–4230 (1988).
19. Lindberg, A. A., Brown, J. E., Stromberg, N., Westling-Ryd, M., Schultz, J. E., Karlsson, K. A., Identification of the carbohydrate receptor for Shiga toxin produced by *Shigella dysenteriae* type 1. *J. Biol. Chem., 262*: 1779–1785 (1987).
20. Eiklid, K., Olsnes, S., Entry of *Shigella dysenteriae* toxin into HeLa cells. *Infect. Immun., 42*: 771–777 (1983).
21. Keusch, G. T., Receptor-mediated endocytosis of shigella cytotoxin. In *Receptor-Mediated Binding and Internalization of Toxins and Hormones* (J. L. Middlebrook, L. D. Kohn, eds.), Academic Press, New York, pp. 95–112 (1981).
22. Eidels, L., Proia, R., Hart, D. A., Membrane receptors for bacteria toxins. *Microbiol. Rev., 47*: 596–620 (1983).
23. Eiklid, K., Olsnes, S., Interaction of *Shigella shigae* cytotoxin with receptors on sensitive and insensitive cells. *J. Recept. Res., 1*: 199–213 (1980).
24. Olsnes, S., Sandvig, K., Entry of polypeptide toxins into animal cells. In *Endocytosis* (I. Pastan, M. C. Willingham, eds.), Plenum Publishing, New York, pp. 195–234 (1985).
25. Hale, T. L., Formal, S. B., Protein synthesis in HeLa or Henle 407 cells infected with *Shigella dysenteriae* 1, *Shigella flexneri* 2a, or *Salmonella typhimurium* W118. *Infect. Immun., 32*: 137 (1981).
26. Brown, J. E., Rothman, S. W., Doctor, B. P., Inhibition of protein synthesis in intact HeLa cells by *Shigella dysenteriae* 1 toxin. *Infect. Immun., 29*: 98–107 (1980).
27. Thompson, M. R., Steinberg, M. S., Gemski, P., Formal, S. B., Doctor, B. P., Inhibition of in vitro protein synthesis by *Shigella dysenteriae* 1 toxin. *Biochem. Biophys. Res. Commun., 71*: 783–788 (1976).
28. Brown, J. E., Ussery, M. A., Leppla, S. H., Rothman, S. W., Inhibition of protein synthesis by Shiga toxin. Activation of the toxin and inhibition of peptide elongation. *FEBS Lett., 117*: 84–88 (1980).
29. Charney, A. N., Gots, R. E., Formal, S. B., Giannella, R. A., Activation of intestinal mucosal adenylate cyclase by *Shigella dysenteriae* 1 enterotoxin. *Gastroenterology, 70*: 1085–1090 (1976).
30. Reisbig, R., Olsnes, S., Eiklid, K., The cytotoxin activity of shigella toxin. Evidence for catalytic inactivation of the 60S ribosomal subunit. *J. Biol. Chem., 256*: 8739–8744 (1981).
31. Endo, Y., Tsurugi, K., RNA *N*-glycosidase activity of ricin-A chain. *J. Biol. Chem., 262*: 8128–8130 (1987).
32. Endo, Y., Tsurugi, K., Yutsudo, T., Takeda, Y., Ogasawara, T., Igarashi, K., *Eur. J. Biochem., 171*: 45–50 (1988).
33. Saxena, S. K., O'Brien, A. D., Ackerman, E. J., Shiga toxin, Shiga-like toxin II variant and ricin are all single-site RNA *N*-glucosidases of 28S RNA when microinjected into *Xenopus* oocytes. *J. Biol. Chem., 264*: 596–601 (1989).
34. Hovde, C. J., Calderwood, S. B., Mekalanos, J. J., Collier, R. J., Evidence that glutamic acid 167 is an active site residue of Shiga-like toxin 1. *Proc. Natl. Acad. Sci. USA, 85*: 2568–2572 (1988).
35. Obrig, T. G., Moran, T. P., Colinas, R. J., Ribonuclease activity associated with the 60S ribosome-inactivating proteins ricin A, phytolaccin and Shiga toxin. *Biochem. Biophys. Res. Commun., 130*: 879–884 (1985).
36. Endo, Y., Huber, P. W., Wool, I. G., The ribonuclease activity of the cytotoxin alpha-sarcin. The characteristics of the enzymatic activity of alpha-sarcin with ribosomes and ribonucleic acids as substrates. *J. Biol. Chem., 258*: 2662–2667 (1983).
37. Obrig, T. G., Moran, T. P., Brown, J. E., The mode of action of Shiga toxin on peptide elongation of eukaryotic protein synthesis. *Biochem. J., 244*: 287–194 (1987).
38. Butler, T., Islam, M. R., Azad, A. K., Jones, P. K., Risk factors for development of the

hemolytic–uremic syndrome during shigellosis: Role of antimicrobial treatment. *J. Pediatr.*, *110*: 894–897 (1987).
39. Raghupathy, P., Date, A., Shastry, J. C. M., Sudarsanam, A., Jadhav, M., Haemolytic uraemic syndrome complicating shigella dysentery in South Indian children. *Br. Med. J.*, *1*: 1518–1521 (1978).
40. Fong, J. S. C., de Chadarevian, J.-P., Kaplan, B. S., Hemolytic–uremic syndrome: Current concepts and management. *Pediatr. Clin. North Am.*, *29*: 835–856 (1982).
41. Anonymous. Unraveling HUS. *Lancet*, *2*: 1437–1439 (1987).
42. Drummond, K. N., Hemolytic uremic syndrome—then and now. *New Engl. J. Med.*, *312*: 116–118 (1985).
43. Karmali, M. A., Infection by verotoxin-producing *Escherichia coli*. *Clin. Microbiol. Rev.*, *2*: 15–38 (1989).
44. Kaplan, B. S., Cleary, T. G., Obrig, T. G., Recent advances in understanding the pathogenesis of the hemolytic uremic syndromes. *Pediatr. Nephrol.*, *4*: 276–283 (1990).
45. Fontaine, A., Arondel, J., Sansonetti, P. J., Role of Shiga toxin in the pathogenesis of bacillary dysentery, studied by using a *tox*$^-$ mutant of *Shigella dysenteriae* 1. *Infect. Immun.*, *56*: 3099–3109 (1988).
46. Richardson, S. E., Karmali, M. A., Becker, L. E., Smith, C. R., The histopathology of the hemolytic uremic syndrome associated with verotoxin-producing *Escherichia coli* infections. *J. Hum. Pathol.*, *19*: 1102–1108 (1988).
47. Morel-Maroger, L., Kanter, A., Solez, K., Sraer, J. D., Richet, G., Prognostic importance of vascular lesions in acute renal failure with microangiopathic hemolytic anemia (hemolytic uremic syndrome): A clinicopathologic study of 20 adults. *Kidney Int.*, *15*: 548–558 (1979).
48. Bridgewater, F. A. J., Morgan, R. S., Rowson, K. E. K., Wright, G. P., The neurotoxin of *Shigella shigae*. Morphological and functional lesions produced in the central nervous system of rabbits. *Br. J. Exp. Pathol.*, *36*: 447–453 (1955).
49. Cavanagh, J. B., Howard, J. G., Whitby, J. L., The neurotoxin of *Shigella shigae*. A comparative study of the effects produced in various laboratory animals. *Br. J. Exp. Med.*, *37*: 272–278 (1956).
50. Eiklid, K., Olsnes, S., Animal toxicity of *Shigella dysenteriae* cytotoxin: Evidence that the neurotoxic, enterotoxic, and cytotoxic activities are due to one toxin. *J. Immunol.*, *130*: 380–384 (1983).
51. Wiley, R. G., Donohue-Rolfe, A., Keusch, G. T., Oeltmann, T. N., Selective destruction of vagal sensory neurons using shigella cytotoxin. *Methods Enzymol.*, *165*: 250–253 (1988).
52. Howard, J. G., Observations on the intoxication produced in mice and rabbits by the neurotoxin of *Shigella shigae*. *Br. J. Exp. Pathol.*, *36*: 439–446 (1955).
53. Gimbrone, M. A., Jr., ed., Vascular endothelium in hemostasis and thrombosis, Churchill–Livingstone, Edinburg (1986).
54. Cotran, R. S., Pober, J. S., Endothelial activation, its role in inflammaatory and immune reactions. In *Endothelial Cell Biology* (N. Simionescu, M. Simionescu, eds.), Plenum Publishing, New York, pp. 335–347 (1988).
55. Colucci, M., Balconi, G., Lorenzet, R., Pietra, A., Locato, D., Donati, M. B., Semeraro, N., Cultured endothelial cells generate tissue factor in response to endotoxin. *J. Clin. Invest.*, *71*: 1893–1896 (1983).
56. Bevilacqua, M. P., Pober, J. S., Majeau, G. R., Cotran, R. S., Gimbrone, M. A., Interleukin-1 induces biosynthesis and cell surface expression of procoagulant activity on human vascular endothelial cells. *J. Exp. Med.*, *160*: 618–623 (1984).
57. Moore, K. L., Andreoli, S. P., Esmon, N. L., Esmon, C. T., Bang, N. U., Endotoxin enhances tissue factor and suppresses thrombomodulin expression of human vascular endothelium in vitro. *J. Clin. Invest.*, *79*: 124–130 (1987).

58. Bevilacqua, M. P., Pober, J. S., Wheeler, M. E., Cotran, R. S., Gimbrone, M. A., Jr., Interleukin 1 (IL-1) activation of vascular endothelium: Effects on procoagulant activity and leukocyte adhesion. *Am. J. Pathol., 121*: 393–403 (1985).
59. Bevilacqua, M. P., Pober, J. S., Majeau, G. R., Friers, W., Cotran, R. S., Gimbrone, M. A., Jr., Recombinant TNF induces procoagulant activity in cultured human vascular endothelium: Characterization and comparison with the actions of IL-1. *Proc. Natl. Acad. Sci. USA, 83*: 4533–4537 (1986).
60. Conway, E. M., Bach, R., Rosenberg, R. D., Konigsberg, W. H., Tumor necrosis factor enhances expression of tissue factor mRNA in endothelial cells. *Thromb. Res., 53*: 231–241 (1989).
61. Crossman, D. C., Carr, D. P., Tuddenham, E. G. D., Pearson, J. D., McVey, J. H., The regulation of tissue factor mRNA in human endothelial cells in response to endotoxin or phorbol ester. *J. Biol. Chem., 265*: 9782–9787 (1990).
62. Loskutoff, D. J., Edgington, T. S., Synthesis of a fibrinolytic activator and its inhibitor by endothelial cells. *Proc. Natl. Acad. Sci. USA, 74*: 3903–3907 (1977).
63. Levin, E. G., Loskutoff, D. J., Cultured bovine endothelial cells produce urokinase and tissue-type plasminogen activators. *J. Cell Biol., 94*: 631–636 (1982).
64. Loskutoff, D. J., van Mourik, J. A., Erickson, L. A., Lawrence, D., Detection of an unusually stable fibrinolytic inhibitor produced by bovine endothelial cells. *Proc. Natl. Acad. Sci. USA, 80*: 2956–2960 (1983).
65. Daniel, T. O., Gibbs, V. C., Milfay, D. F., Garovoy, M. R., Williams, L. T., Thrombin stimulates c-*sis* gene expression in microvascular endothelial cells. *J. Biol. Chem., 261*: 9579–9582 (1986).
66. Waddell, T., Cohen, A., Lingwood, C. A., Induction of verotoxin sensitivity in deficient cell lines using the receptor glycolipid, globotriosyl ceramide. *Proc. Natl. Acad. Sci. USA, 87*: 7898–7901 (1990).
67. Waddell, T., Head, S., Petric, M., Cohen, A., Lingwood, C., Glbotriosyl ceramide is specifically recognized by the *Escherichia coli* verotoxin 2. *Biochem. Biophys. Res. Commun., 152*: 674–679 (1988).
68. Pai, C. H., Kelly, J. K., Meyers, G. L., Experimental infection of infant rabbits with Vero toxin-producing *Escherichia coli*. *Infect. Immun., 51*: 16–23 (1986).
69. Barrett, T. J., Potter, M. E., Wachsmuth, I. K., Bacterial endotoxin both enhances and inhibits the toxicity of Shiga-like toxin II in rabbits and mice. *Infect. Immun., 57*: 3434–3437 (1989).
70. Barrett, T. J., Potter, M. E., Wachsmuth, I. K., Continuous peritoneal infusion of Shiga-like toxin II (SLT II) as a model for SLT II-induced diseases. *J. Infect. Dis., 159*: 774–777 (1989).
71. Wadolkowski, E. A., Sung, L. M., Burris, J. A., Samuel, J. E., O'Brien, A. D., Acute renal tubular necrosis and death of mice orally infected with *Escherichia coli* strains that produce Shiga-like toxin type II. *Infect. Immun., 58*: 3959–3965 (1990).
72. Boyd, B., Lingwood, C., Verotoxin receptor glycolipid in human renal tissue. *Nephron, 51*: 207–210 (1989).
73. Obrig, T. G., Del Vecchio, P. J., Karmali, M. A., Petric, M., Moran, T. P., Judge, T. K., Pathogenesis of haemolytic uraemic syndrome. *Lancet, 1*: 687 (1987).
74. Obrig, T. G., Del Vecchio, P. J., Brown, J. E., Moran, T. P., Rowland, B. M., Judge, T. K., Rothman, S. W., Direct cytotoxic action of Shiga toxin on human vascular endothelial cells. *Infect. Immun., 56*: 2373–2378 (1988).
75. Obrig, T., Lingwood, C., Del Vecchio, P., Moran, T., Brown, J., Branca, A., Rowland, B., Receptor-mediated effects of Shiga toxin on human vascular endothelial cells: A possible cause of hemolytic uremic syndrome (HUS) and hemorrhagic colitis (HC). In *Proceedings of 26th U.S. Japan Cooperative Programs on Cholera and Diarrheal Diseases* (Y. Takeda, et al., eds.), Academic Press, New York (in press; 1991).

76. Obrig, T., Del Vecchio, P., Brown, J. E., Karmali, M., Petric, M., Lingwood, C., Direct cytotoxic action of Shiga toxin and verotoxin on human vascular endothelial cells. Workshop on Verotoxin Producing *E. coli* Infections, Toronto, July 15, Abstr. HUS-5, (1987).
77. Morrison, D. C., Ryan, J. L., Endotoxins and disease mechanisms. *Annu. Rev. Med.*, *38*: 417–432 (1987).
78. Shands, J. W., Jr., Macrophage procoagulants. *Hemostasis, 14*: 373–377 (1984).
79. Cotran, R. S., Pober, J. S., Effects of cytokines on vascular endothelium: Their role in vascular and immune injury. *Kidney Int.*, *35*: 969–975 (1989).
80. Cybulsky, M. I., Chan, M, K. W., Movat, H. Z., Acute inflammation and microthrombosis induced by endotoxin, IL-1, and TNF and their implication in gram-negative infection. *J. Lab. Invest.*, *58*: 365–378 (1988).
81. Harlan, M. D., Harker, L. A., Reidy, M. A., Gajdusek, C. M., Schwartz, S. M., Striker, G. E., Lipopolysaccharide-mediated bovine endothelial cell injury, in vitro. *J. Lab. Invest.*, *48*: 269–274 (1983).
82. Pohlman, T. H., Harlan, J. M., Human endothelial cell response to lipopolysaccharide interleukin-1, and tumor necrosis factor is regulated by protein synthesis. *Cell. Immunol.*, *119*: 41–52 (1989).
83. Nawroth, P. P., Handley, D. A., Esmon, C. T., Stern, D. M., Interleukin-1 induces endothelial cell procoagulant while suppressing cell-surface anticoagulant activity. *Proc. Natl. Acad. Sci. USA*, *83*: 3460–3464 (1986).
84. Bevilacqua, M. P., Schleef, R. R., Gimbrone, M. A., Loskutoff, D. J., Regulation of the fibrinolytic system of cultured human vascular endothelium by interleukin-1. *J. Clin. Invest.*, *78*: 587–591 (1986).
85. Emeis, J. J., Kooistra, T., Interleukin-1 and lipopolysaccharide induce an inhibitor of tissue-type plasminogen activator in vivo and in cultured endothelial cells. *J. Exp. Med.*, *163*: 1260–1266 (1986).
86. Nachman, R. L., Hajjar, K. A., Silverstein, R. L., Dinarello, C. A., Interleukin-1 induces endothelial cell synthesis of plasminogen activator inhibitor. *J. Exp. Med.*, *163*: 1595–1600 (1986).
87. Medcalf, R. L., Kruithof, E. K. O., Scheuning, W. D., Plasminogen activator inhibitor 1 and 2 are tumor necrosis factor/cachectin responsive genes. *J. Exp. Med.*, *168*: 751–759 (1988).
88. Schleef, R. R., Bevilacqua, M. P., Sawdey, M. A., Gimbrone, M. A., Loskutoff, D. J., Cytokine activation of vascular endothelium. Effects on tissue type plasminogen activator and type 1 plasminogen activator inhibitor. *J. Biol. Chem.*, *263*: 5797–5802 (1988).
89. Karch, H., Bitzan, M., Pietsch, R., Stenger, K.-O., von Wulffen, H., Heeseman, J., Dusing, R., Purified verotoxins of *E. coli* O157:H7 decrease prostacyclin synthesis by endothelial cells. *Microb. Pathogen.*, *5*: 215–221 (1988).
90. Rose, P. E., Enayat, S. M., Sunderland, R., Short, P. E., Williams, C. E., Hill, F. G. H., Abnormalities of factor VIII related protein multimers in the haemolytic uremic syndrome. *Arch. Dis. Child.*, *59*: 1135–1140 (1984).

VII
Treatment

29
Treatment of Hemolytic Uremic Syndrome with Antithrombotic Agents

Willem Proesmans and Roger Eeckels *Leuven University Hospital, Leuven, Belgium*

From the first descriptions of thrombotic thrombocytopenic purpura (TTP) and hemolytic uremic syndrome (HUS), thrombotic phenomena were considered to be one of the most striking features of these conditions. In 1925, Moschcowitz (1) published a case of "an undescribed disease," with a unique histological feature of widespread presence of "thrombi in the terminal arterioles and capillaries," "from one to a dozen" in every microscopical field.

More than 25 years later, Symmers (2), reviewing the 33 then known reported cases of TTP, proposed the term thrombotic microangiopathy (TMA) "as a suitable substitute for the names previously used as it indicates the location and the most striking feature of the characteristic histological lesion. . . ." Subsequently, TMA has been generally adopted to describe the vascular lesions of TTP. Gasser et al. (3) stressed the thrombotic nature of the lesion in children with HUS, especially in patient number 3:

> . . . eine thrombotische Mikroangiopathie Symmers mit Befall der kleinen Arterien, Arteriolen und Kapillaren in Myokard, Nieren, Gehirn, Lungen, Dickdarm, Schilddrüse und Nebennieren. [a thrombotic microangiopathy as described by Symmers with involvement of the small arteries, arterioles and capillaries in the myocardium, kidneys, brain, lungs, colon, thyroid, and adrenal glands.]

Habib et al. identified more precisely the pathognomonic lesion of HUS and adopted Symmer's term of TMA (4–6).

Although we consider HUS and TTP as "the opposite ends of a continuum with overlap in some cases" (17), this chapter concentrates mainly on HUS in children.

THE EVIDENCE FOR A THROMBOTIC PHENOMENON IN HEMOLYTIC UREMIC SYNDROME

The evidence for a thrombotic phenomenon in HUS (and TTP) comes from three different sources. First, the authors of the original descriptions of these syndromes (1–6) considered that a thrombotic lesion was the hallmark of the disorders. Second, the majority of subsequent histological studies have confirmed the findings by Moschcowitz, Symmers, Gasser, and Habib. Third, coagulation studies point to an imbalance between coagulation and fibrinolysis, resulting in a procoagulant state.

The Histological Evidence

Almost all studies on the subject show that in HUS microthrombi are found in the glomeruli and the renal arterioles, and that the most severe form of this process is cortical necrosis. The latest in a long series of publications is the report from the Southwest Pediatric Nephrology Study Group dealing with histological features of 24 children with HUS (8). The spectrum of lesions ranges from purely glomerular TMA (". . . thrombosis of capillary lumina was often present in these specimens"), to arterial TMA (" . . . interlobular arteries were narrowed and obstructed by swelling of the endothelium and/or thrombi"), and cortical necrosis. These authors also note

> . . . recent hyaline thrombi . . . in extrarenal arterioles in eight of the nine autopsied patients; They were found in the large bowel of six patients, . . . in the pancreatic islets, . . . in the kidneys (6 patients), brain (3 patients), heart (2 patients), adrenals (1 patient) and lungs (1 patient).

This almost reads like a copy of Gasser et al.'s description. Extrarenal arterial thrombi have also been reported by Upadyaya et al. (9).

Yet, as pointed out by Argyle et al. (8) thrombi are not found in every case of HUS. Two factors might account for this. First, histologial specimens obtained either at autopsy or by biopsy, can never encompass the whole kidney. Second, it seems reasonable to assume a temporal effect. In our experience, children who die in the first few days of the illness have impressive amounts of thrombi in glomeruli and some renal arteries (Proesmans, W., unpublished observations). In contrast, biopsy specimens from our surviving patients taken 3–4 weeks after the onset of HUS only rarely have thrombotic lesions (10).

Immunofluorescence studies add to the evidence. Fibrin deposits are seen in glomeruli and renal arterioles in most specimens from patients with HUS (6, 11). Factor XIII, a fibrin-stabilizing factor, is present in a continuous subendothelial pattern in biopsies from patients with HUS (11). Plasminogen activator inhibitor 1 (PAI-1), which is normally absent, can be demonstrated in kidneys from patients with HUS and TTP (12).

In two experimental models that resemble HUS, fibrin deposits, thrombi, cortical necrosis, or a combination thereof, are found in rabbits challenged with lipopolysaccharide endotoxins from *Escherichia coli* and *Shigella* species, respectively (13, 14).

It thus appears that a thrombotic microangiopathy is a central event in the pathogenesis of HUS. The TMA seems to be the consequence of injury to the vascular endothelium. The most likely causes, at least in classic HUS, are bacterial toxins (15). Damage to the endothelium of the glomeruli and the arterioles exposes the basement membrane collagen, thereby leading to platelet adhesion and activation and local intravascular coagulation with fibrin deposition.

Coagulation Studies

With rare exceptions (8, 16), patients with HUS do not have evidence of disseminated intravascular coagulation (DIC). The coagulation abnormalities observed in HUS are summarized in Table 1.

Thrombocytopenia is a striking and almost constant laboratory abnormality. Bone marrow smears show an abundance of megakaryocytes consistent with peripheral platelet destruction. Platelet survival is reduced (17, 18). Evidence for platelet activation comes from three sources: platelet serotonin content is decreased (19), circulating plasma levels of β-thromboglobulin and platelet factor 4 are increased (20), and a plasma platelet-aggregating factor is present in some children with HUS (21). Finally, the platelets display an impaired response to different aggregating substances and, therefore, appear to be "exhausted" (22). There are two explanations for platelet consumption. Either the platelets are trapped in the damaged vessels, or the etiological factor responsible for HUS directly affects not only endothelial cells, but also platelets and erythrocytes (23).

Coagulation studies (17, 23, 24) yield variable results (see Table 1). The thrombin time is slightly prolonged. The activated partial thromboplastin time and the prothrombin time are either normal or prolonged. Coagulation factors are usually found in normal concentrations. However, levels of factors V and VIII may be slightly higher than normal. The von Willebrand factor (vWF) antigen concentration and activity are normal in mild HUS cases and increased in severe ones (26, 27). In some HUS patients, plasma concentrations of large vWF multimers are decreased (28).

Table 1 Coagulation Findings in Hemolytic Uremic Syndrome

Platelets
Reduced number
Diminished survival rate
Reduced serotonin content
Impaired aggregability
Increased plasma levels of βTG and PF4
Circulating PAF
Coagulation factors
Thrombin time ↑
Activated partial thromboplastin time N/↑
Prothrombin time N/↑
Factor V ↓/N/↑
Factor VIII (concentration and activity) N/↑
vWF antigen (concentration and activity) N/↑
vWF large multimers N/↑
Fibrinogen (↓)/N/↑
Fibrin/fibrinogen degradation products ↑
Fibrinopeptide A N/↑

PF4, platelet factor 4; PAF, platelet aggregating factor; βTG, β-thromboglobulin; vWF, von Willebrand factor; ↓, decreased; N, normal; ↑, increased.

Plasma fibrinogen levels may be slightly low, or they may be within the normal range; however, elevated levels are found in a fair number of patients. All studies agree that titers of circulating fibrinogen/fibrin degradation produces are invariably increased. Fibrinopeptide A levels are elevated in some HUS patients (29).

There is also evidence of defective fibrinolysis in HUS. Bergstein et al. found an inhibitor of fibrinolysis in the serum of HUS patients (30). Gras-Greenwalt et al. found that the levels of functional tissue plasminogen activator were low or unmeasurable in 11 of 12 TTP patients, and levels of the inhibitor of plasminogen activator (PAI) were significantly elevated in all (31). This has been confirmed by Kakishita et al. who found that the elevation of PAI is higher than in patients with overt DIC (32). Bergstein and Bang have also demonstrated that the circulating inhibitor of fibrinolysis is the same PAI-1 (33). These observations complement the demonstration by immunofluorescence of factor XIII and PAI-1 in biopsy specimens (11, 12). Elevated levels of thrombin–antithrombin complexes as well as plasmin–antiplasmin complexes in the serum of ten TTP patients (34) indicate that considerable amounts of thrombin and plasmin are generated in this condition.

There is convincing evidence that the coagulation system is activated in TMA. For reasons that have not yet been determined, the intravascular coagulation seems to be localized and, in HUS, it is mainly limited to the kidneys. Most patients with HUS have, at a minimum, some thrombotic lesions in their kidneys. To which extent these lesions are fully reversible, or contribute to permanent damage to the kidneys, has lately become an important question (see later discussion).

ANTITHROMBOTIC TREATMENT FOR HEMOLYTIC UREMIC SYNDROME

Antithrombotic treatment in HUS could be aimed at (a) preventing further clotting by using anticoagulant drugs, (b) dissolving fibrin deposits by employing fibrinolytic agents, or (c) inhibiting platelet adhesion and activation.

A limited number of drugs have actually been used. Heparin has been the only anticoagulant that has been tried and was popular in the 1960s and 1970s. Urokinase and Streptokinase are fibrinolytic agents that are not without problems; hemorrhage is a frequent complication. Acetylsalicylic acid (aspirin) and dipyridamole, antiplatelet drugs, are safer and have gained some popularity among pediatric nephrologists.

Antithrombotic treatment of HUS has always been controversial. Some believed from the start in the value of early dialysis and other symptomatic measures alone and referred to the early negative experience with heparin in Argentina (35). Others were convinced of the opposite point of view which was supported by our meta-analysis (36). This showed that survival rates of heparin-treated HUS patients were significantly better than those of patients who had not received anticoagulants. The difference was even more striking when only severe cases were taken into consideration. In recognition of the flaws of a retrospective analysis, we concluded that a rigorously controlled, prospective study should be undertaken.

Since then, several retrospective, and mainly uncontrolled, studies have been published (37–42), and the relevant data are summarized in Table 2. With one exception (39), these papers deal with very small groups of patients; this may be another reason for their inconclusive results.

To date, there are only three prospective studies. In the first heparin was used in

Table 2 Antithrombotic Agents for Childhood HUS: Review of the Retrospective Therapeutical Studies

			Outcome		
Ref.	Patients (no.)	Antithrombotic agents[a]	Dead	CRF	Recovered
37	44	None (n=22)	9	5	8
		Hep. (n=14)	5	4	5
		Streptok. (n=8)	2	0	6
38	5	Streptok. + hep.	3	0	2
39	73	Hep. (n=35)	2	3	30
		Streptok. + hep. (n = 38)	3	1	34
40	26	None (n=10)	0	1	9
		Hep. (n=8)	2	2	4
		Streptok. + hep. (n=8)	2	1	5
41	16	None (n=8)	2	0	6
		ASA + dipyrid. (n=8)	1	1	6
42	8	Urokinase (n=8)	3	2	3

[a]ASA, acetyl salicylic acid; CRF, chronic renal failure; dipyrid., dipyridamole; hep., heparin; streptok., streptokinase; (n=), number of cases.

10 of 30 severe cases (35). Patients treated with heparin did worse than the controls, although the differences were not statistically significant. It is now clear that this study does not meet the requirements of a modern prospective, controlled trial. Moreover, heparin was usually started late in the course of the illness and the authors admitted that "appropriate anticoagulation was difficult to obtain in 8 patients who required frequent adjustment of the heparin dosage. . . ." The results of two other prospective studies were, in many respects, more promising (Table 3). Loirat et al. (43) treated 33 children with HUS in a multicenter, controlled study. Fifteen patients received urokinase and heparin, 18 control patients received symptomatic treatment, similar to that offered to the treatment group. The duration of hemolysis, thrombocytopenia, and oliguria were similar in both groups. No differences were seen in terms of renal histological changes and in long-term renal function. This study, however, had its practical problems. In 4 patients, hemorrhage resulted in interruption of antithrombotic therapy after 14–31 hr and, therefore, only 11 patients had no modification of the treatment schedule.

The other prospective, controlled study was undertaken in our department over a 10-year period (10). All patients admitted in the acute phase of HUS were randomly assigned to either symptomatic treatment or to heparin plus dipyridamole plus symptomatic treatment. When dialysis was required, control patients received only peritoneal dialysis, thus avoiding administration of the large doses of heparin that are required for hemodialysis. The evaluation included kidney biopsies and long-term data on renal function. Fifty-eight children were enrolled in the study. There were no differences between the control group and the treatment group insofar as the course of the acute phase of the illness, the outcome, and renal histological changes were concerned.

Both of these latter studies were well designed and properly conducted. However, both have two major flaws: absence of sample-size calculation and a limited

Table 3 Summary of Two Prospective, Controlled Trials with Antithrombotic Agents in Childhood HUS

Loirat et al. (43)			Van Damme Lombaerts et al. (10)	
Multicenter study involving 8 French institutions			Single center (University Hospital, Leuven, Belgium) over 10-yr period	
Patients			All HUS patients entering in acute phase	
Included if serum urea > 25 mmol/L creatinine > 180 umol/L				
Excluded if uncontrollable hypertension, severe hemorrhage or surgery				
Methods	Patients randomized for supportive therapy with or without			
Urokinase: 5000 U/kg first hour 4000 U/kg per hr for 47 hr			Heparin: Starting with i.v. bolus of 200 U/kg; dose according to PTT	
Heparin: Continuous i.v. infusion 200–400 U/kg per 24 hr			Dipyridamole: 0.5 mg/kg i.v., bid	
Renal biopsy at the end of acute phase			Renal biopsy 3 wks after admission	
Results	Controls	Treatment	Controls	Treatment
Number of patients	18	15	28	30
Dead in acute phase	3	0	0	2
Persistent hypertension	0	0	1	0
Late dead	0	0	1	0
Number of biopsies	13	13	26	28
Histological lesions	No differences		No differences	
Conclusions: "Urokinase is of no value in HUS"			"Heparin plus dipyridamole is neither harmful nor beneficial in HUS."	

number of patients. Therefore, although it has not been proved that the use of antithrombotic drugs improves the outcome of children with HUS, it is prudent to state that final conclusions may be derived only after a follow-up period of 10 years.

SUGGESTIONS FOR FUTURE POLICY

The lack of clearcut efficacy of heparin might be explained if the thrombotic event in HUS occurs early in the disease, during one short episode of fibrin deposition in glomeruli and arterioles so that, at the time of diagnosis, anticoagulant intervention is too late. If this were true, fibrinolytic agents should improve the outcome. However, treatment with urokinase has not met our expectations.

One might conclude that thrombosis is not a crucial factor in the outcome of most patients with HUS: thrombosis may be only a lesser, second-rank phenomenon, from which the kidney spontaneously recovers with time or, at worst, the thrombi result in the loss of an insignificant number of nephrons. Cortical necrosis may then be an unusual situation in which thrombosis is associated with severe and possibly permanent damage.

The central question, however, is whether two small prospective studies with inconclusive results, can provide decisive answers. It is our feeling that the last word about antithrombotic agents and HUS has not been written. After all, there are only two reliable studies that together deal with fewer than 100 patients; many had a mild or moderatly severe form of HUS, with a good chance of recovery with symptomatic treatment alone. Moreover, the follow-up period has not been greater than 3–5 years and it is now clear that one needs 10 years, or more, to determine the full impact of HUS on kidney growth, development, and function. Two studies clearly show that ten years after the acute episode sequelae such as decreased renal function are not infrequent (44, 45).

Therefore, there may be a need for more and better designed therapeutic studies. In addition to comparing the fatality rate of the acute disease, irreversible renal insufficiency, the severity of histological lesions, and the prevalence of late sequelae also need to be studied. Patients will have to be followed for at least 10 years after the acute episode.

That it will not be an easy task is shown by the sample-size calculation (Epistat Services, Richardson, Texas). The required sample sizes for three different rates of any study characteristic to be reduced by 50% through a therapeutic agent are shown in Table 4. A far more powerful agent, reducing the rate of the study characteristics to very low levels, would lead to much smaller sample sizes. The best of such studies would be the one that focuses on patients at high risk of an unfavorable outcome, considering known prognostic features (45–47). This approach, combined with a powerful therapeutic agent, might reduce the sample size to amenable figures. Collaboration among many centers will still be required.

Which drug or drugs should be used? The most promising molecule may be the commercially available tissue-type plasminogen activator (t-PA). It is the natural, intrinsic fibrinolytic agent that, in contrast with urokinase and streptokinase, discriminates between free and fibrin-bound plasminogen and, therefore, produces no systemic lytic state. Tissue plasminogen activator is effective in preventing fibrin deposition in rabbits subjected to the Shwartzman phenomenon (48). This preliminary experimental finding suggests that t-PA therapy might be of value in patients with HUS.

FINAL REMARKS

All pediatric nephrologists agree that dialysis has played a major role in the overall spectacular improvement of immediate survival rates in patients with HUS. Many advocate early dialysis. This may mean hemodialysis, except in small infants. Hemodialysis requires large doses of heparin, as does plasmapheresis. For those who cannot give up the idea that antithrombotic treatment is definitely not a dead issue, it

Table 4 Required Sample Size for Rates of Study Characteristic to be Reduced by 50%

Rate of study characteristic		
Control group (%)	Treatment group (%)	Sample size [a]
6	3	2 × 1100
9	4.5	2 × 700
12	6	2 × 500

[a]One control per case; figures rounded to the nearest 100, $(1-\beta) = 90\%$; significance $(1 - \alpha) = 95\%$.

is tempting to speculate that anticoagulation is part of the salutary effect of hemodialysis in HUS patients. It is, however, clear that it is impossible to prove or disprove such a statement. With this hypothesis in mind, it is of note that in an Italian study on the use of fresh frozen plasma in HUS, only those children who needed dialysis were included (49). Not only were there no differences between treated and control patients, but not a single patient died. They all presumably received heparin!

We should endeavor to find the optimal treatment for children with HUS, despite the tremendous progress that has been made over the last 3 decades, for the challenge is still great. In addition to those who die suddenly, between 5 and 10% do not recover renal function and eventually need kidney replacement therapy. Studies on renal function 10 years after HUS indicate that only 60% recover completely (44). A recent study yields even more pessimistic data. O'Regan et al. (50) measured the glomerular filtration rate (GFR), by an isotope clearance technique, in 37 patients, 6–12 years after recovery from HUS. Half of these adolescents had a GFR below 80 ml min^{-1} per 1.73 m^2. Therefore, the best supportive treatment may not be good enough for children with severe forms of classic HUS and for patients with atypical forms.

We clearly still lack the linchpin of the ideal treatment of this disorder, despite impressive progress.

REFERENCES

1. Moschcowitz, E., An acute febrile pleiochromic anemia with hyaline thrombosis of the terminal arterioles and capillaries. *Arch. Intern. Med.*, *36*: 89–93 (1925).
2. Symmers, W. S. C., Thrombotic microangiopathic haemolytic anaemia (thrombotic microangiopathy). *Br. Med. J.*, *2*: 897–903 (1952).
3. Gasser, C., Gautier, E., Steck, A., Siebenman, R. E., Oechslin, R., Haemolytisch–uraemische Syndrome: bilaterale Nierenrindennekrosen bei akuten erworbenen haemolytischen Anaemien. *Schweiz. Med. Wochenschr.*, *85*: 905–909 (1955).
4. Royer, P., Habib, R., Mathieu, H., La microangiopathie thrombotique du rein chez l'enfant. *Sem. Hôp. Paris Ann. Pédiatr.*, *36*: 572–587 (1960).
5. Chaptal, J., Jean, R., Pages, A., Habib, R., Dossa, D., Dumas, R., Forme curable de la microangiopathie thrombotique rénale de l'enfant. *Arch. Fr. Pédiatr.*, *23*: 275–296 (1966).
6. Habib, R., Syndrome hémolytique et urémique. In Néphrologie Pédiatrique (P. Royer, R. Habib, H. Mathieu, M. Broyer, eds.), Flammarion, Paris, pp. 401–413 (1983).
7. Kaplan, B. S., Proesmans, W., The hemolytic uremic syndrome of childhood and its variants. *Semin. Hematol.*, *24*: 148–160 (1987).
8. Argyle, J. C., Hogg, R. J., Pysher, T. J., Silva, F. G., Siegler, R. L., A clinicopathological study of 24 children with hemolytic uremic syndrome. A report of the Southwest Pediatric Nephrology Study Group. *Pediatr. Nephrol.*, *4*: 52–58 (1990).
9. Upadyaya, K., Barwick, K., Fishaut, M., Kashgarian, M., Siegel, N. J., The importance of non-renal involvement in hemolytic uremic syndrome. *Pediatrics*, *65*: 115–120 (1980).
10. Van Damme-Lombaerts, R., Proesmans, W., Van Damme, B., Eeckels, R., Binda ki Muaka, P., Mercieca, V., Vlietinck, R., Vermylen, J., Heparin plus dipyridamole in childhood hemolytic uremic syndrome: A prospective, randomized study. *J. Pediatr.*, *113*: 913–918 (1988).
11. Colossanti, G., Morel-Maroger, L., D'Amico, G., Deposition of fibrin-stabilizing factor (F XIIIA and S), fibrinogen-related antigens, fibrinogen degradation products (FDPd and FDPe) and antihemolytic factor (factor VIII) in renal disease: Analysis of 161 cases by immunfluorescence microscopy. *Clin. Nephrol.*, *28*: 28–34 (1987).

12. Rondeau, E., Mougenot, B., Lecave, R., Peraldi,, M. N., Kruithof, E. K. O., Sraer, J. D., Plasminogen activator inhibitor 1 in renal fibrin deposits of human nephropathies. *Clin. Nephrol., 33*: 55–60 (1990).
13. Bertani, T., Abbate, M., Zoja, C., Corna, D., Remuzzi, G., Sequence of glomerular changes in experimental endotoxemia: A possible model of hemolytic uremic syndrome. *Nephron, 53*: 330–337 (1989).
14. Butler, T., Rahman, H., Al-Mahmud, K. A., Islam, M., Bardhan, P., Kabir, I., Rahman, M. M., An animal model of the haemolytic uraemic syndrome in shigellosis: Leukocyte-mediated renal cortical necrosis in rabbits. *Br. J. Exp. Pathol., 66*: 7–15 (1985).
15. Editorial, Unravelling HUS. *Lancet, 2*: 1437–1439 (1987).
16. Badami, K. G., Srivastava, R. N., Kumar, R., Saraya, A. K., Disseminated intravascular coagulation in post-dysenteric haemolytic uraemic syndrome. *Acta Paediatr. Scand., 76*: 919–922 (1987).
17. Katz, J., Lurie, A., Kaplan, B. S., Krawitz, S., Mets, J., Coagulation findings in the hemolytic uremic syndrome of infancy: Similarity to hyperacute renal allograft rejection. *J. Pediatr., 78*: 426–434 (1971).
18. Riella, M. C., George, C. R. P., Hickman, R. O., Striker, G. E., Slichter, S. J., Harker, L., Quadracci, L. J., Renal microangiopathy of the hemolytic uremic syndrome in childhood. *Nephron, 17*: 188–203 (1976).
19. Edefonti, A., Bettinelli, A., Mondonico, P., Appiani, C. A., Picca, M., Cossu, M. M., Tentori, F., Giani, M., Rossi, E., Intraplatelet serotonin (I5HT) in children with the hemolytic uremic syndrome. *Clin. Nephrol., 23*: 207–211 (1986).
20. Appiani, A. C., Edefonti, A., Bettinelli, A., Cossu, M. M., Paracchine, M. L., Rossi, E., The relationship between plasma levels of the factor VIII complex and platelet release products (beta-thromboglobulin and platelet factor 4) in children with the hemolytic uremic syndrome. *Clin. Nephrol., 17*: 195–199 (1982).
21. Monnens, L., Van de Meer, W., Langenhuysen, C., Van Munster, P., Van Oostroom, C., Platelet aggregating factor in the epidemic form of hemolytic uremic syndrome in children. *Clin. Nephrol., 24*: 135–137 (1985).
22. Fong, J. S. C., Kaplan, B. S., Impairment of platelet aggregation in hemolytic uremic syndrome. Evidence for platelet "exhaustion." *Blood, 60*: 564–570 (1982).
23. Monnens, L., Kleynen, F., Van Munster, P., Schretlen, E., Bonnerman, A., Coagulation studies and streptokinase therapy in the haemolytic uraemic syndrome. *Helv. Paediatr. Acta, 27*: 45–54 (1972).
24. Ekberg, M., Nilsson, I. M., Denneberg, T., Coagulation studies in hemolytic uremic syndrome and thrombotic thrombocytopenic purpura. *Acta Med. Scand., 196*: 373–382 (1974).
25. Rose, P. E., Clark, A. J. B., Haematology of the haemolytic uraemic syndrome. *Blood Rev., 3*: 136–140 (1989).
26. Rose, P. E., Enayat, S. M., Sunderland, R., Short, P. E., Williams, C. E., Hill, F. G. H., Abnormalities in the factor VIII isolated protein multimers in the haemolytic uraemic syndrome. *Arch. Dis. Child., 59*: 1135–1140 (1984).
27. Gill, J. C., Sheth, K. J., Endres-Brooks, J., Leichter, H. E., The predictive value of von Willebrand factor (vWF) in hemolytic uremic syndrome (HUS) [abstract]. *Blood, 72*(Suppl. 1): 1096 (1988).
28. Moake, H. L., McPherson, P. D., Abnormalities of von Willebrand factor multimers in thrombotic thrombocytopenic purpura and the hemolytic uremic syndrome. *Am. J. Med., 87*: 3–9N (1989).
29. Monnens, L., Van Aken, W., De Jong, M., "Active" intravascular coagulation in the epidemic form of hemolytic uremic syndrome. *Clin. Nephrol., 17*: 284–287 (1982).
30. Bergstein, J. M., Kuederli, U., Bang, N. U., Plasma inhibitor of glomerular fibrinolysis in the hemolytic uremic syndrome. *Am. J. Med., 73*: 322–327 (1982).
31. Glas-Greenwalt, P., Hall, J. M., Panke, T. W., Kant, K. S., Allen, C. M., Pollak, V. E.,

Fibrinolysis in health and disease: Abnormal levels of plasminogen activator, plasminogen activator inhibitor and protein C in thrombotic thrombocytopenic purpura. *J. Lab. Clin. Med., 108*: 415–422 (1986).
32. Kakishita, E., Koyama, T., Higuchi, M., Kunitomi, O., Oura, Y., Nagai, K., Fibrinolysis in thrombotic thrombocytopenic purpura. *Am. J. Hematol., 32*: 14–19 (1989).
33. Bergstein, J. M., Bang, N. U., Plasminogen activator inhibitor (PAI-1) is the circulating inhibitor of fibrinolysis in the hemolytic uremic syndrome (HUS) [abstract]. *Kidney Int., 37*: 254 (1990).
34. Takahashi, H., Tatewaki, W., Wada, K., Shibata, A., Thrombin generation in patients with thrombotic thrombocytopenic purpura. *Am. J. Hematol., 32*: 255–257 (1989).
35. Vitacco, M., Sanchez-Avalos, J., Gianantonio, C. A., Heparin therapy in the hemolytic uremic syndrome. *J. Pediatr., 83*: 271–275 (1973).
36. Proesmans, W., Eeckels, R., Has heparin changed the prognosis of the hemolytic uremic syndrome? *Clin. Nephrol., 2*: 169–173 (1974).
37. Powell, H. R., Ekert, H., Streptokinase and antithrombotic therapy in the hemolytic uremic syndrome. *J. Pediatr., 84*: 345–349 (1974).
38. Stuart, J., Winterborn, M. H., White, R. H. R., Flinn, R. M., Thrombolytic therapy in haemolytic uraemic syndrome. *Br. Med. J., 2*: 217–221 (1974).
39. Monnens, L., Van Collenburg, J., De Jong, M., Zoethout, H., Treatment of the hemolytic uremic syndrome. *Helv. Pediatr. Acta, 33*: 321–328 (1978).
40. Diekmann, L., Streptokinase und Heparinbehandlung beim haemolytisch–uraemischen Syndrom. *Klin. Paediatr., 192*: 430–435 (1980).
41. O'Regan, S., Chesney, R. W., Mongeau, J. G., Robitaille, P., Aspirin and dipyridamole therapy in the hemolytic uremic syndrome. *J. Pediatr., 97*: 473–476 (1980).
42. Jones, R. W. A., Morris, M. C., Maisy, M. N., Saxton, H. M., Chantler, C., Endarterial urokinase in childhood hemolytic uremic syndrome. *Kidney Int., 20*: 723–727 (1981).
43. Loirat, C., Beaufils, F., Sonsino, E., Schlegel, N., Guesnu, M., Pillion, G., André, J. L., Broyer, M., Guyot, C., Habib, R., Mathieu, H., Traitement du syndrome hémolytique et urémique de l'enfant par l'urokinase. Essai contrôlé coöpératif. *Arch. Fr. Pédiatr., 41*: 15–19 (1984).
44. Van Dyck, M., Proesmans, W., Depraetere, M., Hemolytic uremic syndrome in childhood: Renal function ten years later. *Clin. Nephrol., 29*: 109–112 (1988).
45. De Jong, M., Monnens, L., Haemolytic uraemic syndrome: A 10-year follow-up study of 73 patients. *Nephrol. Dial. Transpl., 3*: 379–382 (1988).
46. Trompeter, R., Schwartz, R., Chantler, C., Dillon, M. R., Haycock, G. B., Haemolytic uraemic syndrome: An analysis of the prognostic features. *Arch. Dis. Child., 58*: 101–105 (1983).
47. Loirat, C., Sonsino, E., Varga-Moreno, A., Pillion, G., Mercier, J. C., Beaufils, F., Mathieu, H., Hemolytic uremic syndrome: An analysis of the natural history and prognostic features. *Acta Paediatr. Scand., 73*: 505–514 (1984).
48. Bergstein, J. M., Tissue plasminogen activator therapy of glomerular thrombi in the Shwartzman reaction. *Kidney Int., 35*: 14–18 (1989).
49. Rizzoni, G., Claris-Appiani, A., Edefonti, A., Facchin, P., Franchini, F., Gusmano, R., Imbasciati, E., Pavanello, L., Perfumo, F., Remuzzi, G., Plasma infusion for hemolytic uremic syndrome in children: Results of a multicenter controlled trial. *J. Pediatr., 112*: 284–290 (1988).
50. O'Regan, S., Blais, N., Russo, P., Pison, C. F., Rousseau, E., Hemolytic uremic syndrome: Glomerular filtration rate, 6 to 11 years later measured by ^{99m}TcDTPA plasma slope clearance. *Clin. Nephrol., 32*: 217–220 (1989).

30
Treatment of Hemolytic Uremic Syndrome with Fresh-Frozen Plasma or with Plasmapheresis

Chantal Loirat *Hôpital Robert Debré, Paris, France*

The treatment of the hemolytic uremic syndrome (HUS) with infusions of fresh-frozen plasma (FFP) or by plasmapheresis (plasma exchanges; PE) became popular in some centers in the 1980s. The precise indications and rationale for these forms of treatment remain unclear because the pathogenesis of HUS has not been completely elucidated and the prognosis is generally favorable. A good outcome, especially in terms of immediate survival and of renal involvement, is particularly true for patients with the postdiarrheal form of HUS. Although much of the laboratory research that has provided the theoretical basis for using FFP or plasmapheresis has been discussed in Chapters 25–27, this will be reevaluated to support the use of this therapy. Furthermore, the results of two prospective therapeutic trials that assessed the usefulness of FFP for treatment of HUS will be evaluated and an attempt will be made to recommend indications for the use of plasmapheresis. The use of plasmapheresis is also discussed elsewhere in this book.

THEORETICAL BASIS

Numerous factors have been implicated in the pathogenesis of HUS. The more common, typical form is frequently associated with an infection by Shiga-like toxin (SLT)-producing organisms, whereas predisposing factors in atypical cases include a genetic predisposition, drugs, or other agents (1, 2). Most of these factors seem to operate through a final common pathway of endothelial cell injury, with disturbances in platelet–endothelial interactions that may initiate local intravascular coagulation and result in fibrin deposition and further platelet activation (2, 3). Phenomena that may perpetuate platelet adherence, aggregation, and activation include reduced prostacyclin and increased thromboxane production, release of abnormal von Willebrand Factor (vWF) multimers, and platelet-aggregating factors.

Prostacyclin

Plasma from some patients with HUS and thrombotic thrombocytopenic purpura (TTP) may have a reduced ability to stimulate prostacyclin production by endothelial tissues (4–8). This observation resulted in the use of FFP infusions for the treatment of similar patients. Prostacyclin-stimulating activity may improve after infusion of FFP or after PE (4–6, 9–11). Similarly, if one mixes the plasma from a normal individual with that of a patient with HUS, normal activity can be restored in vitro (8, 12). It is possible that FFP prevents the destruction of prostacyclin synthetase and, thereby, restores the normal antioxidant potential of plasma (8). As a result, a vicious cycle that perpetuates the disease is broken. The defect in prostacyclin production has also been ascribed to the presence of an inhibitor of production (13). This inhibitor might be removed by PE. The bioavailability of prostacyclin has been found to be reduced as a result of decreased binding to plasma proteins and rapid destruction (14), which can be corrected by infusion of plasma (15).

However, the defect in prostacyclin has not been found in all patients (16, 17) and appears to be more frequent in adults and in atypical or familial forms of the disease (5, 7, 18) than in typical postdiarrheal cases (8, 19, 20). However, even in atypical forms, it remains to be established whether a missing factor(s) is a primary or a secondary event. Sections of veins from patients with HUS have a reduced ability to produce prostacyclin (4). Plasma concentrations of the 6-keto $PGF_{1\alpha}$ are reduced or undetectable in some patients with HUS and TTP (8), but are elevated in children during the acute phase of HUS (21, 22). These findings suggest that prostacyclin production may increase at the time of the initial insult to the endothelium and that, with ongoing injury, there is a reduced ability to produce enzymes, such as prostacyclin synthetase.

Platelet-Aggregating Activity

Plasma of some adults with TTP has been shown to contain a platelet-aggregating factor (PAF) (23–26), which could be inhibited by normal plasma (23) and normal immunoglobulins (24), but not by the patient's immunoglobulins. Similar findings have been reported in a few children with HUS (19, 27) and TTP (28). We could demonstrate a PAF in only 1 of 16 children with HUS, of whom 7 were atypical. The single case was atypical; HUS occurred 6 months after a bone marrow transplant for neuroblastoma (29). Others (19) have found a PAF of lower potency in children with HUS than that found in adults with TTP; the lower-potency PAF could not be inhibited in vitro by plasma. Despite these conflicting observations, it has been proposed that PAFs may be removed by plasmapheresis, and that, if FFP is given for volume replacement, factors or immunoglobulins may be supplied that inhibit PAFs (26).

von Willebrand Factors

Abnormal ultralarge vWF multimers, apparently released from damaged endothelial cells, have been found in patients with relapsing forms of TTP (30) and in some patients with HUS (31–33), especially if they were atypical cases (34). Because of their role in inducing platelet adhesion (30) and in enhancing PAFs (25), plasmapheresis seems to be a logical method whereby they may be removed.

Shiga-like Toxin-Associated Hemolytic Uremic Syndrome

Commercially available immunoglobulins contain anticytotoxin neutralizing antibodies, which neutralize only Shiga-like toxin type 1 (SLT-1), but not SLT-2 (35, 36). Unfortunately, these preparations have not proved to be of value in the treatment of HUS (35). Despite this misgiving, however, the provision of immunoglobulins by FFP treatment provides another theoretical justification for its potential value, even in patients with typical HUS.

TREATMENT OF HEMOLYTIC UREMIC SYNDROME WITH FRESH-FROZEN PLASMA

In 1977, Byrnes and Khurana proposed that TTP be treated with infusions of FFP (37). A positive effect, mainly on the hematological indexes and neurological course, was found in about 60% of the cases of TTP reviewed by Shepard and Bukowski (38). Apparent benefits (39) and variable benefits (40) were found by Remuzzi's team (39, 40). Although the anemia and thrombocytopenia of children and adults with HUS seemed to benefit from the use of FFP in an uncontrolled trial, there was no demonstrable effect on the renal disease (40). Sheth et al. (41), in a case–control study of infusions of FFP, were unable to demonstrate a positive effect in children with HUS.

Two prospective trials have been performed, one in Italy (17) and the other in France (42) because of the inconclusive findings of these uncontrolled reports. Any controlled study on the treatment of HUS must take into account several important caveats: because the natural history is variable and often favorable with conventional treatment, at least 350 patients may be required to obtain a significant difference in mortality rate and in ultimate renal dysfunction rate (43); fewer cases may require evaluation if the study includes an analysis of the renal pathology, because it is known that patients who recover normal renal function, despite having had cortical necrosis or extensive glomerular thrombotic microangiopathy, may still develop hypertension and chronic renal failure at a later date (44, 45). Therefore, the effect on the renal structural abnormalities must be a prime concern in any well-designed study.

The French Society of Pediatric Nephrology Trial

The trial included 79 patients aged 2 months to 13 years from 19 centers in France (42). Forty patients were randomized to a control (usual treatment) group and 39 to a plasma (FFP infusions, 10 ml/kg per day for 7 days) group. Randomization yielded no significant differences between these groups in age distribution, season of occurrence, incidence of gastrointestinal prodrome, severity of anemia and of renal failure (Table 1). The only difference was seen in the severity of thrombocytopenia, which was slightly worse in the group treated with FFP ($p < 0.05$).

There was no significant difference between the groups in the progression of the hematological changes or renal indexes in the acute phase and during the first month after onset. Renal function was subsequently evaluated by urinary protein and serum creatinine concentrations. The mean serum creatinine concentrations were significantly higher in the control group at 3 and 6 months, but not at 12 months (Table 2). Furthermore, 58% of the control patients, compared with 29% of plasma patients,

Table 1 Clinical and Laboratory Data on Admission

	Rizzoni et al.		Loirat et al.	
	Plasma group (n = 17)	Control group (n = 15)	Plasma group (n = 39)	Control group (n = 40)
Age (yrs)				
Mean	2.7	2.3	2.5	2.5
Range	0.7–6.6	0.4–6.4	0.2–12.4	0.4–13
< 3 yr (%)	66		78	
Occurrence in spring, summer (%)	65	73	72	85
Intestinal prodromes (%)	76	67	82	92
Delay between onset of prodrome and randomization (days)	< 8	< 8	4.5	4.1
Plasma creatinine (μmol/L)	510	518	454	495
Dialysis (%)	100	100	82	85
Hemoglobin (g/dl)	7.8	8.0	6.8	7.0
Platelets (suppress × 103/mm^3)	63,000	67,000	38,000	55,000

had a serum creatinine concentration greater than 60 μmol/L at 3 months ($p < 0.05$). At 6 months, the percentages were 54 and 21%, respectively ($p < 0.02$). The percentage of patients with proteinuria was greater in the control group (46%) than in the plasma group (17%; $p < 0.02$) at 6 months, but not at 1 year. The incidence of arterial hypertension was similar in the two groups at all stages.

The renal histopathological abnormalities were evaluated in 27 patients from each group. Tissue was obtained 24 ± 15 days after onset in the plasma group and 19 ± 14 days after onset in the control patients. Evidence of extensive cortical necrosis was not seen in any of the treated patients, but was apparent in 7 of 27 of the control patients ($p < 0.02$). The frequency of glomerular thrombotic microangiopathy (21 cases), arterial thrombotic microangiopathy (TMA) (4 cases), and polymorphous lesions (16 cases) was similar. Furthermore, the percentage of involved glomeruli did not differ significantly within each of these three categories.

Table 2 Results of The French Trial

	Serum creatinine	(μmol/L mean ± SD)
	Control group	Plasma group
3 mo	66 ± 28	49 ± 14 ($p < 0.02$)
6 mo	63 ± 21	48 ± 13 ($p < 0.005$)

The Italian Study

In this controlled trial the results of 17 patients treated with FFP were compared with those of 15 who were treated conventionally (17). No significant benefits of plasma could be demonstrated during the acute phase or during a follow-up period of about 24 months; nor were there any significant differences in the pathologic appearance of renal biopsy specimens, taken from 11 patients in each group 24–49 days after onset of the HUS. One patient in each group had cortical necrosis, and none had severe arteriolar changes. Ultrastructural studies, however, revealed arteriolar damage and thickening of the lamina rara interna in 5 of 7 control patients; no changes were apparent in any of the plasma-treated patients.

Comparisons Between the French and Italian Trials

It is unclear why none of the French patients treated with FFP had cortical necrosis, whereas the pathologic studies were similar in all the Italian patients. There were no apparent differences between the two populations of patients (see Table 1). However, it is possible that the overall severity of illness in the French was greater than in the Italian patients. Four French patients (two in each group) died in the acute phase; three of these had cerebral, pancreatic, and intestinal involvement. Another four progressed rapidly to end-stage renal failure. None of the Italian patients died or had rapid progression to end-stage renal failure.

Interestingly, the French children entered the trial between February 1983 and February 1985. This period included the summer of 1983 when HUS was most prevalent and severe in the north and west of France (46). A similar epidemic occurred in the West Midlands of England at the same time (47). The Italian patients entered their trial from February 1981 to February 1985 and one could suggest that the pattern was different in Italy, especially in the summer of 1983. In addition, the smaller number of patients in the Italian trial could have affected its conclusions. Furthermore, a different regimen was used in Italy: 30 ml/kg of FFP was given the first day; 10 ml/kg per day was then infused until 3 days after the platelet count had returned to normal. This took a mean of 8.6 days (range 4–25). In contrast, all the French patients received 10 ml/kg per day for 7 days. However, it is unlikely that the difference in quantity of FFP is sufficient to explain the differences observed in the renal histopathological changes.

Cole (48) has noted that a central problem in studying HUS is the need to include patients from different centers. Furthermore, inclusion of different forms of HUS (postdiarrheal, and atypical or inherited cases) can impair the interpretation of the results, because patients with the postdiarrheal form are more likely to recover spontaneously. This may be a specious argument because some of the postdiarrheal cases may develop cortical necrosis and some of the atypical cases may well be the ones who have the most to gain from plasma infusions and, above all, as described in the trial protocol, the proportion of patients with the atypical form of HUS was comparable in both the treated and untreated groups.

In the French trial, the finding that cortical necrosis was significantly more frequent in untreated patients suggested that plasma infusions must be considered as possibly beneficial. However, FFP was discontinued at the beginning of 1985 because of the risk of contamination with human immunodeficiency virus. In addition to the low risk of contamination with hepatitis B virus, two of the Italian patients were infected with hepatitis C.

Infused volumes of FFP larger than 10 ml/kg per day have been proposed for patients with HUS (38) or TTP (37). High doses and prolonged treatment may cause volume overload and nephrotoxicity. Two patients with HUS have had prolonged dialysis-dependent renal failure (74 and 94 days) associated with hyperproteinemia and heavy proteinuria induced by large quantities of FFP given for a long time (20–30 ml/kg per day for 65 days) (49).

Fresh-frozen plasma is also contraindicated in patients with *Streptococcus pneumoniae*-associated HUS. Plasma from adults contains antibodies against the Thomsen–Friedenreich antigen, and these may accelerate polyagglutination and hemolysis (50, 51). These patients should be treated with antibiotics and washed red blood cells. Albumin concentrates should be used for volume repletion, rather than whole blood or plasma.

TREATMENT OF THE HEMOLYTIC UREMIC SYNDROME BY PLASMAPHERESIS (PLASMA EXCHANGE)

Plasma exchange has become the treatment of choice for TTP (38, 52). The following regimen is now generally recommended:

The volume of the exchanges is between 1–1½ that of the plasma volume (40–60 ml/kg)
The replacement fluid is usually FFP
The exchanges are done daily or every other day
Antiplatelet therapy that includes aspirin (acetylsalicylic acid) and dipyridamole or sulfinpyrazone are usually included

Shephard and Bukowski (38) have concluded, from a review of the literature, that the overall response rate was approximately 80%. This is impressive, because TTP has had such high mortality rate. The benefits of PE in the treatment of TTP are discussed in detail elsewhere in this book, but it is pertinent to note that, although there have been improvements in the hematological and neurological course, a similar effect on renal involvement has not been established (53). Despite these caveats, anecdotal evidence suggests that PE may be beneficial in atypical forms of HUS, especially when symptoms of central nervous system (CNS) involvement are present (10, 11, 38, 54–56). This subject has been reviewed in detail in Chapter 10.

We have treated four patients aged 6–8 years with atypical forms of HUS by PE. Volume replacement consisted of 30–40 ml/kg of which two-thirds was FFP and one-third was diluted albumin. The mean number of PEs was nine, and the range was 7–11. One patient was in status epilepticus and coma for 6 days and was anuric. A computed tomographic (CT) scan of the brain was normal. The others had nonoliguric renal failure. Two required dialysis. Plasma exchange seemed to have a beneficial effect on the neurological features of one patient: seizures stopped after the fifth PE, and the coma subsided within 3 weeks and cortical blindness within 6 months. It also appeared to improve the hematological parameters of two patients: PE was associated with an increase in the platelet count and cessation of hemolysis after one and five sessions, respectively. The effect on the renal disease was less encouraging. Three of the patients (one with cortical necrosis, two with glomerular TMA involving all glomeruli) have developed chronic renal failure 1–4 years later. Two have become hypertensive. One patient, whose TMA was less diffuse, has normal renal function after 4 months follow-up. A prospective trial that is now being done in Germany (57) may help clarify the indications and efficiency of PE in patients with HUS.

CONCLUSION: HOW SHOULD THE HEMOLYTIC UREMIC SYNDROME BE TREATED?

Evaluation of the results of many reports and two well-conducted prospective trials suggest that the wisest approach is to adhere to the "First, do not harm" rule in which the natural outcome of the disease versus the benefits, risks, and cost of specific treatment are carefully considered. Currently, the general consensus (1, 20, 58, 59) supports the following approach:

In the typical form of HUS, careful supportive management, without specific treatment, should be carried out until the results of the prospective trials to assess the usefulness of treatments, such as infusions of immunoglobulins, are available.

In the atypical forms of HUS (older children with severe involvement, absent diarrheal prodrome, subacute, or relapsing course, CNS involvement, and familial HUS), FFP infusions can be used, and this can be followed by PE, if necessary. A more aggressive approach in which PE and FFP as the replacement fluid are used from the onset, may be justified in these atypical cases (20).

REFERENCES

1. Kaplan, B. S., Proesmans, W., The hemolytic uremic syndrome of childhood and its variants. *Semin. Hematol.*, *24*: 148–160 (1987).
2. Kaplan, B. S., Cleary, T. G., Obrig, T. G., Recent advances in understanding the pathogenesis of the hemolytic uremic syndromes. *Pediatr. Nephrol.*, *4*: 278–283 (1990).
3. Bergstein, J. M., Glomerular fibrin deposition and removal. *Pediatr. Nephrol.*, *4*: 78–87 (1990).
4. Remuzzi, G., Misiani, R., Marchesi, D., Livio, M., Mecca, G., De Gaetano, G., Donati, M. B., Haemolytic–uraemic syndrome: Deficiency of plasma factor(s) regulating prostacyclin activity? *Lancet*, *2*: 871–872 (1978).
5. Jorgensen, K. A., Pedersen, R. S., Familial deficiency of prostacyclin production stimulation factor in the hemolytic uremic syndrome of childhood. *Thromb. Res.*, *21*: 311–315 (1981).
6. Stuart, M. J., Spitzer, R. E., Coppe, D., Abnormal platelet and vascular prostaglandin synthesis in an infant with hemolytic uremic syndrome. *Pediatrics*, *71*: 120–124 (1984).
7. Turi, S., Beattie, T. J., Belch, J. J. F., Murphy, A. V., Disturbances of prostacyclin metabolism in children with hemolytic uremic syndrome and in first degree relatives. *Clin. Nephrol.*, *25*: 193–198 (1986).
8. Remuzzi, G., Zoja, C., Rossi, E. C., Prostacyclin in thrombotic microangiopathy. *Semin. Hematol.*, *24*: 110–118 (1987).
9. Remuzzi, G., Marchesi, D., Misiani, R., Mecca, G., De Gaetano, G., Donati, M. B., Familial deficiency of a plasma factor stimulating vascular prostacyclin activity. *Thromb. Res.*, *16*: 517–525 (1979).
10. Beattie, T. J., Murphy, A. V., Willoughby, M. C. N., Machin, S. S., Defrein, G., Plasmapheresis in the haemolytic uremic syndrome in children. *Br. Med. J.*, *282*: 1667–1668 (1981).
11. Gillor, A., Bulla, M., Roth, B., Bupmann, K., Schror, K., Tekook, A., Gladtke, E., Plasmapheresis as a therapeutic measure in hemolytic uremic syndrome in children. *Klin. Wochenschr.*, *61*: 363–367 (1983).

12. Stiegler, R. L., Hemolytic uremic syndrome: Clinical observations from the Southwest Pediatric Nephrology Study Group and laboratory findings from the University of Utah Health Sciences Center. In *Recent Advances in Pediatric Nephrology* (K. Murakami, T. Kitagawa, K. Yabuta, T. Sakai, eds.), Elsevier Science, Amsterdam, pp. 581–584 (1987).
13. Levin, M., Elkon, K. B., Nokes, T. J. C., Buckle, A. M., Dillon, M. J., Hardisty, R. M., Barratt, T. M., Inhibitor of prostacyclin production in sporadic haemolytic uraemic syndrome. *Arch. Dis. Child., 58*: 703–708 (1983).
14. Chen, Y. C., McLeod, B., Hall, E. R., Wu, K. K., Accelerated prostacyclin degradation in thrombotic thrombocytopenic purpura. *Lancet, 2*: 267–269 (1981).
15. Wu, K. K., Hall, E. R., Papp, A., Prostacyclin stabilizing factor deficiency in thrombotic thrombocytopenic purpura. *Lancet, 1*: 460–461 (1982).
16. Schlegel, N., Maclouf, J., Loirat, C., Drouet, L., Marotte, R., Scarabin, P. Y., Mathieu, H., Childhood hemolytic uremic syndrome. Absence of deficiency of plasma prostacyclin stimulating activity. *J. Pediatr., 111*: 71–77 (1987).
17. Rizzoni, G., Claris-Appiani, A., Edefonti, A., Facchin, P., Franchini, F., Gusmano, R., Imbasciati, E., Pavanello, L., Perfumo, F., Remuzzi, G., Plasma infusion for hemolytic uremic syndrome in children: Results of a multicenter controlled trial. *J. Pediatr., 112*: 284–290 (1988).
18. Wiles, P. G., Solomon, L. R., Lawler, W., Mallick, N. P., Inherited plasma factor deficiency in haemolytic uraemic syndrome. *Lancet, 1*: 1105–1106 (1981).
19. Walters, M. D. S., Levin, M., Smith, C., Nokes, T. J. C., Hardisty, R. M., Dillon, M. J., Barratt, T. M., Intravascular platelet activation in the hemolytic uremic syndrome. Studies on the typical (epidemic) and atypical (sporadic) sub-groups. *Kidney Int., 33*: 107–115 (1988).
20. Levin, M., Walters, M. D. S., Barratt, T. M., Hemolytic uremic syndrome. *Adv. Pediatr. Infect. Dis., 4*: 51–82 (1989).
21. Stuart, M. J., Spitzer, R. E., Walenga, R. W., Boone, S., Prostanoïds in hemolytic uremic syndrome. *J. Pediatr., 106*: 936–938 (1985).
22. Tonshoff, B., Momper, R., Kuhl, P. G., Schweer, H., Schärer, K., Seyberth, H. W., Increased thromboxane biosynthesis in childhood hemolytic uremic syndrome. *Kidney Int., 37*: 1134–1141 (1990).
23. Lian, E. C. Y., Harkness, D. R., Byrnes, J. J., Wallach, H., Nunez, R., Presence of a platelet aggregating factor in the plasma of patients with thrombotic thrombocytopenic purpura and its inhibition by normal plasma. *Blood, 53*: 333–338 (1979).
24. Lian, E. C. Y., Mui, P. T. K., Siddiqui, F. A., Chiu, A. Y. Y., Chiu, L. L. S., Inhibition of platelet-aggregating activity in thrombotic thrombocytopenic purpura plasma by normal adult immunoglobulin G. *J. Clin. Invest., 73*: 548–555 (1984).
25. Kelton, J. G., Moore, J., Santos, A., Sheridan, D., Detection of a platelet-aggregating factor in thrombotic thrombocytopenic purpura. *Ann. Intern. Med., 101*: 589–593 (1984).
26. Hussey, C. B., Hause, L. L., Gottschall, J. L., Anderson, T., A platelet-aggregating factor in thrombotic thrombocytopenic purpura: Initial activity, fluctuations, and removal by plasma exchange. *Thromb. Res., 44*: 355–364 (1986).
27. Monnens, L., Vandemeer, W., Langenhuysen, C., Van Munster, P., Van Oostrom, C., Platelet-aggregating factor in the epidemic form of hemolytic uremic syndrome in childhood. *Clin. Nephrol., 24*: 135–137 (1985).
28. Viero, P., Cortelazzo, S., Buelli, M., Comotti, B., Minetti, B., Bassan, R., Barbui, T., Thrombotic thrombocytopenic purpura and high dose immunoglobulin treatment. *Ann. Intern. Med., 104*: 282 (1986).
29. Loirat, C., Schlegel, N., Hurtaud, M. F., Pillion, G., Platelet-aggregating activity in hemolytic uremic syndrome [abstract]. *Pediatr. Nephrol., 3*: C182 (1989).
30. Moake, J. L., Rudy, C. K., Troll, J. H., Weinstein, M. J., Colannino, N. M., Azocar, J., Seder, R. H., Hong, S. L., Deykin, D., Unusually large plasma factor VIII–von Wille-

brand factor multimers in chronic relapsing thrombotic thrombocytopenic purpura. *N. Engl. J. Med., 307*: 1432–1435 (1982).
31. Rose, P. E., Struthers, G. S., Robertson, M., Kavi, J., Taylor, C. M., Factor VIII von Willebrand protein in haemolytic uraemic syndrome and systemic vasculitides. *Lancet, 335*: 500–502 (1990).
32. Moake, J. L., Byrnes, J. J., Troll, J. H., Rudy, C. K., Weinstein, M. J., Colannino, N. M., Hong, S. L., Abnormal VIII–von Willebrand factor patterns in the plasma of patients with the hemolytic uremic syndrome. *Blood, 64*: 592–598 (1984).
33. Rose, P. E., Enayat, S. M., Sunderland, R., Short, P. E., Williams, C. E., Hill, F. G. H., Abnormalities of factor VIII related protein multimers in the haemolytic uraemic syndrome. *Arch. Dis. Child., 59*: 1135–1140 (1984).
34. Helmsworth, M., Sherbotie, J., Kaplan, B. S., Abnormal factor VIII: von Willebrand (VIII:Wb) multimers in patients with hemolytic uremic syndrome (HUS) or thrombotic thrombocytopenic purpura (TTP) may predict thrombotic episodes. *Pediatr. Nephrol., 3*: C182 (1989).
35. Ashkenazi, S., Cleary, T. G., Lopez, E., Pickering, L. K., Anticytotoxin neutralizing antibodies in immunoglobulin preparations: Potential use in hemolytic uremic syndrome. *J. Pediatr., 113*: 1008–1014 (1988).
36. Bitzan, M., Klemt, M., Altrogge, H., Immunotherapy for hemolytic uremic syndrome: Different efficiencies of therapeutic immunoglobulins to neutralize Shiga-like toxin I and II [abstract]. *Pediatr. Nephrol., 3*: C182 (1989).
37. Byrnes, J. J., Khurana, M., Treatment of thrombotic thrombocytopenic purpura with plasma. *N. Engl. J. Med., 297*: 1386–1389 (1977).
38. Shepard, K. V., Bukowski, R. M., The treatment of thrombotic thrombocytopenic purpura with exchange transfusions, plasma infusions, and plasma exchange. *Semin. Hematol., 24*: 178–193 (1987).
39. Remuzzi, G., Misiani, R., Marchesi, D., Livio, M., Mecca, G., De Gaetano, G., Donati, M. B., Treatment of the hemolytic uremic syndrome with plasma. *Clin. Nephrol., 12*: 279–284 (1979).
40. Misiani, R., Appiani, A. C., Edefonti, A., Gotti, E., Bettinelli, A., Giani, M., Rossi, E., Remuzzi, G., Mecca, G., Haemolytic uraemic syndrome: Therapeutic effect of plasma infusion. *Br. Med. J., 285*: 1304–1306 (1982).
41. Sheth, K. J., Gill, J. C., Hanna, J., Leichtter, H. E., Failure of fresh frozen plasma infusions to alter the course of hemolytic uremic syndrome. *Child. Nephrol. Urol., 9*: 38–41 (1988–89).
42. Loirat, C., Sonsino, E., Hinglais, N., Jais, J. P., Landais, P., Fermanian, J., Treatment of the childhood haemolytic uraemic syndrome with plasma. A multicenter randomized controlled trial. *Pediatr. Nephrol., 2*: 279–285 (1988).
43. Trompeter, R. S., Schwartz, R., Chantler, C., Dillon, M. J., Haycock, G. B., Kay, R., Barratt, T. M., Haemolytic uraemic syndrome: An analysis of prognostic features. *Arch. Dis. Child., 58*: 101–105 (1983).
44. Habib, R., Levy, M., Gagnadoux, M. F., Broyer, M., Prognosis of the hemolytic uremic syndrome in children. *Adv. Nephrol., 11*: 99–128 (1982).
45. Gagnadoux, M. F., Habib, R., Broyer, M., Royer, P., Pronostic à long terme du syndrome hémolytique et urémique de l'enfant [abstract]. *Clin. Invest. Med., 10*: A67 (1987).
46. Guyot, C., Daniel, M. D., Roze, J. C., Renoult, E., Dubigeon, P., Buzelin, F., Pronostic du syndrome hémolytique et urémique chez l'enfant. Importance de l'atteinte extra-rénale. *Arch. Fr. Pediatr., 43*: 253–258 (1986).
47. Taylor, C. M., White, R. H. R., Winterborn, M. H., Rowe, D., Haemolytic uraemic syndrome: Clinical experience of an outbreak in the West Midlands. *Br. Med. J., 292*: 1513–1516 (1986).

48. Cole, B. R., Plasma infusion therapy in hemolytic uremic syndrome: Is it warranted? *Pediatr. Nephrol.*, *2*: 286–287 (1988).
49. Eddy, A. A., Geary, D. F., Balfe, J. W., Clark, W. F., Baumal, R., Prolongation of acute renal failure in two patients with hemolytic uremic syndrome due to excessive plasma infusion therapy. *Pediatr. Nephrol.*, *3*: 420–423 (1989).
50. Seger, R., Joller, P., Baerlocher, K., Kenny, A., Dulake, C., Leumann, E., Spierig, M., Hitzig, W. H., Hemolytic uremic syndrome associated with neuraminidase-producing microorganisms: Treatment by exchange transfusion. *Helv. Paediatr. Acta*, *35*: 359–367 (1980).
51. McGraw, M. E., Lendon, M., Stevens, R. F., Postlethwaite, R. J., Taylor, C. M., Haemolytic uraemic syndrome and the Thomsen Friedenreich antigen. *Pediatr. Nephrol.*, *3*: 135–139 (1989).
52. Blitzer, J. B., Gran Fortuna, J. M., Gottlieb, A. J., Smith, J. R., Theodorakis, M. E., Zamkoff, K. W., Landaw, S. A., Goldberg, J., Scalzo, A. J., Lamberson, H., Thrombotic thrombocytopenic purpura: Treatment with plasmapheresis. *Am. J. Hematol.*, *24*: 329–339 (1987).
53. Henon, P. R., Treatment of thrombotic thrombocytopenic purpura. First results of a controlled clinical trial. *Plasma Ther. Transfusion Technol.*, *7*: 101–106 (1986).
54. Denneberg, Y., Friedberg, M., Holmberg, L., Mathiasen, C., Nilsson, K. O., Takulander, R., Walder, M., Combined plasmapheresis and hemodialysis treatment for severe hemolytic uremic syndrome following campylobacter colitis. *Acta Paediatr. Scand.*, *71*: 243–245 (1982).
55. Camba, L., Al-Hilali, M. M., Shulji, M. M. H., Joyner, M. V., Feest, T. G., Haemolytic uraemic syndrome with renal failure: The effect of plasmapheresis. *Haematologia*, *70*: 341–344 (1985).
56. Sheth, K. J., Leichter, H. E., Gill, H. C., Baumgardt, A., Reversal of central nervous system involvement in hemolytic uremic syndrome by use of plasma exchanges. *Clin. Pediatr.*, *26*: 651–656 (1987).
57. Muller-Wiefel, D. E., Bulla, M., Klare, B., Balzar, E., Bambauer, R., Tönshoff, B., Therapeutic plasma exchange in hemolytic uremic syndrome [abstract]. *Pediatr. Nephrol*, *3*: C183 (1989).
58. Siegler, R. L., Management of hemolytic uremic syndrome. *J. Pediatr.*, *112*: 1014–1020 (1988).
59. Kaplan, B. S., Remuzzi, G., The hemolytic uremic syndrome. In *Thrombosis and Hemostasis* (G. Remuzzi, E. Rossi, eds.), Butterworths, London, pp. 201–236 (1989).

31
Long-term Outcome of Hemolytic Uremic Syndrome in Children

Margaret M. Fitzpatrick *Institute of Child Health, London, England*

The hemolytic uremic syndromes (HUS) are a heterogeneous group of disorders that can be classified broadly into two major subtypes: the first is common in children and is associated with a diarrheal prodrome (D+ HUS), whereas the second is rare in childhood and not associated with antecedent diarrhea (D– HUS) (1). Over the past decade, there have been significant advances in the understanding of both the etiology and pathogenesis of this disorder (2); however, the long-term outcome in those patients who survive the acute phase of the illness remains incompletely documented. The prognosis for the HUS is known to depend on several factors, most significantly the subtype and predominant histopathological lesion (1, 3, 4). Children with D+ HUS who have a predominant glomerular injury have a much better outcome than those with D– HUS who have arteriolar injury or cortical necrosis. This chapter is based on a study performed at the Hospital for Sick Children, Great Ormond Street (HSC, GOS). The long-term outcome for renal function in 88 infants and children was evaluated 5–21 years after the acute phase of D+ HUS (5). The literature on follow-up in children with HUS has been reviewed.

MORTALITY

Follow-up studies (Table 1) have shown variable results in mortality and renal outcome following an episode of HUS. Before the introduction of dialysis, a high proportion of children with any form of HUS died of fluid overload, metabolic derangement, and uremia (6–10). Once short-term dialysis became a widely available form of treatment, the prognosis for HUS generally improved, and most recent series from Europe and North America report an acute fatality rate of between 4 and 12% (11–14). This decline in mortality is mainly due to a better understanding of how to manage acute renal failure in general and to better identification of less severe cases.

Table 1 Data on Long-Term Follow-up in Infants and Children with HUS: Review of the Literature

Author (Ref.)	Area/ country	Period of study	Number of patients	Number of deaths (%)	Duration of follow up (yr)	Number followed	GFR/creat. clearance > 80 (ml/min per 1.73 m^2)	< 80	H/T	P
Gianantonio et al., 1973 (8)	Buenos Aires, Argentina	1957–1972	679	76 (11)	5–13	124	73	51	18	40
Donckerwolke et al., 1973 (33)	15 West European centers	1970–1971	49	8 (16)	1	40			4	
Tune et al., 1973 (35)	California, United States	1960–1969	27	3 (11)	2–10	21	19	2		
Janssen et al., 1974 (34)	Brussels, Belgium	1957–1972	20	3 (15)	$^3/_{12}$–1	17			1	4
Kaplan et al., 1976 (13)	Johannesburg, South Africa	1969–1975	44	2 (5)	$^6/_{12}$–6	33			3	1
Monnens et al., 1978 (22)	Rotterdam-Nijmegen, Netherlands	1970–1975	73	5 (7)	2	68	64	4	5	10
Sorrenti et al., 1978 (23)	Illinois/ Indiana, United States	1968–1976	19	0	1$^6/_{12}$–8	19	14	5	1	2

Binda ki Mauaka et al., 1981 (24)	Leuven, Belgium	1970–1976	45	4 (9)	3–8	41	38	3	2	2
Trompeter et al., 1983 (11)	London, England	1969–1980	72	3 (4)	2–13	69	50	9	2	2
Loirat et al., 1984 (25)	Paris, France	1974–1981	67	5 (7)	1–7	56	37	8	6	8
Van Dyck et al., 1988 (12)	Leuven, Belgium	1970–1976	54	3 (6)	10	46	32	3	3	5
de Jong et al., 1988	Nijmegen, Netherlands	1965–1977	96	16 (17)	1/12–10	73	66	7	10	6
O'Regan et al., 1989	Montreal, Canada	1977–1982	50	0	6–11	37	16	21		7
Sieniawska et al., 1990 (19)	Warsaw, Poland	1972–1985	73	26 (36)	3–16	46	35	11	6	6
Coad et al., 1991 (14)	Birmingham, England	1970–1987	74	9 (12)	1–18	65	54	10	5	4
Srivastava et al., 1991 (18)	New Delhi, India	1980–1988	73	44 (60)	6/12–2	9	6	3		3
Fitzpatrick et al., 1991 (5)	London, England	1969–1980	103	8 (8)	5–21	88	72	16	3	27

GFR, glomerular filtration rate; H/T, hypertensive; P, proteinuria.

In the HSC series the mortality rate during the acute phase of the disease was 3 of 35 (8.6%) before 1980 and 2 of 68 (3.0%) after 1980. The mortality rate was higher in those presenting with a high polymorphonuclear leukocyte count and in those with severe neurological and gastrointestinal disease. Three children went into end-stage renal failure without recovering function and died between 6 months and 7 years after presentation. Therefore, the overall mortality rate between 1966 and 1985 was 8 of 103 (7.7%). Table 2 provides data on the 8 D+ HUS patients who died.

High mortality rates, up to 60%, have been reported in postdysenteric D+ HUS (15–18). The poor outcome in this form of HUS appears to be because of more profound renal injury. Other factors, including late referral of patients, serious infections, protracted dysentery with resulting malnutrition, and a higher incidence of intestinal complications, could be contributory (15–17). In a recent series from Northern India (17), the mortality rate was higher in those with prolonged anuria and total cortical necrosis. A comparatively more severe form of HUS was recently reported from Poland (18), with a mortality rate of 30% from acute renal failure; these patients had renal cortical necrosis and thrombotic foci in other organs. It is possible that the mortality rates are higher in these countries because milder cases of HUS are not referred to the tertiary centers. Although the mortality rate is high in the acute stage in postdysenteric HUS, most of those who recover appear to regain normal renal function (20).

LONG-TERM PROGNOSIS

Follow-up Studies

The long-term prognosis is less well documented, and follow-up studies (see Table 1) published over the years, from different geographic regions, have produced variable results for renal outcome following an episode of HUS.

The largest series (8) is from Argentina, where HUS is the leading cause of chronic renal failure in childhood and adolescence. Gianantonio et al. (8) produced detailed follow-up data on 124 suvivors followed for at least 5 years. Only 60 children (48%) were reported to have recovered completely, although hypertension was found

Table 2 Data from the HSC, GOS Series on Eight Children with D+HUS Who Died

					Death	
Gender	Year of presentation	Age (yr)	WBC ($\times 10^9$/L)	Duration of dialysis (days)	Time post presentation (mo)	Cause
M	1966	0.6	27.6	14	0.5	Cerebral
F	1966	1.1	32.9	48	1.6	Septicemia
F	1969	0.2	26.7	nil	0.2	Cerebral
F	1971	0.5	14.8	56	6	Cerebral
F	1978	11	22.9	28	5.5	Cardiac
M	1978	1	41.3	28	84	Septicemia
M	1980	2	37.4	6	0.2	Colitis
F	1985	3	22.9	9	0.3	Cerebral

in 10 of them. In 23 cases (18%), a progressive deterioration of renal function was observed. The authors concluded that "survival during the acute phase of HUS has created a new chronic renal disease which is an important cause of chronic uremia in Buenos Aires."

Other groups have published less gloomy results; however, some of these studies suffer from too short follow-up periods, a large number of cases lost to follow-up, and the absence of data on glomerular filtration (21–23).

Binda et al. (24) published a follow-up study on 42 surviving infants and children with HUS. Three patients (7%) had chronic renal failure. Normalization of renal function with no hematuria, proteinuria, or hypertension was documented in 93%. No differences were found when patients were subdivided according to age, severity of disease, or whether or not peritoneal dialysis was required. The same authors reviewed 46 patients 10 years after the acute phase (12). In 3 patients significant late sequelae were discovered: proteinuria, arterial hypertension, and in one, a low glomerular filtration rate. In an additional 14 former HUS patients, one or more mild abnormalities were found. Therefore, only 60% of the total population could be considered to have recovered completely.

In the series from London published in 1983, Trompeter et al. (11) retrospectively analyzed the records of 72 children with HUS to identify prognostic criteria. They identified youth, the presence of diarrhea, and occurrence in the summer months as favorable prognostic features. Furthermore, the duration of the prodromal illness seemed to be important: long prodromes were associated with poor outcome. Of the 37 children who came off dialysis before 2 weeks, only 1 had residual renal disease, whereas of the 16 children needing dialysis longer, only 1 recovered completely.

The Paris experience over the same period shows that children younger than 3 years, patients with oliguria for fewer than 7 days, and patients with fewer than 40% of their glomeruli affected by microangiopathy did better in the long run (25). Bos et al. (26) found that HUS patients with major neurological symptoms associated with dysregulation of breathing do very badly: eight out of nine such children died, and the only survivor had major sequelae. In 1988, Van Dyck et al. (12) compiled data from series in Leuven, Utrecht, London, and Paris, and from a total of 258 patients in Western Europe, drew the following conclusions: acute mortality rate 9%, evolution to end-stage renal failure 9%, chronic renal failure mostly with hypertension 4%, late sequelae 12%, and complete recovery 66%.

More recently, Coad et al. (14), from Birmingham, England, analyzed the changes in the postenteropathic form of the hemolytic uremic syndrome in children who presented between 1970 and 1987. They reported a mortality rate of 12%, development of sequelae in 15%, and recovery in 73% of children following an episode of D+ HUS.

It is apparent from these studies that there is a wide variation in the percentage of children reported as having renal sequelae that include hypertension, proteinuria, a reduced creatinine clearance, or chronic renal failure after an episode of HUS. Two recent publications provide information suggesting that some authors may have underestimated the extent of renal sequelae. Loirat, on behalf of the French Society of Paediatric Nephrology, conducted a multicenter randomized controlled trial (27) on the treatment of childhood hemolytic uremic syndrome with plasma. As part of the protocol, 54 of the 79 children had biopsies taken 1 month postpresentation and 7 cases (7/54; 13%), all from the control group, showed evidence of diffuse cortical necrosis. Perelstein et al. (28) found that children with a history of HUS and normal renal function, as determined by standard diagnostic procedures, had a loss of normal renal functional reserve following a protein load, when compared with normal controls. These two studies suggest there may have been an underestimation of the extent of residual renal problems following D+ HUS.

Follow-up Study from the Hospital for Sick Children of Patients with Diarrhea-Positive Hemolytic Ureamia Syndrome

Patients and Methods

The aim of this study was to assess renal function by using more sensitive methods than had been used previously to produce more reliable data on long-term prognosis, in a large cohort of children after an episode of D+ HUS, with a minimum follow-up of 5 years.

From 1966 to 1985 120 infants and children presented with HUS, 103 had a "typical" enteropathic illness (D+ HUS) and 17 an "atypical" presentation without diarrhea (D– HUS). A follow-up study was undertaken of the D+ HUS children. Of the original 103, 15 were not included in the study (Fig. 1). Eight had died (see Table 2), and 7 other children were unavailable for study because of residence abroad (n = 2), unwillingness to cooperate (n = 2), or inability to locate (n = 3). Of the 88 patients who attended for follow-up investigations, 40 were male and 48 female with a mean age of 11.6 years (range 5.3–22.6). The mean duration of follow-up was 8.5 years (range 5.1–21.3).

The children were reviewed as day cases. They brought with them an early morning urine sample in which the urine albumin/creatinine concentration ratio (UA/UC) was measured in milligrams per millimole. Blood pressure was recorded

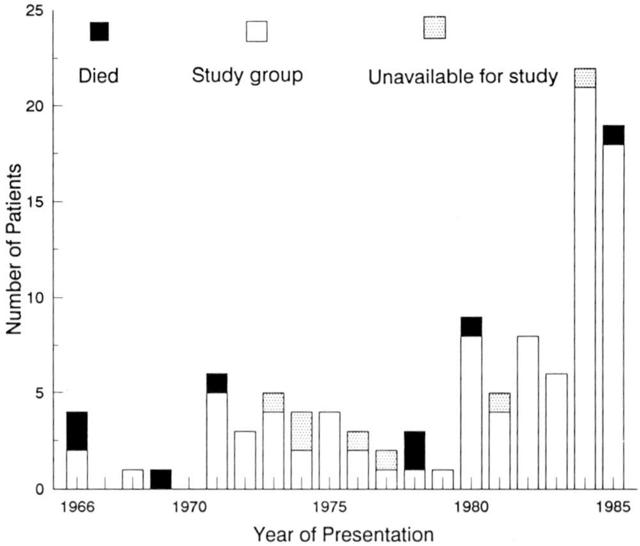

Figure 1 Distribution of the total number of patients with D+ HUS presenting between 1966 and 1985, illustrating those who died, those who were unavailable for study, and the study group.

using a random zero sphygmomanometer, and blood samples were taken for estimation of glomerular filtration rate (GFR) from the plasma clearance of ^{51}Cr-EDTA (29) and for measurement of plasma renin activity (PRA) using a semimicroradioimmunoassay (30).

Results

The children following D+ HUS had a significantly higher UA/UC than normal controls ($t = 5.97$; $p < 0.0001$) (Fig. 2). Twenty-seven of the 88 (31%) children had a UA/UC greater than 2 standard deviations (SD) above the normal mean. The systolic blood pressure (BP) standard deviation score (SDS) for the group was significantly greater than zero ($t = 5.28$; $p < 0.001$), but no child had a systolic BP greater than 2 SDS (Fig. 3). The mean diastolic BP SDS was not significantly different from zero. Data on PRA were available in 42 of the children. The mean PRA SDS was significantly greater than zero ($t = 3.9$; $p < 0.001$), but there was no correlation between systolic BP SDS and PRA SDS in this group of patients. The mean GFR ± SD was 95.1 ± 22.7 ml/min per 1.73m^2 of surface area (SA) ($n = 88$), and 16 had a GFR ≤ 80 ml/min per 1.73m^2 SA (Fig. 4). Significant negative correlations were found between GFR and UA/UC ($r = -0.41$; $p < 0.0001$) and GFR and systolic BP SDS ($r = -0.48$; $p < 0.0001$). A significant positive correlation was found between UA/UC and systolic BP SDS.

The patients were divided into two groups:

1. Poor outcome: those who at follow-up had a GFR ≤80 ml/min per 1.73m^2 SA or who had died of end-stage renal failure
2. Good outcome: those with a GFR >80 ml/min per 1.73m^2 SA at the time of reinvestigation.

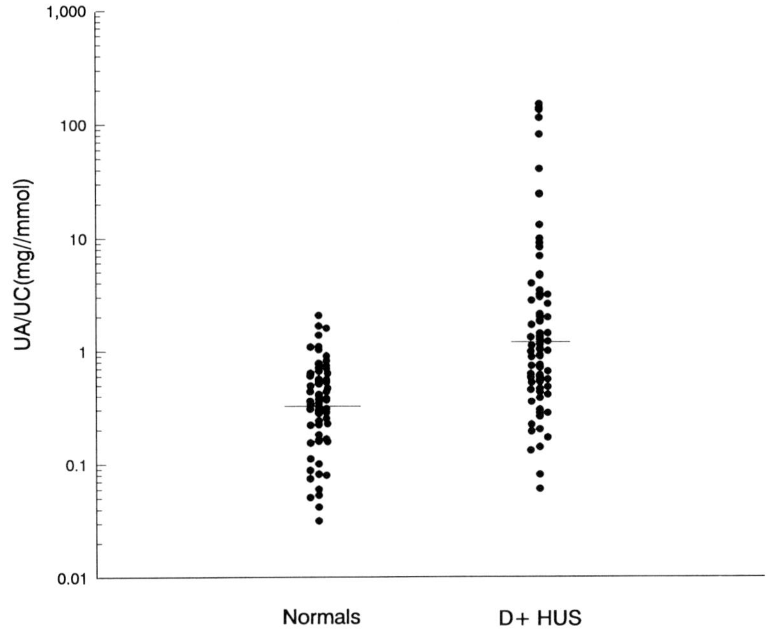

Figure 2 Results of UA/UC ratios in children post D+ HUS and normal controls.

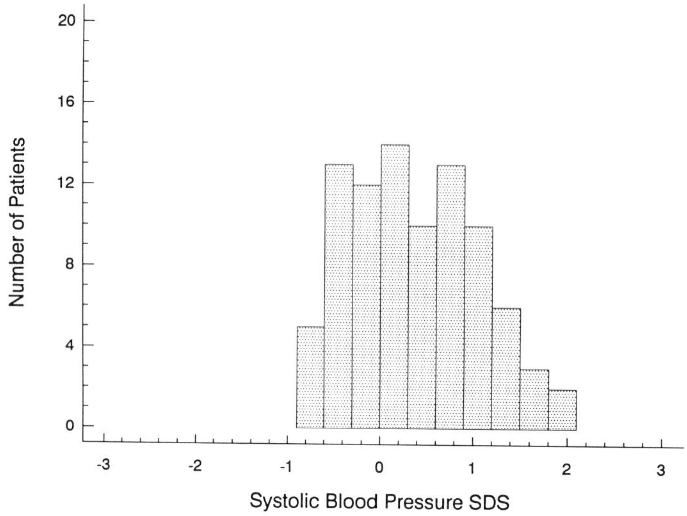

Figure 3 Results of systolic BP SDS at follow-up.

There was no difference in the hemoglobin or platelet count at presentation or in the age of the children when compared between the two groups. However, the children in the poor-outcome group had a significantly higher total white blood cell count (WBC) at the time of admission compared with that recorded for the good-outcome group ($t = -2.4$; $p = 0.01$). A significant negative correlation was found between the WBC at presentation and the GFR at follow-up (Fig. 5). The duration of dialysis was also significantly longer in the poor-outcome group. Eight (57%) of the 14

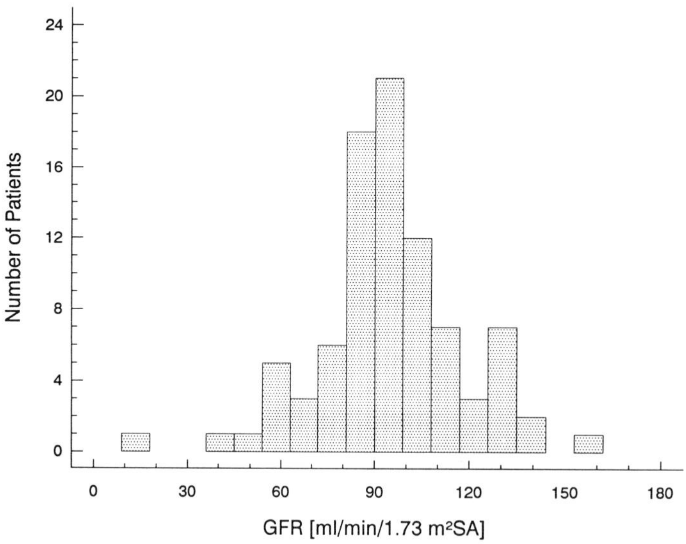

Figure 4 Results of GFR at follow-up.

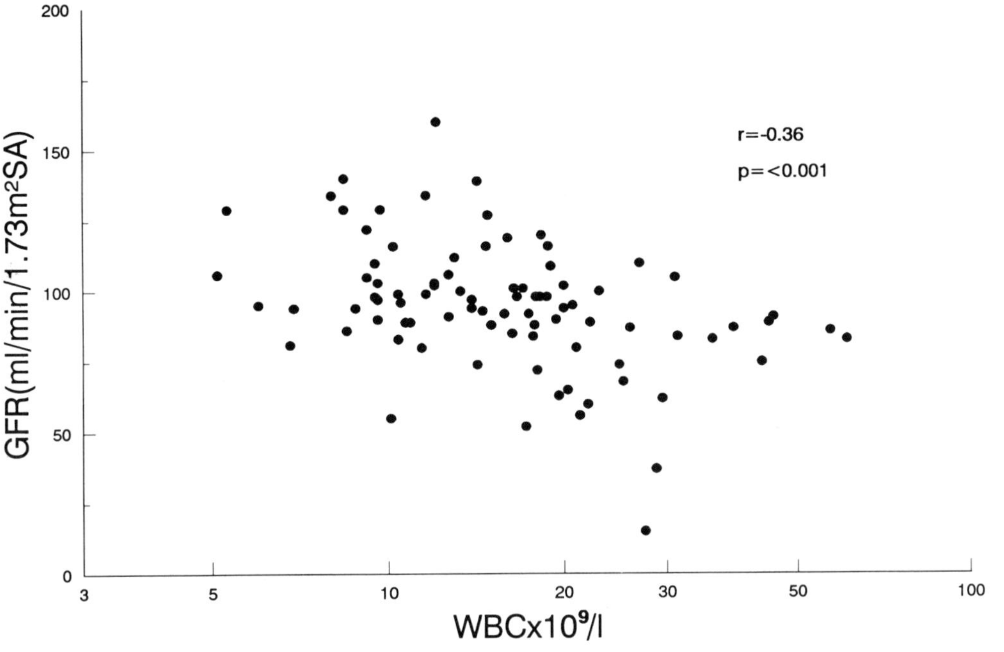

Figure 5 The relation between the total WBC at presentation and the GFR at follow-up.

patients who were dialyzed for 16 days or more had a reduced GFR when reinvestigated, whereas only 11 (14%) of the 74 dialyzed for fewer than 16 days had a low GFR at follow-up.

CONCLUSION

It is increasingly apparent from the literature and, as evidenced by this 5-year follow-up study, that, contrary to a number of earlier reports, D+ HUS is associated with a substantial morbidity. In the HSC, GOS series a significant number of patients had evidence of residual nephropathy at follow-up. Thirty percent of these children had a UA/UC >2 SD above the normal mean, 18% had a GFR ≤80 ml/min per 1.73m^2 SA, and the mean systolic BP SDS for the group was significantly greater than zero. The abnormalities in many of these patients are subtle, and the longer-term implications remain unclear, but it may be that a number of these children will show further decline in renal function with time or have a greater predisposition to the development of hypertension in later adult life.

It has generally been accepted that after recovery from an episode of D+ HUS, children are discharged from hospital follow-up and are not kept under review. However, because of the substantial number of patients with renal sequelae, it is important that children who have had an episode of D+ HUS be kept under general medical review, with blood pressure measurement and urine testing. Because of the positive correlation between UA/UC and systolic blood pressure and the negative correlation between UA/UC and GFR, those patients found to have proteinuria on routine testing then should be referred for further renal evaluation.

REFERENCES

1. Levin, M., Barratt, T. M., Haemolytic uraemic syndrome. *Arch. Dis. Child., 59*: 905–909 (1984).
2. Kaplan, B. S., Cleary, T. G., Obrig, T. G., Recent advances in understanding the pathogenesis of the haemolytic uraemic syndromes. *Pediatr. Nephrol., 4*: 276–283 (1990).
3. Habib, R., Levy, M., Gagnadoux, M. F., Broyer, M., Prognosis of the hemolytic uremic syndrome in children. *Adv. Nephrol.*, pp. 109–128 (1982).
4. Levin, M., Walters, M. D. S., Barratt, T. M., Hemolytic uremic syndrome. *Adv. Pediatr. Infect. Dis., 4*:51–82 (1989).
5. Fitzpatrick, M. M., Shah, V., Trompeter, R. S., Dillon, M. J., Barratt, T. M., Long term renal outcome of childhood haemolytic uraemic syndrome. *Br. Med. J., 303*: 489–492 (1991).
6. Gasser, C., Gautier, E., Steck, A., Siebenmann, R. E., Oeschslin, R., Hamolytisch–uramische Syndrome: Bilaterale Nierenrindennekrosen bei akuten erworbenen hamolytischen Aanamien. *Schweiz. Med. Wochenschr., 85*: 905–909 (1955).
7. Kibel, M. A., Barnard, P. J., The haemolytic–uraemic syndrome: A survey in Southern Africa. *S. Afr. Med. J., 42*: 692–698 (1968).
8. Gianantonio, C., Vitacco, M., Mendilharzu, F., Gallo, G., Sojo, E., The hemolytic uremic syndrome. *Nephron, 14*: 174–192 (1973).
9. Lieberman, E., Haemolytic uremic syndrome. *J. Pediatr., 80*:1–16 (1972).
10. Kaplan, B. S., Katz, J., Krawitz, S., Lurie, A., An analysis of the results of therapy in 67 cases of the hemolytic–uremic syndrome. *J. Pediatr., 78*: 420–425 (1971).
11. Trompeter, R. S., Schwartz, R., Chantler, C., Dillon, M. J., Haycock, G. B., Haemolytic uraemic syndrome: An analysis of prognostic features. *Arch. Dis. Child., 58*: 101–105 (1983).
12. Van Dyck, M., Proesmans, W., Depraetere, M., Hemolytic uremic syndrome in childhood: Renal function 10 years later. *Clin. Nephrol., 3*: 109–112 (1988).
13. Kaplan, B. S., Thomson, P. D., de Chadarevian, J. P., The hemolytic uremic syndrome. *Pediatr. Clin. North Am., 23*: 761–777 (1976).
14. Coad, N. A. G., Marshall, T., Rowe, B., Taylor, C. M., Changes in the postenteropathic form of the hemolytic uremic syndrome in children. *Clin. Nephrol., 35*: 10–16 (1991).
15. Raghupathy, P., Date, A., Shastry, J. C. M., Sudarsanam, A., Jadhav, M., Hemolytic uremic syndrome complicating shigella dysentery in south Indian children. *Br. Med. J., 1*: 1518–1521 (1978).
16. Dedhia, N. M., Shah, B. V., Khanna, U. B., Almeida, A. F., Acharya, V. N., Hemolytic uremic syndrome. *J. Postgrad. Med., 32*: 4–8 (1986).
17. Nammalwar, B. R., Balasubramanian, N., Thangadurai, C., Santhanakrishnan, B. R., Hemolytic uremic syndrome. *Indian J. Pediatr., 54*: 743–752 (1987).
18. Srivastava, R. N., Moudgil, A., Bagga, A., Vasudev, A. S., Hemolytic uremic syndrome in children in northern India. *Pediatr. Nephrol., 5*: 284–288 (1991).
19. Sienawska, M., Korniszewska, J., Gura, C., Welc-Dobies, J., Lewicki, Z., Prognostic significance of certain factors in the haemolytic uraemic syndrome. *Pediatr. Nephrol., 4*: 213–218. (1990).
20. Date, A., Raghupathy, P., Jadhav, M., Pereira, S. M., Shastry, J. C. M., Outcome of the hemolytic–uremic syndrome complicating bacillary dysentery. *Ann. Trop. Pediatr., 2*: 1–6 (1982).
21. Tune, B. M., Leavit, T. J., Gribbe, T. J., The hemolytic uremic syndrome in California: A review of 28 non-heparinized cases with long-term follow-up. *J. Pediatr., 84*: 304–310 (1979).
22. Monnens, L, Van Collenburg, J., De Jong, M., Zoethout, H., Van Wieringen, P., Treatment of the hemolytic uremic syndrome. Comparision of the results of heparin

treatment with the results of streptokinase treatment. *Helv. Paediatr. Acta*, *33*: 321–328 (1978).
23. Sorrenti, L. Y., Lewry, P. R., The hemolytic uremic syndrome: Experience at a center in the Midwest. *Am. J. Dis. Child.*, *132*: 59–62 (1978).
24. Binda ki Muaka, P., Proesmans, W., Eeckels, R., The haemolytic uraemic syndrome in childhood: A study of the long-term prognosis. *Eur. J. Pediatr.*, *136*: 237–243 (1981).
25. Loirat, C., Sonsino, E., Varga Moreno, A., Pillion, G., Mercier, J. C., Beaufils, F., Mathieu, H., Hemolytic–uremic syndrome: An analysis of the natural history and prognostic features. *Acta Paediatr. Scand.*, *73*: 505–514 (1984).
26. Bos, A. P., Donckerwolke, R. A., Van Vugt, A. J., The hemolytic uremic syndrome: Prognostic significance of neurological abnormalities *Helv. Paediatr. Acta*, *40*: 386–389 (1985).
27. Loirat, C., Sonsino, E.,, Hinglais, N., Jais, J. P., Fermanian, J., Treatment of the childhood haemolytic uraemic syndrome with plasma. A multicentre randomized controlled trial. *Pediatr. Nephrol.*, *2*: 279–285 (1988).
28. Perelenstein, E. M., Grunfeld, B. G., Simsola, R. B., Gimenez, M. I., Gianantonio, C. A., Renal functional reserve in haemolytic uraemic syndrome and single kidney. *Arch. Dis. Child.*, *65*: 728–731 (1991).
29. Chantler, C., Barratt, T. M., Estimation of glomerular filtration rate from plasma clearance of 51-chromium edetic acid. *Arch. Dis. Child.*, *47*: 613 (1971).
30. Dillon, M. J., Ryness, J., Measurement of plasma renin activity by semi-microimmunoassay of generated angiotensin 1. *J. Clin. Pathol.*, *28*: 625–630 (1975).
31. de Jong, M., Monnens, L., Haemolytic-uraemic syndrome: a 10-year follow up study of 73 patients. *Nephrol. Dial Transplant.*, *3*: 379–382 (1988).
32. O'Regan, S., Blais, N., Russo, P., Pison, C. F., Rousseau, E. Hemolytic uremic syndrome: glomerular filtration rate, 6–11 years later measured by 99m to DTPA plasma slope clearance. *Clin. Nephrol.*, *32*: 217–220 (1989).
33. Donckerwolke, R. A., Tiddens, H., Kuijten, R. Prospectief onderzoek naar het hemolytisch-uremisch syndroom. *Acta Paediatr. Belg.*, *27*: 284–298 (1973).
34. Janssen, F., Potvliege, P. R., Vainsel, M., Vis, H. L. Le pronostic à court et à long terme du syndrome hémolytic et urèmique. *Arch. Fr. Pediatr.*, *31*: 59–69 (1974).
35. Tune, B. M., Leavitt, T. J., Gribble, T. J. The hemolytic-uremic syndrome in California: a review of 28 non heparinized cases with long-term follow-up. *J. Pediatr.*, *82*: 304–310 (1973).

32
Follow-up of Hemolytic Uremic Syndrome in Argentina

Horacio A. Repetto *Hospital Nacional A. Posadas, Buenos Aires, Argentina*

The idiopathic (classic, enteropathic), form of hemolytic uremic syndrome (HUS) that is endemic in Argentina (1) has been well characterized. More than 95% of patients recover from the acute phase of the disease (2, 3).

Hematological changes occur only during the acute phase. Chronic central nervous system deficits are rare, and sequelae in other organs, for example, diabetes mellitus, are only occasionally described (4–7). As noted by Gianantonio et al., in 1968, more than a quarter of the survivors of the acute phase of HUS had some degree of renal dysfunction (8). As a result, HUS accounts for about 20% of children who enter end stage renal failure programs in Argentina (9, 10).

RENAL FUNCTION AFTER THE ACUTE PHASE

After recovery from acute renal failure, kidney function may follow two patterns. In some patients, the serum creatinine concentration never returns to within a normal range, and there is an inexorable progression to terminal renal failure in a few years (Fig. 1). In most patients, however, renal function returns to normal. In this group, the disappearance of proteinuria is a sensitive index of the absence of residual renal lesions. We have done sequential studies on patients 1 year after the acute phase. Those who had a normal creatinine clearance and no proteinuria in sequential examinations for a period of 6 months thereafter, did not have deteriorating renal function or a recurrence of proteinuria during a follow-up period of up to 12 years (mean period of follow-up 4.7 years) (3).

In accordance with the Brenner hypothesis, it was suggested that some of these patients maintained normal creatinine clearances by glomerular hyperfiltration, and this adaptive mechanism might be detrimental to nephrons that had recovered from the acute injury (11). Therefore, we studied 16 of our patients whose creatinine

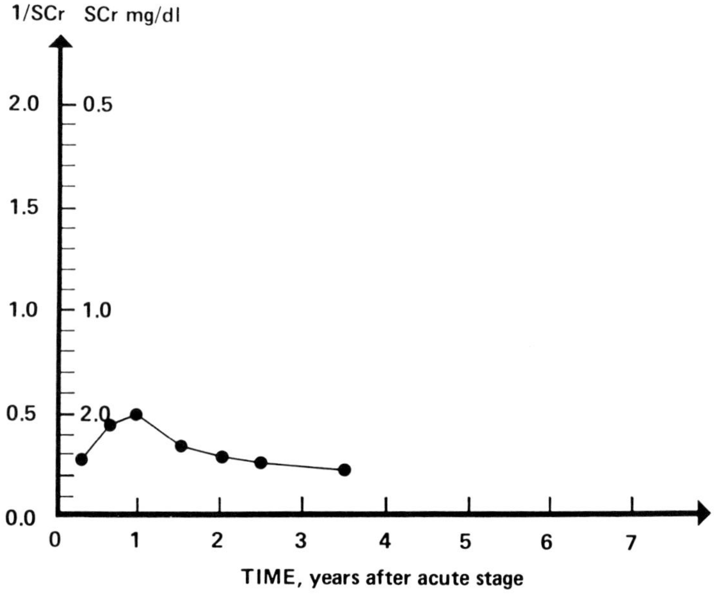

Figure 1 An 8-month-old girl, had severe hemolytic uremic syndrome with 12 days of anuria; she never recovered a normal creatinine clearance, had persistent proteinuria, and was in end-stage renal disease (ESRD) 3½ years after the acute stage.

clearances were normal at a mean time of 6.6 years after the acute phase. Glomerular filtration rates (GFR) were measured by endogenous creatinine clearances and by inulin clearances (12, 13). In general, the mean values for inulin clearance were significantly lower than those for creatinine clearance. Patients with mild involvement in the acute phase (short duration of anuria) had normal inulin clearances, whereas those who had severe involvement had lower clearances.

RENAL FUNCTIONAL RESERVE

The renal functional reserve was assessed in 12 of those 16 patients following ingestion of a defined protein load (14). Four of the 12 patients were unable to increase their prechallenge inulin clearances to the same extent as the other patients and normal controls. The absence of functional reserve may reflect the presence of hyperfiltration in the remaining functioning nephrons.

Within the group of patients who have a normal creatinine clearance, there are some who have persistent proteinuria, with or without hypertension. Therefore, it is possible that some of these may eventually have increasing proteinuria and decreasing glomerular filtration rates that result in end-stage renal failure (Fig. 2) (3). Patients requiring a renal allograft between 1977 and 1988 demonstrated one of the two patterns described earlier. The average time interval between the acute phase and acceptance into a transplant program was, as expected, significantly longer in patients whose creatinine clearances had been normal for at least part of the time (Fig. 3) (10).

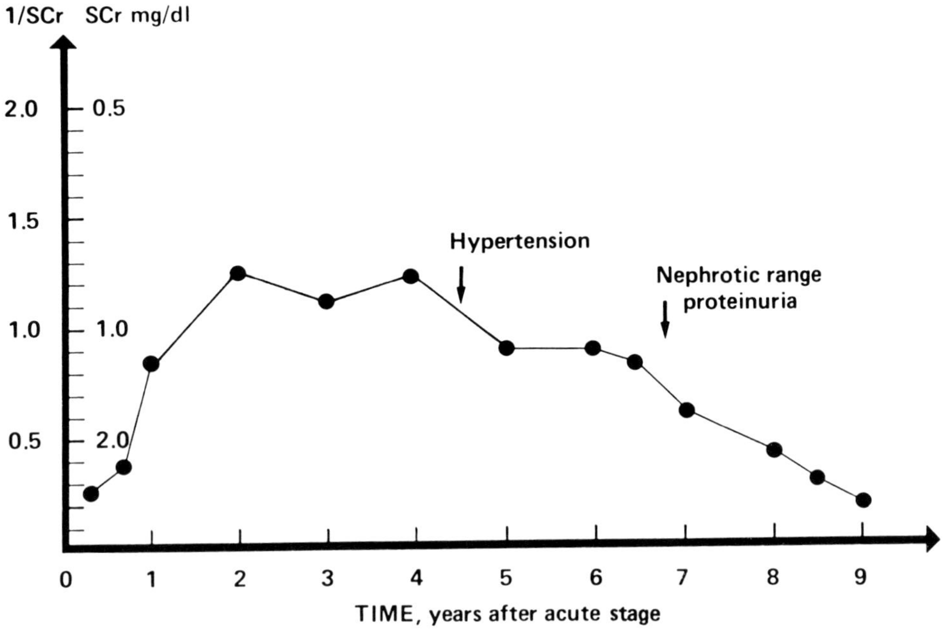

Figure 2 A 9-month-old girl had severe HUS with 8 days of anuria, but she recovered a normal creatinine clearance (ccr) 2 years after the acute stage. She had persistent proteinuria that was intermittent between the third and fourth years and she became hypertensive at 4½ years. Proteinuria increased into the nephrotic range by 6½ years and she developed ESRD 9 years after the acute stage.

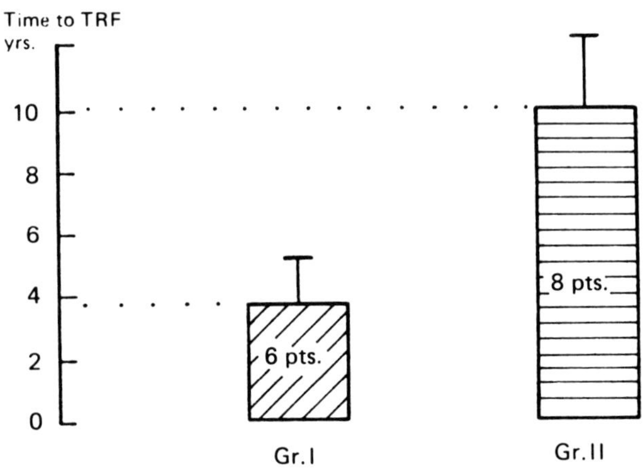

Figure 3 Time to ESRD in 14 patients who received transplants for HUS. Group 1 never recovered normal ccr after the acute renal failure, and they reached ESRD an average of 3.8 years after the acute state. Group 2 recovered a normal ccr, but had persistent proteinuria, ccr decreased after variable periods, and patients progressed to ESRD an average of 10.2 years after the acute stage. Source: Cemic–I.N.B.A. 1975–1988.

The proportion of patients who develop chronic renal failure varies in different reports. This may depend, in part, on the length of follow-up. We did a retrospective review of 208 patients whom we followed from 1 to 14 (mean, 4.7) years after the acute phase: 3% had advanced renal insufficiency; 25% who had persistent proteinuria and some degree of renal insufficiency, were considered to be at risk for progression to end-stage renal failure (3). However, the percentage of patients varied in each group, according to whether the analysis was done at 1 or at 3 years (Fig. 4). As expected, the longer the period of follow-up, the larger is the number of patients whose renal status is more precisely defined in terms of ultimate outcome. Although many still have persistent proteinuria, with or without a decreased creatinine clearance (groups 2 and 3), the group with normal findings has enlarged (group 1).

RENAL TRANSPLANTATION

Renal transplantation has become a routine mode of treatment for patients with HUS who progress to end stage renal failure. We have transplanted kidneys in 15 patients who had originally had HUS. In 1 of these, a recurrence resulted in the loss of the allograft 2 months after transplantation. This was a boy, aged 8 years, who did not have a prodromal illness. His kidneys did not recover, and he was treated by hemodialysis until transplantation. His brother had an equally severe episode of hemolytic uremic syndrome 5 years previously. The other 14 patients had the typical classic infantile form of the syndrome, with a mean age at onset of 10 months (range 3–22 months). They received 12 living, related and 5 cadaveric grafts. At the time of this review, 12 grafts were functioning. Six patients were being treated with cyclo-

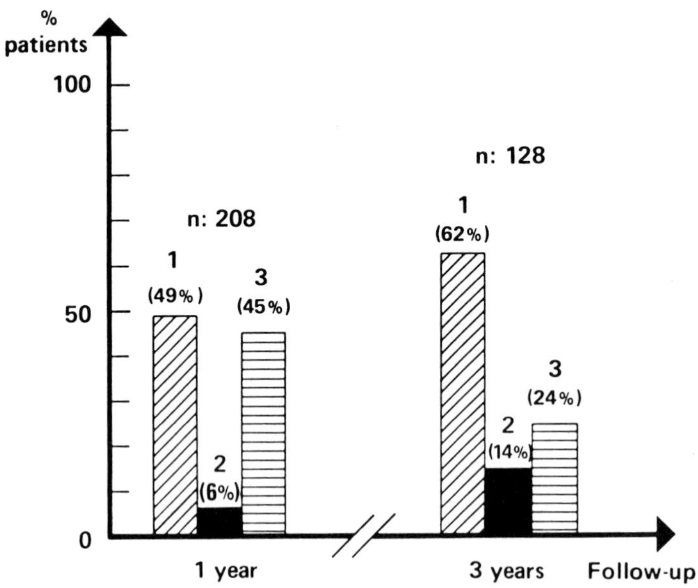

Figure 4 Status of children with classic HUS at 1 and 3 years of follow-up. Group 1: normal ccr, no proteinuria, normal blood pressure. Group 2: normal ccr, proteinuria. Group 3: decreased ccr, proteinuria.

sporine as part of the immunosuppressive protocol. Biopsies were done in 4 of 7 patients who had acute reduction of graft function, and transplant nephrectomies were performed in 3 who lost their grafts: none had clinical, laboratory, or histological evidence of recurrences of HUS. The patients who received transplants for chronic renal failure secondary to HUS had similar prevalences of proteinuria and hypertension and similar levels of graft function and graft survival (80.6% at 1 year and 72.5% at 3 years) when compared with a group of 71 children who received transplants for other causes over the same period (10).

We believe that renal transplantation is clearly indicated for terminal renal failure in patients who have had the typical classic form of hemolytic uremic syndrome. In our experience the risk of recurrence is low and seems to be unaffected by the use of cyclosporine.

REFERENCES

1. Gianantonio, C. A. (1984). Hemolytic uremic syndrome. In *Acute Renal Failure*. Edited by V. E. Andreucci. Martinus Nijhoff Pub. Boston, pp. 327–339.
2. Gianantonio, C. A. (1984). Past and present of hemolytic uremic syndrome in Argentina. In *Renal Emergencies*. Edited by T. Strauss and M. Nyhoff. Boston, pp. 13–20.
3. Repetto, H. A., Bibiloni, N., Spizziri, F. D., Vasquez, L. A., de la Torre, M. C., Orsi, M. C., Rahman, R. C., Deregibus, M. (1989) Long-term follow-up of the renal lesion of the infantile hemolytic-uremic syndrome. Abstract. *Pediatr. Nephrol.* 3: 184.
4. Gianantonio, C. A., Vitacco, M., Mendilaharzu, F., Mendilaharzu, J., Rutty, A. (1964). The hemolytic uremic sydrome. *J. Pediatr.* 64:478–491.
5. Van Rhijn, A., Donckerwolcke, R. A., Kuyten, R. H., (1977). Liver damage in the hemolytic uremic syndrome. *Helv. Pediatr. Acta* 32: 77–81.
6. Andreoli, S. P., Bergstein, J. M. (1982). Development of insulin-dependent diabetes mellitus during the hemolytic uremic syndrome. *J. Pediatr.* 100: 541–545.
7. Burns, J. C., Berman, E. R., Fayne, J. L., Shikes, R. H., Lum, G. H. (1982). Pancreatic islet cell nechrosis: Association with hemolytic uremic syndrome. *J. Pediatr.* 100: 582–584.
8. Gianantonio, C. A., Vitacco, M., Mendilaharzu, F., Gallo, G. (1968). The hemolytic uremic syndrome: Renal status of 76 patients at long term follow-up. *J. Pediatr.* 72: 757–765.
9. Repetto, H. A. (1987). La evolución a largo plazo de la lesion renal del sindrome urémico hemolítico. Editorial. *Medicina (Bs. As.)* 47: 108.
10. Repetto, H. A., Vazquez, L. A., Calvo, P., Palti, G. (1989). Renal transplantation in children with idiopathic "classic" hemolytic uremic syndrome. Abstract. *Pediatr. Nephrol.* 3: 185.
11. Brenner, B. M. (1983). Hemodinamically mediated glomerular injury and the progressive nature of kidney disease. *Kidney Int.* 83: 647–655.
12. Tufro, A., Repetto, H. A., Arrizurieta, E. (1987). Renal functional reserve in children with history of hemolytic uremic syndrome. *Abstracts of the Xth Int. Congress of Nephrology*, London, p. 36.
13. Tufro, A., Arrizurieta, E., Repetto, H. A. (1989). Renal functional reserve in children with history of uremic hemolytic syndrome. *Pediatr. Nephrol.* Accepted for publication.
14. Bosch, J. P., Saccaggi, A., Laner, A., Rouco, C., Belledonne, M., Glabman, S. (1983). Renal functional reserve in humans, effect of protein in take on glomerular filtration rate. *Am. J. Med.* 75:943–950.

VIII
Thrombotic Thrombocytopenic Purpura

33
von Willebrand Factor Abnormalities in Thrombotic Thrombocytopenic Purpura and the Hemolytic Uremic Syndrome

Joel L. Moake *Baylor College of Medicine, and Rice University, Houston, Texas*

Thrombotic thrombocytopenic purpura (TTP) is characterized by intravascular platelet aggregation, profound thrombocytopenia, central nervous system (and other organ) ischemia, and microangiopathic hemolytic anemia (1). The hemolytic uremic syndrome (HUS) is a clinically related entity in which platelet aggregation is predominantly confined to the renal vasculature, with associated acute renal failure (1). Thrombocytopenia and intravascular hemolysis with erythrocyte fragmentation are usually less profound in HUS than in TTP.

Three types of TTP have been recognized: *single-episode TTP*, which may be idiopathic or associated with chemotherapy or immunological disorders and never recurs if the patient recovers; *intermittent TTP*, with occasional episodes at irregular intervals; and the rare *chronic relapsing TTP*, with frequent episodes at regular intervals (1). The HUS almost always occurs as a single, nonrecurrent episode.

VON WILLEBRAND FACTOR (vWF) IN THROMBOTIC THROMBOCYTOPENIC PURPURA

It has been presumed that TTP is a consequence of the intrusion into the systemic circulation of one or more platelet-aggregating agents. This substance has been reported to be a protein of 37,000 (2) or 59,000 (3) Da, or to be vWF after cleavage by a calcium-activated cysteine protease (calpain) (4, 5). We and others have reported that unusually large vWF forms and large vWF multimers may mediate platelet aggregation in the various types of TTP and in HUS (1, 5–13).

The vWF monomers are linked by disulfide bonds into multimers of varying sizes that range into the millions of daltons (14). These multimers are produced within megakaryocytes and endothelial cells and are stored within α-granules and Weibel–Palade bodies, respectively. The predominant source of plasma vWF multimers is, apparently, the endothelial cell.

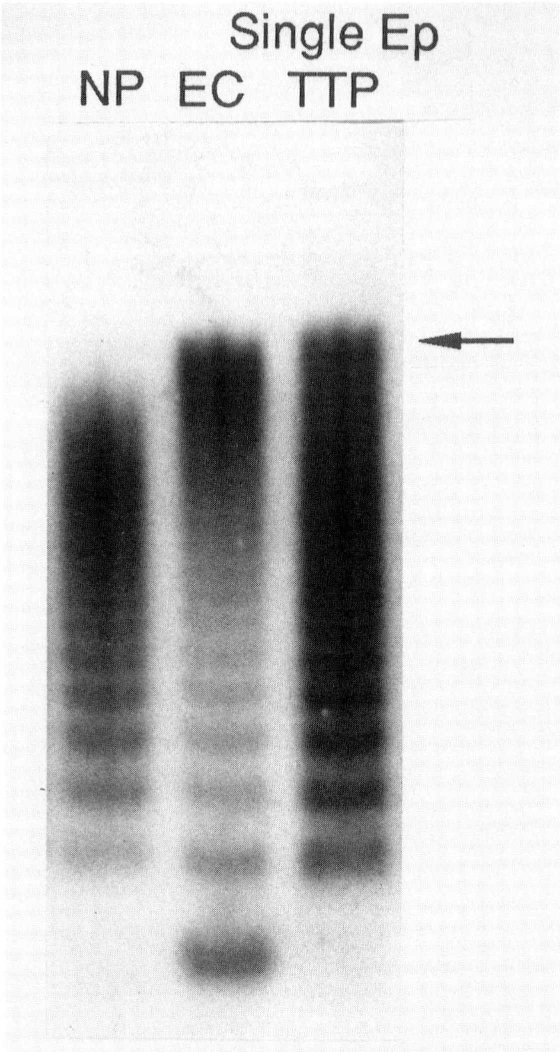

Figure 1 Autoradiogram demonstrating ULvWF multimers in the plasma of an adult patient early during his single episode of TTP. NP, normal pooled EDTA platelet-poor plasma (PPP); EC, supernatant of cultured human umbilical vein endothelial cells (HUVECs) containing ULvWF forms; single Ep TTP, patient EDTA–PPP. Before dilution to 15 U/dl (15%) and mixture with sodium dodecyl sulfate (SDS)–urea–EDTA–Tris for electrophoresis in SDS–1% agarose, vWF antigen level of the patient PPP sample was 147 U/dl (147%). Display of vWF multimers was by incubation with polyclonal rabbit ^{125}I-anti-vWF antibodies, and then exposure to x-ray film. Arrow at right indicates position of ULvWF forms.

The entire constellation of vWF multimers found in the normal circulation is produced within both megakaryocytes and endothelial cells (14). In addition, both cell types construct vWF multimeric forms that are even larger than those found in normal plasma ["unusually large" (UL) vWF multimers] (6, 15). There is evidence that these ULvWF multimers are more active (per unit antigen) than the largest plasma vWF forms in inducing platelet aggregation in the presence of a low concentration (0.3 mg/ml) of ristocetin or in shear fields in the absence of ristocetin (15–18).

A substance in normal plasma, which may be a limited disulfide bond reductase, reduces the size of ULvWF forms from endothelial cells to the somewhat smaller vWF multimers found in normal plasma (19).

In some patients with idiopathic single-episode TTP, ULvWF miltimers have been found in plasma *during* the TTP episodes (Fig. 1). This may be because of systemic endothelial cell injury or intense stimulation. [Platelet aggregation and α-granule release do not result in the appearance of ULvWF multimeric forms in the

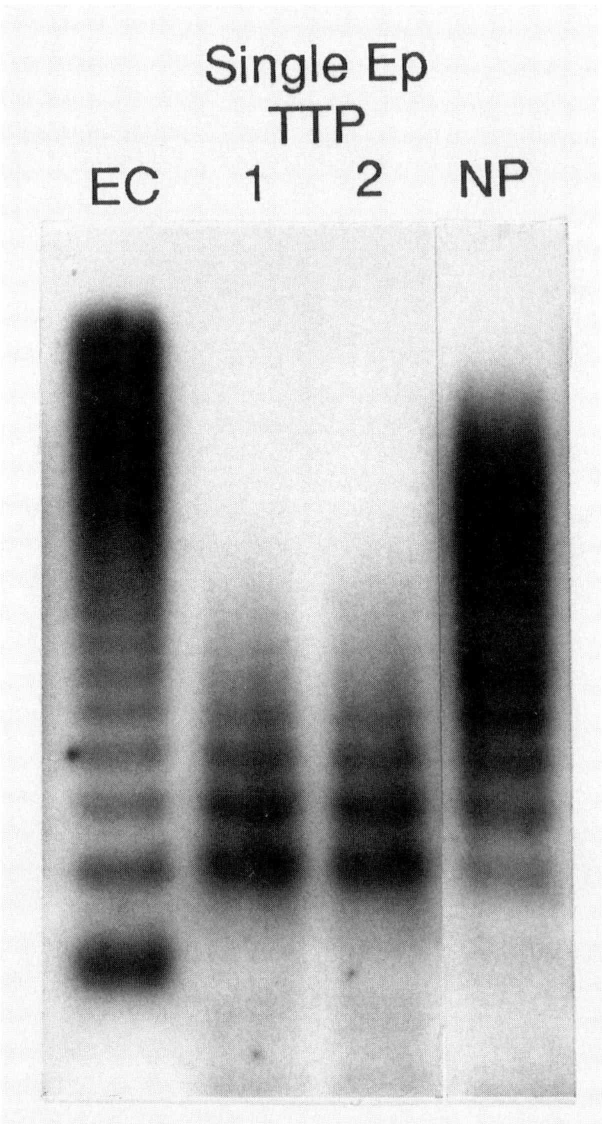

Figure 2 Autoradiogram demonstrating the absence of large plasma vWF multimers in the EDTA–PPP samples of an adult patient on two consecutive days (1 and 2) early during her single episode (single Ep) of TTP. NP and EC are as in Figure 1. Before dilution to 15 U/dl (15%) and mixture with SDS–urea–EDTA–Tris for electrophoresis in SDS–1% agarose, vWF antigen levels were 85 U/dl (85%) and 96 U/dl (96%) on days 1 and 2, respectively.

suspending plasma, probably because the released ULvWF multimers attach tenaciously to vWF receptors on the external surface of the platelet membrane (15).] Serial studies by us of plasma samples from idiopathic single-episode TTP patients have revealed that large vWF multimers may also be absent from patient plasma samples during TTP episodes (Fig. 2) (12). This may be observed even when blood samples are obtained in the presence of EDTA to inhibit calcium-activated proteases, which are capable of cleaving large vWF multimers. Immunohistochemical studies of TTP thrombi by other investigators suggest that the disappearance of large vWF forms may be the result of their attaching to, and aggregating, platelets (20). Therefore, depending on sample timing in single-episode TTP, either the presence of *ULvWF multimers or a decrease in the largest plasma vWF forms may be observed*.

If the patient survives, and suffers no subsequent relapse, vWF multimeric forms in recovery plasma samples are almost always normal (12). We and others have found, however, that if ULvWF multimers are found in plasma samples after

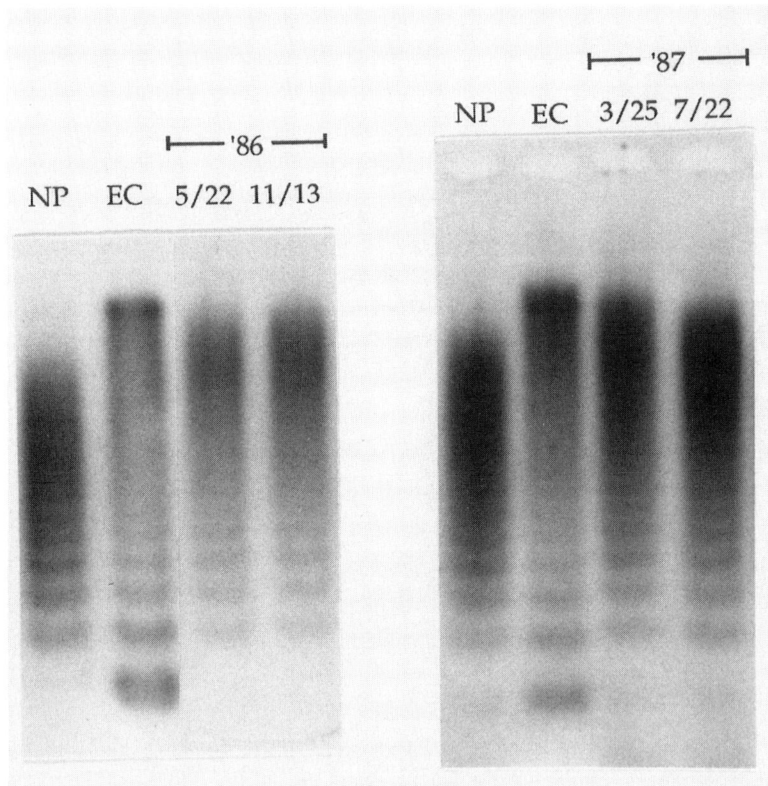

Figure 3 ULvWF multimers in the platelet-poor plasma samples of an intermittent TTP patient between four of her recurrences. These remission samples obtained on May 22, 1986; November 13, 1986; March 25, 1987; and July 22, 1987, all contain ULvWF multimeric forms. NP and EC are as in Figure 1. Before dilution to 15 U/dl (15%) and mixture with SDS–urea–EDTA–Tris for electrophoresis in SDS–1% agarose, vWF antigen levels in patient samples were: May 22, 1986, 126% U/dl; November 13, 1986, 84%; November 25, 1987, 120%; and July 22, 1987, 168%. (From Ref. 12.)

Table 1 Patterns of vWF in Single-Episode TTP

Type of TTP	vWF Patterns during episodes	vWF abnormalities	vWF patterns after recovery
Single-episode TTP	Abnormal in 88% (49/56 patients)	Unusually large vWF multimers or relative decrease in large plasma vWF multimers	Normal in 93% (28/30 patients)

recovery, then there is a considerable likelihood that the patient will have recurrent episodes of TTP (Fig. 3) (6–8, 10–12). During relapses of intermittent or chronic relapsing TTP, the ULvWF multimers decrease or disappear from patient plasma, often in association with the largest plasma vWF multimeric forms (6, 8). In a few of these patients with relapsing TTP, the ULvWF multimers have ultimately disappeared from remission plasma (either "spontaneously" in seven of our unpublished cases, or in association with prednisone–azathioprine therapy; 8), and these patients have not experienced further relapses.

A summary of vWF abnormalities in the different types of TTP is presented in Tables 1 and 2. Table 3 contains a more detailed compilation of vWF observations in single-episode and intermittent TTP patients.

We have proposed that intermittent TTP and chronic relapsing TTP are disorders in the rate of release or the plasma processing of ULvWF multimers from endothelial cells (1, 6, 12). Some cofactor (6, 13) is also apparently necessary in the circulation during TTP episodes to induce the attachment to platelets of ULvWF multimers and large plasma vWF forms. In this vWF–platelet interaction, platelet membrane GPIIb/IIIa complexes may be as (or more) important than the primary platelet vWF receptor, glycoprotein (GP) Ib (21).

The most effective therapy for TTP has been the repeated daily exchange of patient plasma with normal platelet-poor fresh-frozen plasma (FFP) (1, 22, 23) or its cryoprecipitate-poor cryosupernatant fraction (1, 22, 24). The *plasmapheresis* portion of plasma exchange may remove platelet aggregating substances, perhaps including ULvWF forms, large plasma vWF multimers, and a putative vWF cofactor (1, 6, 7). The infusion of normal plasma or cryosupernatant may provide supplemental

Table 2 Patterns of vWF in Intermittent and Chronic Relapsing TTP

Type of TTP	vWF Patterns between episodes	vWF abnormality	vWF patterns during episodes
Intermittent TTP	Abnormal in 14/14 patients	Unusually large vWF multimers	Decrease or disappearance of unusually large vWF multimers
Chronic relapsing TTP	Abnormal in 5/5 patients	Unusually large vWF multimers	Decrease or disappearance of unusually large vWF multimers

Table 3 vWF Multimeric Patterns in TTP

Type of TTP	Total no. of patients (total PPP samples obtained)	Timing of samples	No. of patients in subgroup	Plasma vWF multimeric pattern[c]	Plasma vWF antigen (U/dl)
Single Episode	56 (638)	During episode	17	(1) ULvWFM	222±93[e] (77–474)
M = 21 F = 55			21	(2) Relative decrease in large vWF forms	213±113[e] (54–519)
			11	(3) Patterns (1) and (2) in different serial samples	180±26[e] (134–284)
			7	(4) Normal[d]	211±50[e] (152–280)
	30 (87)	After episode[b]	28	(1) Normal	233±114 (65–500)
			2	(2) ULvWFM	241±26 (220–255)
Intermittent TTP (occasional episodes at irregular intervals)	29[a] (350)	During episode	7	(1) ULvWFM	230±96[e] (84–323)
			3	(2) Relative decrease in large vWF forms	236±125[e] (176–354)
			6	(3) Patterns (1) and (2) in different serial samples	193±68[e] (103–275)
M = 8 F = 21			2	(4) Normal (from ULvWF between episodes)	159[e] (113–204)
		Between episodes	14	ULvWFM	164±64 (83–323)

[a]29 intermittent TTP patients were studied: 10 during an episode only; 7 between episodes only; 7 both during and between episodes; and 5 only after recurrent episodes had ceased.
[b]No recurrences for more than 1 year in 8 single-episode patients; 20 patients were studied only after a single TTP episode.
[c]ULvWFM, unusually large vWF multimers.
[d]Total of 45 samples in these patients.
[e]Pretreatment or earliest sample obtained.

amounts of ULvWF processing activity (7, 19). The transfusion of other substances, including IgG concentrates, are almost always ineffective (1).

At least 10–20% of patients with single-episode TTP do not respond to plasma exchange with FFP (23, 25). In some of these patients, plasma exchange has been rendered effective by the substitution of *cryosupernatant* (plasma that lacks the largest plasma vWF forms, but contains the ULvWF-processing activity) for the whole plasma (Figs. 4 and 5) (24). Purified ULvWF-processing activity may prove useful in the treatment of refractory single-episode and relapsing TTP patients.

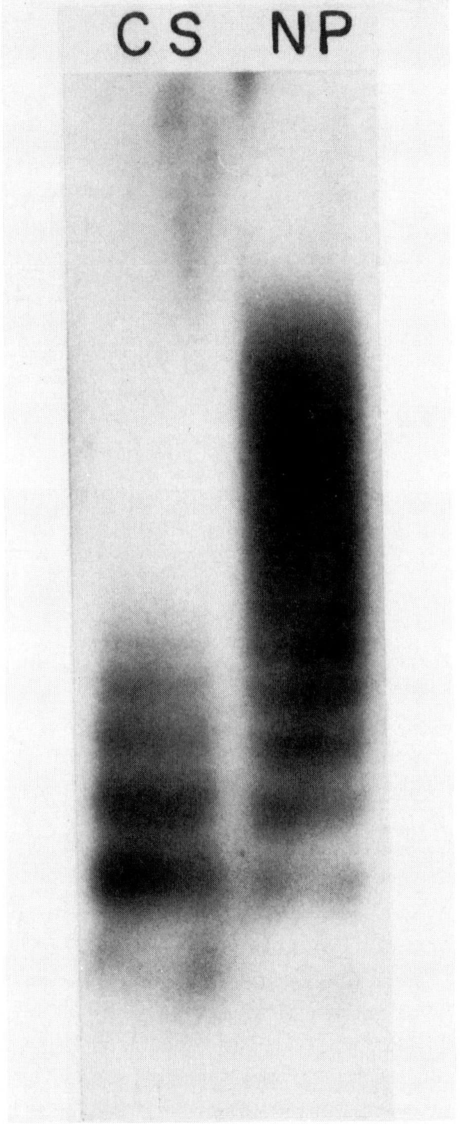

Figure 4 Autoradiogram demonstrating vWF multimeric pattern in normal pooled platelet-poor plasma (NP) and in the cryosupernatant fraction of normal plasma (CS). The vWF antigen levels in NP and CS were diluted to 15 U/dl (15%) and mixed with SDS–urea–Tris–EDTA for electrophoresis in SDS–1% agarose. (From Ref. 24.)

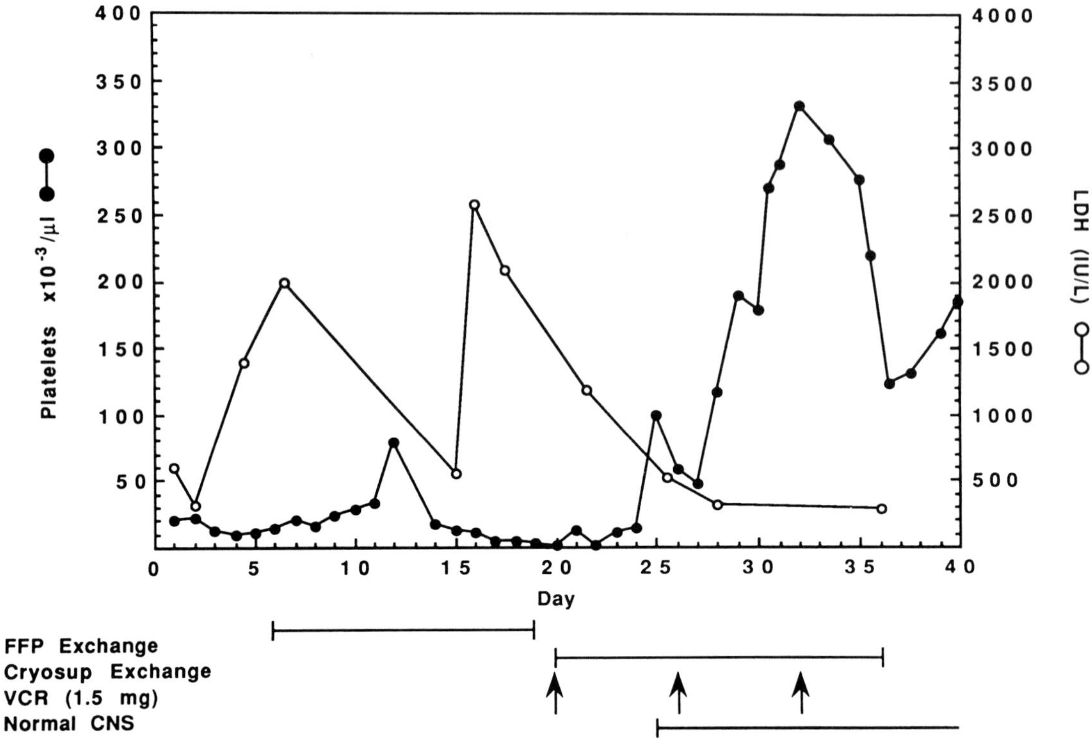

Figure 5 Changes in platelet count in relation to the substitution of the cryosupernatant fraction of plasma for whole fresh-frozen plasma during plasma exchange in a patient with TTP refractory to plasma exchange with FFP. Vincristine (VCR) injections are indicated.

Other patients who have not responded to plasma exchange have benefited from *splenectomy*. Splenectomy may remove a major site for production of autoantibodies directed against the ULvWF-processing activity normally in plasma or, alternatively, for production of the vWF cofactor that may be involved in inducing the attachment of ULvWF multimers and the largest plasma vWF forms to platelets during TTP episodes. This latter explanation may account for the reversion of plasma vWF multimeric patterns to normal in association with clinical cure following splenectomy in one patient recently reported by us (26).

It has been presumed that schistocytosis during TTP episodes is a result of injury to red cells as they flow through areas of the microcirculation that are partially occluded by platelet aggregates. This may not, however, be the entire explanation. We have found that flowing young erythrocytes have surface receptors that are capable of binding to ULvWF multimers (but not to the largest plasma vWF forms) (27, 28). It is possible that reticulocytes and other young red cells that enter the circulation in response to hemolysis during TTP episodes attach to ULvWF multimers secreted onto the external surfaces of intensely stimulated endothelial cells and are then disrupted by fluid shear forces in areas of the microcirculation with the most rapid blood flow.

VON WILLEBRAND FACTOR IN THE HEMOLYTIC UREMIC SYNDROME

About half of the children and adults with HUS thus far evaluated by us and others have had a relative decrease in the largest plasma vWF forms when platelet counts

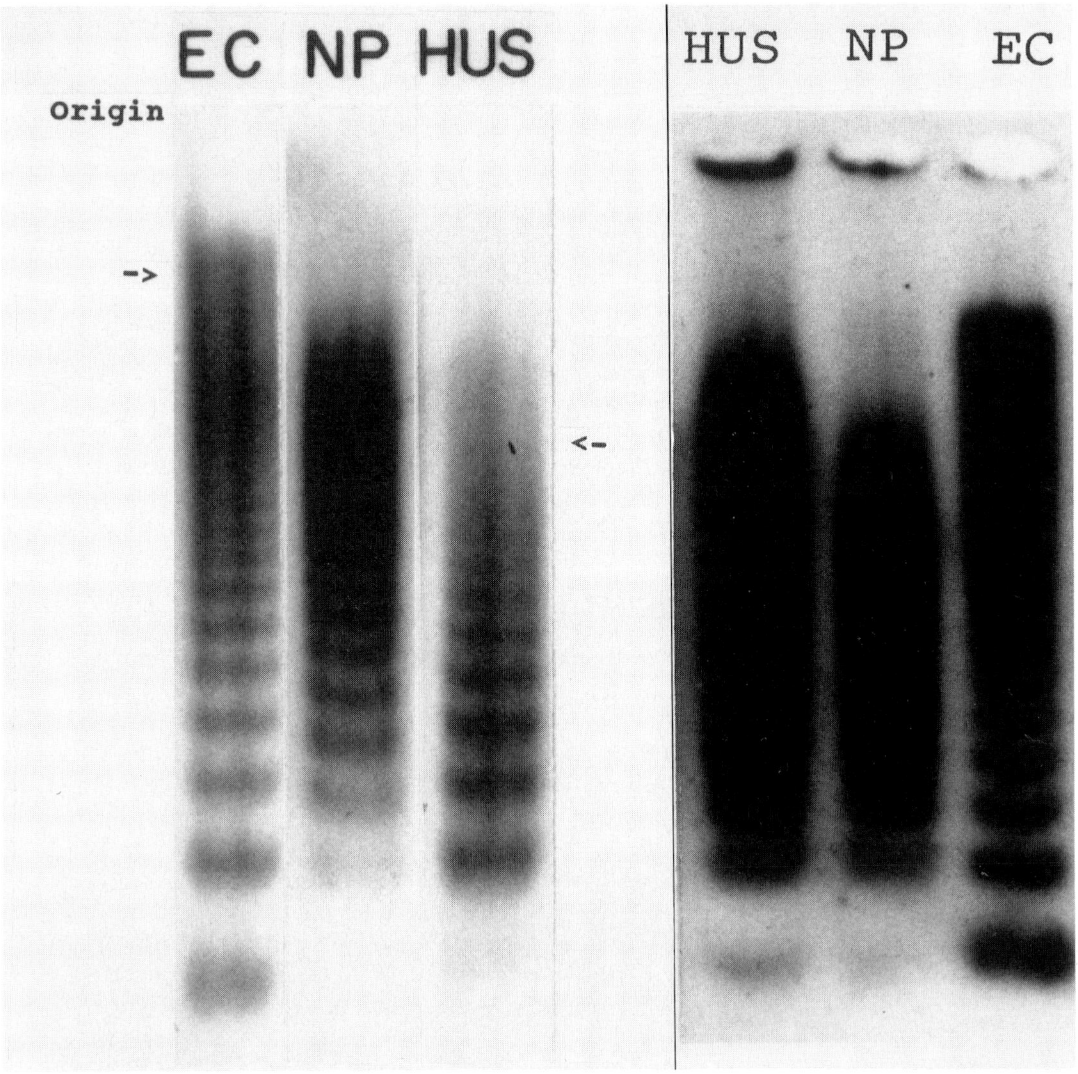

Figure 6 vWF multimeric forms in HUS. vWF multimers were separated in SDS–1% agarose gel electrophoresis, fixed in the gel, and displayed by overlay with ^{125}I-anti-vWF antibody and autoradiography. In the 3 lanes to the left, vWF multimeric patterns in citrated normal (NP) and patient (HUS) platelet-poor plasma samples are compared with ULvWF forms (upper arrow) in the supernatant of human umbilical vein endothelial cells cultured in serum-free medium (EC). The HUS PPP, obtained from a patient during an acute HUS episode, demonstrates a relatively decreased quantity of the largest plasma vWF multimeric forms (lower arrow). In another HUS patient, ULvWF forms are present during the acute episode (HUS, NP and EC lanes to the right).

were low (Fig. 6A and Table 4) (12, 29, 30). A few HUS patients have had ULvWF forms in their plasma during episodes (Fig. 6B and Table 4). These vWF patterns are similar to those seen in plasma samples obtained from most patients during episodes of TTP. In HUS (and TTP) samples that are relatively depleted of the largest plasma vWF forms, no extra bands have been observed at new positions on our sodium dodecyl (SDS)–1% agarose gel autoradiograms. Extra bands would have been expected if proteolysis had occurred either in vivo or ex vivo.

Intravascular platelet aggregation in HUS is predominantly confined to the renal vasculature. A possible explanation for the pathophysiology of HUS is that renal endothelial cell injury (or intense stimulation) results in the release into the renal arterial circulation of ULvWF multimers. These ULvWF multimers, along with the largest plasma vWF forms, may then be induced (possibly by the as yet unidentified cofactor) to attach to platelets and aggregate them in the renal blood. In many patients with HUS, renal arterial endothelial cells may be injured directly by Shiga-like toxin 1 (SLT-1) (31), mitomycin (32), cyclosporine (33), total-body irradiation plus high-dose cyclophosphamide (Cytoxan) (34), or combinations of chemotherapeutic agents. (In patients with drug-induced HUS, ULvWF forms derived from endothelial cells are especially likely to be found in plasma during the episode.) It is also possible that renal arterial endothelial cell antigenic expression may be altered by Shiga toxin from *Shigella* or SLT-1 from certain strains of *Escherichia coli* (e.g., O157 : H7) (31). Autoantibodies produced against renal endothelial cell surfaces that have been altered by SLT-1 may then case HUS (35).

POSSIBLE NEW APPROACHES TO THERAPY

Aurin tricarboxylic acid (ATA) is a polyphenolic polycarboxylated compound that may ultimately prove useful in the treatment of TTP and HUS episodes and in the prophylaxis of relapsing TTP. It reversibly binds to vWF multimers and prevents ULvWF and plasma vWF forms from attaching to platelet GPIb molecules (36). The binding of ULvWF or large vWF forms to platelet GPIb, followed by vWF binding to GPIIb/IIIa complexes, is required for platelet aggregation in fluid shear fields (15–17).

Aurin tricarboxylic acid is capable of inhibiting platelet thrombosis in vivo in the Folts dog model of myocardial infarction (37), and platelet-mediated rethrombosis following fibrinolytic therapy (38). Investigation of ATA in vitro and in vivo in arterial thrombotic models may lead to its trial in refractory TTP, relapsing TTP, and HUS (for which plasma manipulation is relatively ineffective), as well as in myocardial infarction and stroke.

Other new agents of possible future use in the treatment of HUS and refractory

Table 4 vWF and HUS

Patients	Relative decrease in large plasma vWF multimers[a]	Unusually large vWF multimers[a]
51 (37 children, 14 adults)	24 (16 children, 8 adults)	3 children

[a]Pretreatment or earliest sample obtained.

TTP, and in the prophylaxis of relapsing TTP, include a recombinant fragment of the human vWF monomer composed of amino acids 445–733 that contains the platelet GPIb-binding site and competes with large vWF multimers for binding to GPIb (39); and a monoclonal antibody directed against the arginine-glycine-aspartate sequence of the vWF monomer, which is important in binding vWF multimers to platelet GPIIb/IIIa (Also discussed in Chapter 40.).

ACKNOWLEDGMENTS

I am grateful for the excellent technical assistance of Ms. Patsy McPherson, Ms. Margie Harris, and Mr. Jeffrey Massengale, and for the secretarial skills of Ms. Andrea Bethel.

REFERENCES

1. Byrnes, J. J., Moake, J. L., Thrombotic thrombocytopenic purpura and the hemolytic–uremic syndrome: Evolving concepts of pathogenesis and therapy. *Clin. Haematol.*, *15*: 413–442 (1986).
2. Siddiqui, F. A., Lian, E.C.-Y., Novel platelet-agglutinating protein from a thrombotic thrombocytopenic purpura plasma. *J. Clin. Invest.*, *76*: 1330–1337 (1985).
3. Lian, E.C.-Y., Siddiqui, F. A., Platelet agglutinating protein P37 causes platelet agglutination through its binding to membrane glycoprotein IV. *Blood*, *72*(Suppl. 1): 330a (1988).
4. Murphy, W. G., Moore, J. C., Kelton, J. G., Calcium-dependent cysteine protease activity in the sera of patients with thrombotic thrombocytopenic purpura. *Blood*, *70*: 1683–1687 (1987).
5. Moore, J. C., Murphy, W. G., Kelton, J. G., Coelpain proteolysis of von Willebrand factor enhances its binding to platelet membrane glycoprotein IIb/IIIa : an explanation for platelet aggregation in thrombotic thrombocytopenic purpura. *Br. J. Haematol.*, *74*: 457–464 (1990).
6. Moake, J. L., Rudy, C. K., Troll, J. H., Weinstein, M. J., Colannino, N. M., Azocar, J., Seder, R. H., Hong, S. L., Deykin, D., Unusually large plasma factor VIII:von Willebrand factor multimers in chronic relapsing thrombotic thrombocytopenic purpura. *N. Engl. J. Med.*, *307*: 1432–1435 (1982).
7. Moake, J. L., Byrnes, J. J., Troll, J. H., Rudy, C. K., Hong, S. L., Weinstein, M. J., Colannino, N. M., Effects of fresh-frozen plasma and its cryosupernatant fraction on von Willebrand factor multimeric forms in chronic relapsing thrombotic thrombocytopenic purpura. *Blood*, *65*: 1232–1236 (1985).
8. Moake, J. L., Rudy, C. K., Troll, J. H., Weinstein, M. J., Colannino, N. M., Hong, S. L., Schafer, A. I., Therapy of chronic relapsing thrombotic thrombocytopenic purpura with prednisone and azathioprine. *Am. J. Hematol.*, *20*: 73–79 (1985).
9. Moake, J. L., Rudy, C. K., Troll, J. H., Weinstein, M. J., Colannino, N. M., Hong, S. L., Koutcher, J. A., Melaragno, A. J., von Willebrand factor abnormalities and endothelial cell perturbation in acute thrombotic thrombocytopenic purpura. *Am. J. Med. Sci.*, *29*: 47–50 (1985).
10. Miura, M., Koizumi, S., Nakamura, K., Ohno, T., Tachinami, T., Yamagami, M., Taniguchi, N., Kinoshita, S., Abildgaard, C. F., Efficacy of several plasma components in a young boy with chronic thrombocytopenia and hemolytic anemia who responds repeatedly to normal plasma infusions. *Am. J. Hematol.*, *17*: 307–319 (1984).
11. Rowe, J. M., Francis, C. W., Cyran, E. M., Marder, V. J., Thrombotic thrombocytopenic purpura: recovery after splenectomy associated with persistence of abnormally large von Willebrand factor multimers. *Am. J. Hematol.*, *20*: 161–168 (1985).
12. Moake, J. L., McPherson, P. D., Abnormalities of von Willebrand factor multimers

in thrombotic thrombocytopenic purpura and the hemolytic–uremic syndrome. *Am. J. Med.*, *87*: 9N–13N (1989).

13. Kelton, J. G., Moore, J., Santos, A., Sherdan, D., The detection of a platelet-agglutination factor in thrombotic thrombocytopenic purpura. *Ann. Intern. Med.*, *101*: 589–593 (1984).
14. Ruggeri, Z. M., Zimmerman, T. S., von Willebrand factor and von Willebrand disease. *Blood*, *70*: 895–904 (1987).
15. Moake, J. L., Turner, N. A., Stathopoulos, N. A., Nolasco, L., Hellums, J. D., Shear-induced platelet aggregation can be mediated by vWF released from platelets, as well as by exogenous large or unusually large vWF multimers, requires adenosine diphosphate, and is resistant to aspirin. *Blood*, *71*: 1366–1374 (1988).
16. Moake, J. L., Turner, N. A., Stathopoulos, N. A., Nolasco, L. H., Hellums, J. D., Involvement of large plasma von Willebrand factor (vWF) multimers and unusually large vWF forms derived from endothelial cells in shear stress-induced platelet aggregation. *J. Clin. Invest.*, *78*: 1456–1461 (1986).
17. Peterson, D. M., Stathopoulos, N. A., Giorgio, T. D., Hellums, J. D., Moake, J. L., Shear-induced platelet aggregation requires von Willebrand factor and platelet membrane glycoproteins Ib and IIb/IIIa. *Blood*, *69*: 625–628 (1987).
18. Gardner, T. M., Moake, J. L., Unusually large vWF multimers secreted rapidly from stimulated endothelial cells bind to collagen with maximum effectiveness, and agglutinate platelets in the presence of low concentration ristocetin [abstract]. *Circulation*, *78*: II–453 (1988).
19. Frangos, J. A., Moake, J. L., Nolasco, L., Phillips, M. D., McIntire, L. V., Cryosupernatant regulates accumulation of unusually large vWF multimers from endothelial cells. *Am. J. Physiol.*, *256*: H1635–H1644 (1989).
20. Asada, Y., Sumiyoshi, A., Hayashi, T., Suzumiya, J., Kaketani, K., Immunohistochemistry of vascular lesions in thrombotic thrombocytopenic purpura, with special reference to factor VIII related antigen. *Thromb. Res.*, *38*: 469–479 (1985).
21. Kelton, J. G., Moore, J. C., Murphy, W. G., Studies investigating platelet aggregation and release initiated by sera from patients with thrombotic thrombocytopenic purpura. *Blood*, *69*: 924–928 (1987).
22. Moake, J. L., Thrombotic thrombocytopenic purpura (TTP) and the hemolytic–uremic syndrome (HUS). In *Conn's Current Therapy* (R. E. Rakel, ed.), W. B. Saunders, Philadelphia, pp. 339–351 (1989).
23. Rock, G. A., Shumak, K. H., Buskard, N. A., Blanchette, V. S., Kelton, J. G., Nair, R. C., Spasoff, R. A., Canadian Apheresis Study Group, Comparison of plasma exchange with plasma infusion in the treatment of thrombotic thrombocytopenic purpura. *N. Engl. J. Med.*, *325*: 393–397 (1991).
24. Byrnes, J. J., Moake, J. L., Hirsch, R., Klug, P., Periman, P., Effectiveness of the cryosupernatant fraction of plasma in the treatment of refractory thrombotic thrombocytopenic purpura. *Am. J. Hematol.*, *34*: 169–174 (1990).
25. Bell, W. R., Braine, H. G., Ness, P. M., Kickler, T. S., Improved survival in thrombotic thrombocytopenic purpura–hemolytic uremic syndrome. *N. Engl. J. Med.*, *325*: 398–403 (1991).
26. Moake, J. L., McPherson, P. D., von Willebrand factor in thrombotic thrombocytopenic purpura and the hemolytic–uremic syndrome. *Transfusion Med.* *4*: 163–168 (1990).
27. Wick, T. M., Moake, J. L., Udden, M. M., Eskin, S. G., Sears, D. A., McIntire, L. V., Unusually large von Willebrand factor multimers increase adhesion of sickle erythrocytes to human endothelial cells under controlled flow conditions. *J. Clin. Invest.*, *80*: 905–910 (1987).
28. Wick, T. M., Moake, J. L., Udden, M. M., McIntire, L. V., Unusually large (UL) vWF

multimers bind to GPIb-like and integrin receptors on sickle and young non-sickle RBC and on endothelial cells (EC). *Blood, 72*: 76a (1988).
29. Moake, J. L., Byrnes, J. J., Troll, J. H., Rudy, C. K., Weinstein, M. J., Colannino, N. M., Hong, S. L., Abnormal VIII:von Willebrand factor patterns in the plasma of patients with the hemolytic–uremic syndrome. *Blood, 64*: 592–598 (1984).
30. Rose, P. E., Enayat, S. M., Sunderland, R., Short, P. E., Williams, C. E., Hill, F. G., Abnormalities of factor VIII related protein multimers in the haemolytic uraemic syndrome. *Arch. Dis. Child., 59*: 1135–1140 (1984).
31. Karmali, M. A., Petric, M., Lim, C., Fleming, P. C., Arbus, G. S., Lior, N., The association between idiopathic hemolytic uremic syndrome and infection by verotoxin-producing *Escherichia coli. J. Infect. Dis., 51*: 775–782 (1985).
32. Proia, A. D., Harden, E. A., Silberman, H. R., Mitomycin-induced hemolytic–uremic syndrome. *Arch. Pathol. Lab. Med., 108*: 959–962 (1984).
33. Hill, G. S., Drug-associated glomerulopathies. *Toxicol. Pathol, 14*: 37–44 (1986).
34. Chappell, M. E., Keeling, D. M., Prentice, H. G., Sweny, P. Haemolytic uraemic syndrome after bone marrow transplantation: An adverse effect of total body irradiation? *Bone Marrow Transplant., 34*: 339–347 (1988).
35. Leung, D. Y. M., Moake, J. L., Havens, P. L., Kim, M., Pober J. S., Lytic-anti-endothelial cell antibodies in hemolytic–uremic syndrome. *Lancet, 2*: 183–186 (1988).
36. Phillips, M. D., Moake, J. L., Nolasco, L., Turner, N. A., Aurin tricarboxylic acid: A novel inhibitor of platelet–von Willebrand factor association. *Blood, 72*: 1898–1903 (1988).
37. Strony, J., Phillips, M., Brands, D., Moake, J., Adelman, B., Aurin tricarboxylic acid in a canine model of coronary artery thrombosis. *Circulation, 81*: 1106–1114 (1990).
38. Strony, J., Brands, D., Hanners, E., Adelman, B., Platelet thrombus formation following fibrinolytic therapy is dependent upon shear stress and von Willebrand factor. *Clin. Res., 38*: 470a (1990).
39. Sugimoto, M., Ricca, G, Hrinda, M. E., Schreiber, A. B., Searfoss, G. H., Bottini, E., Ruggeri, Z. M., Functional modulation of the isolated glycoprotein Ib-binding domain of von Willebrand factor expressed in *Escherichia coli. Biochemistry, 30*: 5292–5209 (1991).

34
Platelet-Agglutinating/Aggregating Proteins from the Plasma of Patients with Thrombotic Thrombocytopenic Purpura

Eric C.-Y. Lian, Farooq A. Siddiqui, S.-H. Chen, and L.-M. Feng
Veterans Administration Medical Center and University of Miami School of Medicine, Miami, Florida **J.-Z. Li** *Chinese Academy of Medical Sciences, Tianjing, China*

Thrombotic thrombocytopenic purpura (TTP) is pathologically characterized by the presence of platelet thrombi in the arterioles and capillaries. The deposition of platelet thrombi in the small vessels accounts for the clinical pictures of this disorder, including thrombocytopenia, microangiopathic hemolytic anemia, neurological symptoms, and renal abnormalities. The formation of platelet thrombi is triggered by certain stimuli of unknown origin, which may activate or interact with the platelets, endothelial cells, or both. Our laboratory initially demonstrated that the plasmas from three TTP patients during acute disease induce the in vitro clumping of platelets from both normal subjects and patients during remission (1). This platelet-aggregating/agglutinating factor is not dialyzed nor absorbed by $A1(OH)_3$, and it is not inactivated by hirudin or heparin in the presence of normal amounts of antithrombin III. In contrast with the platelet clumping induced by platelet isoantibody, the platelet-clumping activity of TTP plasma diminishes as a function of time when it is incubated with normal plasma at 37°C (Fig. 1). These findings suggest that the substance in the TTP plasma responsible for platelet clumping is not ADP, thrombin, or immunoglobulin. The platelet-clumping activity has also been demonstrated in patients with TTP (2–5) and in the hemolytic uremic syndrome (HUS) (6) by other laboratories. In a different experimental design, Kelton et al. (7, 8) has shown platelet-agglutinating activity in TTP serum after the addition of normal defibrinated cryoprecipitate.

The effect of platelet inhibitors on TTP plasma-induced platelet clumping was examined (9) using plasma from two patients. Aspirin, ibuprofen, sulfinpyrazone, prostaglandin E_1, prostaglandin I_2, dβcAMP, apyrase, creatine phosphate/creatine phosphokinase, antimycin, 2-deoxy-D-glucose, dipyridamole, clofibrate, dextran 40,

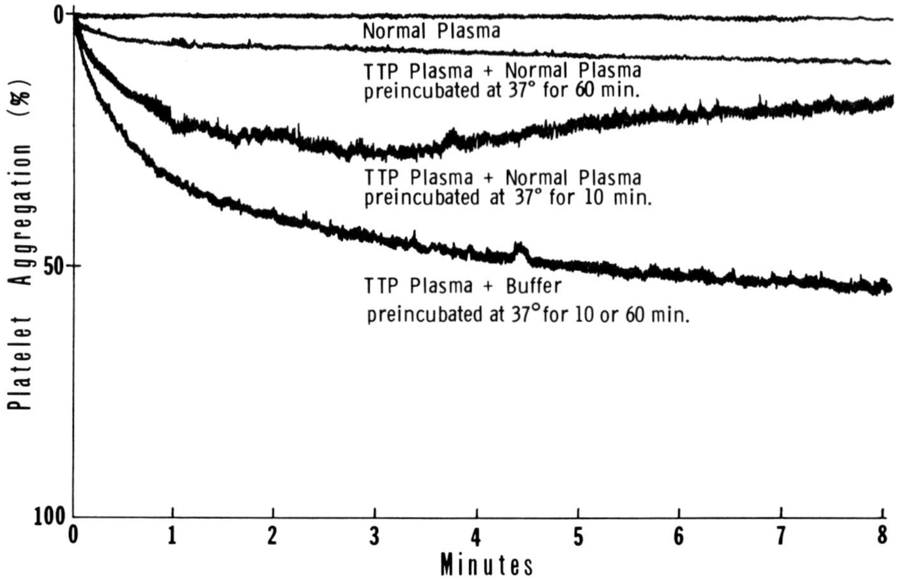

Figure 1 Time-dependent inhibition of TTP–plasma-induced platelet aggregation by normal plasma. (From Ref. 1.)

dextran 70, dibucaine, lidocaine (Xylocaine), methylmaleimide, and ethylene diaminetetraacetic acid (EDTA) had little or no effect. This indicates that the platelet-clumping substance in these two patients was not ADP or collagen, and that, at least in these cases, antiplatelet drugs would be expected to play a limited role in treatment.

One of the substances in normal plasma that is responsible for the inhibition of platelet clumping induced by TTP plasma was purified to homogeneity (10) and identified as IgG (11). The IgG purified from seven normal adults completely inhibited the platelet clumping induced by two TTP plasmas obtained during acute disease. The inhibition of platelet clumping by human adult IgG was concentration-dependent. Similar to intact IgG, the Fab fragments inhibited the TTP plasma-induced platelet clumping, where Fc fragments had no effect (11). Platelet clumping caused by ADP, collagen, epinephrine, or thrombin was not affected by IgG. The IgG obtained from five infants and young children under the age of 4 years did not possess any inhibitory activity. When one of the children reached 3 years of age, his IgG inhibited the clumping induced by one TTP plasma, but not that caused by another plasma. The IgG from the same boy at 4 years of age inhibited the clumping caused by both TTP plasmas. The IgG purified from the TTP plasma during active disease failed to inhibit the clumping caused by the same plasma. After recovery, however, the IgG effectively inhibited clumping. These observations suggest that the platelet-clumping factors present in the TTP plasmas tested were heterogeneous, and possibly derived from infectious agents. The inhibitory activity of IgG is likely acquired through host defense against platelet-clumping factors. Initially the platelet-clumping substance in the plasma of one patient was found to have a relative molecular mass (*M*r) slightly larger than that of IgM, as estimated by molecular sieve chromatography (12). The clumping substance in the plasma of another patient

(H.E.) was purified to homogeneity and had an M_r of 37 kd (p37) (13). Recently, we purified another platelet-clumping protein from the plasma of a third patient, which had an M_r of 59 kd (p59) (14). The properties of platelet-agglutinating protein p37 (PAP p37) will be described in more detail, and those of p59 will be discussed briefly.

PLATELET-AGGLUTINATING PROTEIN p37

Purification and Biochemical Properties

Platelet-agglutinating protein p37 was purified from the plasma of one TTP patient obtained during exchange plasmapheresis by using aluminum hydroxide adsorption, ammonium sulfate fractionation, DEAE-Sephacel chromatography, and cancanavalin A (Con A)–Sepharose affinity chromatography (13). The protein with major platelet-clumping activity bound to DEAE-Sephacel tightly and was eluted only when the salt concentration was increased to 0.3 MNaCl. It also bound tightly to Con A–Sepharose. It was not eluted with 1 M α-methyl-D-glucoside until the buffer was changed to 0.1 M acetate buffer, pH 4.0, containing 0.5 M NaCl. By 0.1% sodium docecyl sulfate–12% polyacrylamide gel electrophoresis (SDS–PAGE), with and without reduction, the protein with platelet-clumping activity was shown to have an M_r of 37 kd. This protein band was absent in the normal and recovery plasma prepared in a similar manner (Fig. 2) (13). It stained with periodic acid-Schiff (PAS) and, therefore, was a glycoprotein.

Platelet-Clumping Properties

Platelet-agglutinating protein p37 induced the clumping of both autologous and homologous platelets in a concentration-dependent manner. The clumping did not require extracellular calcium ions, fibrinogen, or von Willebrand factor (vWF). It was not inhibited by hirudin, heparin in the presence of antithrombin III, phenylmethylsulfonyl fluoride, 2-deoxy-D-glucose, antimycin, apyrase, aspirin, or prostaglandin I_2 (prostacyclin) (13). Consequently, the platelet clumping induced by p37 was an agglutination, rather than aggregation because it was independent of ADP release, energy metabolism, and the cyclooxygenase pathway.

Inhibition of p37-Induced Agglutination by Immunoglobulin G

The platelet agglutination induced by p37 was completely inhibited by IgG procured from normal human adults, as well as from the same TTP patient after recovery (13). The inhibition of p37-induced agglutination by IgG was mediated through complex formation between IgG and p37 (15). This complex formation was demonstrated by (a) the binding of fluid-phase IgG from normal adults and the same TTP patient after recovery to the adsorbed p37 in a microtiter well using an enzyme-linked immunoadsorbent assay; (b) the binding of ^{125}I-p37 to adult IgG covalently cross-linked to Sepharose 4B beads; (c) increase in the sedimentation value of ^{125}I-p37 from 3.5S to 19S after it is mixed and incubated with adult IgG (Fig. 3) (15); and (d) the much earlier elution of ^{125}I-p37 using molecular sieve chromatography when it was incubated with adult IgG. The IgG from a 5-month-old baby and the same TTP patient during active disease did not form a complex with p37. The IgG that was bound to p37 conjugated to Sepharose 4B beads, and later eluted with acidic buffer, inhibited

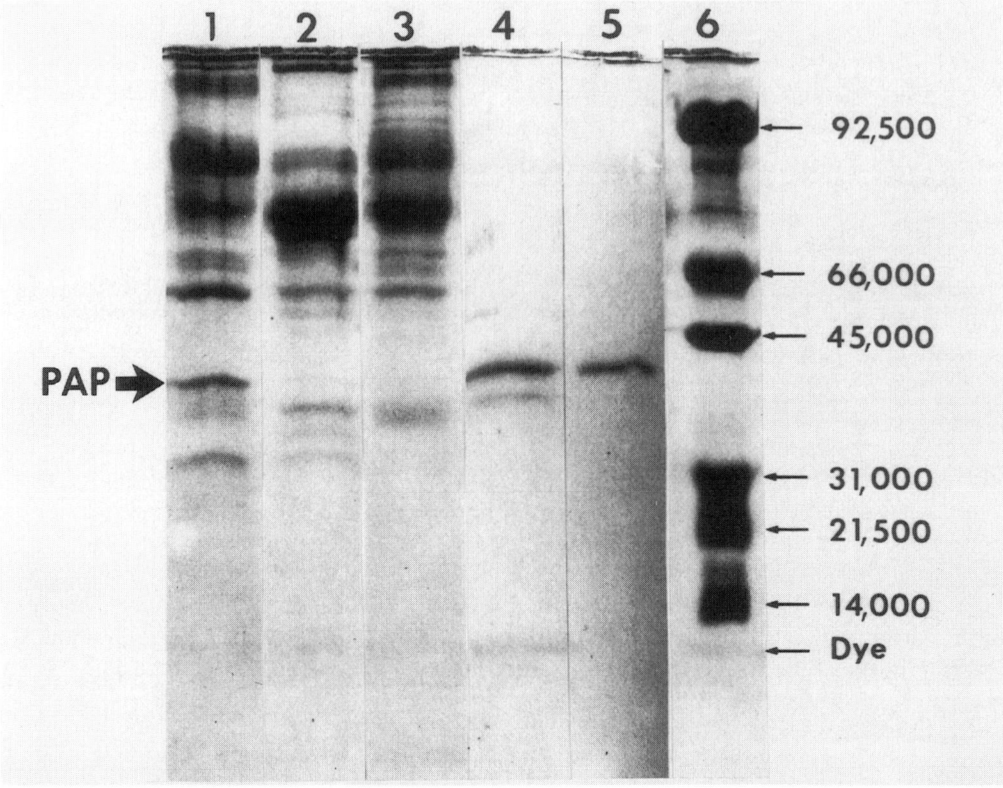

Figure 2 Electrophoretic patterns of the various protein fractions purified from normal, TTP, and TTP recovery plasma, as well as purified PAP, on a 12% sodium dodecyl sulfate (SDS) -polyacrylamide slab gel. Lanes 1–3 show the DEAE–Sephacel fraction III from TTP plasma during active disease (1), after recovery (2), and normal plasma (3). Approximately 12 μg of protein was applied to each lane. Presence of the PAP band is indicated by a thick arrow on the left. Lane 4 shows the gel pattern of 7 μg of Con A fraction IV. The two protein bands were extracted from the gel, and platelet agglutination was checked. Only the 37,000-kd protein (lane 5) agglutinated platelets. Arrows on the right indicate the molecular mass markers. (From Ref. 13.)

the agglutination of washed platelets induced by TTP plasma containing p37, whereas the IgG that was not bound to a p37–Sepharose 4B column did not have a significant inhibitory effect. We conclude that the complex formation between p37 and specific IgG is likely to account for the in vitro inhibition of agglutination induced by this TTP plasma.

Platelet-Agglutinating Protein p37 Is Present Only in a Subset of Patient with Thrombotic Thrombocytopenic Purpura

By using specific rabbit anti-p37 antiserum in Western immunoblotting, p37 was found in three out of five TTP plasmas. The immunoprecipitin band was absent in the plasmas from normal subjects, patients with idiopathic thrombocytopenic purpura, and patients with disseminated intravascular coagulation. The agglutination induced

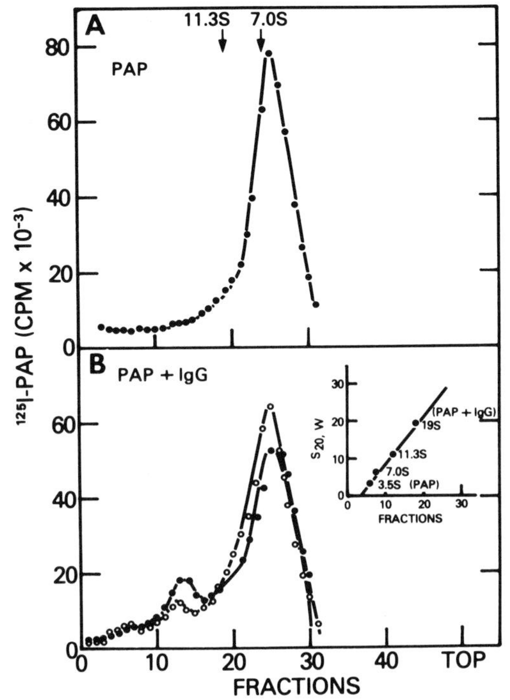

Figure 3 Sucrose density gradient ultracentrifugation of PAP p37 and IgG: ^{125}I-PAP either alone (A) or together with purified human IgG at molar ratios of 1:30 (open circles) or 1:76 (solid dots) (B) was incubated in Tris–saline buffer, pH 7.4, for 1 hr at 37°C. A 0.5-ml portion of the mixture was layered on separate 20–40% linear sucrose gradients (5 ml each) in the same buffer and sedimented at 40,000 rpm in a Beckman SW65 rotor for 14 hr at 4°C. Fractions of 0.16 ml were collected and the radioactivity counted in a gamma counter. Standards used were (a) IgG (7.0S) and (b) catalase (11.3S). The $S_{20}W$ of the PAP and complex formed between PAP and IgG was determined. (From Ref. 15.)

by the three TTP plasmas containing p37 antigenic material was neutralized by the anti-p37 IgG, but that induced by the TTP plasma without p37 was not. These results suggest that p37 is present only in a subset of patients with TTP (13).

Electron Microscopic Study of the Interaction between p37 and Platelets

With a transmission electron microscope in the presence of p37, stirred platelets showed shape change, pseudopod formation, variable degrees of degranulation, dilatation of open canalicular systems, and the formation of agglutinates composed of a few to several hundred platelets. After incubation with p37, platelets were washed and further incubated with rabbit anti-p37 antiserum without stirring, followed by immunostaining. Abundant electron-dense products were bound directly and randomly to the outer surface of the membrane of solitary platelets. When the reaction mixture was stirred, electron-dense particles were also present between the platelet membranes in the agglutinates (16). No staining was observed in control experiments using normal plasma or nonimmune rabbit serum.

Binding Properties of p37 to Platelets

Protein p37 binding to platelets was specific, concentration-dependent, and saturable (17). Scatchard analysis demonstrated about 20,000–27,000 p37-binding sites per platelet, with a dissociation constant of 8×10^{-12} M. Stimulation of platelets with thrombin or ADP did not have any significant effect on the binding. The ^{125}I-p37 also bound to rabbit and rat platelets in a similar manner. Protein p37 did not bind to human erythrocytes. Thiol- and serine-specific protease inhibitors did not inhibit the binding.. Glucose, fructose, mannose, and sialic acid, at a concentration of 40 mM, inhibited p37 binding to platelets by 44, 73, 79, and 91%, respectively, but galactose and amino sugars did not have any significant effect. At 250 μg/ml, concanavalin A inhibited 42% of binding, but phytohemagglutinin-P, potato lectin, and the lectin from *Helix pomatia* did not. As expected, human adult IgG inhibited the binding of p37 to platelets (17).

Platelet Receptor for p37

Monoclonal antibodies to GPIb (6D1) and the GPIIb/IIIa (10E5) complex did not inhibit the binding of p37 to platelets (17) or p37-induced agglutination (18, 19) nor did fibrinogen and vWF affect the binding (17). These results suggest that p37 binds to platelets at sites other than GPIb or the GPIIb/IIIa complex. With use of solubilized platelet membrane proteins from normal donors, it was shown by Western blotting that ^{125}I-p37 binds to a membrane protein of 97 kd under both reducing and nonreducing conditions. The same protein was identified by reverse immunoblotting in which purified p37 was electrophoresed, transferred to nitrocellulose, and incubated with solubilized normal platelet membrane proteins. The complex formed between p37 and the membrane protein was identified by autoradiography using polyclonal and monoclonal (OKM5) anti-GPIV antibodies, but was not detected by polyclonal antibody to GPIIIa. Similar studies with purified platelet GPIV, under both reducing and nonreducing conditions, demonstrated the binding of ^{125}I-p37. Polyclonal and monoclonal antibodies to GPIV completely inhibited platelet agglutination induced by TTP plasma that contained p37. These data indicate that platelet GPIV is the receptor site for PAP p37 (20).

Does p37 Interact with Endothelial Cells?

Endothelial cells have been shown to contain GPIV (CD36) antigen (21). It is possible that p37 can bind to GPIV on endothelial cells and cause injury or mediate the interaction between platelets and endothelial cells.

PLATELET-AGGREGATING PROTEIN p59 AND OTHER PLATELET-CLUMPING PROTEINS

Platelet-aggregating protein p59 was purified from the plasma of one patient with acute TTP, who responded to plasma exchange and infusion (14). The purification procedures included aluminum hydroxide adsorption, polyethylene glycol 6000 fractionation, DEAE cellulose chromatography, lentil lectin–Sepharose 4B chromatography and gel filtration high pressure liquid chromatography. The M_r of this clumping protein was estimated to be 59,000 kd from gel filtration high pressure liquid chromatography and 12% SDS–PAGE, under both reducing and nonreducing conditions. The antiserum produced in a rabbit after repeated injections of p59 forms a single precipitin line against purified p59 by immunodiffusion. Protein p59 induced the clumping of washed platelets from normal subjects, as well as the same patient after recovery. The magnitude of clumping was concentration-dependent. The clumping of washed platelets by p59 was enhanced by adding fibrinogen, but was inhibited by EDTA, prostaglandin I_2, antimycin, 2-deoxy-D-glucose, CV3988, monoclonal antibody (10E5) against the GPIIb/IIIa complex, plasma from healthy adults and the same TTP patient after recovery, or prior incubation at 56°C for 30 min. It was not suppressed by heparin, hirudin, D-phenylalanyl-L-prolyl-L-arginine-chloromethyl ketone (PPACK), apyrase, or aspirin. The p59 antigenic material was present in two of six TTP patients, but absent in seven normal subjects, two patients with disseminated intravascular coagulation, and two patients with idiopathic thrombocytopenic purpura. The anti-p59 antiserum did not react with p37. Apparently, the mechanism of platelet clumping by p59 was different from that induced by p37, requiring energy metabolism, Ca^{2+}, and fibrinogen (14). The clumping caused by p59 was aggregation, rather than agglutination.

Murphy et al. (22) identified, in the plasma of TTP patients, a calcium-dependent cysteine protease that mediated the aggregation of normal platelets. Its activity was not inhibited by serine protease inhibitors; however, it was inhibited by thiol protease inhibitors. This protease disappeared from the plasma of a patient during remission. They suggested that the calcium-dependent protease is important in the functional abnormality of TTP.

Abnormalities of plasma vWF have been reported in patients with TTP and the hemolytic uremic syndrome (HUS). Moake et al. (23) have reported the appearance in plasma of a set of larger-than-normal multimers of vWF during remission of the chronic relapsing form of TTP, and loss of the ultralarge and largest normal plasma multimers during TTP episodes (24). It was postulated that the larger forms of vWF disappeared from TTP plasma because they attach to aggregating platelets and, therefore, play a role in the pathogenesis of TTP (23, 24).

CONCLUSION

Thrombotic thrombocytopenic purpura is a syndrome that may have diverse etiologies. Platelet clumping activity has been demonstrated in TTP plasma during acute disease. Our laboratory has isolated two platelet-clumping proteins from several TTP patients, and found that their mechanisms of platelet clumping are entirely different. Characerization of these proteins and study of their interaction with platelets and endothelial cells may assist us in the further elucidation of this syndrome.

ACKNOWLEDGMENT

This work was supported by National Institutes of Health grant R01HL27007 and the Veterans Administration.

REFERENCES

1. Lian, E. C.-Y., Harkness, D. R., Byrnes, J. J., Wallach, H., Nunez, R., Presence of a platelet aggregating factor in the plasma of patients with thrombotic thrombocytopenic purpura (TTP) and its inhibition by normal plasma. *Blood*, *53*: 333–338 (1979).

2. Ansell, J., Slepchuk, S. I., Pechet, L., Thrombotic thrombocytopenic purpura. *Blood, 54*: 959–960 (1979).
3. Brandt, J. T., Kennedy, M. S., Senhauser, D. A., Platelet aggregating factor in thrombotic thrombocytopenic purpura. *Lancet, 2*: 463–464 (1979).
4. Burns, E. R., Zucker-Franklin, D., Pathologic effects of plasma from patients with thrombotic thrombocytopenic purpura on platelets and cultured vascular endothelial cells. *Blood, 60*: 1030–1037 (1982).
5. Hussay, C., Hause, L., Gottschall, J., A platelet aggregating factor in TTP: Initial activity, fluctuations, and removal by plasma exchange. *Thromb. Haemost., 54*: 138 (1985).
6. Monens, L., van de Meer, W., Langenhauysen, C., et al., Platelet aggregating factor in the epidemic form of hemolytic–uremic syndrome in childhood. *Clin. Nephrol., 24*: 135–139 (1985).
7. Kelton, J. G., Moore, J., Santos, A., Sheridan, D., Detection of a platelet-agglutination factor in thrombotic thrombocytopenic purpura. *Ann. Intern. Med., 101*: 589–593 (1984).
8. Kelton, J. G., Moore, J. C., Murphy, W. G., Studies investigating platelet aggregation and release initiated by sera from patients with thrombotic thrombocytopenic purpura. *Blood, 69*:924–928 (1987).
9. Lian, E. C.-Y., Savaraj, N., Effects of platelet inhibitors on the platelet aggregation induced by plasma from patients with thrombotic thrombocytopenic purpura. *Blood, 58*: 354–359 (1981).
10. Lian, E. C.-Y., Mui, P. T. K., Siddiqui, F. A., Chiu, L. L. S., Purification and some properties of a protein obtained from normal human plasma which inhibits the platelet aggregation induced by thrombotic thrombocytopenic purpura. *Thromb. Res., 33*: 69–76 (1983).
11. Lian, E. C.-Y., Mui, P. T. K., Siddiqui, F. A., Chiu, A. Y. Y., Chiu, L. L. S., Inhibition of platelet-aggregating activity in thrombotic thrombocytopenic purpura plasma by normal adult immunoglobulin G. *J. Clin. Invest., 73*: 548–555 (1984).
12. Lian, E. C.-Y., The role of increased platelet aggregation in TTP. *Semin. Thromb. Hemost., 6*:401–415 (1980).
13. Siddiqui, F. A., Lian, E. C.-Y., Novel platelet-agglutinating protein from a thrombotic thrombocytopenic purpura plasma. *J. Clin. Invest., 76*: 1330–1337 (1985).
14. Chen, S.-H., Lian, E. C.-Y., Purification and some properties of a 59 kda platelet-aggregating protein from the plasma of a patient with thrombotic thrombocytopenic purpura [Abstract]. *Thromb. Haemost., 62*: 568 (1989).
15. Siddiqui, F. A., Lian, E. C.-Y., Platelet-agglutinating protein p37 from a thrombotic thrombocytopenic purpura plasma forms a complex with human immunoglobulin G. *Blood, 71*: 299–304 (1988).
16. Li, J.-Z., Liu, J. W., Benito, G., Siddiqui, F. A., Lian, E. C.-Y., Electron microscopic study of platelet agglutination induced by thrombotic thrombocytopenic purpura plasma containing 37-kda platelet agglutinating protein. *Thromb. Res., 55*: 757–766 (1989).
17. Lian, E. C.-Y., Siddiqui, F. A., Binding of platelet agglutinating protein p37 from the plasma of a patient with thrombotic thrombocytopenic purpura to human platelets. *Thromb. Haemost. 65*: 96–101 (1991).
18. Lian, E. C.-Y., Siddiqui, F. A., Investigation of the role of von Willebrand factor in thrombotic thrombocytopenic purpura. *Blood, 66*: 1219–1221 (1985).
19. Lian, E. C.-Y, Siddiqui, F. A., Role of von Willebrand factor in TTP [letter]. *Blood, 67*: 1524–1526 (1986).
20. Lian, E. C.-Y., Siddiqui, F. A., Jamieson, G. A., Tandon, N. N., Platelet agglutinating protein p37 causes platelet agglutination through its binding to membrane glycoprotein IV. *Thromb. Haemost., 65*: 102-106 (1991).
21. Asch, A. A., Barnwell, J., Silverstein, R. L., Nachman, R. L., Isolation of the thrombospondin membrane receptor. *J. Clin. Invest., 79*: 1054–1061 (1987).

22. Murphy, W. G., Moore, J. C., Kelton, J. G., Calcium-dependent cysteine protease activity in the sera of patients with thrombotic thrombocytopenic purpura. *Blood, 70*: 1683–1687 (1987).
23. Moake, J. L., Rudy, C. K., Troll, I. H., Weinstein, M. J., Colannino, N. M., Azocar, J., Seder, R. H., Hong, S. L., Deykin, D., Unusually large plasma factor VIII: von Willebrand factor multimers in chronic relapsing thrombotic thrombocytopenic purpura. *N. Engl. J. Med., 307*: 1432–1435 (1982).
24. Moake, J. L., Byrnes, J. J., Troll, J. H., Rudy, C. K., Weinstein, M. J., Colannino, N. M., Hong, S. L., Abnormal VIII: von Willebrand factor patterns in the plasma of patients with the hemolytic uremic syndrome. *Blood, 64*: 592–598 (1984).

35
Role of Prostacyclin in the Pathogenesis and Therapy of Thrombotic Thrombocytopenic Purpura

Kenneth K. Wu *University of Texas Medical School, Houston, Texas*

The major pathophysiological feature of thrombotic thrombocytopenic purpura (TTP) and the hemolytic uremic syndrome (HUS) is the deposition of platelet aggregates on the damaged microvascular wall. The pathogenetic mechanisms by which this occurs are not entirely understood. It is generally accepted, however, that enhanced platelet aggregation in this disorder is due to an imbalance between the insulting agents and the defense factors. The latter includes prostacyclin (prostaglandin I_2; PGI_2), a metabolite of arachidonic acid metabolism. Several studies have implied that an aberration in prostacyclin activity may play a role in the pathogenesis of TTP and HUS. The purpose of this chapter is to provide a critical review on basic aspects of prostacyclin biosynthesis and its relevance to this problem.

PROSTACYCLIN BIOSYNTHESIS

Prostacyclin is synthesized primarily by the vascular endothelial cells. Its biosynthesis is catalyzed by several enzymes that are constitutively present in quiescent endothelial cells. Exposure of the cells to the agonists thrombin, histamine, and others leads to activation of phospholipase A_2 (PLA_2), which catalyzes the liberation of arachidonic acid (AA) from membrane phospholipids. The free AA is metabolized in succession to PGG_2 and PGH_2 by prostaglandin endoperoxide synthase (PGH synthase, also called cyclooxygenase), and the PGH_2 is converted to PGI_2 by PGI synthase. Prostaglandin E_2 and $PGF_{2\alpha}$ are also formed through enzymatic and nonenzymatic pathways.

Prostacyclin biosynthesis is controlled at each of these enzymatic steps. The activity of phospholipase A_2 is rate-limiting and controls the availability of free arachidonic acid. On the other hand, PGH synthase and, to a lesser extent, PGI synthase undergo autoinactivation once their respective products—PGH_2 and

PGI_2—are formed. Irreversible inactivation of PGH synthase appears to be the most critical step in controlling PGI_2 production (1). Recent studies reveal that this enzyme has a rapid turnover rate in cultured endothelial cells, with a half-life of about 5 min (2). Stimulation by thrombin, histamine, and calcium ionophore, which are incapable of renewing this enzyme, induces a rapid burst of PGI_2 synthesis that lasts for only 10 min (3, 4). By contrast, cytokines are capable of inducing de novo synthesis of PGH synthase (2, 5). Their stimulation of PGI_2 biosynthesis is, therefore, characterized by a sustained generation of PGI_2, lasting for hours (6, 7). Induction of de novo synthesis of PGH synthase may be the most important step in regulating PGI_2 biosynthesis. These mechanisms must be taken into consideration when elucidating any pathogenetic role for PGI_2 abnormalities in TTP and HUS.

ROLE OF PROSTACYCLIN DEFICIENCY IN THE PATHOGENESIS OF THROMBOTIC THROMBOCYTOPENIC PURPURA AND HEMOLYTIC UREMIC SYNDROME

Deficient Prostacyclin Synthesis

Remuzzi et al. reported on a family with HUS whose serum appeared to elicit a subnormal stimulation of PGI_2 production when incubated with rabbit aortic rings in vitro (8). Subsequent studies implied that serum may contain a prostacyclin-stimulating factor that, if deficient, may lead to a compromised PGI_2 production that is inadequate for defending against excessive platelet aggregation. Although these observations are provocative and interesting, the laboratory data to support this hypothesis are inconclusive. There are several major problems. The foremost is the inability to as yet identify this missing PGI_2-stimulating factor. In fact, recent studies indicate that human serum probably contains a myriad of chemicals capable of stimulating PGI_2 synthesis. These compounds include cytokines, vasoactive kinins, and neutrophil elastase (7, 9, 10). They may be present in the serum in variable quantities, or they may represent in vitro artifacts. The problem is further compounded by the technical difficulty in standardizing a laboratory procedure for determining serum PGI_2-stimulating activity. It is, therefore, questionable whether or not the patients reported have a deficiency of any specific PGI_2-stimulating factor. Recent studies also raise serious doubts about the significance of measurements of serum stimulating activity for PGI_2 synthesis.

An emerging concept is that TTP or HUS may be related to PGI_2 deficiency secondary to the toxic effect of chemical compunds or bacterial toxins on the endothelial cell biosynthesis of PGI_2. The HUS and TTP are increasingly associated with chemotherapeutic agents (i.e., mitomycin, fluorouracil, and cisplatin) (11), the immunosuppressive agent cyclosporine (12), and Shiga-like toxin (SLT)-producing *Escherichia coli* strain O157:H7 (13, 14). Several epidemiological studies have indicated that *E. coli* infection is a common antecedent of HUS in the United States. The SLT-producing *E. coli* release a family of toxins related to those produced by *Shigella* species (Shiga toxins). In fact, type 1 of the *E. coli* toxins is identical with the Shiga toxin (15). These toxins appear to inhibit cellular protein synthesis by interfering with ribosomal polypeptide elongation (16, 17). Studies using purified SLT in the in vitro rat aorta model, revealed that the toxins inhibit endothelial cell PGI_2 production (18).

As the rat aortic segments used in this model were obtained by dissection, mechanical trauma could have activated arachidonic acid metabolism. The model is, as a consequence, unsuitable for studying the mechanism by which SLT inhibits prostacyclin production. We have evaluated the effect of SLT on arachidonic acid metabolism in cultured human umbilical vein endothelial cells. Our preliminary data show that SLT inhibits PGI_2 synthesis, probably by blocking de novo synthesis of PGH synthase (19). Since this enzyme occupies a central position in prostaglandin biosynthesis and has a short half-life, the blocking of its synthesis could rapidly lead to enzyme depletion and reduced PGI_2 synthesis. The inhibition of PGI_2 production appears to occur at low concentrations of SLT. At higher concentrations, cytotoxic effects occur with eventual endothelial cell death (20). It may be the combination of selective inhibition of PGI_2 formation and the general toxic effects on the endothelium that eventually lead to microvascular damage and excessive platelet aggregate formation on the damaged vessel wall. Further studies on the SLT vascular and cellular effects will provide a more precise insight into the pathogenesis of HUS and TTP associated with other inciting agents.

Accelerated Prostacyclin Degradation

Prostacyclin is unstable in aqueous solution at physiological pH and temperature, with a half-life of 3 min (21). Its stability is substantially enhanced in plasma, where its half-life is increased to 40–60 min (22, 23). prostacyclin binds to plasma proteins and, because of this binding, its activity is prolonged (24). The identity of the binding proteins remains controversial. Serum albumin binds PGI_2, but the binding affinity is weak, and its physiological role in protecting PGI_2 activity is uncertain (25). Moreover, albumin would carry PGI_2 into the systemic circulation and dilute PGI_2 activity. I suspect that the mechanisms by which PGI_2 activity is protected, and possibly targeted, are complex. Nevertheless, my colleagues and I have shown that certain patients with TTP exhibit accelerated PGI_2 degradation, accompanied by reduced PGI_2 binding activity in the serum (24). There exist at least two types of binding defects (24), and these defects are mutually corrected (24), further supporting the notion that PGI_2-binding activity is governed by complex mechanisms. The binding defects appear to be due to a reduction in the binding affinity, with the binding capacity unaffected (26). Taken together, these results indicate that the plasma PGI_2 half-life in some patients with TTP is shortened because of defective PGI_2 binding. The exact mechanism at the molecular level remains unclear. Recently Yui et al. have shown that PGI_2 activity is protected in serum by binding to the high-density lipoprotein (HDL), apoprotein A-I (27). Their preliminary results further showed that the binding is defective in patients with coronary artery disease. These findings support the notion that PGI_2 binding plays a pivotal role in regulating PGI_2 activity, which contributes to maintaining the patency of the microcirculation. Defective PGI_2 binding may have broad implications in microvascular thrombosis.

Summary

Prostacyclin is a potent inhibitor of platelet activation and platelet aggregate formation. It acts as an autacoid and works locally at damaged vascular sites. Its production is stimulated by a myriad of physiological and pathological agonists, and stimulation by these agonists is controlled at several enzymatic steps. Furthermore, after its release from the vascular endothelium, its biological activity is regulated by plasma proteins. These biochemical constraints are consistent with the notion that PGI_2 production, its biological half-life, and its platelet targeting are tightly controlled, to carry out its function. Defects in any step of this regulatory chain may lead to PGI_2 insufficiency and unopposed platelet aggregation. At least two types of defects in this regulatory chain have been identified: (a) deficiency in PGI_2 production and (b) defective serum PGI_2 binding. Although we have learned a great deal from these studies, the mechanisms by which these defects occur and their pathophysiological significance are not clear. A very important issue is the lack of understanding at the cellular and molecular level. With availability of powerful analytic and molecular tools, further advances in this field are anticipated. Elucidation of pathogenetic mechanisms at the molecular level may have an important impact on the understanding of microvascular thrombosis, including coronary artery and cerebrovascular diseases.

DETECTION OF PROSTACYCLINE ABNORMALITIES

A common method for measuring the level of PGI_2 is by determination of the plasma level of its stable metabolite, 6-keto-$PGF_{1\alpha}$, by radioimmunoassay. This approach has proved to be inaccurate because of the extremely low levels of 60-keto-$PGF_{1\alpha}$ present in plasma, as well as interference with the assay by plasma proteins (28). By using gas chromatography–mass spectrometry (GC–MS), FitzGerald et al. showed that the plasma concentration of 6-keto-$PGF_{1\alpha}$ in normal subjects is in the low picogram per milliliter range, a value almost below the detection limit of radioimmunoassay (RIA) (28). In most reported studies of TTP and HUS, the suggestion that PGI_2 deficiency occurs is based on a reduced plasma 6-keto-$PGF_{1\alpha}$ level. For the analytical reasons just cited, the reported data were conflicting and difficult to interpret. A different approach is to measure the urinary content of 2,3-dinor-6-keto-$PGF_{1\alpha}$, a metabolite of 6-keto-$PGF_{1\alpha}$, by GC–MS (29, 30). This technique appears reliable for estimating the prerenal systemic producton of PGI_2, and it has been used in determining PGI_2 production in pathological conditions and during pharmacologic alterations. Similar techniques may be used to estimate thromboxane (TX) synthesis. Concurrent measurement of 2,3-dinor-6-keto-$PGF_{1\alpha}$ and 2,3-dinor TXB_2 in the same urine sample will give useful information concerning the relationship between PGI_2 and TXA_2 generation. A study is underway in my laboratory to quantify these metabolites in TTP and HUS patients.

Serum PGI_2-binding activity can be assayed by a method described by Wu et al. (24). A standard concentration of $[^3H]PGI_2$ or its stable analogue $[^3H]$iloprost is incubated with serum samples at 22°C for 3 min, and it is then applied to a Sephadex G-25 column (21.5 × 0.8 cm), preequilibrated with buffer. The fractions are collected, and the radioactivity in each fraction is counted. In the presence of binding proteins, two peaks are noted. The early peak represents the binding component, and the latter peak is the free 6-keto-$PGF_{1\alpha}$ or iloprost peak. The percentage of integrated radioactive counts of peak 1 represents the binding activity. This binding assay is simple and reproducible. The factors that may influence the assay include packing of the column, its size, and its flow rate.

The PGI_2 decay rate in serum is measured by bioassay (24). A known quantity of PGI_2 is incubated with the test sample. At various time intervals, an aliquot is removed, and the PGI_2 activity is determined by testing its ability to inhibit ADP- or U46619-induced platelet aggregation. The extent of inhibition is related to a calibration curve, established for each experiment, that gives the relationship between PGI_2 concentration and inhibition of platelet aggregation. The decay rate and half-life can then be derived.

THERAPEUTIC IMPLICATIONS

Prostacyclin was available (as epoprostenol) for human therapeutic experiments in the late 1970s. Because of the possibility that PGI_2 was deficient in patients with TTP and HUS, it was empirically tried in several patients with TTP. The reported results were conflicting. In some patients, intravenous infusion of PGI_2 was thought to be efficacious in controlling TTP, whereas it failed entirely in others, despite prolonged infusion (31, 32). As only a limited number of patients have been investigated in a noncontrolled manner, it is impossible to ascretain the efficacy of PGI_2. Moreover, there are several inherent problems with PGI_2 as a therapeutic agent. It is unstable in aqueous solutions and, therefore, continuous infusion is required. With continuous intravenous infusion, its systemic side effects include hypotension, headache, and facial flushing (33). Stable analogues of PGI_2 have recently been developed (34). They have shown promise as useful agents for treating arterial thrombotic disorders and tissue injury (35, 36). They are stable and can be easily given. Whether they will be useful in treating TTP and HUS remains to be investigated. A reasonable approach is to identify subgroups of microangiopathic patients who exhibit an underlying defect in prostacyclin production. This subgroup may benefit from PGI_2 therapy.

ACKNOWLEDGMENTS

The author thanks Ms Nancy Fernandez for excellent secretarial assistance. This work was supported by grants from the National Institutes of Health (NS-23327; HL-35387).

REFERENCES

1. Egan, R. W., Paxton, J., Kuehl, F. A., Jr., Mechanism for irreversible self-deactivation of prostaglandin synthetase. *J. Biol. Chem.*, *251*: 7325–7335 (1976).
2. Frasier-Scott, K., Hatzakis, H., Seong, D., Jones, C. M., Wu, K. K., Influence of natural and recombinant interleukin 2 on endothelial cell arachidonate metabolism. *J. Clin. Invest.*, 82: 1877–1883 (1988).
3. Kent, R. S., Diedrich, S. L., Whorton, A. R., Regulation of vascular prostaglandin synthesis by metabolites of arachidonic acid in perfused rabbit aorta. *J. Clin. Invest.*, *72*: 455–465 (1983).
4. McIntire, T. M., Zimmerman, K. S., Prescott, S. M., Cultured endothelial cells synthesize both platelet-activating factor and prostacyclin response to histamine, bradykinin, and adenosine triphosphate. *J. Clin. Invest.*, *76*: 271–280 (1985).
5. Raz, A., Wyche, A., Siegel, N., Needleman, P., Regulation of fibroblast cyclooxygenase synthesis by interleukin-1. *J. Biol. Chem.*, *263*: 3022–3028 (1988).
6. Rossi, V., Breviario, G., Ghezzi, P., Dejana, E., Mantovani, A., Prostacyclin synthesis induced in vascular cells by interleukin-1. *Science*, *229*: 174–176 (1985).

7. Albrightson, C. R., Baenziger, N. L., Needleman, P., Exaggerated human vascular cell prostaglandin biosynthesis mediated by monocytes: Role of monokines and interleukin 1. *J. Immunol.*, *135*: 1872–1887 (1985).
8. Remuzzi, G., Marchesi, D., Misiani, R., Mecca, G., deGaetano, G., Donati, M. B., Familial deficiency of a plasma factor stimulating vascular prostacyclin activity. *Thromb. Res.*, *16*: 517–570 (1979).
9. Alhenc-Gelas, F., Tsai, S. J., Callahan, K. S., Campbell, W. B., Johnson, A. R., Stimulation of prostacyclin formation by vasoactive mediators in cultured human endothelial cells. *Prostaglandins*, *24*: 723–742 (1982).
10. Miller, D. K., Sadowski, S., Soderman, D. D., Kuehl, F. A., Jr., Endothelial cell prostacyclin production induced by activated neutrophils. *J. Biol. Chem.*, *260*: 1006–1014 (1985).
11. Leseane, J. B., Rothchild, N., Erickson, B., Korec, S., Sisk, R., Keller, J., Arbus, M., Wooley, P. V., Chiazze, L., Shein, P., Neefe, J. R., Cancer associated hemolytic uremic syndrome: Analysis of 65 cases from a national registry. *J. Clin. Oncol.*, *7*:781–789 (1995).
12. van Buren, D., van Buren, C. T., Flechner, S. M., Maddox, A. M., Verani, R., Kahan, B. P., De novo hemolytic uremic syndrome in renal transplant recipients immunosuppressed with cyclosporine. *Surgery*, *98*: 54–62 (1985).
13. Karmali, M. A., Petric, M., Lim, C., Fleming, P. C., Arbus, G. S., Lior, H., The association between idiopathic hemolytic uremic syndrome and infection by verotoxin-producing *E. coli*. *J. Infect. Dis.*, *151*: 775–782 (1985).
14. Ostroff, S. M., Kobayashi, J. M., Lewis, J. H., Infection with *E. coli* O157:H7 in Washington State. *JAMA*, *262*: 355–359 (1989).
15. O'Brien, A. D., Holmes, R. K., Shiga and Shiga-like toxins. *Microbiol. Rev.*, *51*: 206–220 (1987).
16. Endo, Y., Tsurugi, K., Yutsudo, T., Takeda, Y., Ogasawara, T., Igarashi, K., Site of action of a verotoxin (VT2) from *E. coli* O157:H7 and of Shiga toxin on eukaryotic ribosomes. RNA *N*-glycosidase activity of the toxins. *Eur. J. Biochem*, *171*: 45–50 (1988).
17. Ogasawara, T., Ito, K., Igarashi, K., Yatsudo, T., Nakabayashi, N., Takeda, Y., Inhibition of protein synthesis by a vero toxin (VT2 or Shiga-like toxin II) produced by *E. coli* O157:H7 at the level of elongation factor 1-dependent aminoacyl-tRNA binding to ribsomes. *Microb. Pathogen.*, *4*: 127–135 (1988).
18. Karch, H., Bitzan, M., Pietsch, R., Stenger, K.-O, Wulffen, H., von Hessemann, J., Dusing, R., Purified verotoxins of *E. coli* O157:H7 decrease prostacyclin synthesis by endothelial cells. *Microb. Pathogen.*, *5*:215–221 (1988).
19. Huang, P. S., Sanduja, R., Sanduja, S. K., Cleary, T., Wu, K. K., Influence of Shiga-like toxins on endothelial cell arachidonate metabolism. *Blood*, *74*(Suppl.): 39a (1989).
20. Obrig, T. G., Vecchio, P. J., Del Brown, E., Moran, T. P., Rowland, B. M., Judge, T. K., Rothman, S. W., *Infect. Immun.*, *56*: 2373–2378 (1988).
21. Wynalda, M. A., Fitzpatrick, F. A., Albumin stabilizes prostaglandin I_2. *Prostaglandins*, *20*: 853–861 (1980).
22. Orchard, M. A., Robinson, C., Stability of prostacyclin in human plasma and whole blood. Studies on the protective effect of albumin. *Thromb. Haemost.*, *46*: 645–647 (1981).
23. Pifer, D. D., Cagan, G. L. M., Chesney, C. M., Stability of PGI_2 in human blood. *Prostaglandins*, *21*: 165–175 (1981).
24. Wu, K. K., Hall, E. R., Rossi, E. C., Papp, A. C., Serum prostacyclin binding defects in thrombotic thrombocytopenic purpura. *J. Clin. Invest.*, *75*: 168–174 (1985).
25. Tsai, A.-L., Wu, K. K., Stabilization mechanism of prostacyclin by human serum: An approach by binding kinetics using a stable PGI_2 analogue, iloprost. *Biochim. Biophys. Acta*, *924*: 67–74 (1987).
26. Tsai, A.-L., Manner, C. E., Rudersdorf, T., Wu, K. K., Quantitation of serum pros-

tacyclin-binding in thrombotic thrombocytopenic purpura. *Thromb. Res.*, *51*: 583–592 (1988).
27. Yui, Y., Aoyama, T., Morishita, H., Takahashi, M., Takatso, Y., Kawai, C., Serum protacyclin stabilizing factor is identical to apolipoprotein A-I. *J. Clin. Invest.*, *82*: 803–807 (1988).
28. Pedersen, A. K., Watson, M. L., FitzGerald, G. A., Inhibition of thromboxane biosynthesis in serum: Limitations of measurement of immunoreactive 6-keto-$PGF_{1\alpha}$. *Thromb. Res.*, *33*: 99–103 (1983).
29. FitzGerald, G. A., Brash, A. R., Falardeau, P., Oates, J. A., Estimated rate of prostacyclin secretion into the circulation of normal man. *J. Clin. Invest.*, *68*: 1272–1276 (1981).
30. FitzGerald, G. A., Pederson, A. K., Patrono, C., Analysis of prostacyclin and thromboxane biosynthesis in cardiovascular disease. *Circulation*, *67*: 1174–1177 (1983).
31. FitzGerald, G. A., Maas, R. L., Stein, R., et al., Intravenous prostacyclin in thrombotic thrombocytopenic purpura. *Ann. Intern. Med.*, *95*: 319–322 (1981).
32. Johnson, J. E., Mills, G. M., Batson, A. G., Cato, A. E., Thornsiard, C. T., Ineffective epoprostenol therapy for thrombotic thrombocytopenic purpura. *JAMA*, *250*: 3089–3091 (1983).
33. Pickles, H., Grady, J. O., Side effects occurring during administration of epoprostenol (prostacyclin). *Br. J. Clin. Pharmacol.*, *14*: 177–185 (1982).
34. Tsai, A.-L., Wu, K. K., Structure-activity relationship between prostacyclin and its platelet receptor. Correlation of structural change and the platelet activity. *Eicosanoids*, 2: 131–144 (1989).
35. de Langen, C. D. J., van Gilst, W. J., Wesseling, H., Sustained protection by iloprost of the porcine heart in the acute chronic phase of myocardial infarction. *J. Cardiovasc. Pharmacol.*, 7: 924–928 (1985).
36. Bitterman, H., Stahl, G. L., Lefer, A. M., Protective effects of CG-4203, a novel stable prostacyclin analog in traumatic shock. *Prostaglandins*, 35: 41–50 (1988).

36
Pathological Features of Thrombotic Thrombocytopenic Purpura

Yujiro Asada and Akinobu Sumiyoshi *Miyazaki Medical College, Miyazaki, Japan*

In 1924, Moschcowitz (1) first described a syndrome in a 16-year-old girl who had an abrupt onset of petechiae, hemolytic anemia, fever, malaise, upper extremity weakness, and microscopic hematuria. Postmortem examination revealed widespread hyaline microthrombi in the terminal arterioles and capillaries of many organs, in particular, the heart, liver, and kidneys. It was postulated that these thrombi were composed of agglutinated and hyalinized erythrocytes caused by a toxin with agglutinating and hemolytic properties. In 1936, Baehr et al. (2) observed four women with severe progressive anemia and thrombocytopenia and, at necropsy, found widespread microthrombi in small arteries and capillaries, without any inflammation. These thrombi were covered with active proliferating endothelial cells. On the basis of Weigert's fibrin and Giemsa stains, the authors contended that the thrombi were composed of agglutinated platelets, with a little fibrin, and suggested that they were caused by widespread vascular injuries. Later, this syndrome was named thrombotic thrombocytopenic purpura (TTP) by Singer et al. in 1947 (3).

Thrombotic thrombocytopenia purpura is a syndrome clinically characterized by five cardinal manifestations: thrombocytopenia, schistocytic, hemolytic anemia, fluctuating neurological signs, fever, and renal abnormalities (4–6). Pathologically, hyaline thrombi and subendothelial hyaline deposits are found in the small arteries, arterioles, and capillaries of many organs (6–12). The thrombotic vascular lesion has been thought to be a cause of clinical manifestations. The pathogenesis of TTP still remains obscure. In some patients TTP has been associated with infection, pregnancy, cancer, or organ transplantation, but most patients have no apparent associated underlying disease (13).

PATHOLOGICAL FEATURES

Light Microscopy

The most striking lesions of TTP are the subendothelial hyaline deposits and multiple occlusive thrombi (6–12) (Fig. 1). These thrombi are periodic acid-Schiff(PAS) and Giemsa stain positive with a finely granular appearance. Staining with phosphotungstic acid– hematoxylin (PTAH) shows either no fibrin or, more commonly, a few

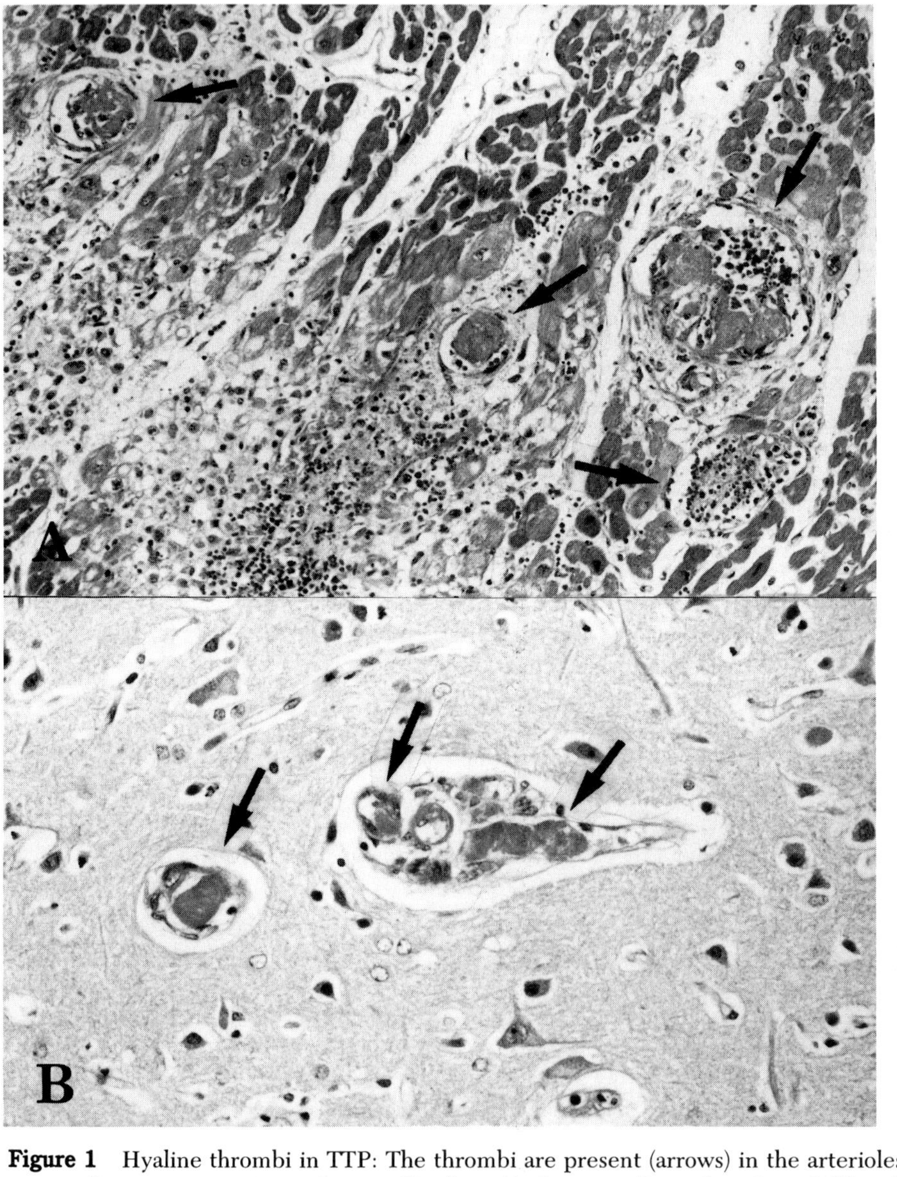

Figure 1 Hyaline thrombi in TTP: The thrombi are present (arrows) in the arterioles of the myocardium in association with a small infarct (A, hemotoxylin and eosin, ×170) and in the capillaries of the cerebral cortex (B, hematoxylin and eosin ×260).

fibrin strands surrounding and sometimes penetrating clumps of amorphous or granular material (Fig. 2). Proliferating endothelial cells are observed covering the thrombi, depending on the age of the lesions. Subendothelial lesions are considered to be of the same nature as the occlusive thrombi, but older. Thrombi in TTP patients who died within several days after onsest, or who received plasma exchange therapy, appear to be smaller (10). Foci of segmental thickening of the intima are observed in small arteries and arterioles in patients with the chronic relapsing type of TTP. These are considered to be healed lesions (Fig. 3).

Thrombotic lesions in TTP are widespread in arterioles and capillaries, sparing venules. The involved vascular walls show no cellular infiltration or inflammation. Dilatation and cylindrical aneurysmal formation at the arteriolocapillary junction have been described (11), but are generally considered nonspecific changes following thrombosis. At autopsy, the most commonly and severely affected organs are the heart, brain (mainly cerebral cortex), kidney, pancreas, liver, spleen, and adrenal glands. Less extensively involved are the lungs, bone marrow, gastrointestinal tract, gallbladder, skeletal muscle, pituitary gland, ovaries, uterus, and testes (7–9, 12). Tissue biopsy samples of the gingiva, skin, and bone marrow may sometimes be useful to confirm the diagnoisis; however, the positive rate is only 30–50% in TTP patients (14–16). Ischemic changes and small infarcts are frequently found near occluded small arteries and arterioles in the heart, brain, pancreas, and spleen (see Fig. 1A). Small foci of hemorrhage are often seen in many organs, especially the brain and heart, adjacent to involved vessels. More extensive hemorrhage may be present in the brain and cause a fatal outcome (12).

Immunohistochemistry

The thrombotic lesions and subendothelial hyaline deposits contain fibrinogen/fibrin (8, 9, 17–19), platelet antigens (8, 18), and von Willebrand factor (vWF) (9). The thrombi formed during episodes of TTP stain strongly for vWF antigen, but only

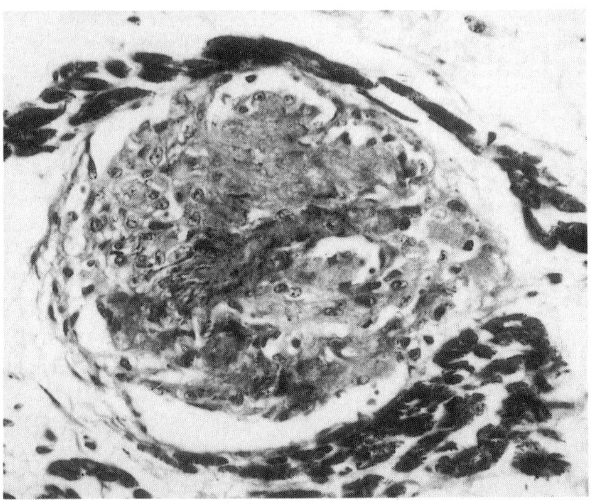

Figure 2 A TTP thrombus in the myocardium: A few fibrin strands penetrate and rim clumps of amorphous or granular material. (PTAH, ×300).

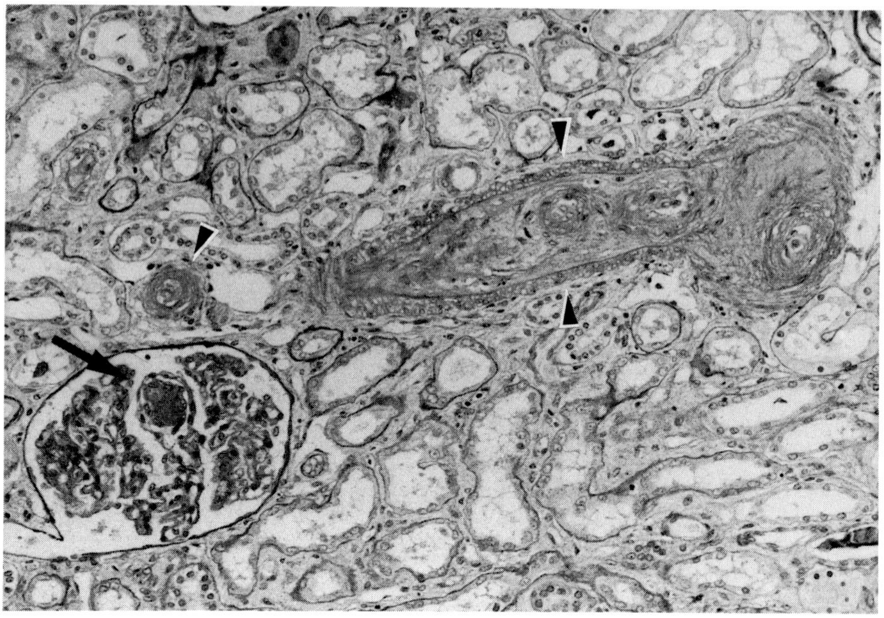

Figure 3 Vascular lesions in the kidney of a patient with the chronic relapsing type of TTP: Foci of prominent intimal thickening of the small artery and arteriole are present (arrow heads). A hyaline thrombus is also noted in the capillary of a glomerulus (arrow). (PAS–alcian blue, ×180).

weakly for fibrinogen/fibrin (Fig. 4). This is in contrast to the opposite immunohistochemical results obtained in thrombi in patients with disseminated intravascular coagulation (9). The immunohistochemical technique for demonstration of vWF antigen is very sensitive and can detect very small TTP thrombi.

Some have reported that IgG, IgM, and complement components are occasionally present in TTP lesions, but others have reported negative results in immunofluorescent studies (8, 16, 17, 19–22). The meaning of these positive results is obscure, because immunoglobulins and complement proteins may be nonspecifically bound or absorbed to exposed Fc and complement receptors after vascular injury (23).

Electron Microscopy

The almost amorphous or granular thrombi and subendothelial hyaline deposits are composed of tightly packed platelets, showing varying degrees of cytoplasmic alteration and degranulation, along with a small amount of interspersed fibrin or amorphous material lacking the periodicity of fibrin (7–9, 19) (Fig. 5). It has been reported that the affected arteriolar wall has electron-dense deposits that are distinct from the subendothelial lesions (19).

PATHOGENIC MECHANISM

Several hypotheses on the etiology of TTP have been proposed; however, the true pathogenic mechanism remains uncertain.

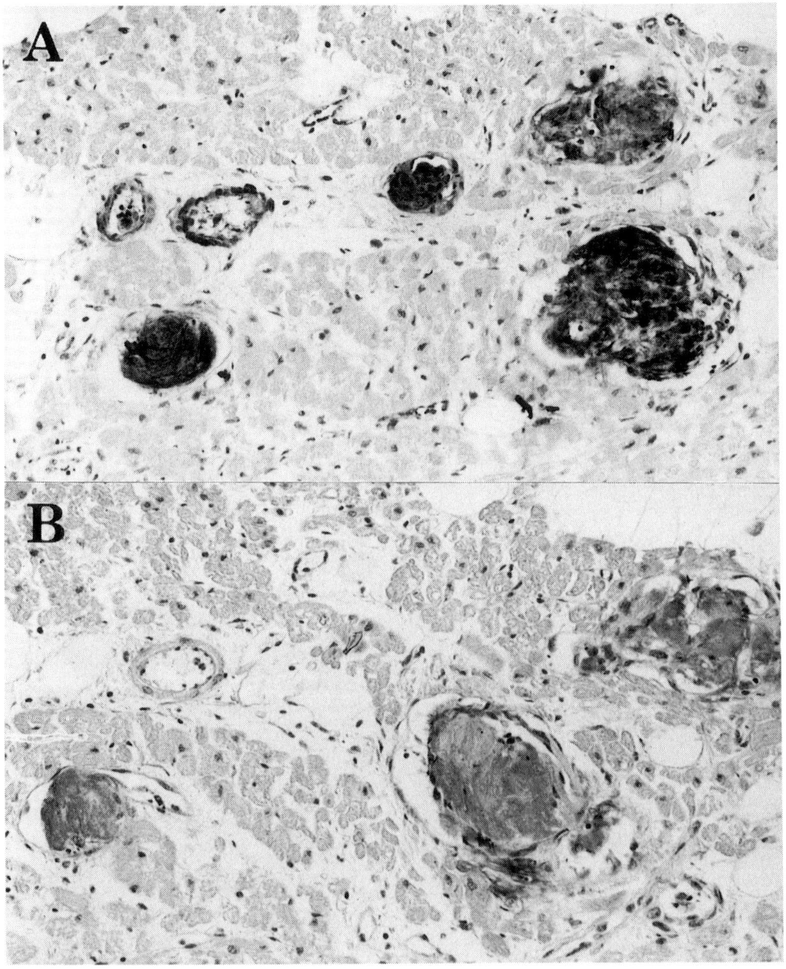

Figure 4 Immunohistochemical staining of TTP thrombi in the myocardium: The lesions show a strongly positive reaction for vWF (A), but only a weakly positive reaction for fibrinogen/fibrin (B). (PAP, ×180) (From Ref. 9.)

The deposition and formation of platelet thrombi in the microvessels are thought to be caused by (a) endothelial cell injury with secondary platelet adhesion and aggregation, (b) disseminated intravascular platelet aggregation or agglutination as a primary event that results in secondary endothelial cell damage, or (c) concurrent occurrence of both processes (24).

From pathological study of the vascular lesions, it is difficult to determine whether the primary event in TTP is endothelial cell injury or disseminated intravascular platelet aggregation or agglutination. However, if vascular injury or increased vascular permeability were to have a primary role in the pathogenesis of TTP, then the subendothelial hyaline deposits would be expected to be strongly positive for fibrinogen/fibrin [similar to the lesions of polyarteritis nodosa (9), in which increased vascular permeability is considered to be part of the pathogenesis (25)].

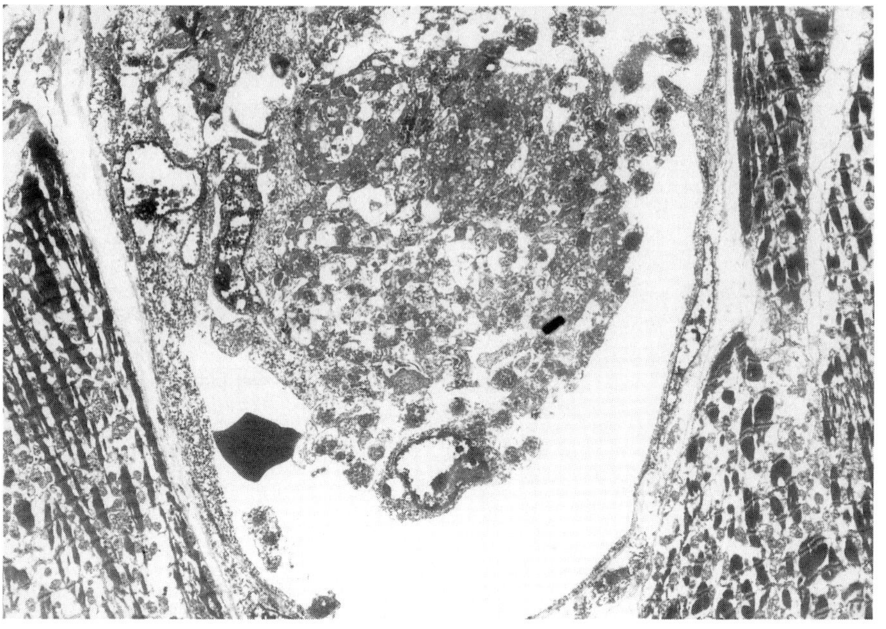

Figure 5 Electron micrograph of a TTP thrombus in an arteriole of the myocardium. The thrombus consists of packed platelets interspersed with amorphous material and is becoming covered with endothelial cells (×2600). (From Ref. 9.)

We suggest that, from the pathomorphological viewpoint, the primary event of TTP may not be primary vascular injury with increased vascular permeability, but rather disseminated intravascular platelet aggregation. Platelet aggregates may lodge as intravascular thrombi in the small arteries, arterioles, and capillaries. Some may become incorporated into the vascular wall as subendothelial hyaline deposits covered with proliferating endothelial cells.

Many etiological factors causing intravascular platelet aggregation have been postulated, including unusually large vWF multimers (26, 27), platelet-agglutinating proteins (28), immune abnormalities (29), impaired fibrinolytic activity of vessels (30), and impaired prostacyclin production (31, 32). These various possibilities are discussed in other chapters. All the vascular lesions in TTP, including subendothelial hyaline deposits, were strongly positive for vWF antigen in our study. This result suggests that vWF multimers may play a role in the pathogenesis of TTP.

REFERENCES

1. Moschcowitz, E., Hyaline thrombosis of the terminal arterioles and capillaries: A hitherto undescribed disease. *Proc. N.Y. Pathol. Soc.*, *24*: 21–24 (1924).
2. Baehr, G., Klemperer, P., Schifrin, A., An acute febrile anemia and thrombocytopenic purpura with diffuse platelet thrombosis of capillaries and arterioles. *Trans. Assoc. Am. Physicians*, *51*: 43–58 (1936).
3. Singer, K., Bornstein, F. P., Wiles, A., Thrombotic thrombocytopenic purpura. *Blood*, 2:542–554 (1947).

4. Petitt, R. M., Thrombotic thrombocytopenic purpura. A thirty-year review. *Semin. Thromb. Hemost., 6*:350–355 (1980).
5. Amorosi, E. L., Ultmann, J. E., Thrombotic thrombocytopenic purpura: Report of 16 cases and review of literature. *Medicine 45*: 139–159 (1966).
6. Umlas, J., Kaiser, J., Thrombotic thrombocytopenic purpura (TTP): A disease or syndrome? *Am. J. Med., 49*: 723–728 (1970).
7. Neame, P. B., Lechago, J., Ling, E. T., Koval, A. Thrombotic thrombocytopenic purpura: Report of a case with disseminated intravascular platelet aggregation. *Blood, 42*: 805–814 (1973).
8. Feldman, J. D., Mardiney, M. R., Unanue, E. R., Cutting, H., The vascular pathology of thrombotic thrombocytopenic purpura. An immunohistochemical and ultrastructural study. *Lab. Invest., 15*: 927–946 (1966).
9. Asada, Y., Sumiyoshi, A., Hayashi, T., Suzumiya, J., Kaketani, K., Immunohistochemistry of vascular lesion in the thrombotic thrombocytopenic purpura, with special reference to factor VIII related antigen. *Thromb. Res., 38*:469–479 (1985).
10. Gordon, L. I., Kwaan, H. C., Rossi, E. C., Deleterious effects of platelet transfusions and recovery thrombocytosis in patients with thrombotic microangiopathy. *Semin. Hematol., 24*: 194–201 (1987).
11. Orbison, J. L., Morphology of thrombotic thrombocytopenic purpura with demonstration of aneurysms. *Am. J. Pathol., 28*: 129–143 (1952).
12. Kwaan, H. C., Clinicopathological features of thrombotic thrombocytopenic purpura. *Semin. Hematol., 24*: 71–81 (1987).
13. Kwaan, H. C., Miscellaneous secondary thrombotic microangiopathy. *Semin. Hematol., 24*: 141–147 (1987).
14. Goodman, A., Ramos, R., Petrelli, M., Hirsh, S. A., Bukowski, R., Harris, J. W., Gingival biopsy in thrombotic thrombocytopenic purpura. *Ann. Intern. Med., 89*: 501–504 (1978).
15. Ruffolo, E. H., Pease, G., Cooper, T. C., Thrombotic thrombocytopenic purpura. Antemortem diagnosis: Use of pariffin sections of sternal bone-marrow aspirate. *Arch. Intern. Med., 110*: 78–82 (1962).
16. Bukowski, R. M., Thrombotic thrombocytopenic purpura. A review. *Prog. Hemost. Thromb., 6*: 287–337 (1982).
17. Craig, J. M., Gitlin, D., The nature of the hyaline thrombi in thrombotic thrombocytopenic purpura. *Am. J. Pathol., 33*: 251–265 (1957).
18. Komori, R., Thrombotic microangiopathy in patients with malignant tumors. *Acta Pathol. Jpn., 12*: 379–405 (1962).
19. Hayasaka, T., Yoshiki, T., Shirai, T., Ninomura, N., Itoh, T., Comparative immunopathologic studies of thrombotic thrombocytopenic purpura, hemolytic–uremic syndrome and disseminated intravascular coagulation. *Acta Pathol. Jpn., 31*: 569–581 (1981).
20. Mant, M. J., Cauchi, M. N., Medley, G., Thrombotic thrombocytopenic purpura: Report of a care with possible immune etiology. *Blood, 40*:416–421 (1972).
21. Weisenburger, D. D., O'Conner, M. L., Hart, M. N., Thrombotic thrombocytopenic purpura with C'3 vascular deposits. Report of a case. *Am. J. Clin. Pathol., 67*: 61–63 (1977).
22. Celada, A., Perrin, L. H., Circulating immune complexes in thrombotic thrombocytopenic purpura (TTP). *Blood, 52*: 855 (1978).
23. Ryan, U. S., The endothelial surface and responses to injury. *Fed. Proc., 45*: 101–108 (1986).
24. Burns, E. R., Zucker-Franklin, D., Pathologic effect of plasma from patients with thrombotic thrombocytopenic purpura on platelets and cultured endothelial cells. *Blood, 60*: 1030–1037 (1982).

25. Rose, A. G., Polyarteritis nodosa. In *Cardiovascular Pathology* (M. D. Silver, ed.), Churchill-Livingstone, New York, pp. 778–779 (1983).
26. Moake, J. L., Rudy, C. K., Troll, J. H., Weinstein, M. J., Colannino, N. M., Azocar, J., Seder, R. H., Hong, S. L., Deykin, D., Unusually large plasma factor VIII:von Willebrand factor multimers in chronic relapsing thrombotic thrombocytopenic purpura. *N. Engl. J. Med., 307*: 1432–1435 (1982).
27. Moake, J. L., von Willebrand factor and the pathophysiology of thrombotic thrombocytopenia: From human studies to a new animal model. *Lab. Invest., 59*: 415–417 (1988).
28. Siddiqui, F. A., Lian, E. C.-Y., Novel platelet-agglutinating protein from a thrombotic thrombocytopenic purpura. *J. Clin. Invest., 76*: 1330–1337 (1985).
29. Lian, E. C.-Y., Mui, P. T. K., Siddiqui, F. A., Chiu, A. Y. Y., Chiu, L. L. S., Inhibition of platelet-aggregating activity in thrombotic thrombocytopenic purpura plasma by normal adult immunoglobulin G. *J. Clin. Invest., 73*: 548–555 (1984).
30. Kwaan, H. C., Role of fibrinolysis in thrombotic thrombocytopenic purpura. *Semin. Hematol., 24*: 101–109 (1987).
31. Remuzzi, G., Rossi, E. C., Misiani, R., Marchesi, D., Mecca, G., Gaetano, G., Donati, M. B., Prostacyclin and thrombotic microangiopathy. *Semin. Thromb. Hemost. ,6*: 391–394 (1980).
32. Machin, S. J., McVerry, B. A., Parry, H., Marrow, W. J. W., A plasma factor inhibiting prostacyclin-like activity in thrombotic thrombocytopenic purpura. *Acta Haematol., 67*: 8–12 (1982).

37
An Animal Model of Thrombotic Thrombocytopenia with von Willebrand Factor Deficiency: The Role of Botrocetin in Studies of Human TTP

William E. Sanders *Duke University, Durham, North Carolina* **Kenneth M. Brinkhous and Marjorie S. Read** *University of North Carolina, Chapel Hill, North Carolina*

GENERAL BACKGROUND

During the last decade, the discovery of specific abnormalities in plasma of patients with thrombotic thrombocytopenic purpura (TTP) and the ultrastructural evaluation of the observed vascular lesions have significantly advanced our understanding concerning the pathophysiology of this rare disease. The clinical manifestations of pronounced thrombocytopenia, microangiopathic hemolytic anemia, and fluctuating mental status are accompanied by the appearance of widely disseminated platelet thrombi in the microcirculation and alterations in circulating von Willebrand factor (vWF) (1–3). Electron microscopic studies of the microthrombi seen in TTP have revealed densely packed platelets, largely devoid of fibrin, and with varying degrees of cytoplasmic alterations (4, 5). The most prominent changes in vWF have involved the multimeric distribution pattern of vWF antigen (vWF:Ag) (6, 7). During evolution of acute-phase TTP, higher relative molecular mass (M_r) forms of vWF are lost from the plasma (8). In contrast, unusually large forms of vWF multimers have been detected in the plasma of patients with chronic TTP in remission (7). These unusually large M_r multimers disappear during acute relapses. This depletion of the higher M_r forms occurs without evidence of release of the platelet α-granule protein, or β-thromboglobulin, and temporally corresponds to periods of circulating platelet agglutinates (9). These findings suggest that vWF, through its interaction with platelet glycoprotein receptors Ib, IIb/IIIa or both, may play a critical role in the pathogenesis of this disorder.

Development of an Animal Model

Selective depletion of plasma vWF and, thereby, the induction of a von Willebrand disease (vWD)-like syndrome has been described in many species after injection of botrocetin (10–12). Recently, we developed animal models (rat, pig, and dog) of thrombotic thrombocytopenia produced by botrocetin administration (12). The acute thrombotic thrombocytopenic state is characterized by thrombocytopenia, loss of higher M_r forms of vWF, and the concomitant appearance of platelet thrombi in the microcirculation of several organs. After platelet recovery, a chronic phase is observed in which abnormally large vWF multimers can be detected in the plasma. This model closely simulates the pathophysiological changes observed in human TTP. In this chapter, we will review the subject of animal models of thrombotic thrombocytopenia induced by botrocetin and present new data on the use of botrocetin in the study of human TTP.

BOTROCETIN

Isolation and Properties

Botrocetin, originally called venom coagglutinin, is a cofactor of vWF, forming a complex that induces platelet agglutination. Botrocetin was first described in 1978 in the venom from several species of snakes, but predominantly from the venoms of the *Bothrops* genus (13). Isolation is accomplished by chromatography on a DEAE-Sepharose column. The thrombinlike material also present in the venom elutes from the column with buffer containing physiological concentrations of salt, whereas the platelet-agglutinating fractions elute with buffer containing high salt concentrations. The material eluting with high salt concentrations agglutinates fixed platelets in normal plasma, but not in plasma that is deficient in vWF. This platelet-agglutinating protein has been named botrocetin, denoting the *Bothrops* venom, from which it was first isolated, and its similarity to ristocetin as a cofactor for vWF-induced platelet agglutination.

Botrocetin has no known enzymatic activity (14); its M_r is 26.5 kd; it is a dimer with no detectable carbohydrate, is stable at room temperature, and does not require calcium for its activity. One unit of botrocetin is defined as that amount in 1 ml that will cause platelet agglutination in 14 sec in a standard four-part assay (10, 14).

Botrocetin-Induced Agglutination of Platelets

Botrocetin is a broad-spectrum probe for vWF. It can be used to detect vWF in plasma resistant to ristocetin (13, 15). This property has provided a method for measuring the vWF content of animal plasma and of plasmas that contain only low M_r multimers of vWF (15–17). In contrast, ristocetin, induces platelet agglutination, dependent on vWF only in the presence of high M_r vWF multimers (18). A more detailed review of the use of botrocetin to identify and study vWD variants, circulating antibodies, and anticoagulants has been published (14).

Mechanism of Action

Unlike many aggregating agents, such as adenosine diphosphate (ADP), botrocetin agglutinates fixed platelets and involves a surface reaction unrelated to platelet activation and release. Botrocetin-induced platelet agglutination requires the platelet membrane receptor glycoprotein Ib (GPIb), and the macromolecular plasma component, vWF. A noncovalent binding of botrocetin to vWF results in a binary complex. This complex initiates the binding of vWF to platelet GPIb (19). The binding of the botrocetin-vWF complex to GPIb apparently forms a ternary complex in which all three components are needed for function. The active complex appears to form bridges between platelets, resulting in the formation of large platelet clumps. Removal of botrocetin from the vWF complex with a rabbit antibotrocetin antibody causes the preformed agglutinates to deagglutinate rapidly (Fig. 1).

The binding of botrocetin to vWF probably results in a conformational change in the vWF protein, exposing active sites on the molecule, which bind to the platelet receptor. When the platelet-agglutinating vWF–botrocetin complex is passed through a chromatography column of Sepharose 2B gel, the complex separates. The vWF elutes in the void volume, and botrocetin elutes in the included volume. The vWF that elutes free of botrocetin will cause platelet agglutination only if botrocetin is again added to the platelet–vWF mixture. There is no evidence that botrocetin produces an asialolike vWF, or that it has any enzymatic action on vWF.

Thus, the vWF–botrocetin reaction can be seen as a three-step reaction:

1. Formation of an activated binary complex

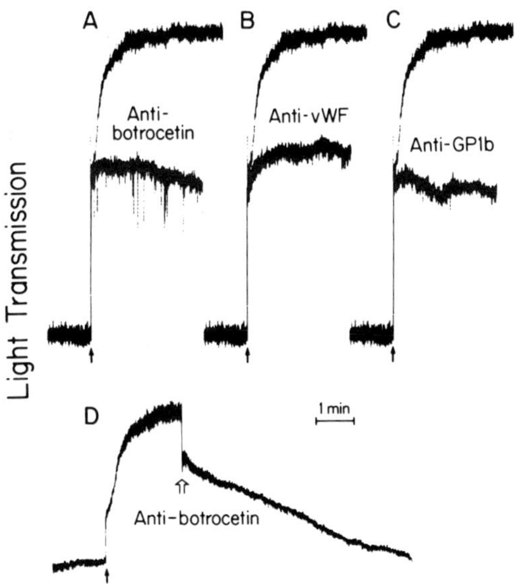

Figure 1 Tracings of vWF-dependent platelet agglutination induced by botrocetin in a Peyton aggregometer. Test mixtures consisted of platelets (0.2 ml, 800,000/μl), buffered saline (0.1 ml), and normal plasma (0.1ml). Solid arrows indicate the addition of botrocetin (0.1 ml, 50 U/ml). The upper tracings (A–C) show positive controls for platelet agglutination. The inhibitory effect of antibotrocetin antibody (undiluted) (A), anti-vWF antibody (undiluted) (B), and anti-GPIb antibody (1:10) (C) on agglutination is shown in the lower portion of each tracing. The antibody was substituted for buffered saline in the test mixtures. (D) Deagglutinating effect of antibotrocetin antibody (0.1 ml, open arrow) on fully formed platelet aggregates. (From Ref. 19.)

vWF + botrocetin → vWF–botrocetin complex

2. Formation of ternary complex

vWF–botrocetin complex + GPIb → vWF–botrocetin–GPIb

3. Formation of large platelet clumps

vWF–botrocetin–GPIb → platelet agglutination

When platelet-rich normal plasma is treated with botocetin, removal of the platelets by centrifugation depletes the plasma of vWF. A similar mechanism is apparently operative in the vWD-like syndrome induced in animals by botrocetin (10) and in animal models of botrocetin-induced TTP (12). When platelets are removed from the circulation by sequestration in the spleen or lung, the plasma is depleted of circulating vWF.

ANIMAL MODELS OF THROMBOTIC THROMBOCYTOPENIA

Acute Murine Thrombotic Thrombocytopenia with von Willebrand Factor Deficiency

Injection of botrocetin into animals results in a decreased platelet count, with depletion of plasma vWF (10–12). A single injection of this reagent into rats produces an animal model that simulates human acute TTP. Intraperitoneal administration of botrocetin (450 units/kg) produces marked depletion of plasma vWF, with activity decreased to <1% (<0.01 units/ml) of the preinjection value (Fig. 2). This plasma vWF deficiency persists for 72 to 96 hr; recovery then occurs rapidly over the following 24 hrs. The botrocetin-induced vWF depletion is accompanied by a tran-

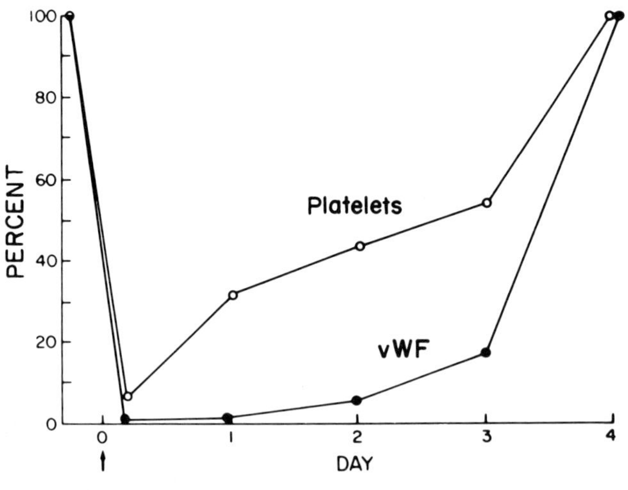

Figure 2 The vWF and platelet response to single botrocetin injection. Dose, 450 U/kg; rat weight, 0.31 kg. vWF (-•-) and platelet count (-o-) are expressed in percent, with 100% being assigned to preinjection levels (vWF 1 unit/ml, and platelet count, 847,000/μl). Postinjection values represent changes from these baselines. Arrow indicates time of botrocetin injection. (From Ref. 12.)

sient thrombocytopenia (65 × 10^9/l), noted at 2-hr postinjection, which persists approximately 5 hr (see Fig. 2). During this period, circulating platelet aggregates (10–50 platelets per aggregate) are observed by phase contrast microscopic examination of blood samples. Platelet recovery to 30–40% that of preinjection levels occurs within 24 hr (see Fig. 2) and is complete at 4 days. Bleeding time is prolonged to >15 min at 5 hr after botrocetin injection and remains prolonged until both vWF and platelet count return to near-normal values.

At 5 hr factor VIII coagulant activity, performed by a modification of the partial thromboplastin time procedure (20), decreases by approximately 50%. Levels recover to preinjection values by 24 hr. These reduced levels of factor VIII are believed to be due to the binding of factor VIII to vWF, which persists in the vWF–botrocetin complex. No hemorrhages have been observed in any animals receiving botrocetin. Botrocetin administration is well tolerated over a wide dosage range (250–2700 units/kg), with the general well-being of the animals maintained, and no adverse reactions noted.

The vWF:Ag, as assessed by the Laurell technique (21, 22), decreases moderately after botrocetin injection, but much less than the vWF activity assayed using a macroscopic aggregation test (23). Crossed immunoelectrophoresis (21, 24) and Laemmli electrophoresis (25, 26) demonstrate a loss of high and intermediate M_r multimers of plasma vWF (Table 1, Figs. 3 and 4).

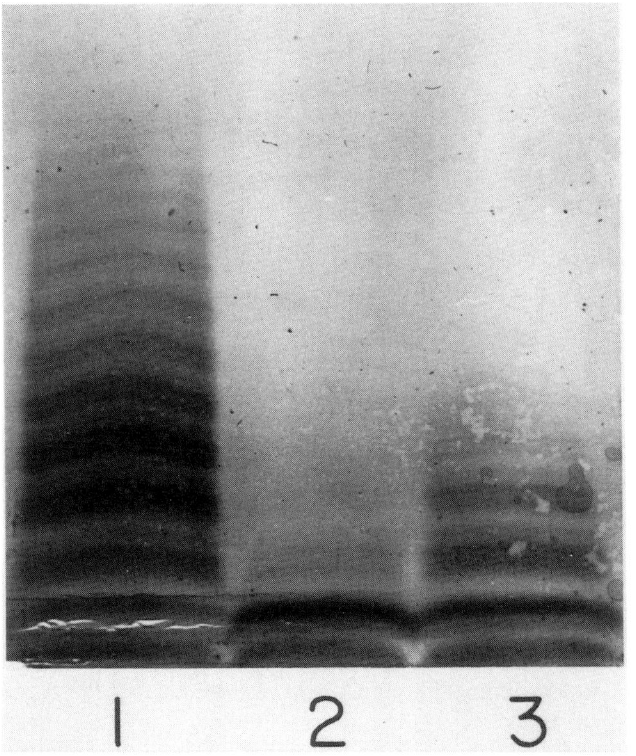

Figure 3 Multimeric distribution of vWF:Ag before and after botrocetin injection. Lane 1, preinjection; lane 2, 24 hr postinjection; lane 3, 48 hr postinjection. (From Ref. 12.)

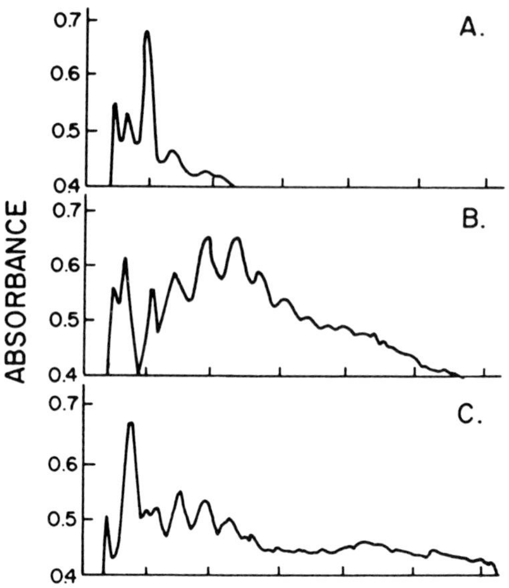

Figure 4 Densitometer scan demonstrating botrocetin-induced changes in multimeric composition of vWF:Ag in rat plasma. (A) Scan of lane 2, Fig. 3, 24 hr after botrocetin injection. (B) Scan of lane 1, Fig. 3, before botrocetin injection. (C) Scan of gel, 8 days after initial botrocetin injection. Left to right, low M_r to high M_r vWF multimers. (From Ref. 12.)

Morphology of Acute-Phase Platelet Microthrombi at Timed Intervals

Two Hours

Two hours after botrocetin injection, platelet aggregates can be seen in the microcirculation of the lung and spleen by light microscopic examination of tissue sections. Similar aggregates are not observed in the liver sinusoids or the capillaries of the renal glomeruli.

Transmission electron micrographs (TEM) of the lung 2 hr postinjection show loose platelet aggregates and occlusive platelet thrombi in vessels of the pulmonary microcirculation (Fig. 5). Platelet organelles are well preserved and dispersed in the cytoplasm. Larger platelet thrombi, consisting of tightly packed discrete platelets, are present in the spleen (Fig. 6). The platelets show little evidence of activation with associated shape change or degranulation.

Twenty-four Hours

Complete resolution of platelet microthrombi in the lung is observed by 24 hr postinjection. A marked reduction in the size and number of aggregates in the spleen is also noted.

Forty-eight Hours

Significant platelet aggregates are not seen in the spleen after 48 hr. Small aggregates, consisting of two to six platelets, are a common feature of the normal histologic appearance of the spleen in many species (27).

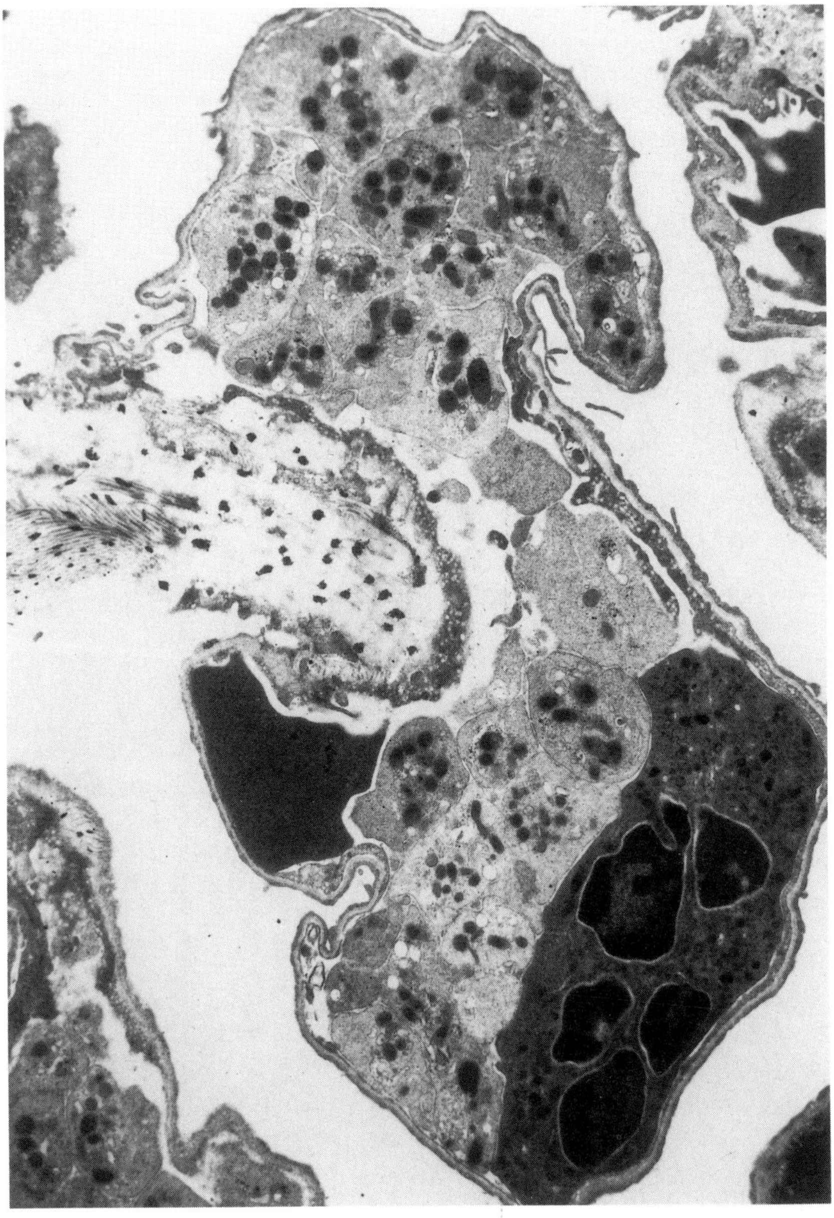

Figure 5 Lung: Platelet microthrombus occluding pulmonary capillary 2 hr postinjection (450 U/kg) (×6388). (From Ref. 12.)

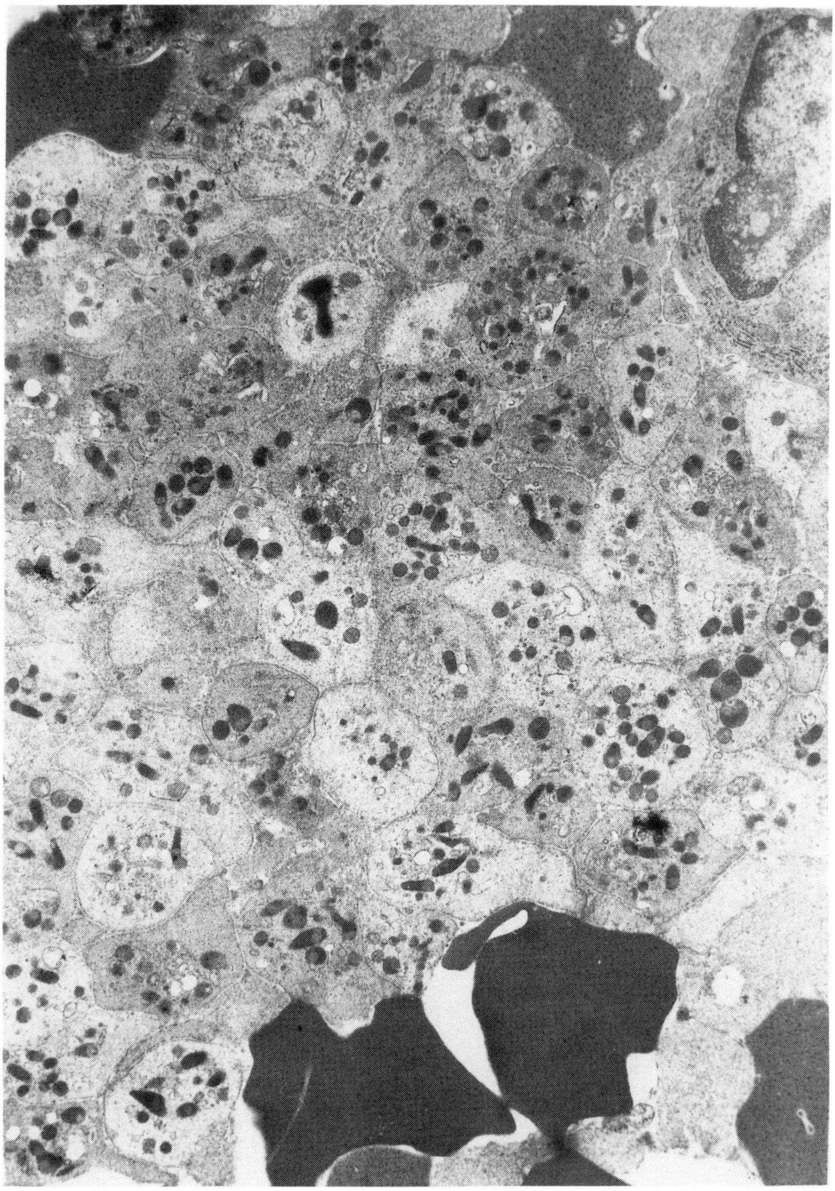

Figure 6 Spleen: Platelet microthrombus in the spleen 2 hr after botrocetin injection (450 U/kg) (×4760). (From Ref. 12.)

Maintenance of Thrombotic Thrombocytopenic State

Prolonged depletion of plasma vWF can be achieved by repeated injections of botrocetin at 48 hr intervals. This sustained deficiency state is characterized by plasma vWF in the range of <1–18% of normal. Limited platelet recovery is observed during the 48-hr period after each botrocetin administration. With cessation of injections, vWF and platelet counts return to preinjection levels within 48 hr. However, vWF:Ag analysis shows not only the return to normal levels of intermediate and high multimers by 24 hr postinjection, but also an increase in the very high M_r forms, compared with preinjection levels (see Fig. 4). Therefore, the immediate recovery period is notable for the presence of increased amounts of very high M_r multimers of vWF.

Porcine and Canine Acute Thrombotic Thrombocytopenia

Intravenous injection of botrocetin has induced a vWD-like syndrome and transient thrombocytopenia in normal pigs and dogs (10). Recently, we have completed studies that further evaluate the action of botrocetin in normal animals. The dose of botrocetin required to produce significant thrombocytopenia (to <25% of preinjection levels) in normal pigs and dogs was determined by a series of graded-dose infusions (range 30–300 units/kg). The maximum effect is seen at a dose of 90–100 units/kg, given intravenously, for both species. The general procedure for intravenous infusion has been described (10). A single botrocetin dose injected into normal pigs or normal dogs resulted in an acute thrombotic thrombocytopenia with vWF deficiency. The acute syndrome is similar to that observed in the rat. The analysis of the multimeric distribution of vWF postinjection in normal animals demonstrates a loss of high and intermediate M_r vWF forms, followed by an increase in lower M_r multimers and the appearance of very high M_r forms not present in the preinjection plasma (unpublished data). The vWF:Ag distribution soon returns to normal.

Transmission electron microscopy of lung sections, following botrocetin injection into normal dogs, reveals occlusive platelet thrombi of the pulmonary microcirculation. Large thrombi consisting of tightly packed discrete platelets can be seen in the spleen. No thrombi could be demonstreated by TEM in the kidney, myocardium, or brain. An acute thrombotic thrombocytopenia with vWF deficiency can be easily induced in normal large animals (pigs and dogs) by intravenous botrocetin administration (unpublished data).

Resistance of Canine Homozygous von Willebrand Disease Animals to Induction of Thrombotic Thrombocytopenia

Botrocetin appears entirely inactive when injected intravenously into severe vWD animals. No thrombocytopenia occurs. No platelet thrombi are present in the pulmonary microcirculation after botrocetin injection, and no platelet thrombi are seen in any other organ examined. Hence, plasma deficiency of vWF conveys protection against the action of botrocetin and, therefore, the induction of a thrombotic thrombocytopenic state (unpublished data).

Table 1 Induced vWF Deficiency in Rats: Response of vWF Activity and vWF:Ag to Botrocetin Injections

Plasma samples	vWF	vWF:Ag	Two-dimensional crossed-immunoelectrophoresis[a]			Distribution of vWF:Ag multimers[b]		
			Migration distances (mm)			M_r		
Postbotrocetin injection (hr)	Botrocetin test (%)	Laurell procedure (%)	Gap	Peak	Total	High	Intermediate	Low
Pre	100	100	1	6	9	+	+	+
6	<1	72	6	10	13	Neg	Neg	+
20–30	<1	ND[c]	ND	ND	ND	Neg	Neg	+
40–50	5	72	8	9	12	Neg	Trace	+
60–72	16	72	2	7	9.5	Neg	+	+
≥96	>100	85	1	6	9	+	+	+

[a]*Gap* is the distance from the center of the well to the beginning of the immunoprecipitation arc. *Peak* is the distance from the center of the well to intercept of a perpendicular from the highest point of the arc. *Total migration* is the distance from the center of the well to the end of the immunoprecipitin arc.
[b]The blood sample used for multimer analysis at 72 hr was obtained by cardiac puncture from a similarly treated rat.
[c]ND, not done.
Source: From Ref. 12.

ACUTE-PHASE HUMAN THROMBOTIC THROMBOCYTOPENIC PURPURA

Comparison of von Willebrand Factor–Botrocetin and von Willebrand Factor–Ristocetin Plasma Levels

We have examined the ability of botrocetin and ristocetin to detect vWF in the acute-phase plasma of patients with TTP (10). Simultaneous analysis of the vWF:Ag multimer distribution was by the Aihara modification (25) of the Ruggeri procedure (26) using 1.5% agarose. Two groups of patients have been studied. Group 1 consisted of three patients who experienced only a single episode of acute TTP. Group 2 contained four patients classified as relapsing TTP by virtue of one or more relapses during a 5-year follow-up period. Plasmas drawn at the time of first presentation of the patients were analyzed in both groups. Plasma samples from one patient with relapsing TTP were obtained and studied during four subsequent recurrences. All patients met stringent clinical criteria for acute TTP, including severe thrombocytopenia, microangiopathic hemolytic anemia, neurological symptoms or signs, and no overt renal failure. None had evidence of a specific inciting event. All plasma samples were obtained concurrent with the height of clinical manifestations and before the initiation of therapy.

A vWF multimer analysis of plasmas from groups 1 and 2 was performed. Plasmas from group 1 showed a loss of high and intermediate M_r forms of vWF. Those from group II showed only a decrease in high and intermediate M_r forms, but not a depletion of these multimers. All plasmas were assayed with botrocetin and ristocetin for vWF activity. Botrocetin detected a plasma vWF activity of at least 60% of normal control in both groups, those with a single acute episode and those with recurrent TTP. The botrocetin activity corresponds to the persistence of lower M_r multimers of vWF:Ag in the acute-phase plasma of TTP in both groups. In contrast, ristocetin, made isochronal to botrocetin, showed minimal or no vWF activity with plasmas in group 1, consistent with the absence of intermediate or high M_r vWF forms in the plasma. Both botrocetin and ristocetin showed significant vWF activity using first presentation plasma samples from relapsing TTP patients and samples of acute-phase plasma drawn at the times of relapse. Laser densitometer analysis of vWF:Ag mulimeric distribution confirmed that moderate amounts of intermediate and, to a lesser extent, high M_r vWF forms remained in the acute-phase plasma of these patients. These intermediate and high M_r forms remain in circulation during subsequent relapse episodes (Read, M. S., Sanders, W. E., Brinkhous, K. M., unpublished data).

Botrocetin Assay as a Screening Tool for Recurring Thrombotic Thrombocytopenic Purpura

A comparison of the botrocetin and ristocetin bioassays of acute-phase plasma allows detection of two distinct groups of TTP patients: namely, single-episode TTP and recurrent chronic TTP. In the first group, vWF–botrocetin was positive, ristocetin–vWF negative. In the recurrent forms both tests were positive. Further studies will be required to evaluate whether this quick and inexpensive method might be used to predict relative risk of patients for subsequent development of chronic relapsing TTP.

DISCUSSION

An animal model of thrombotic thrombocytopenia can be induced by injection of botrocetin, an agent that initiates platelet agglutination only in the presence of vWF. The syndrome is characterized by acute thrombocytopenia, loss of high M_r forms of vWF, and the concomitant appearance of intravascular platelet microthrombi (12). The model can be easily and quickly induced in rats by intraperitoneal injection (12) or in larger animals (pigs or dogs) by intravenous botrocetin administration. The changes observed closely simulate the pathophysiological manifestations seen in patients with TTP. This model should provide a method for further evaluating the pathogenesis of this disorder and may facilitate future testing of therapeutic modalities.

The pathogenesis of TTP is yet to be elucidated with certainty. Many groups have reported "platelet-aggregating factors" in the plasma or serum of TTP patients (2, 8, 28). The characterization of these factors is an area of active investigation (6, 28–30), but their origin remains obscure. Botrocetin, in our animal model, acts as an initiating agent or platelet-aggregating factor that results in vWF consumption and platelet aggregate formation. These aggregates, composed of discrete, primarily nonactivated platelets, are then sequestered in the lungs and spleen where they cause occlusive microthrombi. Homozygous vWD animals (pigs and dogs), severely deficient in plasma vWF, are completely resistant to the action of botrocetin.

The ability of botrocetin to support platelet agglutination only in the presence of vWF has provided a probe for this plasma component. The botrocetin bioassay may be used to quantitate vWF activity, regardless of the mammalian source (13, 15). Classically, ristocetin has been employed to quantitate vWF activity in the clinical setting. Ristocetin is known to require the presence of higher multimeric forms of vWF to initiate platelet agglutination (18). Many animal plasmas are resistant to ristocetin, with no platelet aggregates forming. In contrast, botrocetin has been shown to be reactive with a broad spectrum of high to low M_r vWF multimers (17). Ristocetin, made isochronal with botrocetin (10), fails to detect significant vWF activity in the plasma from patients, during acute-phase TTP, who experience only a single episode. In contrast, botrocetin vWF activity in this group is near normal (>70%). The divergent results of these two assays reflect the persistence of lower M_r multimers and the absence of intermediate and higher forms in the plasma of these patients. However, both ristocetin and botrocetin show substantial vWF activity in plasmas drawn from individuals during acute-phase TTP who subsequently have recurrences, and in acute-phase plasmas obtained at the time of recurrence of TTP. This corresponds to the presence of intermediate and, to a lesser extent, higher M_r vWF forms (analyzed from the electrophoretic patterns seen on SDS–1.5% agarose gels), which remain in the acute-phase plasma of this recurrent group of TTP patients. The comparison of botrocetin versus ristocetin vWF activity in TTP plasma may provide a method for subclassification of patients. Further study will be required to determine if this facile procedure is valuable in predicting the relative risk for subsequent development of relapsing TTP.

CONCLUSIONS

An animal model that closely simulates the pathophysiological changes in thrombotic thrombocytopenic purpura can be induced in normal rats, pigs, and dogs by injection of botrocetin. The acute syndrome is characterized by thrombocytopenia, loss of high M_r multimers of vWF, and the appearance of platelet thrombi in the microcirculation. During the recovery phase, after platelet counts have returned to normal, unusually large vWF multimers are present in the plasma. Similar observations have been reported with relapsing TTP in remission. Further studies employing this animal model may provide additional insights into the pathogenesis of TTP and facilitate evaluation of future therapeutic modalities. A comparison of botrocetin and ristocetin vWF bioassays of acute-phase plasma defines two distinct groups of patients. This may prove useful in subclassifying forms of TTP that carry different prognostic implications. Additional investigations are required to evaluate if this method can be used to predict relative risk of relapsing TTP.

ACKNOWLEDGMENT

This work was supported in part by grant FDR000259 and National Institutes of Health grant HL01648.

REFERENCES

1. Moschcowitz, E., Hyaline thrombosis of the terminal arterioles and capillaries. A hitherto undescribed disease. *Proc. N. Y. Pathol. Soc.*, *24*: 21 (1924).
2. Baehr, G., Klemperer, P., Schifrin, A., An acute febrile anemia and thrombocytopenic purpura with diffuse platelet thrombosis of capillaries and arterioles. *Trans. Assoc. Am. Physicians*, *51*: 43 (1936).
3. Berkowitz, L. R., Dalldorf, F. G., Blatt, P. M., Thrombotic thrombocytopenic purpura: A pathology review. *JAMA*, *241*: 1709 (1979).
4. Feldman, J. D., Mardiney, M. R., Unanue, E. R., Cutting, H., The vascular pathology of thrombotic thrombocytopenic purpura: An immunohistochemical and ultrastructural study, *Lab. Invest.*, *15*: 927 (1966).
5. Neame, P. B., Lechago, L., Ling, E. T., Koval, A. T., Thrombotic thrombocytopenic purpura: Report of a case with disseminated intravascular platelet aggregation. *Blood*, *42*: 805 (1973).
6. Murphy, W. G., Moore, J. C., Barr, R. D., Pai, M. K. R., Kelton, J. G., Relationship between platelet aggregating factor and von Willebrand factor in thrombotic thrombocytopenic purpura. *Br. J. Haematol.*, *66*: 509 (1987).
7. Moake, J. L., Rudy, C. K., Troll, J. H., Weinstein, M. J., Colannino, N. M., Azocar, J., Seder, R. H., Hong, S. L., Deykin, D., Unusually large plasma factor VIII:von Willebrand factor multimers in chronic relapsing thrombotic thrombocytopenic purpura. *N. Engl. J. Med.*, *307*: 1432 (1982).
8. Kelton, J. G., Moore, J., Santos, A., Sheridan, D., Detection of a platelet-agglutinating factor in thrombotic thrombocytopenic purpura. *Ann. Intern. Med.*, *101*: 589 (1984).
9. Moake, J. L., Rudy, C. K., Troll, J. H., Weinstein, M. J., Colannino, N. M., Hong, S. L., Koutcher, J. A., Melaragno, A. J., Manner, C. E., Case report: von Willebrand factor abnormalities and endothelial cell perturbation in a patient with acute thrombotic thrombocytopenic purpura. *Am. J. Med. Sci.*, *291*: 47 (1986).
10. Brinkhous, K. M., Barnes, D. S., Potter, J. Y., Read, M. S., von Willebrand syndrome induced by a *Bothrops* venom factor: Bioassay for venom coagglutinin. *Proc. Natl. Acad. Sci. USA*, *78*:3230 (1981).
11. Sanders, W. E., Read, M. S., Reddick, R. L., Brinkhous, K. M., Induced von Willebrand syndrome in rats [abstract]. *Fed. Proc.*, *46*: 424 (1987).
12. Sanders, W. E., Read, M. S., Reddick, R. L., Garris, J. B., Brinkhous, K. M.,

Thrombotic thrombocytopenia with von Willebrand factor deficiency induced by botrocetin: An animal model. *Lab. Invest.*, *59*: 443 (1988).
13. Read, M. S., Shermer, R. W., Brinkhous, K. M., Venom coagglutinin: An activator of platelet aggregation dependent on von Willebrand factor. *Proc. Natl. Acad. Sci. USA*, *75*: 4514 (1978).
14. Brinkhous, K. M., Smith, S. V., Read, M. S., Botrocetin and von Willebrand factor. In *Hemostasis and Animal Venoms* (H. Pirkle, F. S. Markland, eds.), Marcel Dekker, New York, p. 377 (1988).
15. Read, M. S., Potter, J. Y., Brinkhous, K. M., Venom coagglutinin for detection of von Willebrand factor activity in animal plasmas. *J. Lab. Clin. Med.*, *101*: 74 (1983).
16. Brinkhous, K. M., Fricke, W. A., Read, M. S., Determinants of von Willebrand factor activity elicited by ristocetin and botrocetin: Studies on a human von Willebrand factor-binding antibody. *Semin. Thromb. Hemost.*, *11*: 337 (1985).
17. Brinkhous, K. M., Read, M. S., Fricke, W. A., Wagner, R. H., Botrocetin (venom coagglutinin): Reaction with a broad spectrum of multimeric forms of factor VIII macromolecular complex. *Proc. Natl. Acad. Sci. USA*, *80*: 1463 (1983).
18. Doucet-de Bruine, M. H. M., Sixma, J. J., Over, J., Besser-Visser, N. H., Heterogeneity of human factor VIII. II. Characterization of forms of factor VIII binding to platelets in the presence of ristocetin. *J. Lab. Clin. Med.*, *92*: 96 (1978).
19. Read, M. S., Smith, S. V., Lamb, M. A., Brinkhous, K. M., Role of botrocetin in platelet agglutination: Formation of an activated complex of botrocetin and von Willebrand factor. *Blood*, *74*: 1031 (1989).
20. Langdell, R. D., Wagner, R. H., Brinkhous, K. M., Effect of antihemophilic factor on one-stage clotting tests. *J. Lab. Clin. Med.*, *41*: 637 (1953).
21. Lamb, M. A., Reisner, H. M., Cooper, H. A., Wagner, R. H., The multimeric distribution of factor VIII-related antigen studied by an improved crossed-immunoelectrophoresis technique. *J. Lab. Clin. Med.*, *98*: 751 (1981).
22. Laurell, C.-B., Quantitative estimation of proteins by electrophoresis in agarose gel containing antibodies. *Anal. Biochem.*, *15*: 45 (1966).
23. Brinkhous, K. M., Read, M. S., Use of venom coagglutinin and lyophilized platelets in testing for platelet-aggregating von Willebrand factor. *Blood*, *55*: 517 (1980).
24. Laurell, C. B., Antigen–antibody cross electrophoresis. *Anal. Biochem.*, *10*: 358 (1965).
25. Aihara, M., Sawada, Y., Ueno, K., Morimoto, S., Yoshido, Y., de Serres, M., Cooper, H. A., Wagner, R. H., Visualization of von Willebrand factor multimers by immunoenzymatic stain using avidin–biotin peroxidase complex. *Thromb. Haemost.*, *55*: 263 (1986).
26. Ruggeri, Z. M., Zimmerman, T. S., the complex multimeric composition of factor VIII/von Willebrand factor. *Blood*, *57*: 1140 (1981).
27. Eigjo, R. F., Hovig, T., Ultrastructural studies of platelet activation and aggregation in normal spleen from different species. *Scand. J. Haemateol.*, *9*: 587 (1972).
28. Brandt, J. T., Kennedy, M. S., Senhauser, D. A., Platelet aggregating factor in thrombocytopenic purpura [letter to the editor]. *Lancet*, *2*: 463 (1979).
29. Byrnes, J. J., Moake, J. L., Thrombotic thrombocytopenic purpura and hemolytic–uremic syndrome: Evolving concepts of pathogenesis and therapy. *Clin. Haematol.*, *15*: 413 (1986).
30. Lian, E. C. Y., Pathogenesis of thrombotic thrombocytopenic purpura. *Semin. Hematol.*, *24*: 82 (1987).

38
Treatment of Thrombotic Thrombocytopenic Purpura and Hemolytic Uremic Syndrome: The Role of Vincristine

Lorence A. Gutterman *Riverside Methodist Hospital, Columbus, Ohio*

Thrombotic thrombocytopenic purpura (TTP) is a rare disorder that is fatal without effective therapeutic intervention. Before 1977, approximately 80% of patients with TTP died (1). Since 1977, the survival rate for TTP has improved and is estimated to be between 60 and 80% (1, 2). This statistic is based on retrospective or anecdotal data. Improved survival is usually attributed to the use of exchange plasmapheresis combined with other treatments (1, 2). However, no standardized treatment for TTP has been established, and possibly as many as 40% of patients continue to die of this fulminant disease. Recent experience with vincristine treatment suggests an improved survival rate, with as many as 90% of patients surviving after combined treatment that included plasma and vincristine (3, 4). In this chapter, I will evaluate the data on vincristine-based regimens, discuss future directions of investigation of the pathogenesis and treatment of TTP and othr thrombotic microangiopathies, and speculate on mechanisms of vincristine activity in TTP and hemolytic uremic syndrome (HUS).

CLINICAL EXPERIENCE

Acute Thrombotic Thrombocytopenic Purpura and Hemolytic Uremic Syndrome

Treatment of TTP with vincristine evolved primarily based on our clinical observations that were first reported in 1979 (5) and later in 1982 (3). Five patients consecutively treated with regimens that included vincristine responded successfully. The first patient was treated in 1973 with vincristine, after other treatments had failed. Similar responses in the second and third patients encouraged us to give vincristine as a single agent to the fourth and fifth patients (Figs. 1 and 2). Toxicity

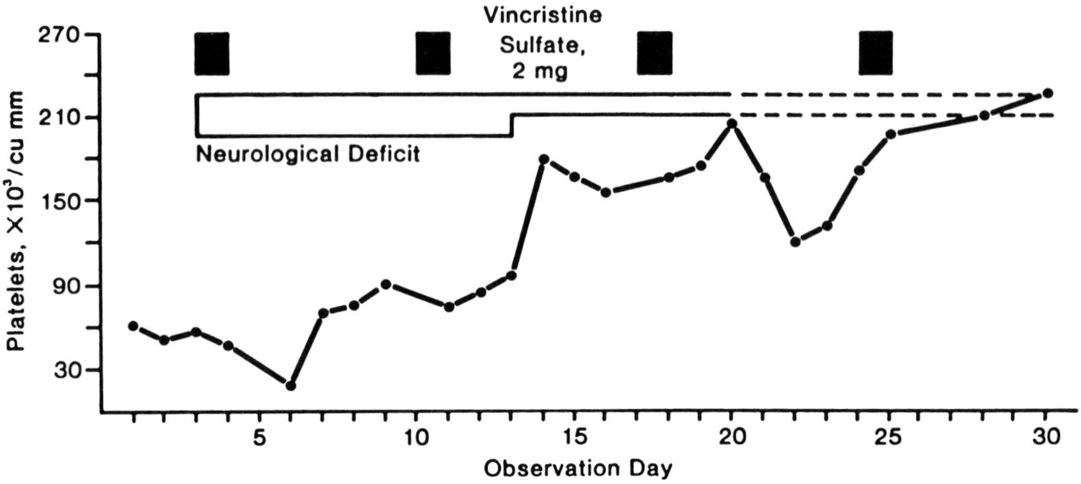

Figure 1 A 19-year-old woman with TTP: Clinical course and response to therapy with vincristine given as a single agent.

was minimal, and responses were prompt. Of these five patients, two relapsed and responded to additional therapy that included vincristine. No additional relapses have been observed over the past 10 years. Subsequently, an adult with HUS was treated and responded to vincristine given as a single agent (6). Relapse has not occurred. The 100% survival rate of these six patients plus Abramson's patient (7), the limited toxicity of vincristine, reasonable time to complete remission, durability of the remissions, and effectiveness as a single agent, prompted other physicians to treat patients with TTP with regimens that included vincristine.

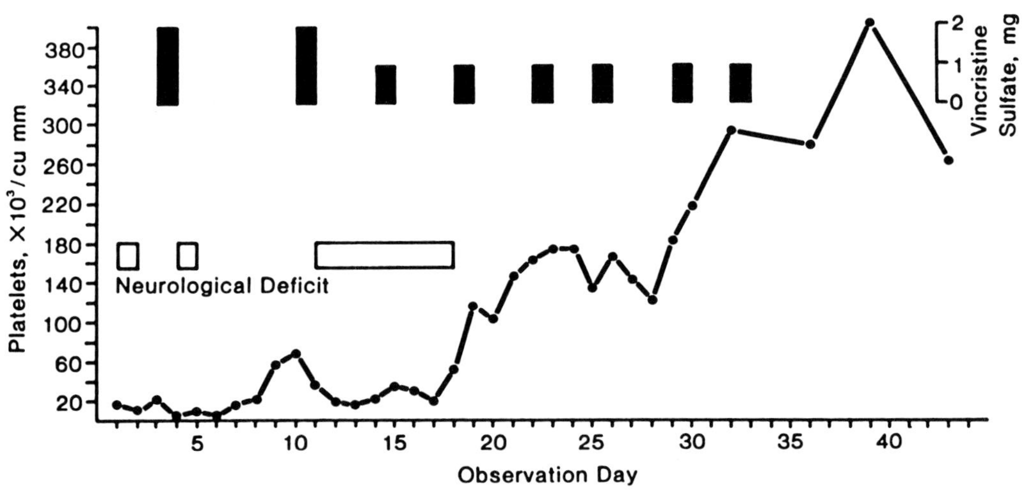

Figure 2 A 36-year-old woman with TTP: Clinical course and response to therapy with vincristine given as a single agent.

A review of the medical literature on vincristine-based therapeutic regimens for TTP reveals that most often vincristine was combined with exchange plasmapheresis, plasma infusion, and usually corticosteroids (3, 6–26). The clinical and laboratory data of these patients indicate most of the patients had neurological manifestations and severe thrombocytopenia (platelet count $< 20{,}000/mm^3$) (Table 1). The amount of plasma exchanged and the dosage of corticosteroids and vincristine varied considerably. In addition, other treatments were sometimes given and included splenectomy, aspirin, dipyridamole, cryosupernatant, and intravenous gamma globulin. Although almost all of the patients in this series survived (48 of 49 patients), bias may have favored reporting only successful outcomes. Also, the data usually did not include information on toxicity of treatment nor follow-up information beyond 1–2 years. Therefore, the true relapse rate is unknown. The results of the accumulated experience suggest that plasma combined with vincristine and corticosteroid is an effective treatment for TTP. However, since these results were based on retrospective and anecdotal data of predominantly combined treatment, which varied considerably, the exact role or influence of vincristine in successfully producing a very high rate of complete responses and survival is difficult to define.

Four other patients received vincristine as part of their treatment for TTP (27, 28), but insufficient data were provided to include them in the series described in Table 1. Three of these four patients survived. Also, personal communications in the form of medical records from several hematologists provided additional data on vincristine-based treatment regimens for TTP. These data are presented in Table 2. Eleven of these 16 patients survived. The variability in treatments and anecdotal data derived from multiple medical centers preclude any meaningful interpretation of these data. These experiences using vincristine-based regimens are presented to show the increasing frequency of treating TTP with plasma combined with vincristine.

Our results with vincristine as a single agent in four patients is summarized in Table 3. The initial neurological response occurred as early as 2 days, whereas the earliest evidence for improvement in the platelet count was 4 days. Complete remission occurred between 17 and 27 days. Two of the four patients relapsed and responded to additional vincristine treatment. Thus, vincristine is an effective treatment for TTP, although relapses did occur. Rose and Eldor point out in their series on relapsing TTP that, although vincristine did not necessarily prevent relapses, the drug may shorten the time to complete remission (27).

Relapsing Thrombotic Thrombocytopenic Purpura

Vincristine has also been effective in stopping cyclic relapses of TTP. We treated a 21-year-old woman with postpartum relapsing TTP with vincristine after other treatments failed to prevent monthly relapses. In the 32nd week of her second pregnancy she developed headaches, petechiae, and edema. Her blood pressure and temperature were normal. Pertinent laboratory test results are in Table 2 (patient 1). After a successful cesarian section her TTP persisted, and she developed bilateral ankle clonus, visual disturbance, and proteinuria. Corticosteroids were given, and then a splenectomy and open renal biopsy were done. Hyaline microthrombi were present in the arterioles of both tissues. A transient response to this treatment was

Table 1 Clinical and Laboratory Data: 49 Patients with TTP and HUS

Patient	Age/sex	Neurol deficit	Plt ct (mm^3)	Hgb/Hct (mg/dl)/%	Retic ct (%)	LDH (U/L)	BUN/Creat (mg/dl)	Outcome	Ref.
1	54/F	Yes	21,000	—/29.0			Normal	S	7
2	45/F	Yes	20,000	—/22.4	7.6		41/1.8	S	8
3	63/M	Yes	20,000	7.0/—			Normal	S	9
4	65/F	No	10,000	Anemia			Normal	S	9
5	29/F	Yes	33,500	Anemia	12.7		Normal	S	3
6	52/M	Yes	55,000	7.5/22.0		460	Normal	S	3
7	19/F	Yes	9,500	7.4/21.0	22.4	1,165	17.0/0.9	S	3
8	19/F	Yes	60,000	11.2/34.0	4.0	Incr.	Normal	S	3
9	36/F	Yes	15,000	8.6/24.0	19.0	1,040	19.0/0.9	S	3
10	64/F	Yes	20,000	6.0/18.0	11.0		—/0.7	S	10
11	33/M	Yes	74,000	11.6/33.6	3.4		23.0/1.9	S	11
12	16/F	Yes	17,000	6.0/17.4	12.4		13.0/1.2	S	11
13	25/F	Yes	21,000	10.2/28.7			21.0/1.6	S	11
14	51/M		Decr.	Anemia				S	12
15	39/F	Yes	Decr.	Anemia				S	12
16	72/F	Yes	8,000	7.6/21.6	9.7		—/0.9	S	13
17	57/F	Yes	25,000	—/20.4	6.6		—/0.8	S	13
18	30/M	Yes	3,500	6.5/21.0			—/0.5	S	13
19	62/M	Yes	19,000	—/27.0	6.1	1,593	28.0/1.3	S	14
20	27/F	Yes	17,000	—/23.0	9.0		Normal	S	14
21	50/M	Yes	16,000	6.9/—		1,050	—/1.6	S	15
22	45/F	Yes	17,000	7.7/21.8		5,560	111.0/7.0	S	6
23	26/F	Yes	5,000	7.1/—			—/2.0	S	16

24	55/F	Yes	13,000	6.2/18.0	13.0	840	15.0/0.8	S	17
25	27/F	Yes	8,000	8.5/25.0	8.4	600	28.0/0.9	S	17
26	57/F	Yes	33,000	6.3/21.0	7.2	2,060	24.0/1.2	S	17
27	55/F	Yes	14,000	6.6/19.0		1,335	99.0/4.4	S	17
28	29/M	Yes	18,000	6.0/20.0	14.0	1,755	49.0/2.2	S	17
29		No	32,000	—/32.0	2.2	600	—/>2.0	S	17
30	18/M	Yes	8,000	6.8/—	10.0	2,062	—/1.6	S	18
31	34/F	Yes	12,000	—/29.0			Normal	S	19
32	49/F	Yes	6,000	—/<30.0	13.0	1,400	—/>2.0	S	20
33	51/M	Yes	4,000	—/<30.0	2.0	1,500	—/>2.0	S	20
34	62/F	Yes	19,000	—/<30.0	10.0	1,205	—/<2.0	S	20
35	59/F	Yes	10,000	—/<30.0	5.0	2,500	—/<2.0	S	20
36	55/F	Yes	<50,000	—/<30.0			—/>2.0	D	20
37	31/F	Yes	<50,000	—/<30.0			—/>2.0	S	20
38	35/F	Yes	25,000	7.2/—	6.0		18.0/1.1	S	21
39	57/M	Yes	28,000	8.4/—	16.0		27.0/1.3	S	21
40	18/F	Yes	18,000	7.8/—	20.0		—/0.9	S	21
41	43/F	Yes	16,000	7.2/—	9.0			S	21
42	49/M		7,000	7.3/19.0	1.0	1,272	9.0/0.9	S	22
43	41/F		5,000	8.6/26.0	22.0	1,136	37.0/1.3	S	22
44	38/F		12,000	7.1/24.2	8.4	1,150	36.0/1.0	S	22
45	46/F		8,000	7.3/22.0	11.4	1,123	33.0/1.3	S	22
46	34/F	No	20,000	7.1/20.3	18.5	2,662	7.0/1.6	S	23
47	33/F	Yes	3,000	7.0/—	7.0	1,145	15.9/0.9	S	24
48	32/F	Yes	4,000	5.6/—		890	—/Normal	S	25
49	40/F	Yes	46,000	Decr.		312	Normal	S	26

Neurol, neurologic; Plt ct, platelet count; Hgb, hemoglobin; Hct, hematocrit; Retic ct, reticulocyte count; LDH, lactate dehyrogenase; BUN, blood urea nitrogen; Creat, creatinine; S, survived; D, died; Incr, increased; Decr, decreased.

Table 2 Clinical and Laboratory Features of 16 Patients with TTP

Patient	Age/sex	Neurol deficit	Plt ct (mm^3)	Hgb/Hct (g/dl/%)	Retic ct (%)	LDH (U/L)	BUN/Creat (mg/dl)	Outcome
1	21/F	Yes	14,000	6.0/18.0	16.0	1350	16.0/1.3	S
2	21/M	Yes	9,000	9.1/27.4	1.2		51.0/1.1	D
3	29/F	Yes	5,000	7.3/21.0	6.8		18.0/0.7	S
4	53/F	No	6,800	8.3/23.0			—/3.5	D
5	36/F	Yes	20,000	5.6/14.7	19.7		18.0/1.0	S
6	41/F	Yes	18,000	11.2/33.2			—/0.7	S
7	43/F	No	19,000	—/25.0	5.9		47.0/3.6	S
8	32/F	Yes	10,000	6.7/21.3	28.0		25.0/1.0	S
9	26/F	Yes	17,000	6.0/21.0	42.0		25.0/1.1	S
10	60/F	Yes	31,500	6.8/—	12.0		Normal	D
11	36/F	Yes	12,000	8.3/23.6	7.6		19.0/0.9	S
12	21/F	Yes	18,000	6.0/17.6	15.6		16.0/1.3	S
13	32/M	Yes	2,000	11.4/38.0			57.0/3.4	D
14	36/M	Yes	18,000	10.4/30.0	11.6		18.0/1.3	S
15	55/F	Yes	7,000	—/25.0	7.0		Normal	D
16	37/M	Yes	15,000	6.8/—	38.0		Normal	S

Neurol, neurologic; Plt ct, platelet count; Hgb, hemoglobin; Hct, hematocrit; Retic.ct, reticulocyte count; LDH, lactate dehyrogenase; BUN, blood urea nitrogen; Creat, creatinine; S, survived; D, died.
Source: Personal communications.

Table 3 TTP and HUS Patients Treated with Vincristine (VCR) Only

Dx	Total dose (mg)	Dose schedule (mg/wk)	Time interval (days) until response		Time to CR (days)	Relapse (mo)	Results of retreatment	VCR toxicity
			Neurologic	Platelet				
TTP	8	2	10	4	22	12	Responded to VCR	None
TTP	10	2 mg/wk for 2 doses then 1 mg q	18	16	27	6	Responded to therapy including	None
		4 days					VCR	None
HUS	4	2		5	23	None		None
TTP	6	2	2	14	17	None		None

Dx, diagnosis; CR, complete remission.

noted, with an increase in the platelet count to 437,000/mm^3. Proteinuria, visual disturbance, and headaches resolved, but clonus persisted. Over the next 7 months a chronic phase of her illness was manifested by petechiae, thrombocytopenia, and hemolytic anemia. Each relapse, occurring every 21–28 days, responded transiently to plasma infusions. After those 7 months, plasma therapy was discontinued, and vincristine treatment was started. She received a total of 8 mg of vincristine given in 1-mg doses every 4 days (Fig. 3). All manifestations of her TTP disappeared. No additional relapses have been observed over the subsequent 7 years.

I have received information about one additional patient with cyclic or frequent relapses of TTP who was eventually treated with an intensive course of vincristine. The relapses ceased promptly (Rosenbaum, D., personal communication). The patient was a 28-year-old man whose initial episode of TTP caused seizures and semicoma. Multiple treatments that included exchange plasmapheresis, corticosteroids, aspirin, dipyridamole, an infrequent dose of vincritstine, and splenectomy, failed to prevent relapses. The relapses, without neurological involvement, occurred approximately every 2 weeks for many months. With an intensive series of vincristine doses, complete remission occurred within 4 weeks, and no further relapses have been observed for the past 10 months. The intensive dose schedule of vincristine chosen for these patients was based on the amount used in the successful treatment of acute TTP (3). The recommended initial dose is 2 mg by intravenous injection, followed by 1 mg intravenously every 4 days until until complete remission is achieved. Vincristine in the second patient was continued for 3 months in less

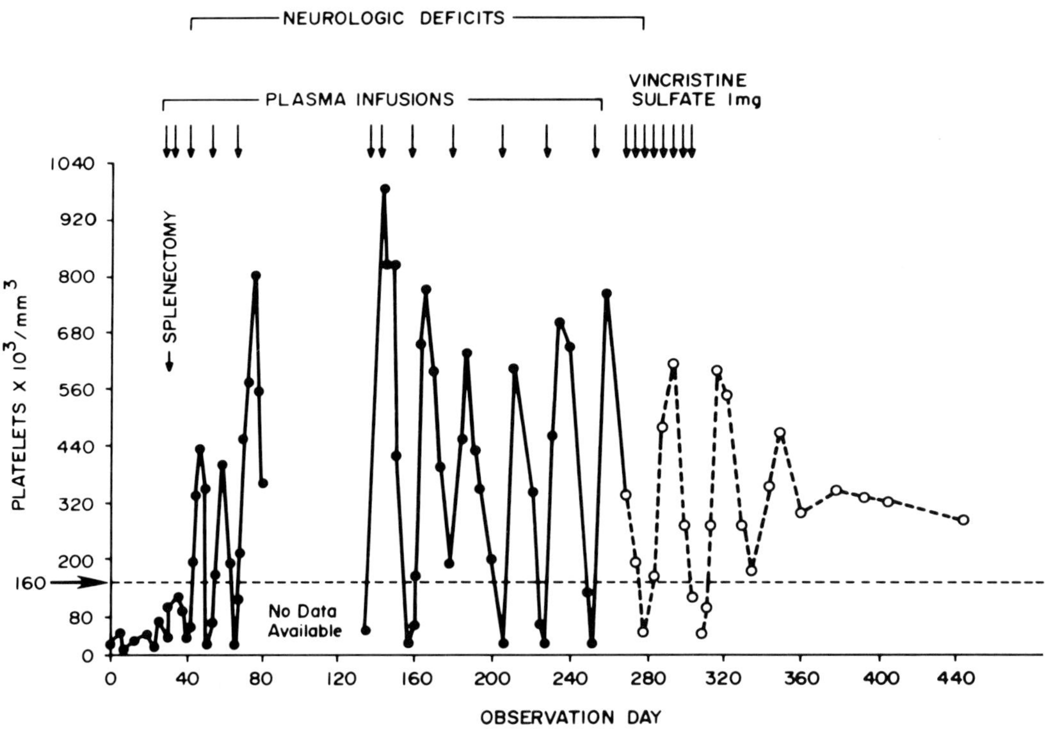

Figure 3 A 21-year-old woman with relapsing TTP: Clinical course and response to therapy.

frequent doses after complete remission occurred. However, treatment probably could have been discontinued much sooner after remission, as was done with the first patient, without resulting in additional relapses.

Hemolytic Uremic Syndrome and Other Related Syndromes

Vincristine has also been effective for the treatment of HUS (6), for a related syndrome, mitomycin-associated microangiopathic hemolytic anemia (29), and for TTP occurring with adenocarcinoma of the breast (unpublished data). When given as a single agent for HUS, vincristine produced a prompt response, as reported by Gutterman et al (6). A 45-year-old woman developed a febrile illness with nausea, vomiting, diarrhea, and jaundice. From a serum creatinine concentration of 7.0 g/dl, schistocytes on the blood smear, platelet count of 17,000/mm^3, anemia, and normal prothrombin and partial thromboplastin times, a diagnosis of HUS was established. Neurological manifestations were absent. She was treated with a total of 4 mg of intravenous vincristine. On day 25, a complete remission resulted, and relapse has not occurred over the subsequent 8 years of observation. The serum creatinine and hemotological values remain normal.

An HUS-like syndrome occurring within a few months of treatment of adenocarcinoma with mitomycin has been described in several patients. Grem et al. (29) reported on two patients wih microangiopathic hemolytic anemia associated with mitomycin treatment. Both patients reveived therapy that included aspirin, dipyridamole, and vincristine for their microangiopathic hemolytic anemia. Their first patient, a 43-year-old woman with metastatic adenocarcinoma of the colon, received two cycles of fluorouracil and mitomycin administered 8 weeks apart. One month after the second course, microangiopathic hemolytic anemia, with renal involvement, was observed and was attributed to mitomycin treatment. In addition to aspirin and dipyridamole, 2 mg of intravenous vincristine was administered weekly for a total of 9.5 mg for treatment of the HUS-like disorder. The hemolytic anemia and renal abnormalities improved, but the platelet count remained slightly low (100,000–110,000 mm^3), possibly secondary to additional fluorouracil therapy for persistent metastatic disease. Microangiopathic hemolytic anemia did not recur.

Their second patient, a 38-year-old woman, was treated with fluorouracil, doxorubicin hydrochloride, and mitomycin for metastatic adenocarcinoma of the gallbladder. After five cycles of chemotherapy, the cancer was in complete remission. Four months later she developed microangiopathic hemolytic anemia with renal involvement, but no evidence of cancer. One month after failure of the hemolytic anemia to respond to aspirin and dipyridamole, intravenous vincristine was administered weekly for a total dose of 9.5 mg. The drug was discontinued because of peripheral neuropathy (muscle weakness). Aspirin and dipyridamole were continued, and the hemolytic anemia resolved within 4 months after initiation of vincristine therapy. Her cancer subsequently recurred, with no evidence of microangiopathic hemolytic anemia.

Treatment for mitomycin related microangiopathic hemolytic anemia–renal dysfunction syndrome usually has been ineffective, although in a few patients the hemolytic anemia has slowly resolved (29). The improvement in the hematological parameters and the stabilization or improvement of renal function in Grem's two patients may have been the result of an unproved synergistic effect of vincristine combined with the antiplatelet drugs. Additional experience in a greater number of patients will be required to determine the effectiveness of vincristine in this situation.

We have observed improvement in TTP associated with metastatic carcinoma of the breast treated with vincristine in two of three patients (unpublished data). One of the responses resulted in a complete remission of TTP, despite eventual progression of the carinoma. The second patient, with stage IV carcinoma, died of her cancer approximately 6 weeks after partial response of her TTP treated only with incristine. In the third patient, no response of TTP to vincristine was observed, and she died of advanced cancer approximately 2 weeks later. Vincristine was administered in combination with other chemotherapy to the first patient, as a single agent to the second patient, and in combination with plasma infusion and corticosteroids to the third patient. The few patients limit the conclusions that can be made, but these data indicate possible benefit from vincristine therapy for TTP associated with adenocarcinoma.

THROMBOTIC THROMBOCYTOPENIC PURPURA MEDICAL RESEARCH GROUP

All of these reported or observed benefits of vincristine without or combined with other treatment for TTP and related thrombotic microangiopathies strongly suggested a role for vincristine in the treatment of these syndromes. However, all of these data were derived retrospectively. Because the need existed for prospective studies on TTP, the TTP Medical Research Group was formed in 1983 by Drs. Lorence A. Gutterman, Michael Rosove and Thomas D. Stevenson. This group now includes 15 hematologists with special clinical and basic science research interests in the disorder. After several meetings, this research group has decided to conduct a prospective pilot study on 100 patients with TTP. The objectives of this pilot study are (a) to compare the clinical and laboratory features of treatment responders and failures; (b) to determine the 5-year survival rate of acute TTP treated with exchange plasmapheresis, vincristine, and methylprednisolone (i.e., a standardized treatment); (c) to determine the incidence and survival rate of relapsing TTP; and (d) to collect plasma samples at various intervals during the study for use in basic research studies on the pathogenesis of TTP. An integral aspect of this study is the establishment of a plasma bank. In this pilot study, patients will receive an initial standardized treatment (Table 4). Fresh-frozen plasma will be used in the exchange.

Table 4 TTP Medical Research Group Treatment Protocol

Exchange plasmapheresis: 60 ml/kg daily
Vincristine: 1.4 mg/m^2 (not to exceed 2 mg) by intravenous push day 1, then 1 mg days 4, 7, and 10 by intravenous push
Methylprednisolone: 0.75 mg/kg by intravenous push every 12 h
(Plasma infusion, 30 ml/kg daily, can be used initially, if exchange plasmapheresis is not immediately available. Within 48 hr start exchange plasmapheresis and discontinue plasma infusion. Patients with caridac or renal failure or coma should receive exchange plasmapheresis starting on day 1).

The decision to combine these three therapies was based on the 60–80% effectiveness of exchange plasmapheresis (1, 2), the apparent benefits of vincristine described in the foregoing, and the observation that most reported successful therapeutic regimens contain a corticosteroid (30).

PROSPECTIVE STUDY

A recent small prospective study done at our 1000-bed hospital in Columbus strengthens the TTP Medical Research Group's decision about the planned initial treatment. Between 1987 and 1989, eight patients with TTP and HUS were evaluated and treated prospectively. The initial treatment given was that recommended by the TTP Medical Research Group (Table 4). The data on patient 4 was subsequently excluded because she died on day 1 before complete therapy was started. The other seven patients survived, six of whom had complete responses to the initial standardized treatment. The one partial responder, patient 6, achieved a complete response with the addition of cryosupernatant infusions. Three patients have had four relapses and responded to additional treatment. Thus, the survival rate was 100% for these seven patients.

The initial clinical and laboratory features (Table 5) indicate that seven of eight patients had neurological manifestations, several of which were moderate to severe and included seizures and coma. Usually, renal involvement was mild, except for patient 3 who had HUS and a serum creatinine level of 13.5 dl. Pulmonary complications were significant and included acute respiratory distress syndrome. Most patients had severe thrombocytopenia (platelet counts below 20,000/mm^3), either initially or shortly after admission to the hospital.

Response to treatment was usually prompt. Improvement in neurological deficits occurred within 2 days in all but one patient. A significant improvement in the platelet count was observed between 4 and 13 days. The time to complete remission ranged from 5 to 29 days, with four of these seven remissions occurring by day 11. Maintenance treatment was not given after complete remission occurred. The specific features of the four relapses are given in Table 6. The treatments given for the relapses varied, but included vincristine in all of these relapses. Longitudinal data indicate that five patients have been observed beyond 1 year. Toxicity of the initial standardized treatment regimen occurred primarily with vincristine and was reversible in all patients. Vincristine caused side effects in four patients and included muscle weakness and alopecia.

Thus, the overall experience of treating TTP and HUS, at our hospital since 1973, with vincristine-based regimen has been successful. All patients received combined or single-agent therapy that always included vincristine. These included the initial five patients with acute TTP reported in 1982 (3), the HUS patient described in 1983 (6), the postpartum patient with chronic relapsing TTP (see Table 2, patient 1), three patients with cancer-associated TTP, and the seven patients with acute TTP and HUS treated prospectively with an initial standardized regimen (see Table 5). Fifteen of these 17 patients responded completely and survived. The two treatment failures occurred in patients who died of their cancer. The larger study proposed by the TTP Medical Research Group will provide further assessment of the effectiveness of the plasma–vincristine treatment combination (see Table 4) and will provide opportunities to study activity mechanisms of these treatment modalities.

Table 5 Initial Standardized Treatment Protocol: Clinical and Laboratory Data on Eight Patients with TTP and HUS

Patient	Age/sex	Neurol deficit	Plt ct (mm^3)	Hgb/Hct (mg/dl/%)	Retic ct (%)	LDH (U/L)	BUN/Creat (mg/dl)	Relapse	Outcome
1	43/F	Yes	11,000	7.1/20.7	3.1	1404	20.0/1.1	Yes	S
2	27/M	Yes	14,000	8.2/24.8	13.9	1060	21.0/1.6	Yes	S
3	55/F	Yes	74,000	7.0/22.0	10.8	2085	134/13.3	No	S
4	67/F	Yes	14,000	10.6/32	2.4	1352	52/2.5		D
5	65/F	Yes	30,000	6.5/18.3	5.6	949	14/0.9	No	S
6	47/M	Yes	54,000	6.6/15.2	3.0	3270	30.0/2.1	No	S
7	40/F	Yes	17,000	6.6/19.8	6.6	1763	28.0/0.8	Yes	S
8	22/M	No	86,000	7.2/21.4	7.7	1097		No	S

Neurol, neurologic; Plt ct, platelet count; Hgb, hemoglobin; Hct, hematocrit; Retic ct, reticulocyte count; LDH, lactate dehyrogenase; BUN, blood urea nitrogen; Creat, creatinine; S, survived; D, died; Incr, increased; Decr, decreased.

Table 6 Initial Standardized Treatment: Relapse Characteristics

Patient	Day of relapse	Neurologic deficit	Renal involvement	Response to treatment
1	128	Yes	No	CR
	198	Yes	No	CR
2	193	Yes	No	CR
7	34	No	Yes	CR
	57	No	No	CR

CR, complete remission.

MECHANISMS OF VINCRISTINE ACTIVITY

How does vincristine effectively reverse the clinical and pathological manifestations of acute and relapsing TTP and related syndromes? Vincristine disassembles the cellular microtubule matrix required for mitosis and cell division and suppresses cellular and humoral immune responses which, perhaps, may alter availability or function of structures or molecules on the surface of platelets and endothelial cells. For example, glycoprotein receptors on platelets may be altered or become less accessible and, therefore, reduce the ability of large von Willebrand factor (vWF) multimers or other agglutinating factors to attach. As a result, platelet aggregation may decrease. Therefore, vincristine may inhibit one of the prime pathological events in TTP, that is, accelerated platelet aggregation, resulting in severe microthrombi formation in arterioles and capillaries.

In our initial report in 1982 (3), we hypothesized that the mechanism of action of vincristine involves the endothelial cell. The initial event in single-episode thrombotic microangiopathies probably is injury to the endothelium, with subsequent formation of thrombotic vascular lesions. Vincristine possibly may directly facilitate repair of or prevent further damage to endothelial cells. Very little data are available that relate to this mechanism, but the following studies may provide support for this hypothesis.

Immune Modulation

Surface events, such as antibody attachment, occur on the endothelial cell. Anti-endothelial cell antibodies, cytotoxic to endothelial cells, have been described in patients with TTP and HUS (31–34). Immune modulation of the endothelial cell, therefore, may be an important mechanism in treating TTP and may be influenced by vincristine. Wall and Harker proposed that the pathogenesis of microvascular injury in TTP may be immune mediated (31). They studied the cytotoxicity of sera from patients with TTP on cultured human endothelial cells by using an endothelial cell ^{51}Cr release assay. Six of the 7 TTP sera produced significant release after the addition of complement. The authors concluded that some patients with TTP may have endothelial cell injury induced by an autoimmune process. They did not evaluate the effect of drugs on the TTP sera.

Burns and Zucker-Franklin found IgG antibodies in the sera of three patients with TTP (33). When the serum was incubated with a culture of human umbilical vein endothelial cells, cytolysis was observed. The IgG fractions of the sera specifically induced immune damage that included the presence of cytoplasmic inclusions and nuclear deterioration. Changes in these cells occurred within 30 min of exposure to the sera and were severe by 24 hr (Figs. 4 and 5). Interestingly, Burns noted that the addition of vincristine to TTP sera before incubation with the endothelial cell culture prevented or reduced cytolysis (personal communication). Further studies on the immune effects of vincristine or other vinca alkaloids on the endothelial cell have not been reported.

Moake et al. (35) and Byrnes and Moake (36) hypothesized that an autoantibody in a patient with frequently relapsing TTP may have interfered with the conversion of unusually large von Willebrand factor (vWF) multimers into smaller vWF forms. They speculated that this antibody may be active on the surface of the endothelial cell. They concluded that this defect in vWF conversion may be immune mediated because the defect was corrected after treatment with two immunosuppressive

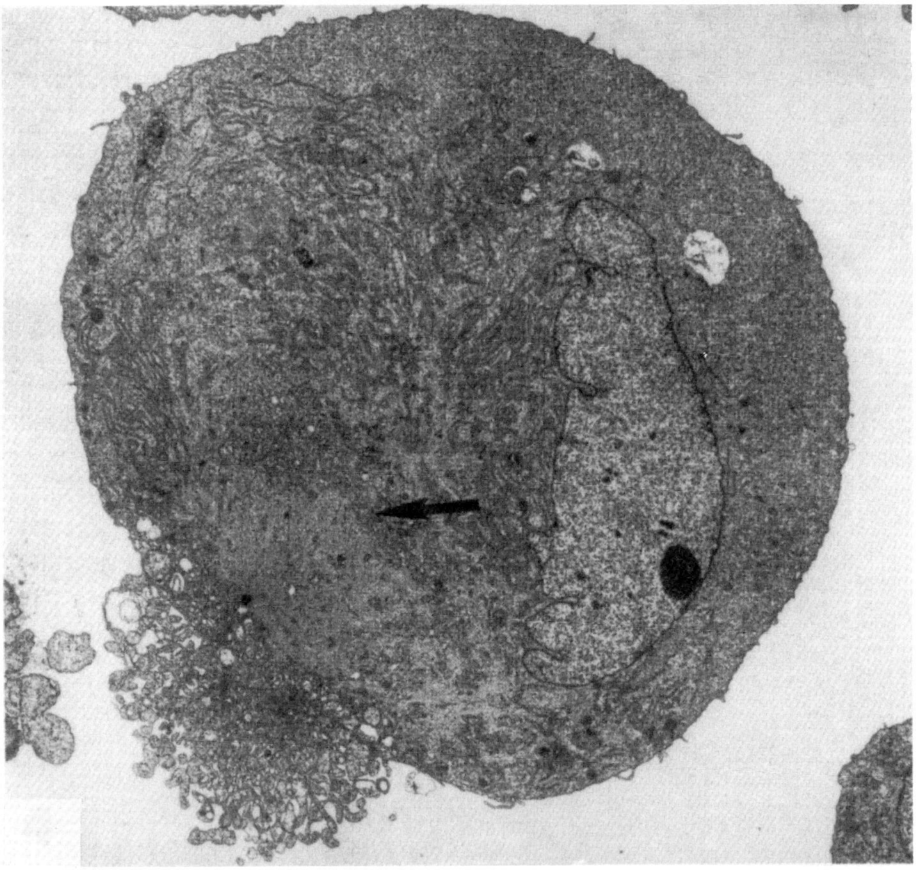

Figure 4 High-power view of a single endothelial cell taken from a specimen that had been incubated with normal serum. Note that the cytoplasmic area, replete with fine fibrils (arrow) often seen in these cells, appears to be well preserved (×2500).

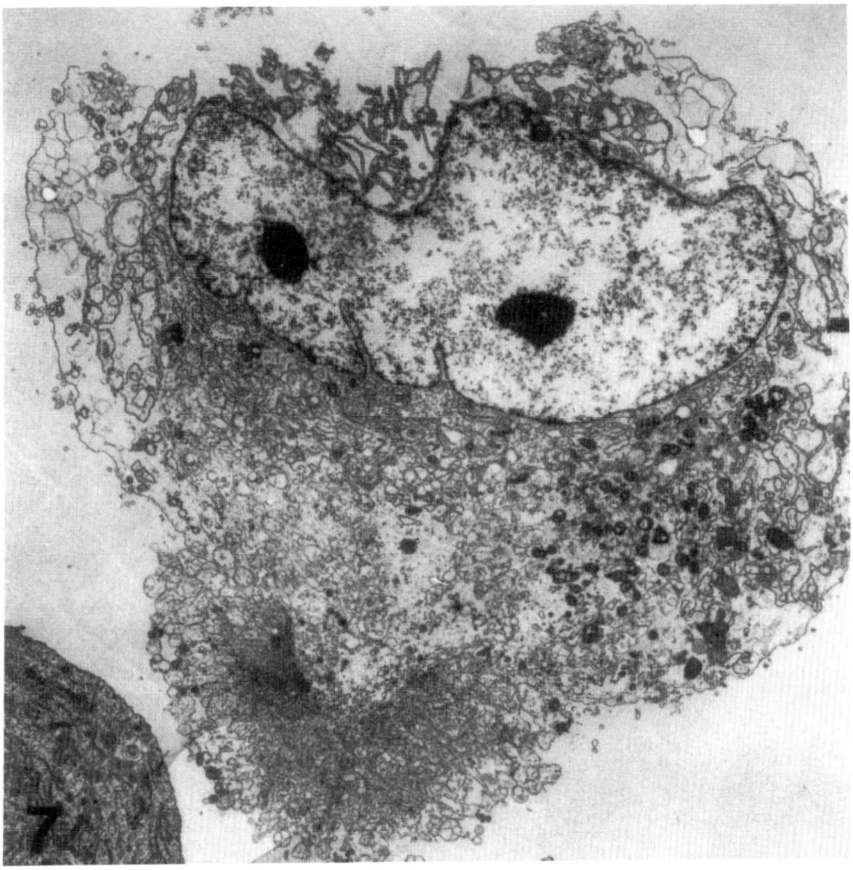

Figure 5 Endothelial cell incubated with TTP serum for 6 hr. The cytoplasm is completely necrotic, and the nucleus appears devoid of chromatin (×4200).

drugs, azathioprine and prednisone. These authors believe that reported responses to other immunosuppressive therapy for patients with TTP who were given vincristine (3) and prednisone plus cyclophosphamide (37), might be similarly explained by invoking effects on the production of autoantibodies or on their capacity to bind to endothelial cells.

In a recent study by Leung et al. (34), the authors found that sera from patients in the acute phase of HUS and TTP contained complement-fixing IgG and IgM antibodies. The cytotoxic damage to endothelial cells caused by these antibodies could be prevented by interferon gamma, especially in the HUS sera. I believe the significance of this study, in addition to detection of antibodies, relates to further evidence of the protective effect of drug on the endothelium. The mechanism of action of interferon or vincristine can only be hypothesized. Thus, the data from Leung's study (34) and the observation by Burns (personal communication) confirm in vitro the inhibitory effects of at least two specific drugs when exposed to TTP or HUS sera.

Other Effects on Endothelium

Immune modulation may be only one of several mechanisms by which vincristine exerts its beneficial effects. Another effect of vincristine on the endothelium is its protective influence on the blood-brain barrier (38). In a study reported by Larsson et al. the hydrostatic pressures of the blood–brain barriers in rats were rapidly increased, causing a reversible opening in the barriers. When the rats were pretreated with vincristine, the barrier damage was significantly reduced. This was attributed to the effect of this antimitotic drug on the intracellular microtubule systems that may be involved in vesicular transport across the endothelial cells of brain microvessels.

The diverse antitubulin effects of vincristine on the endothelium may be better understood by knowing how other antitubulin compounds alter endothelial cell function. In a provocative report, Chaldako suggests a possible furture role for antitubulins to treat atherosclerosis, a disease of the endothelium (39). Colchicine, an antitubulin, appears to interfere with the arterial smooth-muscle cell secretory activity that may be part of the atherogenesis process. In addition, colchicine increases collagenase secretion and "relaxes" hyperactive endothelial cells (40). The hyperactive phagocytic arterial endothelial cells have an increased affinity for the β- and pre-β-lipoproteins that contribute to atherogenesis.

In contrast to apparent beneficial affects of antitubulins on the endothelium, Nicolson et al. describe that vincristine in vitro induced rapid retraction of the endothelial cell (41). This increased platelet and cancer cell binding to exposed subendothelial cell matrix.

These few reported studies of the responses of endothelial cells to vincristine and other antitubulin drugs reveal diverse effects. Without additional studies, definite conclusions cannot be made about the mechanism(s) by which vincristine produces responses in TTP and related syndromes. In general, however, these data indicate beneficial effects on the endothelium when exposed to antitubulin drugs and, therefore, support the clinical data justifying treatment of TTP and the other thrombotic microangiopathies with vincristine. Since multiple etiologies probably account for the variability in TTP, vincristine may be effective through various mechanisms. Scientific investigation of this drug–cell interaction should provide a clearer understanding of the significant role of vincristine in treating patients with TTP and other thrombotic microangiopathies, and it may provide a model for other studies on mechanism and treatment of other diseases of the endothelium.

CONCLUSION

During the past 15 years, many patients with TTP, HUS, and related disorders have been treated with vincristine. This has prompted a critical evaluation of the role of vincristine in the treatment of these thrombotic microangiopathies. The clinical and laboratory features of a large series of patients have been presented. A high response and survival rate was observed in these patients, all of whom were given treatment with vincristine and plasma (as exchange or infusion) or vincristine as a single agent. Given these current data, a reasonable initial treatment regimen for TTP is one that combines exchange plasmapheresis, vincristine, and corticosteroids. Speculation about mechanisms of action of vincristine on the endothelium have been discussed.

As an antitubulin drug, vincristine alters endothelial cells and platelets. Future studies should clarify many of the issues concerning the role of vincristine in TTP.

REFERENCES

1. Bukowski, R. M., Thrombotic thrombocytopenic purpura: A review. In *Progress in Hemostasis and Thrombosis*, T. H. Spaet, ed., Grune & Stratton, New York, p. 287 (1982).
2. Shepard, K. V., Bukowski, R. M., The treatment of thrombotic thrombocytopenic purpura with exchange transfusions, plasma infusions, and plasma exchange. *Semin. Hematol.*, *24*: 178 (1987).
3. Gutterman, L. A., Stevenson, T. D., Treatment of thrombotic thrombocytopenic purpura with vincristine. *JAMA*, *247*: 1433 (1982).
4. Gutterman, L. A., Meek, L. E., Stevenson, T. D., Treatment of thrombotic thrombocytopenic purpura and hemolytic uremic syndrome with vinca alkaloids. *Blood*, *60*: 186A (1982).
5. Gutterman, L. A., Stevenson, T. D., Vincristine in the treatment of thrombotic thrombocytopenic purpura. *Blood*, *54*: 242A (1979).
6. Gutterman, L. A., Levin, D. M., George, B. S., Sharma, H. M., The hemolytic uremic syndrome: Recovery after treatment with vincristine. *Ann. Intern. Med.*, *98*: 612 (1983).
7. Abramson, N., Treatments for thrombotic thrombocytopenic purpura: Plasma, vincristine, hemodialysis, and exchange transfusions. *N. Engl. J. Med.*, *298*: 971 (1978).
8. Frankel, A. E., Rubenstein, M. D., Wall, R. T., Thrombotic thrombocytopenic purpura: Prolonged coma with recovery of neurologic function with intensive plasma exchange. *Am. J. Hematol.*, *10*: 387 (1981).
9. Ahn, Y. S., Harrington, W. J., So, A. G., Vinca alkaloids in the treatment of thrombotic thrombocytopenic purpura. *Blood*, *58*: 187A (1981).
10. Rosove, M. H., Ho, W. G., Goldfinger, D., Ineffectiveness of aspirin and dipyridamole in the treatment of thrombotic thrombocytopenic purpura. *Ann. Intern. Med.*, *96*: 27 (1982).
11. Grosbach, A. B., Brown, S. R., Bowen, L. M., et al., Treatment of thrombotic thrombocytopenic purpura and adult hemolytic uremic syndrome with vincristine and plasma exchange. *Blood*, *60*: 186A (1982).
12. Makary, A. Z., Kough, R. H., Thrombotic thrombocytopenic purpura. *Penn. Med.*, *86*: 50 (1983).
13. Pisciotto, P., Rosen, D., Silver, H., et al., Treatment of thrombotic thrombocytopenic purpura. *Vox Sang.*, *45*: 185 (1983).
14. Schreeder, M. T., Prachal, J. T., Successful treatment of thrombotic thrombocytopenic purpura by vincristine. *Am. J. Hematol.*, *14*: 75 (1983).
15. Thompson, H. W., McCarthy, L. J., Thrombotic thrombocytopenic purpura. *Arch. Intern. Med.*, *143*: 2117 (1983).
16. Caggiano, V., Fernando, L. P., Schneider, J. M., et al., Thrombotic thrombocytopenic purpura: Report of fourteen cases—occurrence during pregnancy and response to plasma exchange. *J. Clin. Apheresis.*, *1*: 71 (1983).
17. Evans, T. L., Winkelstein, A., Zeigler, Z. R., et al., Thrombotic thrombocytopenic purpura: Clinical course and response to therapy in eight patients. *Am. J. Hematol.*, *17*: 401 (1984).
18. Stoffner, D., Banthien, F. C. A., Habersetzer, R., et al., Plasma exchange and concomitant therapy in TTP. *Int. J. Artif. Organs*, *7*: 223 (1984).
19. Stein, R. S., Flexener, J. F., Idiopathic thrombocytopenic purpura during remission of thrombotic thrombocytopenic purpura. *South. Med. J.*, *77*: 1599 (1984).
20. Schneider, P. A., Rayner, A. A., Linker, C. A., et al., The role of splenectomy in

multimodality treatment of thrombotic thrombocytopenic purpura. *Ann. Surg.*, *202*: 318 (1985).
21. Sennett, M. L., Conrad, M. E., Treatment of thrombotic thrombocytopenic purpura. Plasmapheresis, plasma transfusion, and vincristine. *Arch. Intern. Med.*, *146*: 266 (1986).
22. Blitzer, J. B., Granfortuna, J. M., Gottlieb, A. J., et al., Thrombotic thrombocytopenic purpura: Treatment with plasmapheresis. *Am. J. Hematol.*, *24*: 329 (1987).
23. Finn, N. G., Wang, J. C., Hong, K. J., High-dose intravenous gamma immunoglobulin infusion in the treatment of thrombotic thrombocytopenic purpura. *Arch. Intern. Med.*, *147*: 2165 (1987).
24. ter Borg, E.-J., Houtman, P. M., Kallenberg, C. G. M., et al., Thrombocytopenia and hemolytic anemia in a patient with mixed connective tissue disease due to thrombotic thrombocytopenic purpura. *J. Rheumatol.*, *15*: 1174 (1988).
25. Weidemann, G., Kantner, I., Schenke, M., et al., Platelet factor 4 and the response to plasma exchange in the treatment of thrombotic thrombocytopenic purpura. *Klin. Wochenschr.*, *67*: 551 (1989).
26. Neubauer, R. L., Thrombotic thrombocytopenic purpura. *Alaska Med.*, *31*: 57 (1989).
27. Rose, M., Eldor, A., High incidences of relapses in thrombotic thrombocytopenic purpura: Clinical study of 38 patients. *Am. J. Med.*, *83*: 437 (1987).
28. Wurzel, J. M., TTP lesions in placenta but not fetus. *N. Engl. J. Med.*, *301*: 503 (1979).
29. Grem, J. L., Merritt, J. A., Carbone, P. P., Treatment of mitomycin-associated microangiopathic hemolytic anemia with vincristine. *Arch. Intern. Med.*, *146*: 566 (1986).
30. Ridolfi, R. L., Bell, W. R., Thrombotic thrombocytopenic purpura: Report of 25 cases and review of the literature. *Medicine*, *60*: 413 (1981).
31. Wall, R. T., Harker, L. A., The endothelium and thrombosis. *Ann. Rev. Med.*, *31*: 361 (1980).
32. Foster, P. A., Anderson, J. C., Effects of plasma from patients with thrombotic thrombocytopenic purpura on cultured human endothelial cells. *Blood*, *54*: 240A (1979).
33. Burns, E. R., Zucker-Franklin, D., Pathologic effects of plasma from patients with thrombotic thrombocytopenic purpura on platelets and cultured vascular endothelial cells. *Blood*, *60*: 1030 (1982).
34. Leung, D. Y. M., Moake, J. L., Havens, P. L., et al., Lytic antiendothelial cell antibodies in haemolytic–uremic syndrome. *Lancet*, *2*: 183 (1988).
35. Moake, J. L., Rudy, C. K., Troll, J. H., et al., Therapy of chronic relapsing thrombotic thrombocytopenic purpura with prednisone and azathioprine. *Am. J. Hematol.*, *20*: 73 (1985).
36. Byrnes, J. J., Moake, J. L., Thrombotic thrombocytopenic purpura and the haemolytic–uraemic syndrome: Evolving concepts of pathogenesis and therapy. *Clin. Haematol.*, *15*: 413 (1986).
37. Wallach, H. W., Oren, M. E., Herskowitz, A., Treatment of thrombotic thrombocytopenic purpura with plasma infusion and cyclophosphamide. *South. Med. J.*, *72*: 1346 (1979).
38. Larsson, B., Skarby, T., Edvinsson, L., et al., Vincristine reduces damage of the blood-brain barrier induced by high intravascular pressure. *Neurosci. Lett.*, *17*: 155 (1980).
39. Chaldakov, G. N., Antitubulins—a new approach for atherosclerosis? *Atherosclerosis*, *44*: 385 (1982).
40. Shimamoto, T., Hidaka, H., Moriya, K., et al. Hyperactive arterial endothelial cells: A clue for the treatment of atherosclerosis. *Ann. N. Y. Acad. Sci.*, *275*: 266 (1976).
41. Nicolson, G. L., Custead, S. E., Effects of chemotherapeutic drugs on platelet and metastatic tumor cell–endothelial cell interactions as a model for assessing vascular endothelial integrity. *Cancer Res.*, *45*: 331 (1985).

39
Antiplatelet Agents in Thrombotic Thrombocytopenic Purpura

Martin D. Phillips *Baylor College of Medicine and Rice University, Houston, Texas*

Platelet thrombi in arterioles and smaller vessels are the characteristic pathological finding in biopsies taken from patients with thrombotic thrombocytopenic purpura (TTP) (1). It is logical, therefore, that antiplatelet therapy has been attempted in this disorder. However, it is difficult to draw conclusions about therapy from published reports, because all of the clinical data are from case reports and small retrospective series. Although frequently a positive outcome has been ascribed to antiplatelet therapy, most reports have not demonstrated unequivocally any benefit. In virtually all cases, multiple therapeutic modalities were used both simultaneously and sequentially. Nevertheless, the temporal association of antiplatelet therapy and recovery has been dramataic in a few instances. In addition, many practitioners have anecdotal evidence that inhibition of platelet function appeared to have been beneficial in some patients. Conversely, some authors have documented progressive disease while patients were taking antiplatelet drugs (2–4). Others have shown deleterious effects of inhibiting platelet function in these acutely ill, thrombocytopenic patients (5). There is no systematic evidence proving or disproving an effect of antiplatelet agents in TTP. Hemorrhagic complications have been associated with these agents, but thrombocytopenic hemorrhages are a part of the pathogenesis of the disease. The drugs currently available for inhibiting platelet function should not be used to the exclusion of plasma exchange, which is an effective therapy, nor should they be used when there is evidence of intracerebral or gastrointestinal hemorrhage. These conclusions are generally in agreement with two other recent reviews (3, 6).

ROLE OF VON WILLEBRAND FACTOR

von Willebrand factor (vWF) is likely to have a role in the intravascular platelet aggregation of TTP. Characteristic abnormalities have been documented in the size of the largest vWF multimeric forms present in the plasma of patients with active TTP, depending on the stage of the disease at the time the plasma is sampled (see Chap. 33). Frequently the platelet thrombi in TTP have a positive histochemical stain for vWF (1). Other putative platelet aggregating proteins of 37 and 59 kd (7, 8) have been isolated from some patients with TTP. In addition, it is likely that fluid shear stresses in narrowed arterioles perpetuate platelet aggregation (9–11).

Fluid shear stress can induce platelet aggregation that is dependent upon platelets with intact surface glycoproteins Ib and IIb/IIIa, large plasma vWF multimers [or the "unusually large" (UL) vWF multimers secreted from intensely stimulated or damaged endothelial cells], calcium, and adenosine diphosphate (ADP) (11). There is in vitro evidence that aspirin does not inhibit shear stress-induced, vWF-mediated platelet aggregation (10). A dye compound, aurin tricarboxylic acid (ATA), has been shown to inhibit shear stress-induced, vWF-mediated platelet aggregation in vitro (12), and in an in vivo (13) canine model of coronary artery thrombosis. This agent may be a prototype "antiplatelet" agent for use in TTP. Further studies are planned to determine if ATA can prevent platelet aggregation in animals with a syndrome like TTP induced by botrocetin (14).

USE OF SPECIFIC ANTIPLATELET DRUGS

Several drugs in addition to aspirin have been used in an attempt to inhibit platelet aggregation in patients with TTP. These include dipyridamole, ticlopidine, sulfinpyrazone, PGI_2 and its analogues, dextrans, and nifedipine. Defective fibrinolysis has been postulated as a pathogenetic mechanism of TTP (15, 16); however, the use of fibrinolytic agents would be extremely hazardous in a thrombocytopenic patient. Defibrotide, a biologic extract with multiple-proposed antithrombotic and fibrinolytic properties, has also been employed with reported success (17, 18). Controlled studies of this agent are needed before it can be recommended.

Several authors have noted the difficulty in assessing the efficacy of any of these agents because the data are mostly from case reports and small retrospective series. Frequently, there is insufficient detail to evaluate the diagnosis and the therapeutic regimen. Invariably, multiple modes of therapy were used. Corticosteroids and splenectomy have been included in some combination therapies. Many practitioners have observed cases in which steroids attenuated the disease until more definitive therapy could be instituted, or a remission occurred. Rarely is detailed information reported about the use of blood products. This is noteworthy, because plasma exchange or infusion definitely has been shown to be an effective therapeutic modality in this disease (3, 19, 20). In addition, as noted by Byrnes and Lian (3), it is not possible to discern from most case reports how many blood products were given during splenectomy to these thrombocytopenic patients. Frequently, the volume of blood administered is equivalent to one or more blood volume exchanges. From this inhomogeneous background it is unwise to attempt to draw firm therapeutic recommendations, as many of the authors of these small series point out.

Aspirin and Dipyridamole

Aspirin has been used in many reported cases of TTP. The main effect of aspirin on platelets is irreversible acetylation of cyclooxygenase, with a resultant loss of ability to generate prostaglandins (PGs) from arachidonic acid (21). Aspirin also inhibits endothelial cell cyclooxygenase, with the resultant loss of production of prostacyclin (PGI_2). There is considerable speculation about the dose of aspirin needed to inhibit platelet function in vivo, and the higher dose required for the inhibition of endothelial cell PGI_2 production. Fifty milligrams of aspirin taken orally by an adult is sufficient to prolong the bleeding time and severely depress the amount of thromboxane A_2 (TXA_2) metabolites excreted in the urine; the dose required to inhibit the generation of prostacyclin is probably higher (22). In every study of TTP in which aspirin was used, the dose was greater than 325 mg. If a relative PGI_2 deficiency is part of the pathogenesis of TTP, the use of a dose of aspirin sufficient to inhibit endothelial cell cyclooxygenase paradoxically may have contributed to a prothrombotic state.

Several of the reports of antiplatelet agents in TTP have noted a temporal association between the administration or increase in dosage of dipyridamole and recovery from the disease. In addition to the difficulty in interpretation of these data, owing to the administration of other drugs and blood products, there has been little documentation of the efficacy of dipyridamole in other arterial thrombotic disorders (23). Randomized trials in clinical diseases comparing dipyridamole with aspirin or placebo have not demonstrated any superiority of dipyridamole. Although dipyridamole is proposed to raise the platelet intracellular concentration of cyclic adenosine monophosphate (cAMP), this effect cannot be demonstrated at physiologically attainable concentrations of the drug. The use of dipyridamole in thrombotic disorders is largely based on historical bias and precedent, not on carefully performed, randomized comparison studies.

Table 1 is a summary of reports of the use of aspirin, dipyridamole, or both, in TTP (a similar table appears in Ref. 6). It demonstrates that, in most cases, several therapeutic modalities were in use, although the authors frequently attributed a treatment success to aspirin or dipyridamole. Conversely, in several reports, the patients were receiving aspirin in their multidrug therapy, but the authors attributed success to other agents. In one reported case, a patient with TTP improved while taking only aspirin and dipyridamole (37). There are several reports of progressive disease while the patients were regularly taking these antiplatelet agents (2–4, 43). Taken together, these reports do not provide strong support for the use of aspirin and dipyridamole in TTP.

Ticlopidine

The use of ticlopidine has been limited in TTP (44–46). Ticlopidine is comparable with aspirin in prophylaxis of cerebrovascular embolic phenomena (47). Several days are required for its antiplatelet effect to develop in vivo (48). It remains to be shown whether or not it is effective in acute arterial thrombotic disease or in TTP.

Sulfinpyrazone

Sulfinpyrazone is mostly of historical interest. This drug has not shown enough antithrombotic efficacy to be retained in current use.

Prostinoids

The support for the use of prostaglandins and prostaglandin inhibitors in the treatment of TTP is not compelling. It has been proposed that either a deficiency in

Table 1 Summary of Reports on Therapy and Drug Use for TTP

	No. of patients										
Ref.	R	NR	CS	ASA	Dip	Slf	Dex	Spl	PGI	Hep	Bld
24		1	*	+	+			*		*	*
25[a]		12	*	*			*	*		*	
		1		*	*	*			*		
26[b]	1		*	*	+			*			*
27	18	2	+(20)	*(3)	*(4)		+(15)	+(18)			*(3)
28	2		*	*	+	*		*			*
20[c]	5			+	*(1)	*(1)			+		*
20[c]		2	*					*(1)			
30	1		*	+	+						*
31	1		*	+	+					*	
32	1				+			d		*	
33	1		*	*			+				*
5		14	+	-	-		*(1)			+	
34	1		*				+				*
35	9		*(1)	+(4)	+(4)			*(1)			+(8)
36[e]	1		*	+							*
37	1			+	+						*
38	1		*	+	+						
39	1		*	+	+		+				
40	2		+					+			*
41	1	4	*	*	*			*		*	
43				+	+	+					+

Abbreviations: CS, corticosteroids; ASA, aspirin; Dip, dipyridamole; Slf, sulfinpyrazone; Dex, dextrans; Spl, splenectomy; PGI, PGI_2; Hep, heparin; Bld, Blood products.
Explanation of Symbols: *, therapy was used; +, therapy was used and authors ascribe clinical benefit to this agent; −, therapy was used and authors ascribe clinical deterioration to this agent; (n), number of patients receiving this therapy; R, number of patients who responded to therapy; NR, number of patients who did not respond to therapy.
[a]Three of 12 patients had disseminated intravascular coagulation (DIC) as well as TTP. The authors state that ". . . no 'cure' has withstood the test of time, and no claims should be made on the basis of one case."
[b]The patient also received cyclophosphamide.
[c]The patients also received 6-mercaptopurine.
[d]The patient had a prior splenectomy.
[e]The patient also received azathioprine.

prostacyclin (49), a decrease in serum prostacyclin binding (50, 51), or a plasma factor that inhibits prostacyclinlike activity (52) is present in TTP. Two independent groups of investigators have used the vascular ring assay of Moncada (53) for generation of PGI_2 by endothelial cells in the presence of sera from patients with TTP. One set of experiments was interpreted to demonstrate a serum inhibitor of PGI_2 (52); the other experiments showed no difference between TTP and normal sera (54). Plasma levels of $PGF_{1\alpha}$ (the stable metabolite of PGI_2) and thromboxane B_2 (the stable metabolite of thromboxane A_2) have been measured in the sera of TTP patients and shown to be normal (55) or abnormal (49). These variable results may be an indication of the difficulty of performing these measurements on clinical samples.

Intravenous PGI_2 infusion (with and without other agents) has been associated with clinical response (56, 57) and with lack of response (55–59) in advanced TTP. Although an insufficient dosage has been cited as the reason for the treatment failures, 8–16 ng/kg per min (a high dose) has been documented to be ineffective. Nafazatrom (Bay g 6575) is reported to raise the plasma level of PGI_2 by various mechanisms. The reported use of nafazatrom in TTP is inconclusive (60, 61). In a recent review of prostaglandins in thrombotic microangiopathy, Remuzzi (49) contends that a lack of therapeutic efficacy of PGI_2 replacement does not rule out a role for abnormal prostaglandin metabolism in the pathogenesis of TTP. However, aspirin administered at doses sufficient to profoundly decrease the endogenous production of PGI_2 has not appreciably worsened the outcomes of TTP patients (62).

Dextrans

Dextrans have also been used as antiplatelet therapy of TTP. Dextrans may interfere with reactions of the humoral coagulation cascade (63), and may also bind to vWF in vitro (64, 65) or alter vWF multimer size distribution in vivo (66). In several case reports, there has been a temporal association of the administration of dextrans with improvement of TTP (27, 67), and dextrans have been part of the drug regimen administered to other patients who had good outcomes (see Table 1). Some authors strongly advocate their use. However, the same cautions that apply to the interpretation of data in the use of other antiplatelet agents also apply to the retrospective interpretation of clinical data in the use of dextrans.

Calcium Channel Blockers

The calcium channel blocking drug nifedipine has been proposed as an antithrombotic agent owing to its effect on platelet calcium levels (68). Verapamil and nifedipine, like dipyridamole, can modestly decrease platelet deposition on polytetrafluoroethylene arterial grafts in dogs (69), but it is uncertain how well this model reflects the events in human arterial thrombosis. There is some evidence that dihydropyridones can singly or synergistically affect in vitro tests of platelet function after several days of administration (4), but these effects are not universally accepted (70). In addition, calcium channel blocking drugs do not have a clinically recognized effect on platelet function, nor do they alter the template bleeding time (4, 71).

SIDE EFFECTS OF ANTIPLATELET AGENTS

With the potential therapeutic efficacy of antiplatelet agents, there is also the potential for adverse side effects. In any reporting of case material, there is a bias against negative results. Therefore, antiplatelet agent failures may be underrepresented in the literature. However, there is a published series (5) in which it was demonstrated that the hemorrhagic complications were worse in those TTP patients in whom antiplatelet agents were used. These findings are also retrospective analyses of patient data and are subject to the same flaws in interpretation as the positive outcomes. In addition, it is the nature of thrombocytopenic patients to hemorrhage. However, the potential worsening of hemorrhage induced by inhibiting the function of those platelets remaining in the circulation must be considered.

CONCLUSIONS

A large prospective study of therapy of TTP has recently been published that agrees with the conclusions presented here (72). One hundred eight patients were treated according to a protocol over a 10-year period. Aspirin was administered to these patients early in the study, but its use was discontinued when it was demonstrated to be ineffective. In addition, it is important to note in the interpretation of historical data that 28% of these patients achieved a remission on corticosteroids alone.

Although the events initiating platelet aggregation in TTP are unknown, the disease is likely perpetuated by elevated fluid shear forces causing platelet aggregation in partially occluded arterioles. Fluid shear stress-induced platelet aggregation has been modeled in vitro, and the necessary components have been demonstrated to be metabolizing platelets with intact glycoprotein Ib and IIb/IIIa surface receptors, large (or endothelial cell-derived unusually large) vWF multimers, calcium ions, and ADP (9). In vitro, fluid shear stress-induced platelet aggregation is not impeded by aspirin treatment of the platelets (11). Although it is likely that factors other than shear stress contribute to the intravascular platelet aggregation in TTP, the failure of aspirin to inhibit shear stress-induced aggregation in vitro may partially explain the failure of aspirin to affect unequivocally the clinical course of TTP.

There is evidence that vWF, at least in part, mediates the intravascular platelet clumping in TTP. We have demonstrated that a dye compound, aurin tricarboxylic acid (ATA), is an effective inhibitor of both fluid shear stress-induced and ristocetin-induced, vWF-mediated platelet agglutination (12). The ATA binds to vWF multimers, and likely causes a change in the tertiary structure of the molecule near the GPIb binding domain. The ATA forms complex polymers during its synthesis, and the polymers of several thousand daltons are the most effective platelet aggregation inhibitors (73–75). This agent has been demonstrated to be a very potent inhibitor of platelet thrombus formation in the arterial circulation in vivo in the Folts model of canine coronary arterial thrombosis (13). It is the only agent yet reported that inhibits vWF-mediated platelet aggregation. ATA will soon be tested in an animal model of TTP (14). Because of the involvement of vWF in the platelet thrombi of TTP, if ATA or one of its analogues is suitable for administration to humans, then this agent will be a useful antiplatelet aggregatory agent in the therapy of TTP.

REFERENCES

1. Asada, Y., Sumiyoshi, A., Hayashi, T., Suzumiya, J., Kaketani, K., Immunohistochemically of vascular lesion in thrombotic thrombocytopenic purpura, with special reference to factor VIII related antigen. *Thromb. Res.*, *38*: 469 (1985).
2. Holdrinet, R. S. G., Namdar, Z., Haanen, C., Thrombotic thrombocytopenic purpura: Clinical course and response to therapy in twelve patients. *Neth. J. Med.*, *33*: 113 (1988).
3. Byrnes, J. J., Lian, E. C. Y., Recent therapeutic advances in thrombotic thrombocytopenic purpura. *Semin. Thromb. Hemost.*, *5*: 199 (1979).
4. Lindquist, J. R., George, R. P., Thrombotic thrombocytopenic purpura: Onset during dipyridamole therapy. *JAMA*, *246*: 2577 (1981).
5. Rosove, M. H., Ho, W. G., Goldfinger, D., Ineffectiveness of aspirin and dipyridamole in the treatment of thrombotic thrombocytopenic purpura. *Ann. Intern. Med.*, *96*: 27 (1979).
6. del Zoppo, G. J., Antiplatelet therapy in thrombotic thrombocytopenic purpura. *Semin. Hematol.*, *24*: 130 (1987).

7. Siddiqui, F. A., Lian, E. C., Novel platelet-agglutinating protein from a thrombotic thrombocytopenic purpura plasma. *J. Clin. Invest.*, *76*: 1330 (1985).
8. Kelton, J. G., Moore, J. C., Murphy, W. G., Studies investigating platelet aggregation and release initiated by sera from patients with thrombotic thrombocytopenic purpura. *Blood*, *69*: 924 (1987).
9. Moake, J. L., Turner, N. A., Stathopoulos, N. A., Nolasco, L. H., Hellums, J. D., Involvement of large plasma von Willebrand factor (vWF) multimers and unusually large vWF forms derived from endothelial cells in shear stress-induced platelet aggregation. *J. Clin. Invest.*, *78*: 1456 (1986).
10. Hellums, J. D., Peterson, D. M., Stathopoulos, N. A., Moake, J. L., Giorgio, T. D., Studies on the mechanism of shear-induced platelet activation. In *Cerebral Ischemia and Hemorheology* (A. Hartmann, W., Kuschinsky, eds.), Springer-Verlag, Berlin, p. 80 (1987).
11. Moake, J. L., Turner, N. A., Stathopoulos, N. A., Nolasco, L., Hellums, J. D., Shear-induced platelet aggregation can be mediated by vWF released from platelets, as well as by exogenous large or unusually large vWF multimers, requires adenosine diphosphate, and is resistant to aspirin. *Blood*, *71*: 1366 (1988).
12. Phillips, M. D., Moake, J. L., Nolasco, L. H., Turner, N. A., Aurin tricarboxylic acid: A novel inhibitor of platelet–von Willebrand. *Blood*, *72*: 1898 (1988).
13. Strony, J., Phillips. M. D., Brands, D., Moake, J. L., Adelman, B., Aurin tricarboxylic acid in a canine model of coronary artery thrombosis. *Circulation*, *81*: 1106 (1990).
14. Sanders, W. E., Read, M. S., Reddick, R. L., Garris, J. B., Brinkhous, K. M., Thrombotic thrombocytopenia with von Willebrand factor deficiency induced by botrocetin. An animal model. *Lab. Invest.*, *59*: 443 (1988).
15. Glas-Greenwalt, P., Hall, J. M., Panke, T. W., Kant, K. S., Allen, C. M., Pollak, V. E., Fibrinolysis in health and disease: Abnormal levels of plasminogen activator, plasminogen activator inhibitor, and protein C in thrombotic thrombocytopenic purpura. *J. Lab. Clin. Med.*, *108*: 415 (1986).
16. Kwaan, H. C., Role of fibrinolysis in thrombotic thrombocytopenic purpura. *Semin. Hematol.*, *24*: 101 (1987).
17. Vangelista, A., Frasca, G. M., Raimondi, C., Liviano-D'Arcangelo, G., Bonomini, V., Effects of difibrotide in acute renal failure due to thrombotic microangiopathy. *Haemostasis*, *16*: 51 (1986).
18. Bonomini, V., Vangelista, A., Frasca, G., A new antithrombotic agent in the treatment of acute renal failure due to hemolytic–uremic syndrome and thrombotic thrombocytopenic purpura. *Nephron*, *37*: 144 (1984).
19. Moake, J. L., Rudy, C. K., Troll, J. H., Weinstein, M. J., Colannino, N. M., Azocar, J., Seder, R. H., Hong, S. L., Deykin, D., Unusually large plasma factor VIII: von Willebrand factor multimers in chronic relapsing thrombotic thrombocytopenic purpura. *N. Engl. J. Med.*, *307*: 1432 (1982).
20. Bukowski, R. M., King, J. W., Hewlett, J. S., Plasmapheresis in the treatment of thrombotic thrombocytopenic purpura. *Blood*, *50*: 413 (1977).
21. Roth, G. J., Stanford, N., Majerus, P. W., Acetylation of prostaglandin synthase by aspirin. *Proc. Natl. Acad. Sci. USA*, *72*: 3073 (1975).
22. Fitzgerald, G. A., Oates, J. A., Hawiger, J., Maas, R. L., Roberts, L. J., Lawson, J. A., Brash, A. R., Endogenous biosynthesis of prostacyclin and thromboxane and platelet function during chronic administration of aspirin in man. *J. Clin. Invest.*, *71*: 676 (1983).
23. Fitzgerald, G. A., Dipyridamole. *N. Engl. J. Med.*, *316*: 1247 (1987).
24. Amir, J., Krauss, S., Treatment of thrombotic thrombocytopenic purpura with antiplatelet drugs. *Blood*, *42*: 27 (1973).
25. Jaffe, E. A., Nachman, R. L., Merskey, C., Thrombotic thrombocytopenic purpura—coagulation parameters in twelve patients. *Blood*, *42*: 499 (1973).

26. Woodruff, R. K., Castaldi, P. A., Treatment of TTP with high-dose dipyridamole. *Blood, 52*: 856 (1978).
27. Cuttner, J., Splenectomy steroids, and dextran 70 in thrombotic thrombocytopenic purpura. *JAMA, 227*: 397 (1974).
28. Eckel, R. H., Crowell, E. B., Waterhouse, B. E., Bozdech, M. J., Platelet-inhibiting drugs in thrombotic thrombocytopenic purpura. *Arch. Intern. Med., 137*: 735 (1977).
29. Goldenfarb, P. B., Finch, S. C., Thrombotic thrombocytopenic purpura. A ten year survey. *JAMA, 226*: 644 (1973).
30. Rossi, E. C., Redondo, D., Borges, W. H., Thrombotic thrombocytopenic purpura–survival following treatment with aspirin, dipyridamole, and prednisone. *JAMA, 228*: 1141 (1974).
31. Giromini, M., Bouvier, C. A., Dami, R., Denizot, M., Jeannet, M., Effect of dipyridamole and aspirin in thrombotic microangiopathy. *Br. J. Med., 1*: 545 (1972).
32. Howard, D. J., Roberts, A. B., Page, F. T., Late recurrence of thrombotic thrombocytopenic purpura after splenectomy. *Br. J. Med., 2*: 317 (1975).
33. Faguet, G. B., King, M. B., Thrombotic thrombocytopenic purpura: Treatment with anti-platelet agents. *Am. J. Med., 268*: 113 (1974).
34. Lerner, R. G., Rappaport, S. L., Meltzer, J., Thrombotic thrombocytopenic purpura. Serial clotting studies, relation to the generalized Swartzman reaction, and remission after adrenal steroid and dextran therapy. *Ann. Intern. Med., 66*: 1180 (1970).
35. Myers, T. J., Wakem, C. J., Ball, E. D., Thrombotic thrombocytopenic purpura: Combined treatment with plasmapheresis and antiplatelet agents. *Ann. Intern. Med., 92*: 149 (1980).
36. Jobin, F., Delage, J. M., Aspirin and prednisone in microangiopathic hemolytic anemia. *Lancet, 2*: 208 (1970).
37. Gundlach, W. J., Tarnasky, R., Thrombotic thrombocytopenic purpura. Remission following treatment with aspirin and dipyridamole. *Minn. Med., 60*: 20 (1977).
38. Zacharski, L. R., Walworth, C., McIntyre, O. R., Anti-platelet therapy for thrombotic thrombocytopenic purpura. *N. Engl. J. Med., 285*: 408 (1971).
39. Birgens, H., Ernst, P., Hansen, M. S., Thrombotic thrombocytopenic purpura: Treatment with a combination of anti-platelet drugs. *Acta. Med. Scand., 204*: 437 (1979).
40. Schwartz, J., Rosenberg, A., Cooperberg, A. A., Thrombotic thrombocytopenic purpura: Successful treatment of two cases. *Can. Med. Assoc. J., 106*: 1200 (1972).
41. Neame, P. B., Hirsh, J., Browman, G., Denburg, J., D Souza, T. J., Gallus, A., Brain, M. C., Thrombotic thrombocytopenic purpura: A syndrome of intravascular platelet consumption. *Can. Med. Assoc. J., 114*: 1108 (1976).
42. Updike, S. J., Bozdech, M. J., Johnson, C. A., Zimmerman, S. W., Management of fulminating thrombotic thrombocytopenic purpura. *Semin. Thromb. Hemost., 7*: 33 (1981).
43. Breckenridge, R. L., Solberg, L. A., Pineda, A. A., Petitt, R. M., Dharkar, D. D., Treatment of thrombotic thrombocytopenic purpura with plasma exchange, antiplatelet agents, corticosteroid, and plasma infusion. *J. Clin. Apheresis, 1*: 6 (1982).
44. Itoh, Y., Taniguchi, T., Takagi, D., Takeyama, N., Soga, T., Tanaka, T., Thrombotic thrombocytopenic purpura (TTP) associated with chromosomal aberration and treated with plasma exchange. *Jpn. J. Clin. Hematol., 30*: 546 (1989).
45. De Pasquale, A., Venturoni, L., Paterlini, P., Cretara, G., Di Francesco, A., Quaglino, D., Possible usefulness of ticlopidine in combined treatment of thrombotic thrombocytopenic purpura. *Haematologica, 71*: 53 (1986).
46. Ishii, Y., Ebata, H., Satoh, K., Ueda, H., Harada, M., Mashiko, N., Nouno, R., Tanikawa, K., Hidaka, T., Case of thrombotic thrombocytopenic purpura. Successful treatment with ticlopidine. *Jpn. J. Clin. Hematol., 25*: 1097 (1984).
47. Hass, W. K., Easton, J. D., Adams, H. P., Pryse-Phillips, W., Molony, B. A., Anderson, S., Kamm, B., A randomized trial comparing triclopidine hydrochloride with

aspirin for the prevention of stroke in high-risk patients. *N. Eng. J. Med., 321*: 501 (1989).

48. Defreyn, G., Bernat, A., Delebassee, D., Maffrand, J.-P., Pharmacology of ticlopidine: A review. *Semin. Thromb. Hemost., 15*: 159 (1989).
49. Remuzzi, G., Zoja, C., Rossi, E. C., Prostacyclin in thrombotic microangiopathy. *Semin. Hematol., 24*: 110 (1987).
50. Tsai, A.-L., Manner, C. E., Rudersdorf, T., Wu, K. K., Quantitation of serum prostacyclin-binding in thrombotic thrombocytopenic purpura. *Thromb. Res. 51*: 583 (1988).
51. Wu, K. K., Hall, E. R., Rossi, E. C., Papp, A. C., Serum prostacyclin binding defects in thrombotic thrombocytopenic purpura. *J. Clin. Invest., 75*: 168 (1985).
52. Machin, S. J., McVerry, B. A., Parry, H., Marrow, W. J. W., A plasma factor inhibiting prostacyclin-like activity in thrombotic thrombocytopenic purpura. *Acta Haematol., 67*: 8 (1982).
53. Moncada, S., Higgs, E. A., Vane, J. R., Human arterial and venous tissues generated prostacyclin, a potent inhibitor of platelet aggregation. *Lancet, 1*: 18 (1977).
54. Pini, M., Manotti, C., Megha, A.a, Poli, T., Poti, R., Normal prostacyclin-like activity and response to plasma exchange in thrombotic thrombocytopenic purpura. *Acta Haematol., 67*: 8 (1982).
55. Lee, S. H., Wainscoat, J. S., Zeitlin, H., Bolton, F. G., Leaver, H. A., Seawright, A., Preece, J. M., Prostacyclin and thromboxane A_2 in thrombotic thrombocytopenic purpura. *Br. J. Med., 283*: 1351 (1981).
56. Fitzgerald, G. A., Maas, R. L., Stein, R., Oates, J. A., Roberts, L. J., Intravenous prostacyclin in thrombotic thrombocytopenic purpura. *Ann. Intern. Med., 95*: 319 (1981).
57. Payton, C. D., Belch, J. J. F., Boulton Jones, J. M., Successful treatment of thrombotic thrombocytopenic purpura by epoprostenol infusion. *Lancet, 1*: 927 (1985).
58. Cocchetto, D. M., Cook, L., Cato, A. E., Niedel, J. E., Rationale and proposal for use of prostacyclin in thrombotic thrombocytopenic purpura therapy. *Semin. Thromb. Hemost., 7*: 43 (1981).
59. Johnson, J. E., Mills, G. M., Batson, A. G., Cato, A. E., Thornsvard, C. T., Ineffective epoprostenol therapy for thrombotic thrombocytopenic purpura. *JAMA, 250*: 3089 (1983).
60. Williams, H. J. H., Myatt, L., Young, K. D., Thrombotic thrombocytopenic purpura: Treatment with nafazatrom. *Clin. Lab. Haematol., 6*: 199 (1984).
61. Durrant, S. T. S., Joosten, P., Gordon-Smith, E. C., Nafazatrom in treatment of thrombotic thrombocytopenic purpura. *Lancet, 2*: 842 (1985).
62. Byrnes, J. J., Moake, J. L., Thrombotic thrombocytopenic purpura and the haemolytic–uraemic syndrome: Evolving concepts of pathogenesis and therapy. In *Clinics in Haematology: Thrombosis and the Vessel Wall* (C. N. Chesterman, ed). W. B. Saunders, London, p. 413 (1986).
63. Raasch, R. H., Effects of Dextran 70 on factor VIII activity. *Am. J. Hosp. Pharm., 36*: 89 (1979).
64. Harrison, P., Saundry, R. H., Savidge, G. F., Chromatography of the VIII/vWF complex on dextran sulphate Sepharose. *Thromb. Res., 50*: 295 (1988).
65. Saundry, R. H., Harrison, P., Savidge, G. F., Chromatography of vWF on dextran sulphate Sepharose. *Thromb. Res., 48*: 641 (1987).
66. Batlle, J., del Rio, F., Lopez-Fernandez, M. F., Martin, R., Effect of dextran on factor VIII/von Willebrand factor structure and function. *Thromb. Haemost., 54*: 697 (1985).
67. Liu, E. T., Linker, C. A., Shuman, M. A., Management of treatment failures in thrombotic thrombocytopenic purpura. *Am. J. Hematol., 23*: 347 (1986).
68. Ahn, Y. S., Jy, W., Harrington, W. J., Shanbaky, N., Fernandez, L. F., Haynes, D. H., Increased platelet calcium in thrombosis and related disorders and its correction by nifedipine. *Thromb. Res., 45*: 135 (1987).

69. Pumphrey, C. W., Fuster, V., Dewanjee, M. K., Chesebro, J. H., Comparison of antithrombotic action of calcium antagonist drugs with dipyridamole in dogs. *Am. J. Cardiol., 51*: 591 (1983).
70. Walley, T. J., Woods, K. L., Barnett, D. B., Effects of calcium channel blockers on in vitro platelet function in whole blood using single platelet counting. *Thromb. Haemost., 61*: 137 (1989).
71. Cremer, K. F., Pieper, J. A., Joyal, M., Mehta, J., Effects of diltiazem, dipyridamole, and their combination on hemostasis. *Clin. Pharm. Ther., 36*: 641 (1984).
72. Bell, W. R., Braine, H. G., Ness, P. M., Kickler, T. S., Improved survival in thrombotic thrombocytopenic purpura—hemolytic uremic syndrome—clinical experience in 108 patients. *N. Engl. J. Med., 325*: 398 (1991).
73. Weinstein, M. J., Phillips, M. D., Turner, N. A., Vosburgh, E., Moake, J. L., Both monomeric and polymeric aurin tricarboxylic acid (ATA) compounds inhibit von Willebrand factor (vWF)-mediated platelet aggregation. *Blood, 74*(Suppl. 1): 667 (1989).
74. Strony, J., Phillips, M. D., Moake, J. L., Adelman, B., Aurin tricarboxylic acid in a canine model of coronary artery thrombosis. *Circulation, 81*: 1106 (1990).
75. Weinstein, M. J., Vosburgh, E., Phillips, M. D., Turner, N., Chute-Rose, L., Moake, J. L., Isolation from commercial aurintricarboxylic acid of the most effective polymeric inhibitors of von Willebrand factor interaction with platelet glycoprotein Ib. Comparison with other polyanionic and polyaromatic polymers. *Blood, 78*: 2291 (1991).

40
An Update on the Therapy of Thrombotic Thrombocytopenic Purpura

Joel L. Moake *Baylor College of Medicine and Rice University, Houston, Texas*

Recommendations for the treatment of TTP episodes are based on studies of small numbers of patients by many different investigators, and on two large series that included a total of more than 200 patients published in 1991 (1, 2). The various observations have led to considerable progress over the past two decades in the treatment of this once inevitably fatal disorder.

PLASMA EXCHANGE AND SUPPORTIVE THERAPY

In about 70–90% of patients, initial TTP episodes (as well as severe recurrences in relapsing TTP patients) can be reversed by intensive plasma manipulation 1–15. A 3- to 4-L plasma exchange (i.e., the combination of plasmapheresis and plasma infusion) with normal fresh-frozen, platelet-poor plasma is the single most effective therapeutic maneuver and should be initiated as soon as practical in severely ill TTP patients. It is presumed that a platelet-aggregating substance or substances, perhaps unusually large von Willebrand factor (ULvWF) multimers and a putative vWF cofactor (16–18), are being removed by plasmapheresis; and that normal plasma is providing some antiaggregating agent, perhaps an ULvWF "depolymerase (19)," that is present in patient plasma in inadequate amounts. Transfusions or exchange transfusions with fluids other than plasma, the cryosupernatant fraction of plasma, or whole blood (e.g., with albumin or IgG concentrates) are almost always ineffective (4, 7, 14, 15, 17, 20, 21).

Immediately after diagnosis, infusion of normal fresh-frozen plasma at the rate of about 30 ml/kg per day should be started and continued until plasma exchange can be arranged (7, 14, 17). This is usually within 24–48 hr. TTP patients in coma, or with cardiac failure or renal dysfunction should receive plasma exchange commencing immediately after diagnosis, if practical.

Relapses in infants, children,and adult patients with the chronic relapsing type of TTP often respond to, or are prevented by, transfusion of 1 to several units of normal fresh-frozen plasma alone (i.e., without the need for concurrent plasmapheresis) (5, 7, 14, 17, 22, 23).

Some patients have recovered from TTP episodes without receiving glucocorticoids (11). Other patients, with less severe TTP, were recently reported to have recovered in association with glucocorticoid therapy alone (2). On the basis of this latter series (2), it can be concluded that glucocorticoids are probably useful in the treatment of TTP episodes (24). In some patients, the apparent effectiveness of glucocorticoids in TTP may relate to an underlying autoimmune pathogenesis. This may be the production of autoantibodies against endothelial cells in the single-episode type of TTP, or against the ULvWF depolymerase in relapsing types of TTP (intermittent TTP and chronic relapsing TTP) (17, 18, 24). Unless glucocorticoids are contraindicated in an individual patient, it is probably advisable for methylprednisolone to be started immediately after diagnosis in a dosage of about 0.75 mg/kg intravenously every 12 hr (or prednisone orally at about 1.0 mg/kg), and continued until the patient recovers (14, 17, 24).

Depending on the hemoglobin level and intensity of hemolysis, red blood cell transfusions may be required. If the platelet count is very low and bleeding is a primary problem, or if intracranial bleeding is demonstrated by computerized tomography or magnetic resonance imaging, then platelet transfusions will be necessary. In an increasing number of patients, however, the transfusion of platelets has been temporally associated with exacerbation of the thrombotic process in the cerebrovascular (2, 25) or coronary microcirculation.

Plasma exchange should be continued until responding patients attain a normal neurological status, a platelet count higher than 150,000/μl, a rising hemoglobin level, and a normal serum lactate dehydrogenase (LDH) value. Plasma exchange should then be continued for at least 2–3 additional days. Prompt relapse is, nevertheless, common (2). If this occurs, the same treatment protocol should be repeated. In patients who achieve a partial response without deterioration in their clinical condition, plasma exchange should be continued for a few to many additional days in an effort to achieve a complete remission (14, 17).

OTHER TREATMENT OPTIONS

If a patient does not respond within the first 5 days of treatment, or deteriorates within the first 3 days, other forms of therapy should be tried. Options include: addition of vincristine, in a dosage of 1.4 mg/m^2, but not exceeding 2 mg total dosage, given by intravenous push on day 1, followed by 1 mg on days 4, 7, and 10 (14, 26); substitution in the plasma exchange procedures of cryosupernatant (plasma depleted of the cryoprecipitate fraction that contains the largest plasma vWF multimeric forms, as well as fibrinogen and fibronectin) for fresh-frozen plasma (15, 17, 21); splenectomy (14, 17, 27); or addition of another immunosuppressive agent (e.g., azathioprine) (28).

The apparent usefulness of vincristine in some patients may be because its depolymerizing effects on platelet microtubules produce secondary alterations in the exposure of surface receptors. It is not known whether splenectomy is sometimes effective in refractory TTP because it removes a major site of synthesis of an autoantibody or of a vWF cofactor. It should be emphasized, however, that refractory TTP does not always respond to splenectomy (2), and that TTP has been reported in splenectomized patients (29).

The use of aspirin and dipyridamole is controversial (1, 2, 30–34). Neither would be predicted to be effective if the pathogenesis of systemic platelet clumping involves ULvWF multimers, which can clump even metabolically inert platelets (17, 35). Aspirin may exacerbate hemorrhagic complications in TTP patients with severe thrombocytopenia (33), although this was not reported as an important problem in a recent large series (1). Neither drug has been unequivocally demonstrated to be useful in TTP.

Intravenous dextran, fibrinolytic agents, and epoprostenol (prostacyclin; PGI_2) also have not convincingly been shown to be effective therapy in TTP (14, 17). Fitzgerald et al. (36) treated a young man with intravenous epoprostenol after he had deteriorated clinically while receiving aspirin, dipyridamole, sulfinpyrazone, prednisone, and plasma exchange. Although improvement in mental status occurred within 24 hr, remission required an additional 18 days of treatment. Other patients have not responded to epoprostenol (37–39).

Heparin in therapeutic dosages is considered to be contraindicated, based on anecdotal experiences.

RELAPSING TTP

When a patient achieves remission and the plasma exchanges (or infusions) have been discontinued, platelet counts should be obtained on a reasonably frequent schedule. Patients with a protracted initial episode who do not attain a complete remission, as well as patients with the chronic relapsing form of TTP, usually relapse within a few weeks after discontinuation of therapy. In the intermittent type of TTP, the disorder may not recur for months or, occasionally, years. If ULvWF multimers are demonstrated in patient EDTA–plasma samples *after recovery* from an initial episode of TTP, and if the ULvWF forms then persist in subsequent samples, the patient has about a 90% probability for TTP recurrence (16–18, 28, 40).

INVESTIGATIONAL AGENTS

Aurin tricarboxylic acid (ATA) is a polyphenolic polycarboxylated compound that may ultimately prove useful in the treatment of TTP and severe hemolytic-uremic syndrome (HUS) episodes, and in the prophylaxis of relapsing TTP. Polymeric ATA binds reversibly to vWF multimers and prevents ULvWF and plasma vWF forms from attaching to platelet glycoprotein Ib (GPIb) molecules (41). The binding of ULvWF or large vWF forms to platelet GPIb, followed by vWF binding to GPIIb/IIIa complexes, is required for platelet aggregation in fluid shear fields (35, 42, 43). Use of ATA inhibits this shear-induced, vWF-mediated aggregation. ATA is also capable of inhibiting platelet thrombosis in vivo in the Folts dog model of myocardial infarction (44), and in platelet-mediated rethrombosis following fibrinolytic therapy in the same animal model (45).

If either ATA polymers, recombinant fragments of the vWF monomer that competitively block the binding of vWF multimers to GPIb (46), or monoclonal antibodies to the arginine-glycine-asparate (RGD)-binding region for glycoprotein

IIb/IIIa on vWF monomeric subunits of vWF multimers (47) should prove to be successful in treating refractory TTP or severe gastroenteritis-associated or drug-associated HUS, then compelling additional evidence would be provided for the role of vWF in the pathogenesis of these thrombotic microangiopathies (24) (See Chapter 33.)

REFERENCES

1. Rock, G. A., Shumak, K., Buskard, N. A., et al., Comparison of plasma exchange with plasma infusion in the treatment of thrombotic thrombocytopenic purpura. *N. Engl. J. Med., 325:* 393–397 (1991).
2. Bell, W. R., Braine, H. G., Ness, P. M., and Kickler, T. S., Improved survival in thrombotic thrombocytopenic purpura–hemolytic uremic syndrome. Clinical experience in 108 patients. *N. Engl. J. Med., 325:* 398–403 (1991).
3. Rubinstein, M. A., Kaga, B. M., MacGillvinary, W. H., et al., Unusual remission in a case of thrombotic thrombocytopenic purpura syndrome following fresh blood exchange transfusions. *Ann. Intern. Med., 51:* 1409–1419 (1959).
4. Byrnes, J. J., and Khurana, M., Treatment of thrombotic thrombocytopenic purpura with plasma. *N. Engl. J. Med., 297:* 1386–1389 (1977).
5. Schulman, I., Pierce, M., Lukens, A., et al., Studies on thrombopoiesis. I. A factor in normal human plasma required for platelet production; chronic thrombocytopenia due to its deficiency. *Blood, 16:* 943–957 (1960).
6. Ansell, J., Beaser, R. S., and Pecket, L., Thrombotic thrombocytopenic purpura fails to respond to fresh frozen plasma. *Ann. Intern. Med., 89:* 647–649 (1978).
7. Byrnes, J. J., Plasma infusion in the treatment of thrombotic thrombocytopenic purpura. *Semin. Thromb. Hemost., 7:* 9–14 (1981).
8. Byrnes, J. J., and Lian, E. C.-Y., Recent therapeutic advances in thrombotic thrombocytopenic purpura. *Semin. Thromb. Hemost., 5:* 199–215 (1979)
9. Taft, E. G., and Baldwin, S. T., Plasma exchange transfusion. *Semin. Thromb. Hemost., 7:* 15–21 (1981).
10. Gottschall, J. L., Pisciotta, A. V., and Darvin, J., Thrombotic thrombocytopenic purpura: Experience with whole blood exchange transfusion. *Semin. Thromb. Hemost., 7:* 25–32 (1981).
11. Petitt, R. M., Thrombotic thrombocytopenic purpura—a thirty year review. *Semin. Thromb. Hemost., 6:* 350–355 (1980).
12. Bukowski, R. M., Hewlett, J. S., Reimer, R. R., et al., Therapy of thrombotic thrombocytopenic purpura: An overview. *Semin. Thromb. Hemost., 7:* 1–8 (1981).
13. Shepard, K. V., and Bukowski, R. M., The treatment of thrombotic thrombocytopenic purpura with exchange transfusions, plasma infusions, and plasma exchange. *Semin. Hematol., 24:* 178–193 (1987).
14. Moake, J. L., Thrombotic thrombocytopenic purpura (TTP) and the hemolytic-uremic syndrome (HUS). In *Conn's Current Therapy* (R. E. Rakel, ed.), W. B. Saunders, Philadelphia, pp. 339–341 (1989).
15. Byrnes, J. J., Moake, J. L., Klug, P. et al., Effectiveness of the cryosupernatant fraction of plasma in the treatment of refractory thrombotic thrombocytopenic purpura. *Am. J. Hematol., 34:* 169–174 (1990).
16. Moake, J. L., Rudy, C. K., Troll, J. H., et al., Unusually large plasma factor VIII:von Willebrand factor multimers in chronic relapsing thrombotic thrombocytopenic purpura. *N. Engl. J. Med., 307:* 1432–1435 (1982).
17. Byrnes, J. L., and Moake, J. L., Thrombotic thrombocytopenic purpura and the haemolytic-uraemic syndrome: evolving concepts of pathogenesis and therapy. *Clin. Haematol., 15:* 413–442 (1986).

18. Moake, J. L., and McPherson, P. D., Abnormalities of von Willebrand factor multimers in thrombotic thrombocytopenic purpura and the hemolytic uremic syndrome. *Am. J. Med., 87:* 9N–15N (1989).
19. Frangos, J. A., Moake, J. L., Nolasco, L., et al., Cryosupernatant regulates accumulation of unusually large vWF multimers from endothelial cells. *Am. J. Physiol., 256:* H1635–H1644 (1989).
20. Kelton, J. G., Moore, J. C., and Murphy, W. G., Studies investigating platelet aggregation and release initiated by sera from patients with thrombotic thrombocytopenic purpura. *Blood, 69:* 924–928 (1987).
21. Moake, J. L., Byrnes, J. J., Troll, J. H., et al., Effects of fresh-frozen plasma and its cryosupernatant fraction on von Willebrand factor multimeric forms in chronic relapsing thrombotic thrombocytopenic purpura. *Blood, 65:* 1232–1236 (1985).
22. Chintagumpala, M., Hurwitz, R., Moake, J., Mahoney, D., and Steuber, C., Thrombotic thrombocytopenic purpura in two children: fresh frozen plasma prevents recurrence. *J. Pediatr.,* (in press, 1991).
23. Upshaw, J. D., Congenital deficiency of a factor in normal plasma that reverses microangiopathic hemolysis and thrombocytopenia. *N. Engl. J. Med., 298:* 1350–1352 (1978).
24. Moake, J. L., TTP—desperation, empiricism, progress. *N. Engl. J. Med., 325:* 426–428 (1991).
25. Harkness, D. R., Byrnes, J. J., Lian, E. C.-Y., et al., Hazard of platelet transfusion in thrombotic thrombocytopenic purpura. *JAMA, 246:* 1931–1933 (1981).
26. Gutterman, L. A., and Stevenson, T. D., Treatment of thrombotic thrombocytopenic purpura with vincristine. *JAMA, 247*: 1433–1436 (1982).
27. Cuttner, J., Thrombotic thrombocytopenic purpura: A ten year experience. *Blood, 56:* 302–306 (1980).
28. Moake, J. L., Rudy, C. K., Troll, J. H., et al., Therapy of chronic relapsing thrombotic thrombocytopenic purpura with prednisone and azathioprine. *Am J. Hematol., 20:* 73–79 (1985).
29. Zacharski, L. R., Lustad, D., and Glick, J. L., Thrombotic thrombocytopenic purpura in a previously splenectomized patient. *Am. J. Med., 60:* 1061–1063 (1976).
30. Faguet, G. B., and King, M. D., Thrombotic thrombocytopenic purpura: Treatment with anti-platelet agents. *Am. J. Med. Sci., 268:* 113–116 (1974).
31. Birgens, H., Ernst, P., and Hansen, M. S., Thrombotic thrombocytopenic purpura: treatment with a combination of antiplatelet drugs. *Acta Med. Scand., 205:* 437–439 (1979).
32. Gundlack, N. J., and Tarnasky, R., Thrombotic thrombocytopenic purpura—remission following treatment with aspirin and dipyridamole. *Minn. Med., 60:* 20 (1977).
33. Rosove, M. H., Ho, W. G., and Goldfinger, D., Ineffectiveness of aspirin and dipyridamole in the treatment of thrombotic thrombocytopenic purpura. *Ann. Intern. Med., 96:* 27–33 (1982).
34. del Zoppo, G. J., Antiplatelet therapy in thrombotic thrombocytopenic purpura. *Semn. Hematol., 24:* 130–139 (1987).
35. Moake, J. L., Turner, N. A., Stathopoulos, N. A., et al., Shear-induced platelet aggregation can be mediated by vWF released from platelets, as well as by exogenous large or unusually large vWF multimers, requires adenosine diphosphate, and is resistant to aspirin. *Blood, 71:* 1366–1374 (1988).
36. Fitzgerald, G. A., Maas, R. L., and Stern, R., Intravenous prostacyclin in thrombotic thrombocytopenic purpura. *Ann. Intern. Med. 95:* 319 (1981).
37. Johnson, J. E., Mills, G. M., and Batson, A. G., Ineffective epoprostenol therapy for TTP. *JAMA, 250:* 3089–3091 (1983).
38. Hensby, G. N., Lewis, P. J., Hilgard, P., et al., Prostacyclin deficiency in TTP. *Lancet, 2:* 748 (1979).

39. Budd, G. T., Bukowski, R. M., Lucas, F. U., et al., Prostacyclin therapy of TTP. *Lancet, 2:* 915 (1980).
40. Moake, J. L., and McPherson, P. D., von Willebrand factor in thrombotic thrombocytopenic purpura and the hemolytic-uremic syndrome. *Transfusion Med., 4:* 163–168 (1990).
41. Phillips, M. D., Moake, J. L., Nolasco, L. H., et al., Aurin tricarboxylic acid: A novel inhibitor of platelet–von Willebrand factor association. *Blood, 72:* 1898–1903 (1988).
42. Moake, J. L., Turner, N. A., Stathopoulos, N. A., et al., Involvement of large plasma von Willebrand factor (vWF) multimers and unusually large vWF forms derived from endothelial cells in shear stress-induced platelet aggregation. *J. Clin. Invest., 78:* 1456–1461 (1986).
43. Peterson, D. M., Stathopoulos, N. A., Giorgio, T. D., et al., Shear-induced platelet aggregation requires von Willebrand factor and platelet membrane glycoproteins Ib and IIb/IIIa. *Blood, 69:* 625–628 (1987).
44. Strony, J., Phillips, M., Brands, D., et al., Aurin tricarboxylic acid in a canine model of coronary artery thrombosis. *Circulation, 81:* 1106–1114 (1990).
45. Strony, J., Brands, D., Hanners, E., and Adelman, B., Platelet thrombus formation following fibrinolytic therapy is dependent upon shear stress and von Willebrand factor [abstr.]. *Clin. Res., 38:* 470 (1990).
46. Sugimoto, M., Ricca, G., Hrinda, M. E., et al., Functional modulation of the isolated glycoprotein Ib binding domain of von Willebrand factor expressed in *Escherichia coli*. *Biochemistry, 30:* 5202–5209 (1991).
47. Berliner, S., Niiya, K., Roberts, J. R., Houghten, R. A., and Ruggeri, Z. M., Generation and characterization of peptide-specific antibodies that inhibit von Willebrand factor binding to GPIIb/IIIa without interacting with other adhesive molecules: selectivity is conferred by Pro^{1743} and other amino acid residues adjacent to the sequence Arg^{1744}-Gly^{1745}-Asp^{1746}. *J. Biol. Chem., 263:* 7500–7505 (1988).

Index

About the Editors

BERNARD S. KAPLAN is Director of Nephrology, Children's Hospital of Philadelphia, Pennsylvania, and Professor of Pediatrics and Medicine, University of Pennsylvania, Philadelphia. The author or coauthor of over 70 professional papers and more than 50 book chapters, editorials, and reviews, he is a member of the International Society of Nephrology, the International Society of Pediatric Nephrology, the European Society of Pediatric Research, the American Society of Pediatric Nephrology, and the American Society of Nephrology, among other organizations. Dr. Kaplan received the M.B. and B.Ch. degrees (1964) from the University of the Witwatersrand, Johannesburg, South Africa.

RICHARD S. TROMPETER is Consultant Pediatric Nephrologist to the Hospitals for Sick Children, London, England, and Senior Lecturer in Pediatric Nephrology, the Institute of Child Health, London. A Fellow of the Royal College of Physicians, he is the author of numerous professional papers and book chapters on renal transplantation, the management of chronic renal failure, and the nephrotic syndrome. Dr. Trompeter received the M.D. B.S. degree (1970) from Guy's Hospital Medical School, London.

JOEL L. MOAKE is Professor of Medicine and Director, Medical Hematology Section, Baylor College of Medicine, and Associate Director, Biomedical Engineering Laboratory, Rice University, Houston, Texas. He is a member of the American Society of Hematology, the American Federation for Clinical Research, the American Society for Clinical Investigation, and the Association of American Physicians, among other organizations, and the author or coauthor of more than 110 professional papers. Dr. Moake received the M.D. degree (1967) from Johns Hopkins University School of Medicine, Baltimore, Maryland.